ALLE · ZEIT · WACH · 1842

Psychiatry Series 43

Edited by
H. Hippius, München · W. Janzarik, Heidelberg
C. Müller, Prilly-Lausanne

K.W. Bash J. Bash-Liechti

Developing Psychiatry

Epidemiological and Social Studies in Iran 1963–1976

With 141 Tables, 4 Maps, 1 Plate,
and 4 Diagrams

Springer-Verlag
Berlin Heidelberg New York
London Paris Tokyo

K. W. BASH †
Formerly Associate Professor at the University of Bern

J. BASH-LIECHTI †
Stäfa, Switzerland

ISBN-13:978-3-642-82917-8 e-ISBN-13:978-3-642-82915-4
DOI: 10.1007/978-3-642-82915-4

Library of Congress Cataloging-in-Publication Data. Bash, K. W. (Kenower Weimar) Developing psychiatry. (Monographien aus dem Gesamtgebiete der Psychiatrie : Bd. 43).
Bibliography: p. 1. Mental illness—Iran. 2. Mental health surveys—Iran. 3. Psychological tests —Iran. 4. Psychiatric epidemiology—Iran. I. Bash-Liechti, J. II. Title. III. Series: Monographien aus dem Gesamtgebiete der Psychiatrie ; 43.
RC451.I7B37 1987 362.2'0955 86-26013
ISBN-13:978-3-642-82917-8 (U.S.)

Softcover reprint of the hardcover 1st edition 1987

Typesetting: Fotosatz & Design, 8240 Berchtesgaden

2125/3130-543210

Foreword

This book is a bequest. The author, K. W. Bash, did not live to see its appearance. Though of American parentage, he spent most of his life in Switzerland, where his last professional appointment before his retirement was that of Associate Professor of Psychiatry in Bern. Professor Bash made a lasting name for himself with his textbook of psychopathology, his research on Rorschach interpretations and his eminent position in the Jung school of psychological thought. In his last years, however, it was Iranian psychiatry that claimed his main interest. As an expert in the field who also spoke the language, he spent several long periods in Iran, working in an advisory capacity. This book is the product of intensive cross-cultural and epidemiological research, which unfortunately had to be broken off because of the political events in Iran. Nevertheless, editor and publisher count themselves fortunate indeed that it was possible to save the important material that the author had already accumulated from oblivion and to make it accessible to others interested in the field.

Prilly-Lausanne C. MÜLLER

Preface

The conception of this book originated in our Shiraz Mental Health Survey of 1969/70 when, after we had begun epidemiological studies in the villages in 1963, we for the first time gained comparable data from a city. The course of the village studies is described under "Origins", Part A, Chap. II, and in the chapters on local surveys in Part B. Because of great initial delays field work occupied us practically to the day of our departure from Shiraz, leaving no time for any but the most superficial evaluation. Thereafter the first author's clinical, administrative and teaching duties reasserted their claims so that it was possible to prepare only a few articles up to a precious fellowship year in Holland in 1973/74. Much of this year was needed for coding and processing the data. In the remainder roughly the first half of the book was drafted, after which the same situation as before intervened until the first author was emerited from the University of Bern in 1978. In the meanwhile both authors had returned to Iran almost every year, in 1965 for four months for the Khuzestan Mental Health Survey and in 1976 three weeks for the resurvey of Qassemabad. Concrete plans had been made for further resurveys following the first author's retirement in September, 1978. What has happened since then is a part of contemporary history.

This cataclysmic turn of events confronted us not only with frustrations over the impossibility of the intended resurveys, but with the problem of how to present our findings. For each survey and the one resurvey we have attempted to describe succinctly conditions as they were at the given time, with references backward and a few forward. The latter were needful especially for the earlier surveys, as the changes between 1963 and 1976, though not cataclysmic, were by no means slight or insignificant. Could we bring our descriptions, including that of Shiraz, up to date? We have been forced to recognize that at present there are no means of doing so. The first author did indeed return to Iran in March, 1984, on a short term assignment for the WHO, but time did not permit him to revisit all localities (part of which were within the war area) or to collect even at second hand information of a sufficiently detailed character. What he was able to glean is presented in Annex II. Many of our former sources have become inaccessible. As it did not seem practical or useful to rewrite the manuscript with ever recurring reference to indefinable alterations of circumstance, we have allowed present tenses to stand. They must be read with the understanding that they apply at the very latest to the conditions of 1978 unless otherwise stated, but mostly to about 1976, when the authors last carried out surveys in Iran.

To the execution of the surveys and the making of this book have contributed many institutions, organizations and persons. Among the former two the World Health Organization, especially its Regional Office for the Eastern Mediterranean in Alexandria, Egypt, and its lately deceased Director Dr. A.H. Taba must take first place. All surveys (though not the Qassemabad Resurvey) were conducted under its auspices, the first author acting as Adviser or Consultant to the Organization, and with its financial support together with that of the Iranian Government and many of its subsidiary institutions such as Provincial Health Offices, the Khuzestan Water and Power Authority and the University of Shiraz. The WHO has also performed the larger part of the data processing. Besides Dr. Taba, who made possible the Shiraz Mental Health Survey, the first author wishes to thank personally his immediate chief during his four and a half years as Senior Adviser for Mental Health in Tehran, Dr. Tigani el Mahi, the deceased former Regional Adviser for Mental Health in Alexandria, for his patience, understanding and unflagging support. At the Geneva Headquarters of the WHO he has enjoyed similar encouragement and aid from two past Chiefs of the Division (then only a Section) of Mental Health: Drs. E. Krapf and P. Baan and from the present incumbent Dr. N. Sartorius. The statisticians Mr. K. Uemura and Mr. W. Gulbinat have provided generous assistance and technical advice for processing the data.

The Iranian officials of all ranks, colleagues and friends are numerous beyond count, and our debt to them is incalculable. After conversations with several of them and after weighing the circumstances past and present we have come regretfully to the conclusion to mention no names and simply to record here our gratitude to all. Their names are in our hearts, and we trust they will understand. Neither does it seem expedient to name any non-Iranian governmental and semi-governmental organizations to which we are indebted, though some will be found in our earlier publications.

Though work never ceased and was sustained over intervals mainly by the second author, it did proceed slowly in the period from 1970 to 1973, when a year's fellowship at the Netherlands Institute for Advanced Studies in the Humanities and Social Sciences in Wassenaar enabled the first author, with the constant co-operation of the second, to devote his entire time to it. While that magnificent institution, one of the few refuges of unstinted academic freedom in the world today, ordinarily does not grant fellowships to medical scientists, it stretched its rules with characteristic liberality to accept him as a social psychiatrist. In this period the WHO Headquarters took over the processing not only of the Shiraz Survey data, but also of certain additional material from the villages needed in order adequately to standardize the intelligence test. Therein we benefited from the advice of Dr. C. Hamaker of the Psychological Laboratory of the University of Amsterdam. Data processing had been performed hitherto by hand count, in which we were aided greatly by Iranian colleagues and students living in Europe.

With the exception of the Qassemabad resurvey of 1976, progress was again slow from 1974 to 1978. Seeking to gain some knowledge about the prevalence of mental illness in connection with the National Census of 1976 a semi-official agency invited both authors back to Iran and entrusted them jointly with the resurvey. After the data had been organized and coded in Switzerland they were to be processed in Tehran. The first task was approximately completed by the fall of 1978. We were left with masses of data on our hands for which no one then would assume responsibility. A portion of them relating to a thesis for the licentiate at the University of Bern was handled by the Psychological Institute there; we thank Mr. P. Ballinari. After the first author's retirement from that institution in the same year it was the Research Department of the Psychiatric University Hospital of Zürich with its Director Prof. J. Angst and Vice-Director Prof. Chr. Scharfetter that unhesitatingly, generously and understandingly brushed aside all red tape and came to our rescue. With lively gratitude we note also the names of their two sociologist-statisticians: Mrs. A. Dobler and Mr. J. Binder. Both this Department and the WHO Headquarters possess a tape record of our coded data (incomplete for Marvdasht, Khuzestan and the Qashqai, the larger part of whose data were tabulated by hand only).

Some notes on the formal aspects of our presentation may be desirable. We have considered and rejected the decimal system of classification for headings and subheadings. It has the advantages of impeccable logic and limitless expansibility, but is perceptually unfavorable. The eye does not as easily grasp nor memory retain the difference between e.g. 1.1.2.1 and 1.2.1.1 as it does between, say, A I 2 a and A II 1 a, as the reading experience of a professional lifetime has shown us. A not insurmountable difficulty can arise when the number of categories exceeds four, but we have seen no necessity for them to do so. Fragmentation of a text into a vast number of categories and subcategories, each with its extensive decimal cipher, sometimes may serve a purpose. It can also be a tattered cloak for incoherent writing.

Transcription from the Persian or Farsi is as nearly phonetical as the ordinary Latin alphabet permits and custom sanctions. We have not attempted a scientific transcription for linguists and Iranists, to whom it is superfluous. Place names have their usual English forms with the exception of Tehran, which is spelled here as it is pronounced there: with two syllables. The second is long and carries the accent, as is true for Shiraz also. We have retained the Farsi locative adjectival ending in i for ease and convenience. It serves for both singular and plural.

Translations from the German are by the present authors unless otherwise noted.

Bibliographic references have been arranged by alphabet and numbered consecutively throughout. Our bibliography does not pretend to be exhaustive. The range of subjects is so wide that it would have required another book to quote and even briefly to discuss the principal literature on each. No reader but will miss some favorite author or source. Much of the literature quoted is European. Since this is treated as practically nonexistent by all but a few Anglo-American authors, we concede the rest no ground for criticism or complaint.

In respect to the several local surveys it would be natural to look for data on the magnitude and composition of the population at the beginning or close to the beginning of each respective chapter. In order to avoid needless repetition we have placed them instead in the section called "Tests" (except for Shiraz, where they are to be found under "Demography and Social Psychiatry", Chap. IV 1 of Part B). Apart from a few discrepancies caused by drop-outs or untestable subjects and recorded as such, the number tested in one way or another agrees with the number of subjects scrutinized. These can be found again for all surveys in Table D III 1.

One set of the handwritten Persian original records is deposited for Marvdasht and the Qashqai in the Fars Ostan Department of Public Health, Shiraz, for Khuzestan in the Khuzestan Ostan Department of Public Health, Ahwaz (we do not know whether it has survived the war), for Shiraz and Qalandari in the Psychiatric Out-Patient Department, Fars Ostan Department of Public Health, Shiraz, and for the Qassemabad Resurvey in the archives of the Ministry of Health, Tehran. The authors have retained in their possession a full set of original records from all surveys and a copy of the aforementioned tape. It is intended to deposit these in the Research Department of the University Psychiatric Hospital, Zürich.

Part A of the manuscript was typed in the Netherlands Institute for Advanced Study, most of Part B and some of Part C by the first author's faithful secretaries at the University Psychiatric Hospital in Bern: Mrs. U. Ortelli-Strickler, Miss E. Hänni and Mrs. N. Aeschlimann; the rest by himself. He has copied or redrawn maps from Gremliza [86] and Petrossian, Shayan, Bash and Jessup [166] and thanks Mrs. A. Jessup for permission to use her aerial photographs in Plate B I. The general map of Iran with administrative divisions has been taken from the Sahab Geographic and Drafting Institute, Tehran.

References will be noted here and there to groups of data that have not been evaluated, calculations that have not been performed, questions that might, but have not been answered. The reasons should be apparent from the foregoing and from circumstances related in more detail in the appropriate chapters. Another circumstance is still more cogent. The first author, possessing a longer familiarity with the English language, undertook writing the text. In all the rest the second author, almost always without corresponding official position, title or reward has borne her full share. Having read and approved the completed text (though not the Foreword or the Annexes), she died on December 18, 1980. Abandoning the no longer applicable plural, I let serve in place of a dedication to my wife the sketches of our Persian subjects and friends on the title page that she left in her field notebooks.

"Go thou forth, my booke, though late;
Yet be timely fortunate.
It may chance good-luck may send
Thee a kinsman, or a friend,
That may harbour thee, when I,
With my fates neglected lye.
If thou know'st not where to dwell,
See, the fier's by: Farewell."

K. W. BASH

Contents

Tables

Part D: Comparisons and Conclusions

I. Differential Psychology

II. Indicators of Psychopathology

III. General Psychiatric Epidemiology

Maps, Diagrams, Plate

Abbreviations and Formulae

A	ambiequality
A.D.	Anno Domini
Ad., Adult.	adult(s)
A.H.l.	Anno Hedjrae lunari
A.H.s.	Anno Hedjrae solari
Ar.	arithmetic
AV	attitudinal value
AV_p	attitudinal value, practical notation
AV_t	attitudinal value, theoretical notation
Bl.	block (design)
BM	best memory
Ch., Child.	child(ren)
D	difference
DIPA	Dez Irrigation Pilot Area
Dr	reactively disordered
E, e	extraversion
EPI	Eysenck Personality Inventory
Epi.	epilepsy
EPQ	Eysenck Personality Questionnaire
f	female(s)
FPI	Freiburg Personality Inventory
i., ill.	illiterate(s)
I, i	introversion
ICD	International Classification of Diseases
IQ	intelligence quotient
KWPA	Khuzestan Water and Power Authority
KZ	Khuzestan
m	male(s)
MD	manic-depressive
MMPI	Minnesota Multiphasic Personality Inventory
MPI	Maudsley Personality Inventory
MMQ	Maudsley Medical Questionnaire
N	number; neuroticism (Eysenck)
nc	not counted, not classifiable
ND	non-disordered
Neur.	neurosis, neurotic
NIAS	Netherlands Institute for Advanced Study
ns	not significant
P	pathological
P_1	pathological in mild degree
P_2	pathological in medium degree
P_3	pathological in severe degree
p.	per
perc.	per cent
Pop.	population
PP	Psychiatric Survey Population
Q	question, questionnaire
QL	Qalandari
QQ	Qashqai
Ro.	Rorschach (Test). Signa for this and the Z Test are given in Part C, Chap. II 3 b.
Reac.	reactive
Ref.	reference
RS	raw score
SAD	senile-arteriosclerotic dementia
Schiz.	schizophrenia
SD	standard deviation
SES	socio-economic status
SH	Shiraz
sign.	significant, significance
SP	Shiraz Survey Population
WHO	World Health Organization
WM	worst memory
WS	weighted score
X	examiner(s)
Z	Zulliger Test

Note on Presentation of Statistics

The generally used Snedecore convention for indicating the significance of differences by means of crosses or asterisks, the number of which corresponds to the degree of significance from * for $p < 0.10$ to *** for $p < 0.001$, can serve for two rows of data, though even there it is not altogether satisfactory because it does not show in which direction the difference lies. It is altogether inexpedient where one row must be compared with several or many others, especially when these lie on different pages, for the reader must then carry the absolute numbers in his head or constantly leaf, or at least glance, back and forth. Yet a large part of our data have had to be compared in this way. We have been forced to adopt another expedient. It rests upon the assumption that the reader is hardly ever interested in the numerical value of the χ^2 or the critical ratio, but only in whether, under the given conditions, number of cases, degrees of freedom, etc. a critical confidence level is reached or not, that is, whether the zero hypothesis, again by convention, can be rejected. We have therefore omitted such values except in a few cases where the context seemed to demand them. The reader's real need, when he has columns of data to compare, is to see whether an apparent difference between pairs of data is significant and, if it is, in what direction the difference lies. If $a \neq b$, is $a > b$ or $b > a$? By the Snedecore method he cannot ascertain the latter except by looking at both a and b, which in many cases may be separated by several pages and the comparison of which even on the same page is cumbersome. We have therefore introduced chevrons, the usual signs of inequality, in a special sense to indicate both the direction of the difference and the degree of its statistical significance. If this is less than 10% ($p < 0.10$) no sign appears. For levels of confidence better than this the number of chevrons corresponds to the number of asterisks according to Snedecore, but now it is not necessary to write each time the numbers, rates or percentages being compared or to carry them – an impossible task– in one's head. If we wish to compare for example the scores of males and females on a number of test items or the frequency with which they affirm a list of questions, we set m : f at the head of the table and the items one below the other to the left. A chevron pointing to the left against a certain item then implies that the males scored lower on it and that $p < 0.05$. Two chevrons pointing to the right mean that the males scored higher and that the level of confidence is 0.01, etc. Differences are to be understood in usual reading order: what is to the left or above as antecedent, what is to the right or below as consequent. Where chevrons are employed simply to indicate inequality as above it is presumed that this will be clear from the context.

All fourfold χ^2 tables contain a correction for continuity. Critical ratios have been calculated with the help of the formula

$$SD_D = \sqrt{p\,q\left(\frac{1}{N_1} + \frac{1}{N_2}\right)}$$

as given by McNemar [157], in which p and q are the proportions for the two groups N_1 and N_2 combined. Thus proportions of 1.0 or 0.0 can be handled, such as do in fact not infrequently occur.

" از دریچه چشم مجنون بایستی درجمال لیلی نظر کردن "

"To esteem Leila's beauty one must see her through the port of Madjnoun's eyes".

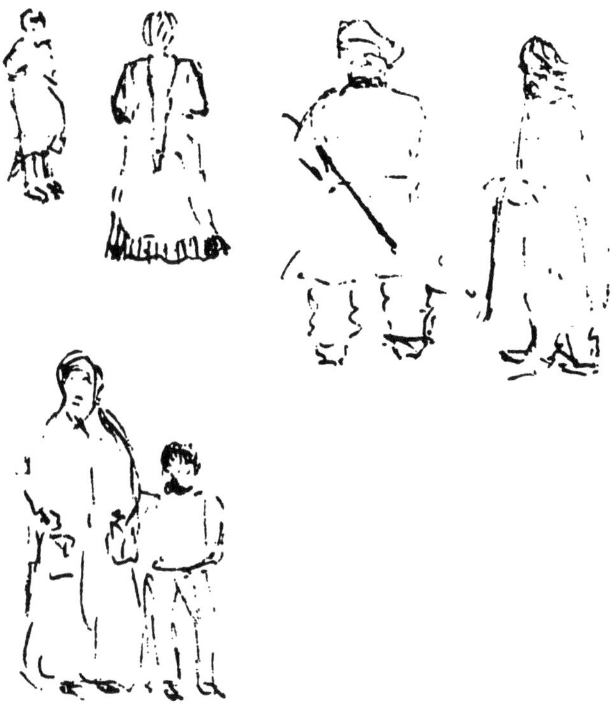

Part A Introduction

I. Background

Though it cannot be our object to write a medical or psychiatric history of Iran or a comprehensive account of hygiene and medical epidemiology at the time our work began, a few salient facts must be stated as points of reference from which these surveys and their results better can be understood. Fortunately, medical history up to the inception of "modern" medicine in Iran has been well covered by Elgood [66]. Some more recent events and appraisals are quoted in the following, mainly from the first joint survey report of Petrossian, Shayan, Jessup and Bash from Fars Ostan (Province) in 1964/1343[1] [166].

Iran covers an area of 1630000 square kilometers, equal roughly to the area of Great Britain, France, Italy and Germany combined, within which is comprised an almost continental diversity of climate, vegetation, altitude and, to a somewhat less degree, of ethnological groups. Population density varies greatly and is concentrated along the edges and foothills of the two mountain ranges, the Elborz and the Zagros, which converge in Azerbaijan in the north-west toward the Russian and Turkish borders. Their outer slopes fall to the Caspian Sea and the Persian Gulf respectively, their inner to the great and nigh empty central plain and desert, into which the water from the southern and eastern mountain slopes flows and evaporates. Another fringe of inhabitants follows the coasts. Figures for the population are given below. The majority of it always has been and still is engaged in agriculture directly or indirectly, though industrialization is making rapid strides, and the petroleum industry occupies large numbers at the head of the Gulf and on up into Khuzestan. No small part of the agricultural population in the wider sense is pastoral and migratory, a point to which we shall return.

The people of Iran adhere almost unanimously to Islam (98.4 %) and to its Shia division (95 %), which is the state religion. Religious minorities did not enter into our surveys except in Shiraz, where they will be mentioned. Religious toleration obtained, however, as it traditionally has, and religious minorities received representation in the parliament (Madjlis).

Administration is highly and up to 1962 was extremely centralized in Tehran after the French and Italian model. Since then the tendency has been increasing to delegate authority first to the ostans or provinces, thence to the administrative districts (sharestans) and municipalities. The local units generally have administrative, but not legislative councils. When the Adviser began work in Iran in 1960 there were thirteen ostans. In 1984 there were twenty-four.

---

[1] In double yearly dates, the first refers to the Gregorian, the second to the Iranian solar calender, which begins with the Hedjra (622 A.D.), but does not coincide with the lunar calender used in other Islamic countries. By this latter 1980 = 1400 H.l. (Hedjra lunaris) or by the Iranian calender 1359 H.s. (Hedjra solaris).

Each of these has a centrally appointed Governor-General (Ostandar), whose rank is equal to that of a cabinet minister, but who is also responsible to the Minister of the Interior. The Ostandar wields great authority in his province. Among his council is a Director-General of Health for the Ostan, responsible to the central Minister of Health. It is worth noting that this Minister and the Directors-General of Health in the ostans are always physicians.

L. E. Burney wrote in 1963 [53]: "Health services began in Iran about 1904 as a branch of the Ministry of Education. In 1921 the Health Department became a ministry, but responsible to the Minister of the Interior. The Ministry of Health as an autonomous unit was established in 1941. Prior to 1952 the Ministry of Health was concerned almost totally with curative medical care. Public health and preventive medicine programs began in 1952 with the assistance of the United States" and, the present authors should like to add, of the World Health Organization (WHO). American assistance in public health and preventive medicine was still playing a substantial role when the first author took up his duties as WHO Senior Adviser in Mental Health in 1960 but did not extend to his special field. It was to all purposes, except for a few residual projects, terminated in 1962. Up to then and even thereafter the government health services were split vertically into curative and preventive divisions, the split extending into provincial and local health administration, with two directors in each ostan and often in smaller units. In 1963 it was decided to coalesce the two services, a process which took several years to complete and was finished about 1965. Technically, mental health services, so far as they were rendered by the central government, were a responsibility of the curative division, though actually the majority of the psychiatric beds in the entire country were in a hospital belonging to the Municipality of Tehran.

Concerning general health conditions Overseas Consultants, Inc., reported in 1949 to the Plan Organization of the Imperial Government of Iran [165]: "The birth rate in Iran is about 20 per thousand . . . the infant death rate is believed to be over 500 per thousand . . . Malaria is not only the most important disease . . ., but is also the most important public health problem in Iran". At the time of writing it has been brought under control, eliminated over great areas and is still present only in some remote and endemic pockets thanks to energetic efforts by the Ministry of Health working in close co-operation with the World Health Organization. Trachoma and smallpox, both often with resultant blindness, as well as tuberculosis were widespread: smallpox has disappeared meanwhile after vigorous vaccination campaigns, and trachoma and tuberculosis are on the wane. "Two major causes of death are . . . completely unskilled midwifery . . . and failure on the part of mothers to safeguard the young infants from infection."

Surveying 9030 persons in 2053 families in 173 villages in a "typical agricultural area" south west of Tehran a year later Mashayekhi and Hayes [134] found that "43.2 % of the population is 14 years or younger; birth rate is 51.4 per 1000 population; stillbirth rate is 20.0 per 1000 live births; neonatal mortality rate is 86.5 per 1000 live births . . . Malnutrition appears to be a fundamental problem in Iran . . . 85.1 % of the population (excluding children under 5 years) totally illiterate . . . 66 % of the families lived in one room . . . less than one per cent of all the observed water supplies could be considered potentially free of contamination".

In 1961 Moayyed [152], reporting on *Rural Health Organization in Iran*, reviewed data from surveys done in the intervening years. "Life in Iran is short; the life expectancy from birth is 35–40 years . . . Mortality rate of children under 5 years was 311 per 1000 in Shiraz (and) . . . infant mortality rate for Shiraz rural areas was 146 per 1000", being even higher in villages near Tehran. In the same year Dr. Ch. M. H. Mofidi in a paper on the "Health Status of Iran" [153] given before a CENTO conference in Shiraz mentioned: "With the improvement of the general environmental sanitary conditions, and with the increase of campaigns against communicable diseases, the growth of population in Iran already has shown its implications on food supply . . . The growth rate of population is estimated as 2.5 per hundred per year with a crude birth rate of 28.8 per thousand in 1948 and 37.4 per thousand in 1957 . . . In the rural areas the following factors are added to the background of landscape, epidemiology and ecology: absence of communications and roads; the close association of man with the farm, pasture and domestic animals; the scarcity of water, which is always saved for agriculture and animal use; illiteracy and deficient health education . . . ; overwhelming patriarchy; social habits and superstitions; difficult life for securing food and income – because of erosion of land, absence of fertilizers" and other factors besides.

It has been necessary to recapitulate briefly this picture of poverty, distress and disease because it characterizes the environment in which the adult population and older children had grown or were growing up and because many of our findings can only be understood against this background. On the sixth of the Iranian month of Bahman 1341 (26th January 1963) Reza Shah Pahlavi promulgated far-reaching reforms covering the following six points:

1. Abolition of the landlord-serf system,
2. Stock sales in government-owned factories,
3. Worker profit sharing,
4. Nationalization of the forests,
5. Women's suffrage,
6. The Literacy Corps (followed soon after by the Health Corps).

They have marked a turning point that has entered into modern Iranian history under the name of the "White Revolution". Besides the central measure of land reform, reflected in the villages in which we worked, major direct effects consisted in the institution and subsequent expansion of the Health Corps and the Literacy Corps. Under the former Iranian medical graduates were conscripted into the army and sent, after brief military training, into the countryside to work for a year and a half as village physicians, supported by regional and provincial medical centers. Under the latter graduates of secondary schools, also in the form of military service, were sent into the villages as primary teachers, functioning at the same time as communal advisers and social workers insofar as a brief but intensive training prepared them. It is not our province as psychiatrists to trace the social and economic, still less the political development of Iran over the last decades. A wealth of relevant and objective information can be found in the files of the United Nations and its special agencies, to which the World Health Organization belongs. Such a study as this would be well-nigh meaningless, however, without reference to the profound and still continuing changes in Iranian life, the effective beginnings of which nearly coincided with our first field investigations.

Aspects of the ongoing changes are debated both within and without the country. We will simply record that we have been acquainted with conditions before the reforms and during the ten or more years following them, that we have witnessed ourselves step by step how effective medical care and prevention have been carried into numberless villages near and remote that were hitherto destitute of them, have been intensified in the towns and cities likewise and have altered and brightened to an encouraging degree the doleful picture of Iranian public health sketched above. We have witnessed, too, a corresponding upsurge in public education, have sat in schoolrooms and school tents remote from the beaten tracks, seen eager youngsters trudging far over the deserts to classes, shared their own and their parents' enthusiasm for a new world of knowledge revealing itself to them and, in our travels into every ostan of Iran, have been able to assure ourselves that we were observing not sporadic or isolated occurrences on display to the foreign visitor, but a transformation in the fields of general medicine and education that is nation-wide and far more than skin-deep.

The transformation is reflected already in newer public health data and in medical facts. Reference has been made to the eradication of malaria and smallpox. The same holds more recently of another scourge, poliomyelitis, which has been drastically reduced by systematic immunization (as late as 1963 poliomyelitis was still considered a relatively minor problem as compared with other, more urgent ones). Epidemics of cholera still strike, usually over the eastern border, but are kept in check. Trachoma and tuberculosis require more time, but are coming under control. The enormous infant and child mortality has been reduced within a relatively short time by the training of rural midwives, better sanitation and the intervention of the Health Corps to the point at which the population problem is beginning to emerge. Iran did not wait until it was hopelessly overpopulated to tackle this, but began already in 1967 to introduce and propagate family planning, which remained a major department of the public health services up to 1978. A family planning seminar held in Meshed in 1973 offered facts and forecasts. The total population, determined by the national census of 1966/1345 to 25788722 persons, was projected to 31–32 millions by 1972–3 and expected to reach 48 millions by 1993. It was hoped to reduce the rate of population increase from 3.2 % a year in 1973 to only one percent over the next two decades. Life expectancy had risen during the period 1960–1973 from about forty years for both sexes to 56.2 years for women and 54.5 years for men.

The most recent figures available, though far from complete, are those of Nahapetian and Khezaneh [155] published in 1977 as a first summary and projection of samples taken from the 1976 census. They are mostly given separately for urban und rural areas and point out the immense difference between them. The most important are tabulated below:

	Urban	*Rural*	
Crude birth rate	25.1	40.5	per 1000
Crude death rate	6.1	10.0	per 1000
Neonatal mortality (< 1 month)	18.3	45.0	per 1000
Infant mortality (1–12 months)	43.3	76.8	per 1000

Population from 0 through 14 years of age	42.9 per cent
Growth rate of population in 1976	2.8 per cent
Sex ratio m : f	107.5 : 100.0
Life expectancy	51–52 years

Turning briefly to origins and development of mental health and psychiatry in Iran, there is evidence that the term "mental health" in contradistinction to mental illness was first used there, having been introduced (if not already current before) by a certain Imami from Herat in an ode commanded by the registrar Shams'ud-Din Mohammed and written in the year 1268/667, wherein it is called szehat-e-äqli, صحت عقلی. It is well known that the Arab Moslem world could boast of mental hospitals in which patients were humanely treated centuries before such institutions could be found in Europe, whither Arab civilization brought them by way of North Africa and Spain. The earliest mental hospital of which we have record was apparently founded in Baghdad in 765 A.D., the earliest in Europe in Valencia in 1409 A.D. Considering how closely Persian and Arab medicine are interwoven and that no small part of the latter actually derives from the former, one must surmise that mental hospitals in which patients were kindly and understandingly treated existed in Iran at an early date. The traces, however, are few. Dr. M. H. Sahebo'z-Zamani, the first author's Persian counterpart, discovered a reference to such an one built as a division of a general hospital by the munificence of the aforementioned Shams'ud-Din Mohammed in Yazd in 1267/666 and lovingly described by the poet Imami [172]. Of it only half an arch still stands. History then becomes silent up to the opening of the present century, from which exist horrifying accounts of custodial institutions in which the "mad" were chained and abused. The mental hospitals of newer history have all been founded within recent decades, the first in Tehran in 1917, followed probably by Isfahan in 1930. A short summary of them is presented in Annex II. All the medical faculties in Iran, of which there were seven in 1973, teach psychiatry as a discipline separate from neurology.

It would be a satisfaction to us if we could state that psychiatric care in Iran has proceeded along the lines laid down so long ago in Yazd and that advances in it have kept pace with those in other fields of medicine such as we have just sketched. Such, however, has been no more the case than it has been in Europe and in the Anglo-Saxon countries up at least to very recently. It would require another treatise to analyze why, even in international health perspectives, mental health with dismaying regularity is assigned the last place [18]. Rather do we attempt here to record observations, hoping that these will speak for themselves and stimulate much-needed efforts.

II. Origins

The work hereafter to be described took its inception with the appointment of the first author as Senior Adviser to the World Health Organization Mental Health Project in Iran and therewith to the Iranian Ministry of Health in January, 1960. Commissioned to plan and promote mental health endeavors at all levels in Iran, he was soon concerned by the absence of basic information essential for planning. His prime, obvious task was to make an inventory of the facilities and resources actually available. A first step had been taken in 1954 by his distinguished predecessor G. Kraus [117], who surveyed the larger part of the Middle East for the Eastern Mediterranean Regional Office (EMRO) of the World Health Organization, yet in spite of the thoroughness, conscientiousness and exceptional detail of Kraus's report it covered only Tehran. G. C. Tooth [190] in 1958 and a visiting team of WHO medical teachers [203] a year later added some comments, but the picture remained, in every respect, cloudy. Though in sequel to Kraus's report the Government had begun to request a Mental Health Adviser as early as 1954, there had been difficulties in filling the position, documents and their recommendations drifted into obsolescence and were only rescued by the creation in 1959/1337, at the insistence of the then Minister of Health, of a Mental Health Unit within that ministry.

After having gathered by circular letter to the Departments of Health of all ostans information as to what institutions and facilities, both public and private, might be found, the Adviser set off to acquaint himself with them at first hand and to acquire such statistical information as he could. This was meager enough and hardly ever went beyond the number of beds in psychiatric hospitals together with the number of admissions and discharges during the past year. Counting the staff members presented little difficulty, much more an attempt to discover how the mental hospitals and their patients subsisted. Here is not the place to enter into detailed descriptions of Iranian psychiatric institutions and mental health facilities, a compilation of documents on which is presented in Annex II, but a few remarks, sketching the background, may not be amiss.

In the early nineteen-sixties Iran, with a census population then of just over twenty million [2], possessed some 2700 psychiatric beds in ten public, semi-public or charitable psychiatric hospitals besides an insignificant and fluctuating number of such beds in hospitals of private character, thus attaining the minimum of one bed per ten thousand population which the WHO has recommended for the care of the most urgent psychiatric disorders in developing countries. Yet over half of these beds were concentrated in Razi Mental Hospital in Rey near Tehran, leaving the remainder of the vast country with scanty psychiatric provision. At that time, one single psychiatrist was engaged in private practice outside the capital, and an endeavor to estimate the number of physicians with some specialized training in psychiatry did not carry beyond forty.

Auxiliary professions existed hardly, psychiatric nurses not at all. Of psychiatric outpatient services, mental health centers and the like certain rudiments could be found, tending to appear and disappear with equal suddenness, but nearly devoid of stabilizing influence and of impact upon the enormity of the felt, but not yet defined need.

Data to assist in even a rough estimate of the real requirement did not exist. The Adviser, summoned to plan, could work only upon the conviction that a mere copy of the Central European system of psychiatric care familiar to him was not appropriate. Even before the question of the kind of care and training therefore lay the question of the kinds of presumptive patients and their number. The holder of a university chair achieved some notoriety by proclaiming that ninety percent of Iranians were mentally disordered. On the other hand, when the Adviser expressed his interest in the three-quarters of the population that were agricultural and rural (the proportion had lessened to some 62 percent by the census of 1966 [164]), he was scoffed at by both Iranians and foreign residents convinced that the country people were too simple at the best, at the worst too dull to entertain mental conflicts. It seemed necessary to find out.

The resources of the WHO Mental Health Project consisted of one psychiatrist and one (foreign) psychiatric nurse, those of the Mental Health Unit in the Ministry of Health of its Chief, himself a psychologist, his secretary and his driver, with hardly any budget to speak of and no more in sight, so there was ample opportunity for cogitation upon methods that might be used in an epidemiological survey, the execution of which to all appearances lay if anywhere in the remote distance. The institutional structure described together with other peculiarities concerning the use of, stay in and discharge from psychiatric hospitals made hospital statistics, even when obtainable, as they slowly became, useless as indices of morbidity and prevalence. Suggestions repeatedly proferred for a pilot study of one or another kind in Tehran impressed the Adviser as rather worse than valueless because of the size and many-layered diversity of the city (then of over one million, in 1984 variously estimated as between 9 and 14 millions), the absence of any means for representative sampling, but above all because of the basic and overwhelming preponderance of the rural areas and population which, and not the capital city, must be considered to represent Iran.

An early information-gathering trip to Ahwaz, capital of the oil-rich but then arid Ostan of Khuzestan at the head of the Persian Gulf, opened a first door. The Health Department itself could do nothing, but introduced the Adviser to the Director of Village Health and Sanitation, Dez Irrigation Pilot Area, Khuzestan Water and Power Authority, Plan Organization of Iran, Dr. F. G. L. Gremliza. In preparation for the construction of the Dez Dam and for the development of the area to be irrigated by its waters, the Khuzestan Water and Power Authority through its contractor, the Resources and Development Corporation of New York, was conducting a health survey of a pilot area within the larger (Greater Dez) region subsequently to be affected and had placed Dr. Gremliza, a man of long experience in the Iranian Health Services in the remotest parts of Khuzestan, in charge. Mental health had not been accorded a place in the survey. Dr. Gremliza, while aware of its importance, was skeptical about finding any practical and moderately objective ways of determining it, but kindly invited the Adviser to return to the Pilot Area and try out the methods he had in mind. He did so in 1961, made informal field trials in government dispensaries in the vicinity of Isfahan and Tehran as well as in Tehran itself, improved his instruments and was able to convince both Dr. Gremliza and himself that these did demonstrate both individual and group differences such as between residents of marginal urban areas and those of remote country settlements of the south. For reasons beyond the control of both, however, regular field work in Khuzestan could not be carried out before the spring of 1964.

Meanwhile, however, another door had opened. The newly appointed Director-General of Public Health to the Ostan of Fars in 1963 determined to open a rural dispensary in the Marvdasht District. His able head of the Department of Maternal and Child Health and a visiting Professor of Hygiene at the University of Shiraz conceived the idea of a preliminary public health survey in the three rural villages the dispensary was intended mainly to serve with the threefold aim of collecting basic data, establishing terms of reference for the dispensary's effectiveness and conducting a field exercise in public health and preventive medicine for the training of students and staff. As in Khuzestan, mental health had not been considered, but at the Adviser's suggestion was immediately and enthusiastically included, and he was invited to supervise that section of the survey. The principal field work was performed in the summer of 1963 with follow-ups on into the spring of 1964. Included in the Marvdasht Survey, though relevant to a different population, was a study by the same principles, methods and staff of a sub-tribe of Qashqai nomads encamped for three days in the desert at a negotiable distance from Shiraz. Results are presented in [17].

In the spring of 1964 circumstances permitted a trial survey (unpublished) in Khuzestan. In the summer of that year the Adviser left Iran to go to the University of Bern, but was able to return on leave in the last quarter of 1965 as WHO Short Term Consultant to execute the actual Khuzestan Survey together with his wife, a psychiatrist and former Director of the Psychiatric Policlinic in Winterthur, Switzerland. In 1966 and 1967 he was in Iran again for short term consultantships that did not include epidemiological investigation directly but served to pave the way for a larger project directed toward an urban sample. As two rural and one nomad studies had led to confirmatory rather than contradicting results and had given us confidence in our methodology, we felt that, our primary responsibility to the agricultural and rural population having been discharged, comparison with an urban population was needed and justified, both for itself and for what light it might shed upon mental health problems of groups exposed to change more intense and rapid than that taking place in the more conservative countryside. The Iranian Government agreed and presented a corresponding request to the World Health Organization's Office of Research, Planning and Co-Ordination, which rejected it. The Eastern Mediterranean Regional Office took a different view, obtained a pledge of the Iranian Government for local expenses and re-appointed the first author as Short Term Consultant from October 1, 1969, to the end of August, 1970, in order to carry out, again together with the second author, the Shiraz Mental Health Survey. An account of the main neuropsychiatric epidemiological findings has been given in [31]. A happy, unforeseen by-product of this was the opportunity to survey the village of Qalandari some 80 km distant from the city on the Shiraz-Kazerun road. This village was of particular interest to us because it had been founded eight years before by Qashqai nomads who determined to settle there, so that a direct comparison was possible between truly nomadic and sedentary members of the same tribe. The first full account thereof appears here.

The purpose of this volume is to offer a comprehensive and coherent report not only on all the epidemiological investigations the authors have performed up to 1976 in Iran, with reference to such findings as others have recorded, but also on their background psychological studies, published hitherto only in small part.

III. General Principles

As indicated in the preceding chapter the authors – clinical psychiatrists in public service with an interest in depth psychology, one holding also a degree in general psychology, the other in chemistry – entered the field of epidemiology late and almost fortuitously. From their own thinking, from the pressure of circumstantial necessities, from experience and from growing acquaintance with the literature and practitioners of their new discipline certain considerations have emerged that have guided their work throughout and thus appropriately may be presented here, as they hold for all the several studies that follow. A few seem to possess general validity over and above the special circumstances under which our work in Iran was performed, and these we shall try to articulate at the beginning.

The WHO project went under the head of "mental health", and from the very first we were interested in the well as much as the ill – an interest that surely requires no special explanation or justification. It had, however, its practical grounds as well. To judge what one should count as ill, one must know the well, as between the two in most fields of medicine, though conspicuously so in psychiatry, the boundary is not sharp. The large body of psychological data, especially test data, on the well such as exists in most Western countries and is often taken for granted as a basis for comparison did not exist in Iran up at least to 1970 and has not grown to comparable dimensions since then. While the first author was working as WHO Adviser in the country not a few rumors of test projects reached his ears, but, with few exceptions to be mentioned in their appropriate places, no useable, suitably standardized and generally accessible data met his eyes. Neither did they do so on most of his subsequent missions to Iran, though he was constantly on the search for them. This is not to say that psychological tests were not in use. They were, in troubling diversity, little or not at all adapted and never restandardized, usually translated out of the language of the psychologist's training and applied by rule of thumb, with such adjustment in presentation and evaluation as experience suggested to the user. We recognize that preliminary stage in the development of test psychology in Iran as unavoidable and do not aim to criticize it, but merely to remark that it offered us no instruments ready for our use.

A not inconsiderable body of descriptive ethnological and socio-economic studies on many diverse aspects of Iranian life existed and continues to multiply. Interesting as they were and are, they could assist us regrettably little in our specific purpose, and therefore we have drawn upon them in this volume sparingly. Rather it will be for our successors to correlate the psychological and psychiatric findings with the ethnological facts. Gladly would we and our colleagues in Iran have welcomed an ethnologist to our team, especially in the rural areas, but with our limited resources we could not even earnestly think of trying to find one. On the other hand, our Iranian colleagues were familiar enough with their own people to guide us and shield us from grosser errors, though they are acquitted of course of all responsibility, and our own accumulating experience stood us in good stead. Even more gladly would we have added a sociologist in Shiraz and did then make efforts to do so, but without result.

Our aims in gathering test data therefore were several: 1. to obtain basic information on the normal psychology of the Iranian people; 2. to standardize certain numerical tests for future general use; 3. to decide whether a projective test of personality not essentially numerical in character could be used transculturally and, if so, to extract from it again as much information as possible on the normal psychology of the people studied; 4. to use our small test battery as a screening device for the identification of subjects suspect of psychopathology. Since we were nearly without trained interviewers or enjoyed their assistance only sporadically and in insufficient numbers, such a screening device was essential if any sample of even moderate size was to be investigated. The tests had to be simple enough so that medical and educated lay persons could be prepared in a brief course in the field to administer, though not to score them. A short questionnaire was added. If a suspicion of pathology rising from any source whatever was clinically confirmed, it was checked against the test findings, but no diagnosis was made on the basis of test findings alone. Conversely, assured clinical findings could be used to refine the interpretation of tests conceived and in part standardized in other climes.

While it may be taken as a truism that the counting of sick people has little epidemiological meaning unless the well ones also are counted, it seems too often to be forgotten and sometimes even to be denied that the kind and degree of illness from which they suffer are of hardly less importance. In any other field of medical epidemiology beside the psychiatric the importance at least of kind would be indisputable. While "diseases of the eye" may form in one sense a meaningful entity, what ophthalmologist would lump together a conjunctivitis and an amotio retinae? While the classification of ophthalmological disorders may be more precise, the divisions between them sharper than in psychiatry, to affirm that there is no workable or valid classification of psychiatric disorders at all is to magnify slight differences, often of phraseology only, at the expense of larger, general ones, practicable agreement on which has been demonstrated by recent WHO studies on the diagnosis of schizophrenia and affective psychoses and by similar endeavors [179, 205]. While we are still far from an altogether satisfactory classificatory system, those systems that we have, and upon which a moderate agreement prevails, seem infinitely superior to chaos. There is more to this than a mere craving for order. Returning to the ophthalmological comparison, a conjunctivitis is usually a banal, an amotio retinae a grave disorder with different priorities and methods of treatment and with potentially very different consequences. The same holds for a transitory reactive depression and e.g. a catatonia. Diseases differ not only in their etiology and pathology, but also in their social consequences both immediate and remote. This may impress itself especially upon the adviser laboring with scant resources in a country just emerging into Anglo-European conceptions of medico-social care. He must set priorities as best he can, and the first priority will not necessarily pertain to the severest disorders, but to those which can be treated fairly effectively with restricted means. Thus, catatonia and imbecility are both crippling diseases, but the former is frequently amenable to therapy, while the latter is not. For such simple and practical reasons besides scientific curiosity we decided at the outset that psychiatric diagnoses were indispensable, though well aware of the difficulties inherent in and the controversies waged about them. We agree with Strotzka's [188] sharp criticism of psychiatric surveys without diagnoses. These include some of the most extensive and expensive on record, the effort on which, we feel regretfully, has been only partially rewarded.

Another aspect to be considered is that of the interrelationships of psychiatric and other diseases among themselves. Leaving the non-psychiatric, non-neurological disorders aside, it is a question of great interest for psychiatry itself whether the distribution of psychiatric disorders within the total remains more or less constant, even though the sum may vary, and if it does not (as indeed in our findings it does not), what shifts appear, to what putative causes may they be ascribed, and how is their variance related to that of other disorders? Surveys of one disease only such as schizophrenia, affective psychoses, epilepsy or the like lead unavoidably to the question of interrelationship, but stop short of it. The survey of global psychiatric or personality disorder circumvents it, leaving the psychiatrist frustrated and furnishing mainly fuel for futile socio-political arguments, the so-called "factual" basis of which is dubious in the extreme. That not all psychiatric disorders are sharply set off one from the other is a fact only too painfully familiar to the clinician plagued by problems of differential diagnosis, yet we hold this to be no excuse for begging the problem or legislating it, as is were, out of existence. On the other hand, here is not the place to enter into a discussion of the thorny question of psychiatric disease entities. Fashions in regarding them change from decade to decade, while clinicians since Kraepelin's time continue to work, not altogether ineffectively, with groups of patients, common formal characteristics of whose disorders and their courses, abetted sometimes by knowledge of etiology or reasonable hypotheses about pathogenesis, remain recognizable, more or less definable and constitute a disease picture if not an entity. This basis, upon which we have elected to work, possesses at all events the advantages of a fairly general, though not universal agreement and of comprehensibility to the great majority of our colleagues and to scientists in related fields. When we speak, as we sometimes shall, of a psychiatric "disease", it is in this sense that we intend it to be understood.

Thus it was clear from the outset that our surveys were not to be directed to one disease or one class of diseases, e.g. the psychoses, but were to embrace all ascertainable psychiatric disorders of significant degree – the organic, the functional, the reactive and the constitutional. The overlapping of neurological and psychiatric disorders implied that the former must be included as well as for their own sake. Our survey could be called neuropsychiatric. For brevity and convenience, however, we shall generally speak only of a psychiatric survey, reserving the term "neuropsychiatric" for those cases which actually showed a combination of neurological and psychiatric features, etiology or symptoms. The inclusion of purely neurological cases had another reason besides. Most developing countries, especially those influenced by British medical tradition, tend to institute chairs and departments of neurology before those of psychiatry, to train their students accordingly and to relegate psychiatry, if recognized at all, to a Cinderella-like marginal existence. In such situations, specialists prefer to be addressed as neurologists while mostly earning their livings from the prescription of psychopharmaceuticals. It therefore becomes a matter of interest to ascertain the relative prevalences of neurological, neuropsychiatric and psychiatric disorders together with their degrees of severity or disablement.

These basic decisions entailed others, two of which are interrelated: what was to be considered a "case", and what kinds of cases were to be rubricated, i.e. what nosological system was to be employed? As implied above, the general Kraepelinian classification common, with variations, to the majority of Anglo-European psychiatrists and to their pupils scattered about the world was accepted as a working basis. A reasonable conclusion from this seemed to be to regard as a "case" a person whose mental health was disturbed to such a degree that he would be regarded as a "case" by ordinary Central European out-patient clinic standards such as were familiar to us and will be, we may presume, to a large proportion of our readers, leaving aside minor deviations of little or no consequence to their bearers. Such can indeed be discovered and registered even in distant and to some extent foreign countries, but their compilation to the point where nigh upon three quarters of a population is declared to be disordered or at any rate "deviant" can imply hardly anything but deviation from a highly questionable ideal norm. Easy though it is to argue that the decision upon such a basis as to whether or not a given individual represents a "case" is arbitrary and subjective, this is in truth far less the fact than it seems to be upon the surface, at least if the decisions are made, as they were here made, by colleagues trained in similar schools and with similar backgrounds of experience. Other, newer epidemiological surveys [178, 188] bear out this point. The oft advocated criterion of willingness to consult a physician or of actually being under medical treatment is clearly inapplicable in a situation wherein psychiatrists and psychiatric hospitals or policlinics are extremely few, not to mention a widespread lack of knowledge about them at the time we began our work. Where knowledge of a sort existed, it was accompanied by a prejudice against them as representatives of custodial care. The recommendation of a WHO Expert Committee in 1960 [205] to use absence from work or the application of legal or social measures as criteria of disturbances serious enough to constitute a "case" is, if anything, still less feasible, since absence from work in unindustrialized countries seldom can be controlled objectively, is indulged in (*sit venia verbo!*) the more sparingly the harder is the struggle for existence and is, except in rare instances, nearly impossible to ascertain objectively or even to define among the vast majority of the female population. Where social and legal measures are only seldom and sporadically taken, this criterion is not only insufficient, but deceptive. Reliance upon indigenous criteria or opinions of what is "sick" or "abnormal" has been advocated with some fervor, but their actual application presents difficulties hardly surmised by epidemiological strategists theorizing in their studies. Our Iranian colleagues, for the most part Western trained, who should have been competent if anybody was, protested their inability to make other than highly conjectural use of them, and we did not esteem ourselves more knowledgeable than they. Complicated interview techniques with abundant questioning of informants from the presumably disordered person's environment might conceivably have led to results, but it would have necessitated far more skilled local staff than we had at our service as well as a much greater expenditure of time for many fewer persons, thus narrowing the statistical basis precariously. In general the reflection seems justified that the application of highly various indigenous standards of what is well and ill the world over, while of undoubted ethno-sociological interest and sometimes illuminating in regard to pathogenesis, is of questionable medical value. This holds especially where one is looking, as here, for comparative statistics. One cannot compare meters of different length. From a more practical point of view countries in transition such as Iran with an ancient and highly developed traditional culture behind them are shifting ineluctably in medical concepts and patterns of medical care toward Anglo-European standards (themselves in a process of slow change, to be sure, but to a degree stable and for much of the rest of world still exemplary), so it is only reasonable that they be measured by these standards. Here lies no question of preference and no judgment of value. The direction in which secular transition was moving in the nineteen-sixties and -seventies was that of convergence with the Western socio-economic system in its larger sense, which lies beyond and behind political controversies. Stated Iranian policy at that time called for such convergence. Medical concepts developed within the frame of reference of that system are therefore, we opine, relevant, applicable, appropriate and above all suitable for international discourse. In the discussion of our test results we shall return to this question.

If we are to employ Western nosology, then, we must ask ourselves which nosology? At the time the Adviser began his epidemiological studies the seventh revision of the WHO's International Classification of Diseases and Causes of Death (ICD) was in force. Its psychiatric section was generally admitted to be unsatisfactory. In some respects it was over-simplified, in others too complicated and detailed for the collection of simple mental hospital statistics, to which he set himself at about the same time. To this aim he devised a deliberately simplified schema based on his own experience and on then current Swiss practice, which was utilized subsequently by the Mental Health Unit of the Iranian Ministry of Health, modified and expanded it slightly for his first two epidemiological surveys in rural areas and has retained it for the Shiraz Survey and for this book in the interests of comparability. As against previously published articles some small additions have been made to it in order to include and specify disorders encountered in the larger urban sample but too sparingly represented in the rural groups to have deserved there a rubric unto themselves. The framework and all principal categories remain the same. The introduction of the eighth revision of the ICD in 1969 altered little. The ninth revision, introduced in 1979, obviated a number of its predecessor's disadvantages, especially in regard to the classification of the reactive disorders, and might have served as a basis for our tables if its glossary had not appeared too late, just after these had been compiled and cast into their final form. Nevertheless, we have utilized it in a number of auxiliary tables which did not imply complete reclassification and for coding exemplary cases, have prepared a table of equivalents between ICD-9 and our classification (D IV 5) and a tabulation of all cases according to ICD-9 (Table D IV 6). Except where otherwise stated, the definitions of mental disorders given in the *Glossary and Guide to their Classification in Accordance with the Ninth Revision of the International Classification of Diseases* [207] apply.

In the first paragraphs of this chapter a distinction between degree as well as kinds of psychiatric illness was implied. Rather curiously it has received little consideration in most epidemiological studies up to now, though it is essential for planning psychiatric services. These will tend to be directed, as mentioned above, toward the more severe forms, but restricted to those which are either amenable to treatment or, if not, imperatively require custodial care. Apart from this it makes a substantial difference in socio-economic terms whether a given segment of a population is mainly subject to psychiatric disorders that are of lighter or graver degree. Even if total prevalence remains the same in different segments or strata, differences in the severity of affliction may cast light upon questions of etiology and pathogenesis. An obvious example is the deficiency diseases with psychiatric effects. We have therefore distinguished throughout between three degrees of psychiatric, neuropsychiatric and neurological disorder and defined them as follows:

1. *Mild.* These comprise borderline and milder cases suffering more than trifling inconvenience, but not gravely impaired or likely to become gravely impaired in their social adjustment or economic productivity. They will be designated as P_1.
2. *Medium.* Individuals with unquestionable psychiatric, neuropsychiatric or neurological pathology and need of specialized medical aid, socially and economically significantly impaired, but not wholly or largely incapacitated or likely to become so, designated P_2.
3. *Severe.* Severely diseased individuals who have required, require or seem likely to require hospitalization, institutionalization or some form of long-continuing medico-social assistance presuming that such facilities are available, designated P_3. (Often they were not. The assumption was made by conscious comparison with and adjustment to Central European standards for the same reasons as set down above in regard to diagnoses and case determination). All idiocies, but not all major psychoses are included in this group, the psychoses being graded partly by their present status, partly by their presumptive prognosis.

Judgments of severity were clinical, made as they are from day to day in practice, with all the complexities, sources of error and subjectivities therein implied. For this we make no apologies. Far-reaching objectification and quantification were out of the question under field conditions and for sociological reasons. There were questions that could not be asked, verifications that could not be undertaken without jeopardizing the survey. If such judgments be made on the one hand with explicit, conscious reference to Central European standards, on the other hand they can only be made with some modest claim to validity by investigators familiar with the field under investigation, though not necessarily indigenous to it. In this respect we had the advantage, besides Iranian counsel, of the circumstance that the first author had lived and traveled in Iran for several years before beginning epidemiological field work.

In judging severity anamnesis and prognosis were taken duly into account as far as feasible (regarding restrictions see above). *Clinical diagnosis,* while buttressed by anamnesis as in all medicine, *referred to the condition at time of examination.* Past illnesses from which full recovery had taken place were not counted. If recovery had not been complete the residues were assigned their proper diagnostic position, e.g. pseudo-psychopathy after meningo-encephalitis. Obvious as this procedure seems, it could have far-reaching consequences, as when one person who had clearly suffered several attacks of schizophrenia did not figure as schizophrenic in our sample because he had fully remitted. Since field work continued over half a year in Shiraz, two and a half months in Khuzestan, and in Marvdasht also more than half a year when all follow-ups are included, what we can offer are *period prevalence rates.* Nothing in our experience suggests that for such a period they would differ substantially from point prevalence rates if these could be obtained. This became particularly clear in Khuzestan, where we were in constant close contact with the entire population under study in a clearly circumscribed area throughout the whole period of field work and did not observe the emergence or disappearance of any psychiatric illness. Our overview in Shiraz naturally was less close, but neither did we observe there in households which we visited repeatedly any incidence of previously unrecorded disorders.

Standards of diagnostic precision, following our general guide lines set down above, were those of out-patient clinical practice in Central Europe, though we had more psychological test material at our disposal than many policlinics do. We did not strive to obtain full case histories in every instance, but contented ourselves for imperious economic reasons with as much information as was necessary to establish a diagnosis beyond reasonable doubt. This was sought freely from household members and, where the adult proband agreed, from other informants, in the case of school children nearly always from their teachers, when possible from hospital or policlinic records, occasionally from private physicians and from diverse other sources. The hospitals and out-patient services of the Health Department and of the Shiraz University generously carried out special examinations and laboratory tests where necessary and where the patient consented, both in the Shiraz and Marvdasht studies, while in Khuzestan we had the able and ready assistance of Dr. Gremliza's efficient mobile laboratory. With a handful of exceptions the two authors themselves saw, severally or together, diagnosed and rated in respect to severity every case subsequently classified as pathological in Khuzestan and Shiraz. In Marvdasht and in the Qashqai camp the first author saw all suspected cases and assessed them together with one or another of his Iranian colleagues. The exceptions mentioned were formed by a few neurological cases in Marvdasht examined by an Associate Professor of Neurology in Shiraz University, and a very small number of children with behavior disorders whom an experienced nurse visited and of whom she delivered unambiguous descriptions. This exception we were forced to make as time toward the end of our permissible stay in the field became scant. Where her accounts of certain other suspected cases left room for doubt, we returned ourselves for an examination. Practically the entire material here presented has the advantage of having been diagnosed and judged finally according to agreed criteria and common experience by at least one of the responsible authors and in the overwhelming majority by both. Thus within the bounds of human subjectivity and error a certain constancy and consistency in its evaluation is guaranteed and therewith a better comparability of the several samples studied between each other.

After our initial experiences in Marvdasht we adopted the principle of tabulating only a single psychiatric or neurological diagnosis per person. Combined neuro-psychiatric cases received one each. The reason for this was, of course, the difficulty of treating multiple diagnoses statistically, especially when, as in Shiraz, larger groups were under consideration. The diagnosis chosen for tabulation was the one judged to be of the first importance for the pathological picture, of the greatest severity and also, other things being equal, of the highest specificity. Thus, for example, psychoses or acquired, symptomatic psychiatric disorders received in general priority over primary lack of intelligence, primary psychopathy and secondary neuroticism unless the proportions in which such factors contributed to the clinical picture were manifestly reversed (e.g. severe neuroticism after minor cerebral trauma or general illness without indication of significant organic complication). Inevitably this led to an attenuation of the figures for such secondary (in point of importance, not of time) conditions in our general diagnostic tables, but we have preferred to err upon the side of parsimony. Also we have added outside our main tables comprehensive data, including secondary and tertiary diagnoses, for groups of basic disorders such as the oligophrenic, psychopathic and reactive. Overlapping occurs in the case of the mixed neuropsychiatric disease pictures, which appear in two tables, the psychiatric and the neurological, but in estimating total prevalence are counted only once. As the psychiatric cases were much more numerous than the neurological ones, whereas the majority of these presented some psychiatric complications (in other words were neuropsychiatric by our terminology), we have adopted the expedient of including the psychiatric diagnoses of the neuropsychiatric cases in the psychiatric diagnostic tables without comment, but of listing such combined cases in the neurological tables together with mention of the attendant psychiatric complications, their kind and frequency, in each neurologic group.

Comment is required upon our use and estimation of certain diagnostic categories, taking them in the order in which they appear throughout our tables. The first major category, that of the functional psychoses, hardly requires explanation, being central to clinical psychiatry nearly everywhere. The number of cases in it is small, as must be expected from the size of our combined samples. As we did not encounter schizo-affective psychoses we did not include any (empty) sub-category for them. From the emptiness of the second major category, acute symptomatic psychoses, of course does not follow that such do not occur in Iran. They do indeed, as elsewhere, but none happened to fall into our sample during the period of our field work. Even though empty, it seemed proper to mention this important class to reassure readers that it had not been forgotten. The like holds for the sub-category general paralysis under main category III, subchronic and chronic symptomatic psychoses and residual states. It is agreed by all local neuropsychiatrists to be a very rare disease in Iran and is hardly encountered outside the southern port areas and the nearby urban settlements (e.g. Ahwaz). Within this main category it is most difficult to arrive at precise differential diagnoses, which had to be assigned to some cases of unquestionable organic origin more on the basis of likelihood than of satisfying proof.

Contrary to frequent practice category IV, reactive disorders, has been thrice subdivided instead of twice or not at all. The distinction between the neuroses and the psychosomatic disorders will be conceded by the majority. Since detailed somatic investigations seldom could be performed under survey conditions, diagnoses of psychosomatic illnesses often were made according to probability where typical subjective complaints coincided with a neurotic anamnesis and personality structure. They seemed most problematical in cases of gastrointestinal troubles, such being all too common by themselves, particularly in rural areas, by reason of inadequate diet, unsanitary living conditions and parasitic and other infestation.

Less often made, but illuminating and important in our opinion, is the distinction between simple and neurotic pathological developments. In this and in other respects within category IV we follow Binder [35, 36], whose classification of reactive and psychopathic disorders we find to be the clearest hitherto advanced. Briefly, the criteria of the neurosis by this are that the pathogenic psychic content is both dissociated from the remainder of the conscious and repressed. In the simple development dissociation, but not repression may occur: the pathogenic factor remains known, even if not constantly present in the individual's awareness. It is a component of the conscious. While some others hold that the distinction, though theoretically interesting, cannot be carried out in practice, both our clinical and survey experience convince us that it generally can be to a degree that is practically useful and not more subject to error than other diagnostic differentiations in common use. Its application in the field, where time is limited and the language foreign, requires frequently besides the ordinary exploration of the subject the aid of a test that can indicate with reasonable reliability the presence or absence of neurotic structure and can often point to the sources of repressed conflict. For this we have found the Zulliger Test in the field like its parent, the Rorschach Test in the clinic, to be invaluable. The importance of the distinction lies in the information that it conveys about the tendency to repress – a valuable piece of information when mental hygiene measures must be considered as well as of substantial scientific interest. The reader is asked to note the word "development", to which in the text both the adjectives "simple" and "neurotic" apply (in the tables for the sake of brevity only we use the heading "neuroses" instead of "neurotic pathological developments"). It is intended to imply, following again Binder, a more than momentary or transitory disorder such as a fleeting reactive depression or an isolated fit of anger, but rather the development, out of an initial psychic trauma or conflict, of a disorder that becomes a lasting or recurring, though not by any means necessarily permanent, source of discomfort or even of suffering. All cases here diagnosed under "reactive disorders" are in this sense developments. We regard their differentiation from simple pathological reactions such as may occur once or rarely in a lifetime as essential, particularly for epidemiological purposes. Since we are all subject occasionally to simple or neurotic pathological reactions, as when we weep or rage over trifling causes, those are nearly insignificant for epidemiology and for the planning of psychiatric services, even though the practicing psychiatrist may be and not seldom is confronted with them. They can be so serious as to lead to crimes of violence, but they are ephemeral. Furthermore, the inclusion of the transitory pathological reactions, whether simple or neurotic, together with the pathological developments of both kinds and the over-inclusive labeling of them all as "neurosis" has led in psychiatric and especially in psychotherapeutic circles to regrettable misunderstandings and to superfluous, sometimes acrimonious debate over the duration, course and tendency to remission or self-healing of the "neuroses" and over the efficacy of psychotherapy in general. Agreement remains impossible so long as the word "neurosis" is employed now in a very wide, now in a restricted sense and concepts are not defined. Following Binder's exemplary theoretical clarification, the empirical studies of Ernst [69] and of Cremerius [59] have done much to place discussion upon a more solid basis. The first author of this volume has summarized some of the more important results [19].

Under the main heading of "reactive disorders" we thus have three secondary headings ordered according to the degree of repression encountered in each. The simple pathological developments show dissociation, but not repression; the true neuroses are characterized by dissociation and repression of the pathogenic content, usually a complex; and in the psychosomatic disorders the theory of double or two-phased repression advanced by Mitscherlich [151] has at all events much to recommend it. The tertiary headings mostly correspond to those in common use, from which a selection was made empirically, our guiding principle being that no separate heading was to be used for a category represented only by a single case. Therefore the subheadings in our several journal publications are not the same throughout. The list had been revised again for this book in such a way that, while a tertiary category may remain vacant in one or another survey, each category comprises at least two cases from the total, whereas single cases (e.g. psychosomatic cholecystopathy) were placed in the group of "other and polymorphous." They are usually mentioned in the text. The truly polymorphous cases we find both in epidemiological field work and in clinical practice to be more numerous than most classificatory schemes, especially the ICD, concede and agree with Jung [110, p. 92] "that the classification of the neuroses is a very unsatisfactory affair and therefore . . . a specific diagnosis (sc.: of a neurosis) only seldom really means anything". Elsewhere he writes [110, p. 44]: "About a third of my cases do not suffer from any clinically definable neurosis".

Certain sub-headings under the reactive disorders and their secondary categories may need definition and comment. The "anxious" and "depressive" developments and neuroses speak for themselves. "Phobic" implies here the irrational fear of a specific object or situation in contrast to diffuse objectless anxiety. "Hysteric" is used strictly in the sense of a conversion neurosis. When applied to every kind of demonstrative and tendentious behavior it tends to become an almost meaningless and all too often simply abusive term. "Hypochondric" and "neurasthenic" are related to it and to each other by the preoccupation with the body, a preoccupation that becomes diffuser as one proceeds from hysteria over hypochondria to neurasthenia. The distinction between the two latter impressed itself upon us the more strongly as our experience grew and we were better able to compare societal levels, peasants and townsmen. We shall return to this when commenting upon the results. There follows under the "neuroses" (IV 2 g in the diagnostic tables) an ad hoc created concept that we introduced to avoid minimal categories on the one hand or the obliteration of them in the mixed category on the other: the concept of neuroses of self-insufficiency. The English term is cumbersome: the German *Unzulänglichkeit* would be both handier and more precise. It is intended to cover cases of neurotic withdrawal or holding back, of adjustment or performance below the objective level of capability because of imagined or exaggerated self-insuffiency, a relatively common instance of which is neurotic pseudo-debility. Other instances not uncommon in Iran are a similar withdrawal and refusal or inability to function at true capacity because of partial paralysis or paresis (often from poliomyelitis) or impaired vision (often from trachoma), the reaction being disproportionate to the defect. Such patients are not primarily depressive and indeed may not be depressive at all and characteristically react, e.g., to a paretic limb, by a smiling refusal of any attempt to exercise or use it. That such behavior is frequent in pseudo-debility is well known. In many girls and women it has been encouraged hitherto by tradition and constitutes, when not extreme, a "normal" pattern, as we shall see in connection with the test findings. Neither does it fit the case, we believe, to call such behavior "hysterical", especially when hysteria is restricted, as it is here, to a conversion neurosis. The paresis or amaurosis is not a product of conversion: it is objectively present and organically based. Together with the following group of the negativistic neuroses (*Trotzneurosen*) the neuroses of self-insufficiency account for a substantial share of such neuroses of childhood as we have observed in Iran, though of course they are not confined to children.

Again for empirical reasons we have distinguished between migrainoid and other types of psychosomatic headache (mostly tension headaches) as from the very first the difference between the sexes impressed us. Because true hemicrania was rare we have preferred the term migrainoid, implying most or all the other usual symptoms of migraine.

The constitutional disorders we have divided into two groups, the predominantly intellectual and the predominantly affective. The title "clinically manifest oligophrenia" speaks for itself. Though we were using intelligence tests, they were far from being standardized on the population under study, their standardization being one of the purposes of this book. We took their results as adjuvant indications of oligophrenia only when performance on them was zero or very close to zero and never made a diagnosis of mental deficiency upon this basis alone. We demanded direct or indirect (anamnestic) evidence of congenital or early acquired inability to perform intellectually up to the level of relatively independent subsistance as defined by the social and economic pattern in the case of adults, with the appropriate modifications for age in the case of children, confirmed wherever possible by the familiar clinical, physical and physiognomic signs. Our diagnoses applied, in other words, mostly to what is ordinarily called imbecility or idiocy (ICD 318–319) but did not exclude milder cases, often called feeble-minded or moronic, where the patient's inability to cope with the environment was impressive. The tendency to diagnose only the lower grades accords with the recommendations of the WHO and is surely more practical and realistic in field work unless well validated tests are available. We have chosen "oligophrenia" as a designation because of its advantages as a single and relatively neutral word, the other current terms being cumbersome and generally loaded with pejorative connotations. The common "mental deficiency" does not state what kind of mental deficiency and could be (though it is not) applied equally well to psychopathy, whereas "mental subnormality" is long and awkward and "mental retardation" carries an implication that it is preferable to avoid. Finally, diagnosis of the genetic forms of oligophrenia was made clinically as we had no facilities for karyotyping or for elaborate metabolic and endocrinological examinations.

Constitutional affective disorders or psychopathies were diagnosed parsimoniously for a number of reasons which include abuse of the term in the past, increasing knowledge about the organic or somatic bases of such disorders which enables us to assign more and more of them to the symptomatic category III as pseudo-psychopathies, and the desire to avoid as far as possible confusion with the reactive disorders. The ICD places psychopathies and "abnormal personalities" in the same category. Depending upon the case, we have assigned the abnormal personalities sometimes to the inveterate neuroses, sometimes to the psychopathies in our classification. We have not restricted the meaning of psychopathy as mainly Anglo-Saxon schools of psychiatry do to the so-called "sociopathies", i.e. the antisocial, frequently criminal or in older parlance "morally insane". Rather we have employed it as is generally done in Central European practice to refer to any kind of congenital, continuing affective anomaly lacking both ascertainable somatic cause and process character, but grave enough to engender suffering upon its bearer, the environment, or both. Beside antisocial or asocial psychopaths we thus find irritable, schizoid, sensitive and even hypomanic cases and regret that the German *haltlos*, which describes adequately and precisely one of the commonest groups, has not only no equivalent in English but appears practically untranslatable (it denotes a person incapable of forming durable affective ties, but lacks a corresponding adjective in English).

IV. General Procedures

Insofar as procedure was the same in all five fields of investigation it will be described here, variations due to special needs and circumstances in the respective chapters. Care was taken to keep it as nearly uniform as possible.

Circumstance had its hand in the choice of sites, as is clear from the first chapter, but the sites can be taken as largely representative in the view both of numerous competent Iranians and of the authors. To search for one "representative" site, village or city in a country as large and multifarious as Iran would be, in any case, to chase after an illusion. Iran possesses large ethnic and linguistic (Turkish, Kurdish, Armenian and Arab) minorities. Except for the nomad groups and what sprinkling might occur in predominantly Persian regions these were excluded, not without the hope that they will be studied soon. Focussing first on the rural population as the backbone of the country, it was inevitable that comparison should be sought with the two other principal constituents of the nation, the cities and the tribes.

Having fixed upon a site, our next step was to decide, always in council with local authorities and colleagues and with the aid of as much preliminary information as we could get, whether a census or a sampling study or a mixture of both was to be performed. Either decision implied a fresh local population census, which in each case was carried out shortly before the beginning of the survey itself. General census had been performed in 1956 and 1966, but we could not trust to extrapolation of local figures and needed in any case identifying numbers. Census and later sampling were done by households, the natural sociological unit, using the Iranian National Census' definition of a household [157, page b], which "consists of one or several individuals residing in one place and sharing expenses and principal meals". Not all members of a household must be related under this definition – an important point, as servants and other employees not seldom live together with the employer. Each household was assigned a number, and for sampling purposes every n-th number was taken. All persons living together in a household (including naturally those temporarily absent) were registered, but for survey purposes those under six years of age were eliminated. It was decided to do so because hardly any known tests, if any at all, register reliably from adulthood or late childhood to and below an age under six, and because the assessment of psychiatric disorder becomes increasingly difficult, calling for special training and experience, as one regresses from school age to the cradle. Neither our collaborators nor we ourselves possessed such training. In this way some early, severe and not infrequently fatal neurological disorders undoubtedly were missed, but a minute search for them among the near quarter of the census population aged below six would have made claims upon our limited resources and time that we felt in general to be disproportionate (an exception was made in Marvdasht: see [20]), and that would have forced us to neglect other aspects of the survey. The survey population constitutes the census population or a randomly selected sample of it less all children below five and half years. There was no upper age limit. In all that follows, age in years implies half a year to either side of the birthday marking the completion of the year specified.

The definition just given sounds very much more precise than it really is, as every epidemiologist knows, so a word must be added about determination of age. In 1918 a decree of the Council of Ministers "urged" all Iranians to hold an identity card, but not until 1952 was the Civil Registration Bureau established and the registration of births and deaths begun. Identity cards were not issued everywhere simultaneously, on the whole sooner in the cities than in the country, and were still not universal in 1970. Numbers of middle aged to elderly people in the countryside had none, nor was the date of their birth anywhere recorded. Many among the illiterate knew neither their birth date nor their age. Some, upon being pressed, would hazard a wild guess, others not even that. Elderly persons might prefer to exaggerate to more than patriarchal dimensions and even claim over a century. Here the testimony of offspring, comparison with these and their neighbours' ages, recollection of events and the like were our resources. In some cases on the land we were forced to fall back upon medical criteria, general appearance and more or less informed guess work. A sequel of this was to make our age groups beyond adulthood comprehensive, of twenty years span, as persons generally could be allotted roughly to one of the three groups from 20–39, 40–59 and 60 or more, errors on either side tending to cancel each other out. The younger the subject the easier, as a rule, it was to ascertain the age – a fortunate circumstance since we aimed at age-scale testing. Children's or youths' identity cards nevertheless could lull one in specious security, as our co-workers explained, for the parents could omit registering their child or the registry official could neglect preparing the card for remarkable lengths of time, upon which a card might be issued bearing the current date as the date of birth! Only in the Dez Irrigation Pilot Area (Khuzestan), where the entire population had been under continuous scrutiny for a number of years and was registered in Dr. Gremliza's excellent files, could the ages of young children at least be taken as accurate. Elsewhere we strove by interrogation and the help of available documents after a reasonable approximation to accuracy but are aware of unavoidable shortcomings.

The next step, sometimes coinciding with census taking as in Marvdasht, sometimes following upon it as in Shiraz, was for an Iranian worker to prepare a household sheet with the names and ages of all persons in the household and their relationship (not necessarily of blood) to the head of the household, who was to be identified as such. Children below six were listed for the possible benefit of future workers, but were not further investigated. A set of forms with places for personal and demographic data, psychological tests, questionnaire and notes was then allotted to each proband of the psychiatric survey.

For the rural and nomad studies (Marvdasht, Khuzestan, Qashqai) we recorded the following personal characteristics: family name and forename (both required by law in Iran and in fact everywhere used), age in years (but see above), sex, literacy, household number and number of house or tent by local census list. All persons in these surveys were engaged directly or indirectly in agriculture. Socio-economic differences were slight with the exception of village headmen of the chief of the sub-tribe. The city survey called for more detailed data, which will be described and commented upon in the relevant chapter.

The personal and family data having been filled out, testing was performed either immediately or by appointment, often in stages, as it seldom happened that all members of a larger household could be assembled at one time. They were, indeed, tested and interrogated wherever and whenever circumstances dictated: at home, schools, places of work or business, in nomad tents or in the open fields and desert (herdsmen), hospitals, institutions and dispensaries, in groups or singly. While they were enjoined not to tell one another about the tests, the questions put, the answers given or the difficulties encountered, we have no illusions about the effectiveness of this instruction. More often than not, testing and interviewing had to be performed among onlookers, in courtyards or in single rooms where not only the family but the neighbors congregated by the shine of a petroleum lamp, or outdoors in a village where anyone was free to come and go. Attempts to test in uninfluenced isolation, as all good books of instruction require, would not only have created a situation totally alien to the vast majority of our subjects and therefore in its own way productive of falsification, but also led, as we quickly realized, to resentment that had to be avoided at whatever cost. The spectators and especially the interested relatives abundantly displayed the world wide tendency to kibitz but usually could be held in check by repeated friendly admonitions coupled with the assurance that their turn was coming. In family or neighborhood groups a spirit of cheerful rivalry often emerged. As a rule to which only rare exceptions were necessary because of refusal midway, fatigue, illness or interference the test battery and questionnaire were completed in an average of half an hour or less per person. This time limit had been set for practical reasons at the beginning and the battery designed to meet it. Younger children required less time in general, pathological subjects more, especially when interrogated about answers to the questionnaire.

Questions of access, acceptance and motivation are implied in the last paragraph, but as they themselves and their solutions varied from site to site they can be discussed more appropriately under local headings. On the whole, they presented less difficulties and frustrations than we had feared. Outright refusals were rare; initial protestations of unwillingness, shyness or distrust nearly always could be overcome. Though in certain cases of unsurmountable refusal its pathological origin seemed evident, these were not reckoned to the pathological cases. In the very few instances in which probands accepted the test but rejected a follow-up examination the test results were included, but no clinical evaluation was made (in a memorable case the psychiatrist and his associate were turned from the door by man and wife so volubly and with such copious, frenetic expostulation of the refusal (encouraged by the psychiatrist) that the exploration took place while the subjects were unaware of it and laid their diagnoses open for the heartily abused physician to read. They were naturally included, and when the psychiatrist laughingly told the story to an Iranian colleague the latter, to whom the couple were known, verified them). Other, happily rare causes of drop-outs from the psychiatric samples were departure of a household member shortly after census taking or after testing until after completion of field work, e.g. on a long journey or on military service elsewhere, removal to a locality that could not reasonably be reached or (in the city) to a new residence that could not be discovered, intercurrent severe and prolonged illness or, in one single case, death. Persons normally belonging to the household but absent from the beginning to the end of our stay at the site (mostly for military service) were not included in the sample. Those away for a briefer time were sought out later at home or, where practicable, in the vicinity, including villages and areas not in our sample, and usually found by patience and pertinacity. In particular, ill members were traced to general and mental hospitals and examined there. None, fortunately, as far as we learned were institutionalized or hospitalized in remote and inaccessible places, e.g. abroad.

Faulty or incomplete testing and questioning sometimes had to be corrected by a revisit, to which probands in general submitted with remarkable lack of complaint. The authors strove to be present themselves at as much testing as they could. The degree to which this was in fact possible again varied considerably from site to site and will be mentioned in the respective chapters. Even the preparation of the examiners, though basically the same, had to be carried out somewhat differently from time to time and will also be described locally.

An interrupted test battery was completed whenever possible. Only a handful of refractory cases had to be given up. A different cause for an incomplete battery could be sensory defect such as blindness (especially in trachoma-ridden Khuzestan) or deafness; therefore differences sometimes occur in the total number of single tests performed at a given site.

In order to carry out this program tests of intelligence and personality were desired that, together with a questionnaire, could serve during field work even before standardization or restandardization for screening marked deviates. The data obtained during field work would form the basis for standardization, after which the same tests should be applicable to the general population and the indications of deviancy that they had suggested could be checked against the newly established norms. Their choice was limited by a number of considerations:

1. The tests (including the questionnaire) had to be administered in general by lay persons after relatively brief specific training.

2. The entire battery should not require on the average more than half an hour per subject.

3. While there are no "culture-free" tests, the cultural bias should be kept as low as possible.

4. Verbal tests requiring the subject to read and either to mark or write answers were not suitable for a largely illiterate population.

5. Group tests, which usually involve some kind of written response, were unsuitable for the same reason, but even more to individualistic Iranian customs and mentality and to our basic practice of individual examination and interview.

6. Tests could not be used that depended upon a regular supply of expendable material from abroad (e.g. maze tests).

7. Tests should have a very wide age range, if possible from six upward, and if not designed for such a range should be capable of interpretation, even though less exact, outside the designated range.

8. Since we had begun with rural populations the great majority of whom were illiterate, it would be desirable to employ tests that could be used later in predominantly literate urban areas also or could be supplemented there without being supplanted.

Our selection ultimately fell upon:

1. An *arithmetical reasoning test* in two forms (one for illiterates, another for literates), aimed primarily at abstract intelligence.
2. A *block design test,* also in two forms, aimed primarily at practical or concrete intelligence. Both are described in Part C, Chap. I.
3. The *Zulliger Inkblot Test* or Z Test, requiring only three cards as against ten for its progenitor, the Rorschach Test. This was chosen as a short and relatively culture-free test of personality, free also from the thorny problems of translation out of a Western language into Persian. It is described in Part C, Chap. II 3.
4. The self-constructed *questionnaire* mentioned above and described in Part C, Chap. II 1–2.

After completion of each test battery with questionnaire, the examiner was required to characterize non-technically, in his or her own words, the impression the proband had made ("Describe him briefly as you would a new acquaintance in a letter to a friend"). Professionally trained co-workers of course enjoyed full freedom to write what they liked, including a diagnosis, to which however we did not bind ourselves and which we revised freely when reason appeared for doing so. Furthermore and more important, the examiner was obliged by marking an affirmative or negative response to answer strictly alternatively the question whether the person just examined in his opinion needed further, professional psychiatric-psychological examination for whatever reason or did not. An affirmative answer was always a signal for us to explore, whereas we disregarded a negative one and explored nonetheless when any other indicator was suspicious, the indicators being test results, replies to questionnaires that led to suspicion of pathology, or any other direct or indirect information pointing in this direction.

Such information was gathered where it could be found, from heads of households or more often from housewives about their members, from relatives and sometimes from neighbors, from headmen (kadkhodas) of villages and tribes, schoolteachers, physicians and (more rarely and unwillingly) from administrative officials. Its usefulness and reliability varied through a wide range and will be discussed, together with the reliability of other indicators, subsequently.

Completed forms were gathered at the end of each day, counted and roughly checked. Detailed checking and evaluation were carried out as soon as possible, generally within days, though enforced delays might occur for many reasons such as sheer load of work, administrative duties, necessity of translation, etc. Here it should be mentioned that records were hand written by the examiners in Persian with one carbon copy which was always deposited in an appropriate Iranian archive for the use of later investigators and for protection against loss. Persian rapidly hand written under field conditions with a board teetering on the examiner's knee presents its problems to one who can read the language in print, so that delays were inevitable until decipherment, with friendly aid, could be accomplished.

Training of examiners usually took place in groups or classes and lasted two to three weeks. After the general plan and purpose of the survey had been explained, our Persian colleagues and we ourselves demonstrated the various methods of examination, gave each examiner (or in Shiraz each pair) his kit, had them test each other, then patients of a dispensary, finally outside persons (not in the sample or geographically near it) or anybody who could be found, checked and discussed their recording both individually and collectively until a useable level had been attained. For the much more extensive Shiraz survey we prepared a stencilled book of instructions in English und Persian that was given to every examiner. Though some of our examiners, and not always the most highly educated among them, did excellent work, we make no claim that the general level of accuracy and reliability was equal to that which we should have desired and in the case of a group of trained technicians or professional psychologists expected. The results are offered, in full consciousness of their inherent deficiencies, as what could be obtained with the resources at hand in a first effort of this kind in a land to which psychiatric epidemiology was new.

When forms and other sources of information had been appraised and cases suspect in any way of pathology identified, these latter were subjected to individual psychiatric (and, where called for, neurological) examination by ordinary open techniques. This constituted the second phase of the survey, usually overlapping in time with the first. With the exceptions noted above, the authors performed or were present at all examinations, accompanied as a rule by a Persian co-worker able to act as a translator. This co-worker seldom was a physician, as in no case did we have a Persian physician attached full time to our project. The aid that many kind colleagues nevertheless did render, some more or less officially, some from sheer interest and good will, stealing time from other duties and from private practices, was an indispensable asset for which we remain deeply grateful. The former WHO Adviser spoke, read and wrote Persian with admitted limitations of vocabulary and his co-author acquired a fair conversational knowledge of the language so that, while sometimes needing interpretation, we were independent of it to a degree that greatly facilitated our work and enhanced, we believe, the validity of our results. If we could not frame all questions as nuancedly as desireable, we could fall back upon our interpreters and could above all understand the greater part of the answers, so that we could guide, extend and deepen an interview or terminate it when the information sufficed even though we might not be able to conduct it independently. We enjoyed furthermore the priceless advantage of being able to observe directly psychomotor reactions, expressions, attitudes, gestures – the whole behavior of the proband in his own environment such as written records can at best poorly and crudely convey.

As a check upon the effectiveness of our two-phased method, we performed census studies of sub-areas in Marvdasht and Shiraz and compared their results with those of our sampling.

Diagnoses and judgments of severity were made provisionally in the field, but all were reappraised before publication.

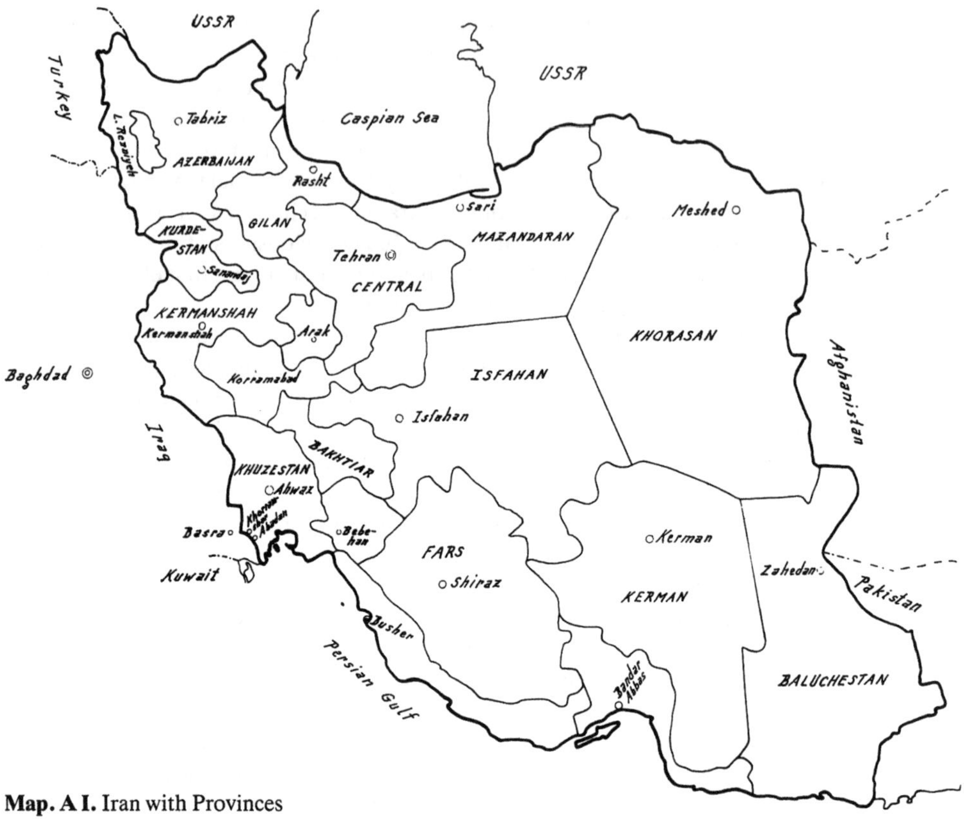

Map. A I. Iran with Provinces

Part B Local Surveys

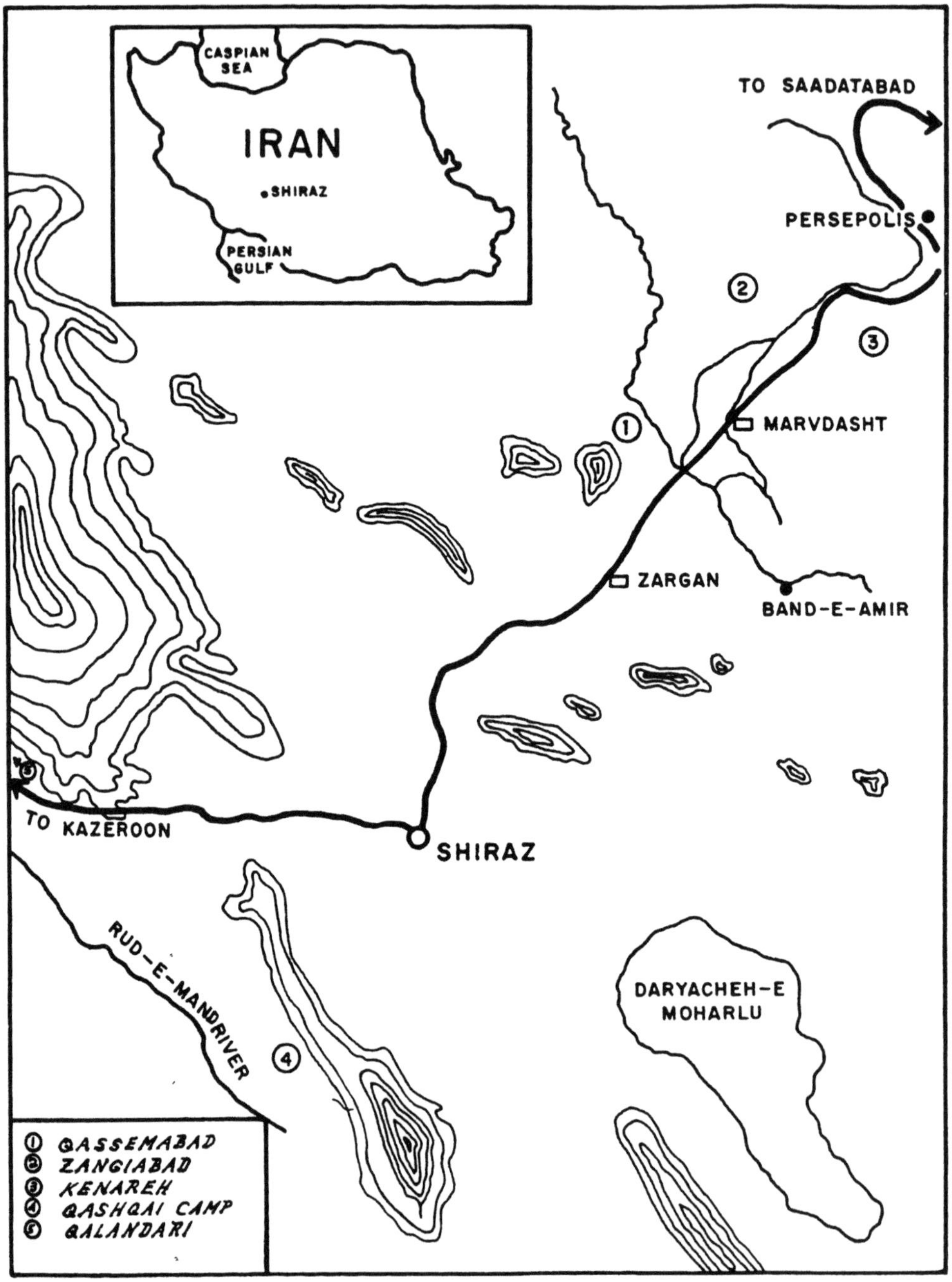

Map B I. Marvdasht and Qashqai Survey Region

I. Marvdasht

1. General[1]

Marvdasht or the Grassy Plain is a mostly fertile, level, wide expanse at an altitude of some 2000 m, hedged about by outrunners of the Zagros chain and extending at the east to the very foot of the platform of Persepolis. It has been under cultivation almost continually since the time of Cyrus the Great. Occasional floods from the Sivand River have interrupted this and in places destroyed fertility through salt deposits. The pylons and pillars of Persepolis mount guard over it from the east, a chain of abandoned watch towers on outcropping rocky ridges from the west, while on a huge butte to the north the remains of a Sassanian fortress await exploration. The plain has given its name to the district and city of Marvdasht (population about 25500 by census of 1966) lying roughly in its midst. This is a center of administration, distribution and local trade, possesses primary and secondary schools and a beet sugar refinery that provides occupation for part of the city population and for some people from the villages round about. Nevertheless, the village economies in 1963 were almost exclusively agricultural, wheat, barley and sugar beet being the most important crops. Rice, sesame, cotton and vegetables are grown in small quantities; some sheep, cattle and poultry are raised; a few villages have fruit orchards. Cultivation and animal husbandry at the time of the survey were mostly by primitive traditional methods. Yields were far below what agricultural experts estimated could have been obtained and had been still further reduced by eight preceding years of drought (average rainfall in normal years about 35 cm, but in 1962 only 16 cm and in 1963 24 cm). Temperatures range between –4° and +40° C. Relative humidity is generally low.

The recently appointed Director-General of the Department of Public Health, Province of Fars, had obtained funds for a new general policlinic in the city of Marvdasht, some 50 kilometers distant from Shiraz and 11 from Persepolis by asphalted road. From this district center a physician was to hold regular consultations in the three villages of Qassemabad, Zangiabad and Kenareh. As explained in the introductory chapter, this afforded a most welcome opportunity for a public health survey, into which mental health came to be included.

The greater part of the way to the three villages could be traversed by paved highway, but the final access was by dirt road or track. None of the villagers owned an automobile. They made the trip to Marvdasht by foot, donkey or bicycle and in winter might be almost mired in (snow falls only once every few years on the plains of Fars, but the wind and rain can make movement across them an ordeal). Many had never in their

---

[1] Briefer accounts have been published in 1964 [166] and 1967 [18].

lives been to the provincial capital Shiraz, an hour's drive distant. Too late we realized that it would have been interesting to put this question systematically. Dwellings, with few exceptions, were mud brick huts, usually of one room and one story, often clustered several to a courtyard, in which cooking was done, fowls had their run and cattle were folded for the night. Roofs were of beams covered with hard rolled clay, served for sleeping in the hot nights and very seldom supported a second story of like construction. Water generally came from shallow wells or was fetched in goatskins from a stream, seldom from qanats (artificial underground water courses, typical for Iran) or springs, not from deep wells and was practically always contaminated by the time is was used, even when drawn from a (rare) uncontaminated source. Uncovered pit privies were the rule. Other refuse was cast into the street. When its accumulation has nearly engulfed the village, this is abandoned and rebuilt on a new site, as one could see well in the immediate vicinity of Qassebad.

The type of settlement as of house was that which prevails through nearly all Iran with the exception of the Caspian area. There are no isolated farm houses. Peasants huddle together for protection against robbers (whose incursions in the years just preceding our survey had caused severe losses to the villagers), beasts and harsh weather in qalehs (قلعه) or fortified towns surrounded by a high wall of baked clay and sometimes surmounted by watch towers, admission to which is by a single massive wooden gate that is barred at nightfall. If there is a communal orchard, it is usually surrounded by another wall. Thousands of such villages (in Fars about 5000) of sizes varying from a few hundred to a couple of thousand people dot the Iranian plains and hillsides. There are few shops or handworkers in them. The women in some houses knotted carpets on horizontal frames pegged into the ground and sold them in Marvdasht or Shiraz. Occasionally an itinerant peddler might come by with thread, needles, candles, tea and the like. There were no telephones. For their other needs people go to the nearest small city, in this case Marvdasht. The villager is his own builder and repairman. From this structure of life and commerce on the one hand and on the other from the then very new land reform it followed that within such villages there were but small differences of occupation, all being mixed agriculturalists and husbandmen, and few and relatively slight differences of socio-economic status. To assert that there were none would be misleading, for they were unmistakeable in the livestock, the appointment of the houses, in clothing, in the presence of a bicycle, a cheap clock or a transistor radio etc., but they were rather the differences between the poor and the very poor. The village headman or kadkhoda is likely to stand out, though not conspicuously, before the rest. Accordingly, we have not attempted in our village studies to classify minimal socio-economic or occupational differences or to rate them as we have in our later urban investigation, except in Table B I 2.

This general description in the past tense held and still holds structurally for the vast majority of Iranian villages to the present day, though the dark picture painted therein of poverty, lack of elementary sanitation, isolation and ignorance has been brightening year by year. It may be applied to our other village studies also, with modifications to be noted in the appropriate places. Our purpose is to depict conditions as they then existed, not as they have become in the subsequent decade or may become in the next, as a frame of reference within which our findings are to be understood.

In the original public health survey report [166] the three villages were treated separately with the aim of making concrete recommendations for each. In our first publication on neuropsychiatric epidemiology in Marvdasht [20] we gave separate prevalence figures but pooled all other data and shall do so here. Nevertheless, a tabular presentation of demographic, social and occupational data (cf. Tables B I 1 and 2) together with a brief note on each village will serve to illustrate the variety beneath a superficial monotony and to acquaint the reader with a number of measures for social, economic, educational and agricultural reform that in 1963 were beginning to play a part and have played a greatly increased one since that time. Their specific and local enumeration, we believe, will be more instructive than a general description and at the same time more precise.

Table B I 1. Demographic Data

	Qassemabad	Zangiabad	Kenareh	Total
Census population	321	1336	2327	3984
Sample size (percent)	100	20	10	
Pop. studied by public health survey	321	250	249	820
Pop. previsaged by mental health survey (≥ 6 years)	239	184	175	598
Number of families	57	53	49	159
Mean family size	5.6	4.8	5.1	5.2
Percent ≥ 15 years	57	48	55	53
Percent literate[a] (> 5 y.)	20	15	10	21
Birth rate per 1000	62	68	68	
Crude death rate per 1000	22	16	12	
Infant mortality per 1000 live births	152	174	122	

[a] The public health survey took as its lower limit for this group five years of age, the mental health survey six. The figure under "Total" is calculated from the data of the mental health survey and includes a certain number of children who had entered school at six and were therefore classed as "literate", as explained in Chap. C I. The percentage of literates thus comes out slightly higher.

Table B I 2. Social and Occupational Data of Survey Population

	Qassemabad	Zangiabad	Kenareh	Total
Percent of families owning their own houses	95	40	96	72
Percent of families living in one room	67	41	43	51
Gainfully occupied males				
Farmers	53	27	38	118
Skilled laborers	0	10	14	24
Unskilled laborers	10	18	7	35
Pedlars (men and women)	2	5	3	10
Teachers, demonstration agents, etc. (men and women)[a]	2	5	3	10
Women doing carpet weaving or other skilled work	23	24	41	88

[a] Not included in survey population.

1. *Qassemabad,* in 1963–4 still 8.7 km from the nearest connection with the asphalted highway from Shiraz to the towns of Marvdasht, Persepolis, Isfahan and Tehran and much the smallest of the three villages, was selected for census study both by the public health and the mental health survey. In the heart of the Marvdasht, it stands on the historic site of one of the caravanserais of Shah Abbas the Great that linked Shiraz with Isfahan four centuries ago and beneath a butte atop which stand the remains of a Sassanian fortress. With its approximately 1600 hectares of land it had been the property of a Shirazi landlord who, before he was dispossesed by the Land Reform Act of 1963, had begun construction of six rows of hard brick and cement houses, then left them unfinished. They stood unoccupied at either side of the village gate but outside its wall, have been completed since and are now in use. In Plate 1 they are to be seen at center left. This aerial view shows Qassemabad as an in all other respects typical village with its wall and watch towers, its mostly one-story houses around a courtyard and a larger area just behind the main gate, which serves more as a distributor than as a social center. People meet in the courtyards, during inclement weather in their houses. Further to the left center is the abandoned village, at the top the neatly laid out orchard with the irrigation channel running to it from the center right. The village water supply was by qanat.

Except for the communal orchard and the new houses just mentioned, the village holdings had been divided among the inhabitants a year before the survey. Each farmer was working about 6 hectares of land. A joint co-operative had just been organized together with the adjacent village (not surveyed) of Fakhrabad. A school, staffed by two Literacy Corps teachers, had been opened a year ago. Not far from the village construction of a phosphate fertilizer factory had just been completed, but the factory was not yet operating. It now is, has been connected by a paved road with the highway and provides work for many people from Qassemabad itself and from the villages round about.

2. *Zangiabad,* 3 km from the highway, lies midway between Persepolis and near-by Naqsh-e-Rustam with its empty rock tombs of Darius and other Achaeminian kings. The village and its approximately 4400 hectares of land had belonged to two absentee landowners. At the time of the survey the land had passed through a trust to the Mosque and was being rented to the farmers, whose average holdings were about 12 hectares. The holdings were reallocated by lot each year. Water was drawn from the Sivand River. Two home demonstration agents, a man and a woman, were assisting the Zangiabad families. A school with three teachers had existed already for ten years and offered night classes in agricultural and industrial subjects that were attended by pupils from other villages as well. The Red Lion and Sun Out-Patient Clinic had been available to the villagers hitherto. Most houses were of the usual mud brick, but a few, including the former landlords', had cement foundations, hard floors and windows and some even had two stories. The bath house urgently needed essential revisions.

3. *Kenareh,* 2.5 km from the highway, the largest and most prosperous of the three, with some 2800 hectares adjoining, presented a more varied property structure. The villagers who received land under the Reform Act controlled 40 % of the total. The rest was divided between village resident landowners (before reform), burgess absentee owners, and owners of the irrigation water supply, the Ali Abad Qanat. Water is also drawn from shallow wells and the Sivand River. The four groups named share in the

profits from the thirteen farms that composed the estate of Kenareh before land reform. The village had a co-operative, since five years a home demonstration agent of the Ministry of Agriculture and since eight years a school, from which several pupils had gone on to secondary education in Marvdasht or Shiraz. As in Zangiabad, the Red Lion and Sun Out-Patient Clinic at Persepolis had served the villagers.

Officials of the Department of Public Health called on headmen and their associates, explained to them the purpose and nature of the survey and gained assurance of their co-operation long before field work began. As the time approached, evening out-door talks and health film demonstrations were held in the respective villages. A small group surveyed these, plotted and enumerated houses and households and took a careful census. Meanwhile the larger part of the field staff had been undergoing training in Shiraz for the task ahead. One week was devoted to interviewing, to the definition of questions and items and to the proper way of filling out forms, a second week to giving and recording psychological tests and questionnaires. Biological measurements, samplings and tests were performed by specialists or their technicians. Field work proper was carried out very intensively from early morning until about two o'clock in the afternoon for approximately a week each in Kenareh and Zangiabad and during a few days in the much smaller Qassemabad. Family interviews, mental testing and laboratory procedures were performed in the sequence named for the sake of better acceptability. Interview teams were composed of one man and one woman, the latter being responsible for taking histories of pregnancies, etc. At all times a physician was on hand to give treatment. Several emergency or grave chronic cases could be referred to the Shiraz hospitals. Acceptance and co-operation on the whole were excellent, but subsequently revealed themselves as more of a problem for the mental health survey than we had supposed at first. Because of the considerable number of persons, cars and resources from the most variegated instances involved it was impossible to keep the field force or any large part of it together beyond the few weeks in July and August, 1963, after which the WHO Adviser had to return to Tehran. Despite a reasonably satisfactory response to the mental health survey some villagers, especially men busy in the fields, had been reluctant, while other cases that seemed suspicious could not be cleared up adequately in the short time that the main survey endured. Over several months and on into early 1964 the stragglers were pursued as far as time and resources allowed, in part by kindly Shiraz colleagues, in part by the Adviser, who returned ever and again to Shiraz and Marvdasht as his work in Tehran allowed. Even then the drop-out from all causes was larger than in other surveys that could be conducted with greater continuity.

Before progressing to the proper matter of the mental health or psychiatric survey a few results of the public health survey may be summarized. They confirmed what has been said about the state of Iranian public health in the fifties and early sixties in Part A, Chap. I. Inadequate, generally contaminated domestic water supply and environmental sanitation were taking their toll. Mal- and undernutrition with grossly insufficient amounts of protein (the standard summer diet was rice, bread and tea, with a few vegetables and almost no meat) led to significantly lowered plasma protein and hemoglobin levels in large groups of the population. Gastrointestinal, infectious eye diseases and various handicapping conditions were rife, and infestation with intestinal parasites was presumed to be general, although for the most part only single stool specimens could be taken. For the first time, as far as known, a dental survey was performed in Iran: over 10 % of the youngest and 75 % of the oldest subjects had signs of dental decay; none had fillings. Echinococcus skin tests (Casoni) were positive in 4 % to 8 % of village populations. A fraction of the population had been vaccinated against smallpox, the rest were for the most part on the spot. The problem of tuberculosis, common in Iran, did not assume the dimensions that had been feared. On the positive side, the results of the rigorously executed DDT spraying campaigns against malaria, formerly a scourge, proved highly satisfying, as only a single positive thick smear was found.

Already the still debated question of the effects (if any) of zinc deficiency had arisen, so the public health survey took and analyzed several dozen hair specimens. The Adviser has seen in other places in Fars cases of hypogenital dwarfism such as Prasad and Halsted [168] have ascribed to zinc deficiency, but none of them has fallen into any of his survey samples, and none were encountered in Marvdasht.

2. Tests

From the 500 individuals actually scrutinized in the Marvdasht Survey eight (3 male, 5 female) were afflicted by defects of vision to such a degree that they could not perform the block design or Z tests. Three were omitted therefore also from the arithmetic test (which possessed its visual component in the three exercises with coins), leaving 497 test subjects.

Males outnumber females as nearly throughout Iran, and illiterates outnumber literates, except for boys of school age, as in most rural areas of the country. The low numbers of both sexes in the age classes 13–14 puzzled us until Dr. Z. Ghorban, then

Table B I 3. Distribution of Test Subjects by Sex, Age and Literacy

Age	lm	im	m	lf	if	f	m + f
6	1	4	5	0	1	1	6
7	10	7	17	0	9	9	26
8	12	3	15	1	8	9	24
9	6	4	10	2	7	9	19
10	8	4	12	2	8	10	22
11	7	2	9	0	8	8	17
12	11	4	15	0	11	11	26
13	2	2	4	1	4	5	9
14	4	5	9	1	3	4	13
Sub-total children	61	35	96	7	59	66	162
15–19	10	11	21	1	29	30	51
20–39	16	72	88	0	95	95	183
40–59	6	31	37	2	31	33	70
60 +	3	16	19	0	12	12	31
Sub-total adults	35	130	165	3	167	170	335
Total	96	165	261	10	226	236	497

Dean of the Faculty of Medicine in Shiraz and the first western trained physician to practice there, provided us with the probable explanation. Thirteen to fourteen years ago in the Ostan of Fars there had been such a catastrophic epidemic of malaria that over long periods nobody could be found in the city who was able to bring medicines to the stricken in the countryside, and the mortality had been correspondingly high. The contrast to the single positive blood smear found in the public health survey was impressive.

Mean raw scores on the arithmetic test were listed in our earlier publications but are omitted here for most classificatory groups because these comprise singly rather few individuals, leaving the means dubious and the standard deviations large. The illiterates up to age 14 have been included in the standardizing population described in Chap. C I 3. The illiterate adult groups of both sexes were larger: mean raw scores for these are shown in Table C I 8. A glance at this reveals the enormous discrepancies between the illiterate males and females, the latter tending to score only about half as high as the former. The sex differences proved by the t-test to be highly significant for all adult age groups and for the adults as a whole ($p < 0.001$).

Here and throughout we have taken the age of beginning adulthood to lie at fifteen years, mainly for sociological reasons. Neither the Marvdasht Public Health Survey nor or other studies in Iran, so far as we know, indicate that biological maturity (leaving aside the question of acceleration) is attained earlier in Iran than in western countries. The modal age at onset of menses in Marvdasht, for example, was found to be 13–14 years. Very soon thereafter, for the girl, marriage follows. The bridegroom may or may not be a few years older. Often the couple remains living for a while with the bridegroom's family but there too is swiftly integrated into the adult world. School, on the land, terminates after six grades, in the city usually after six or nine, and since again outside of the cities few proceed to secondary schools, formal education, if received, tends to have been finished at about fifteen or before. A village "spinster" of eighteen may worry, not without reason, lest she remain unwed. Furthermore the mental growth curve (gained, to be sure, on western subjects, but not contradicted at least by any of our Iranian findings) flattens out around fifteen, larger age classes comprising more than a single year can be formed, and statistical comparison becomes more reliable. For this technical reason too we have adopted fifteen as the threshold of adulthood, realizing that any boundary is to a degree arbitrary.

As the numbers even in the adult age groups are still relatively small, we shall postpone discussion of the age-performance curve until larger collectives are available. A comment on the apparent sex difference seems required already, however. As intelligence test studies in Anglo-European countries generally show no sex differences or, if any, slight ones in favor of the female population, it would be strange to find a difference in its disfavor, and of such an order, in Iran. The reason for it cannot be deduced from test statistics but is obvious to the observer. By the Iranian-Islamic tradition of centuries it is unseemly for the girl or woman to be as clever as her brother or husband, and still less does it beseem her inquisitively and boldly to approach a new problem (we do not affirm that this attitude is confined to the tradition just named). To do this is the province of the lords of creation. It struck every examiner over and over again as obvious that female subjects either did not try at all to solve the test problems or abandoned their efforts after a half-hearted beginning, as soon as even a minimal difficulty occurred, and took flight into lame excuses, inattention, silence or frequently into feigned giggling embarrassment. This seemed to hold equally whether the examiner was a man or a woman. Lavishly given encouragement availed little, somewhat more in tests without time limits (arithmetic, Z). It was noticeable too that the performances of the few school girls in Marvdasht did not remain as far behind that of their brothers as did the performance of the few literate women behind that of the literate men.

The response to the block design test was very poor, with a low ceiling and high variability, so that no data on it are given here. Only later, when platelets were substituted for blocks, did it become a useful instrument: Cf. Chap. C I.

3. Psychiatry and Neurology

Out of 500 subjects actually examined (from 598 intended) in the first phase of the survey, 66 or 13 % had been identified by various criteria as suspect of psychopathology and 50 or 10.0 % were finally adjudged to exhibit it in a more than casual degree. Tables B I 5–8 show their distribution by sexes, major psychiatric categories, diagnoses and degree of severity. The reader is asked to bear in mind that these tables differ in respect to numbers and percentages of diagnoses from the corresponding tables in the original publications [20, 166], in which multiple diagnoses were admitted, though not in number of cases. They have been rewritten and recalculated on the basis of a single principal diagnosis per case.

Among the 50 cases, 18 or 36 % were male, 32 or 64 % female, whereas the population surveyed was composed of 261 males and 239 females = 500, i.e. 52.2 % males and 47.8 % females, corresponding to a sex ratio of 109:100. The excess of female patients is statistically significant ($X^2 = 5.144$, $0.05 > p > 0.02$), this being the only one of our surveys in which it proved to be so. We suspect that the difference is none the less spurious, as is probably another difference (in the prevalence rate for mild cases) which we shall discuss further below. Circumstance prevented an immediate follow-up of suspect persons not clinically examined during the few days allotted to each village. Returning from time to time from Tehran to Shiraz, the Adviser could more easily find the women at home, whereas the suspect males were more likely to be away in the fields at some distance from the villages or in another town, whither he could not trace them. Ultimately, endeavors to track them had to be abandoned due to the pressure of other work and the Adviser's impending departure. The subjective suspicion of a meaningless "significance" approaches conviction when we regard the results from the sociologically similar Khuzestan sample (Part B, Chap. II) and notice that the shares of the sexes in psychopathology there were equal.

In the field of the major psychoses we encountered one case of chronic paranoid schizophrenia, unproductive at the time of examination but with typical alteration of character and a supporting anamnesis that included hospitalization for acute catatonic episodes, none of affective and none of acute symptomatic psychosis. Another case, a woman of some thirty years, could have been regarded easily as a schizophrenic according to the psychopathological picture, but a history of trauma and later recurrent vegetative crises with probable dreamy states led us to classify it as a psychomotor epilepsy even though there was no record of major fits. Such were present in another, almost certainly posttraumatic case of psychomotor type. We did not meet with obvious psychoses of old age, but it is probable that milder cases of dementia may have been missed, as we shall see below. A rather severe endocrine psychosyndrome (P_2) was represented by an 18 year old stunted, but otherwise well-proportioned youth without beard or secondary hair, whose voice had broken. Testicles of hazel-nut size could be palpated on both sides. He denied erections, erotic interests and sexual dreams, complained about spells of lacrimose self-pity and mental confusion to the point that "the world went 'round" and he "did not know where he was", but questioning did not elicit indications of epilepsy or true syncope. He fidgeted, played with his fingers and did not appear more than 12–14 years of age in his habitus and demeanor. There was hypotension (100/70) and dyspnea, but no clinical cardiac finding. Beatings by his father and step-mother contributed to a persistent mood of hopelessness. Further endocrinological examination regrettably was not possible, as the family was uncooperative. Of the three cases under III.7 "other", one was an eight year old boy suffering from severe malnutrition; the second was a 32 year old prematurely aged woman who claimed she felt ill since the birth of her first child 15 years ago, had aborted twice, suffered from oligo- and dysmennorhea and was undergoing constant abdominal pain. A reactive component was obvious, but the chronic condition was such that we assumed a gynecological somatosis of unknown origin to be basic. The third case, a woman of 35, was anemic, complained of dyspepsia and turned out upon routine examination to have a positive Casoni reaction to echinococcus, but circumstances did not allow a diagnostic clarification sufficient to justify a single unequivocal diagnosis, for which reason we included her among the "other".

Space forbids a case by case discussion of the 36 reactive disorders. In Marvdasht as elsewhere not a few of the reactive depressions were due to illness or disability (carcinoma, cataract, trachoma, paralysis, etc.). As there was much of both, with corresponding opportunity for comparison, it was not insurmountably difficult to distinguish those cases in which the depressive reaction stood out as pathological by its degree, persistence or manner of expression. One case illustrated with exemplary clarity, because of its familial background, the distinction we have tried to make:

Table B I 4. Mean Raw Point Scores on Block Design Test by Age, Sex and Literacy

Age	lm	im	m	lf	if	f	f + m
6	2.0	0	0.4	–	0	0	0.3
7	1.0	0.7	0.9	–	0	0	0.6
8	1.9	0.7	1.7	0	0.5	0.4	1.2
9	1.5	1.8	1.6	0.5	0	0.1	0.9
10	3.4	1.5	1.8	3.5	1.3	1.7	2.3
11	3.7	2.0	3.3	–	1.3	1.3	2.3
12	3.6	2.2	3.3	–	0.6	0.5	2.1
13	2.0	1.0	1.5	0	2.0	1.6	1.5
14	3.7	1.4	2.4	0	0.3	0.2	1.8
15–19	9.6	2.9	6.1	2.0	1.6	1.6	3.5
20–39	8.1	3.7	4.5	–	1.3	1.4	2.8
40–59	7.5	2.4	3.2	1.0	1.0	1.0	2.3
60 +	3.7	1.0	1.4	–	1.1	1.1	1.3

Table B I 5. Psychiatric Diagnoses of Mild Cases (P_1)

Diagnoses	Number of cases					p. 100 of 50 cases					p. 1000 of 500 subjects				
	m	f	m + f			m	f	m + f			m	f	m + f		
I. Funct. psychoses			0					0					0		
1. Schizophrenia															
2. Affect. psychoses															
II. Acute symptomatic psychoses			0					0					0		
III. Subchronic & chron. sympt. psychoses & residual states			0					0					0		
1. Epilepsy															
a. cryptogen.															
b. symptomatic															
2. Sen. & arterioscl.															
3. post-infectious															
4. post-traumatic															
5. endocrine															
6. addiction															
7. other															
IV. Reactive disorders	3	10	13			6.0	20.0	26.0			6.0	20.0	26.0		
1. Simple path. dev.	1	5		6		2.0	10.0		12.0		2.0	10.0		12.0	
a. anxious		1			1		2.0			2.0		2.0			2.0
b. depressive	1	3			4	2.0	6.0			8.0	2.0	6.0			8.0
c. irritable															
d. neurasthenic		1			1					2.0					2.0
e. other															
2. Neuroses	2	3		5		4.0	6.0		10.0		4.0	6.0		10.0	
a. anxious		1			1		2.0			2.0		2.0			2.0
b. phobic															
c. depressive	1	1			2	2.0	2.0			4.0	2.0	2.0			4.0
d. hysterical															
e. hypochondriac															
f. neurasthenic	1				1	2.0				2.0	2.0				2.0
g. self-insuff.															
h. negativistic															
i. other & polym.		1			1		2.0			2.0		2.0			2.0
3. Psychosomatic		2		2			4.0		4.0			4.0		4.0	
a. headache															
migrainoid															
other															
b. gastro-intest.		1			1		2.0			2.0		2.0			2.0
c. asthmatic															
d. other & polym.		1			1		2.0			2.0		2.0			2.0
V. Constitutional disord.	1		1			2.0		2.0			2.0		2.0		
1. Clin. oligophrenia	1			1		2.0			2.0		2.0			2.0	
a. cryptogenetic	1				1	2.0				2.0	2.0				2.0
b. genetic															
2. Psychopathy				0					0				0		
a. irritable															
b. anti-social															
c. schizoid															
d. other															
Total	4	10	14	14		8.0	20.0	28.0	28.0	28.0	8.0	20.0	28.0	28.0	28.0

Table B I 6. Psychiatric Diagnoses of Medium Cases (P_2)

Diagnoses	Number of cases					p. 100 of 50 cases					p. 1000 of 500 subjects				
	m	f	m + f			m	f	m + f			m	f	m + f		
I. Funct. psychoses			0					0					0		
1. Schizophrenia															
2. Affect. psychoses															
II. Acute symptomatic psychoses			0					0					0		
III. Subchronic & chron. sympt. psychoses & residual states	2	2	4			4.0	4.0	8.0			4.0	4.0	8.0		
1. Epilepsy															
a. cryptogen.															
b. symptomatic															
2. Sen. & arterioscl.															
3. post-infectious															
4. post-traumatic															
5. endocrine	1			1		2.0			2.0		2.0			2.0	
6. addiction	1	2		3		2.0	4.0		6.0		2.0	4.0		6.0	
7. other															
IV. Reactive disorders	7	15	22			14.0	30.0	44.0			14.0	30.0	44.0		
1. Simple path. dev.	1	2		3		2.0	4.0		6.0		2.0	4.0		6.0	
a. anxious															
b. depressive	1	1			2	2.0	2.0			4.0	2.0	2.0			4.0
c. irritable															
d. neurasthenic		1			1		2.0			2.0		2.0			2.0
e. other															
2. Neuroses	3	6		9		6.0	12.0		18.0		6.0	12.0		18.0	
a. anxious	3	1			4	6.0	2.0			8.0	6.0	2.0			8.0
b. phobic															
c. depressive		3			3		6.0			6.0		6.0			6.0
d. hysterical		1			1		2.0			2.0		2.0			2.0
e. hypochondriac		1			1		2.0			2.0		2.0			2.0
f. neurasthenic															
g. self-insuff.															
h. negativistic															
i. other & polym.															
3. Psychosomatic	3	7		10		6.0	14.0		20.0		6.0	14.0		20.0	
a. headache					5					10.0					10.0
١. migrainoid	1	4				2.0	8.0				2.0	8.0			
ب. other															
b. gastro-intest.	1	2			3	2.0	4.0			6.0	2.0	4.0			6.0
c. asthmatic															
d. other & polym.	1	1			2	2.0	2.0			4.0	2.0	2.0			4.0
V. Constitutional disord.	2	2	4			4.0	4.0	8.0			4.0	4.0	8.0		
1. Clin. oligophrenia	2	2		4		4.0	4.0		8.0		4.0	4.0		8.0	
a. cryptogenetic	2	2			4	4.0	4.0			8.0	4.0	4.0			8.0
b. genetic															
2. Psychopathy			0					0					0		
a. irritable															
b. anti-social															
c. schizoid															
d. other															
Total	11	19	30	30		22.0	38.0	60.0	60.0		22.0	38.0	60.0	60.0	

Table B I 7. Psychiatric Diagnoses of Severe Cases (P_3)

Diagnoses	Number of cases					p. 100 of 50 cases					p. 1000 of 500 subjects				
	m	f	m + f			m	f	m + f			m	f	m + f		
I. Funct. psychoses	1		1			2.0		2.0			2.0		2.0		
1. Schizophrenia	1			1		2.0			2.0		2.0			2.0	
2. Affect. psychoses															
II. Acute symptomatic psychoses			0					0					0		
III. Subchronic & chron. sympt. psychoses & residual states	1	2	3			2.0	4.0	6.0			2.0	4.0	6.0		
1. Epilepsy				2					4.0					4.0	
a. cryptogen.															
b. symptomatic	1	1			2	2.0	2.0			4.0	2.0	2.0			4.0
2. Sen. & arterioscl.															
3. post-infectious															
4. post-traumatic		1		1			2.0		2.0			2.0		2.0	
5. endocrine															
6. addiction															
7. other															
IV. Reactive disorders	1		1			2.0		2.0			2.0		2.0		
1. Simple path. dev.	1			1		2.0			2.0		2.0			2.0	
a. anxious															
b. depressive	1				1	2.0				2.0	2.0				2.0
c. irritable															
d. neurasthenic															
e. other															
2. Neuroses															
a. anxious															
b. phobic															
c. depressive															
d. hysterical															
e. hypochondriac															
f. neurasthenic															
g. self-insuff.															
h. negativistic															
i. other & polym.															
3. Psychosomatic															
a. headache															
١. migrainoid															
ب. other															
b. gastro-intest.															
c. asthmatic															
d. other & polym.															
V. Constitutional disord.		1	1				2.0	2.0				2.0	2.0		
1. Clin. oligophrenia		1		1			2.0		2.0			2.0		2.0	
a. cryptogenetic		1			1		2.0			2.0		2.0			2.0
b. genetic															
2. Psychopathy			0					0					0		
a. irritable															
b. anti-social															
c. schizoid															
d. other															
Total	3	3	6	6		6.0	6.0	12.0	12.0		6.0	6.0	12.0	12.0	

Table B I 8. Psychiatric Diagnoses of All Cases

Diagnoses	Number of cases					p. 100 of 50 cases					p. 1000 of 500 subjects				
	m	f	m+f			m	f	m+f			m	f	m+f		
I. Funct. psychoses	1	0	1			2.0		2.0			2.0		2.0		
1. Schizophrenia	1			1		2.0			2.0		2.0			2.0	
2. Affect. psychoses															
II. Acute symptomatic psychoses			0					0					0		
III. Subchronic & chron. sympt. psychoses & residual states	3	4	7			6.0	8.0	14.0			6.0	8.0	14.0		
1. Epilepsy				2					4.0					4.0	
a. cryptogen.															
b. symptomatic	1	1			2	2.0	2.0			4.0	2.0	2.0			4.0
2. Sen. & arterioscl.															
3. post-infectious															
4. post-traumatic		1		1			2.0		2.0			2.0		2.0	
5. endocrine	1			1		2.0			2.0		2.0			2.0	
6. addiction															
7. other	1	2		3		2.0	4.0		6.0		2.0	4.0		6.0	
IV. Reactive disorders	11	25	36			22.0	50.0	72.0			22.0	50.0	72.0		
1. Simple path. dev.	3	7		10		6.0	14.0		20.0		6.0	14.0		20.0	
a. anxious		1			1		2.0			2.0		2.0			2.0
b. depressive	3	4			7	6.0	8.0			14.0	6.0	8.0			14.0
c. irritable															
d. neurasthenic		2			2		4.0			4.0		4.0			4.0
e. other															
2. Neuroses	5	9		14		10.0	18.0		28.0		10.0	18.0		28.0	
a. anxious	3	2			5	6.0	4.0			10.0	6.0	4.0			10.0
b. phobic															
c. depressive	1	4			5	2.0	8.0			10.0	2.0	8.0			10.0
d. hysterical		1			1		2.0			2.0		2.0			2.0
e. hypochondriac		1			1		2.0			2.0		2.0			2.0
f. neurasthenic	1				1	2.0				2.0	2.0				2.0
g. self-insuff.															
h. negativistic															
i. other & polym.		1			1		2.0			2.0		2.0			2.0
3. Psychosomatic	3	9		12		6.0	18.0		24.0		6.0	18.0		24.0	
a. headache					5					10.0					10.0
1. migrainoid	1	4				2.0	8.0				2.0	8.0			
ب. other															
b. gastro-intest.	1	3			4	2.0	6.0			8.0	2.0	6.0			8.0
c. asthmatic															
d. other & polym.	1	2			3	2.0	4.0			6.0	2.0	4.0			6.0
V. Constitutional disord	3	3	6			6.0	6.0	12.0			6.0	6.0	12.0		
1. Clin. oligophrenia	3	3		6		6.0	6.0		12.0		6.0	6.0		12.0	
a. cryptogenetic															
b. genetic															
2. Psychopathy			0					0					0		
a. irritable															
b. anti-social															
c. schizoid															
d. other															
Total	18	32	50	50		36.0	64.0	100	100		36.0	64.0	100	100	

Four brothers had pooled their meagre savings and had a pump installed to irrigate a field that they worked in common (it may be recalled that in the hot, parched Iranian landscape the farmer's well-being depends on water). A year ago the pump broke down. The four brothers had no money left to repair it, lost both their modest capital and the leased land and had to support themselves and their families by odd jobs. Three of them were able to bear their worries and come to terms with their hard lot. The fourth fell into a fairly severe depression and had not recovered from it. He was nervous, irritable, sleepless, could not abide the noise his own children made, had no interest in anything and was unable to perform the odd jobs that came his way. Upon closer questioning we learned that several times before this calamity he had suffered pronounced depressive reactions, e.g. after minor quarrels with neighbors, in family difficulties and even in military service, which he had liked and in which he had been a good soldier and marksman. After he had been struck by lightning (?) in a thunderstorm his right hand and left foot by his own account had remained paralysed for some time. Two years ago, when things were going well and the crops were good, he could not sleep for happiness: now he was depressed by his financial failure, want and the high cost of living. On the arithmetic test his intelligence quotient was 103. The Z Test protocol follows (signa see Chap. C II 3 b). ICD-9 300.4.

Z Test Protocol

Subject from household 131, house 14, Kenareh, male 39 years old, tested autumn 1963. Unschooled, but able to read and write.
Beginning 10:02 o'clock

Card I.	Initial time 2 sec.	
1. a.	Butterfly	WF+ A
2. a.	Shape of a cloud (lateral)	DFChia– N
Card II.	10:05 o'clock, initial time 105 sec.	
3. d.	Shape of a fish (brown)	DF– A red shock
4. c.	The white in the center of the red seems like a lamp in a shrine	DSFC– Obj
Card III.	10:10 o'clock, initial time 120 sec.	
5. d.	A mouse and a cat (both smaller black)	DF– A O–
6. d.	The red center has the shape of a fan	DF+ Obj
7. d.	The red at the side has the shape of a camel	DF+ A

End 10:14 o'clock.

Total time 12 min., total responses 7, mean reaction time 1 min. 42 sec.

W	1	F	5	H	0	P	0
D	6			A	4		
	—	F+	3			f%	86
	7	F–	2	Obj	2		
						F+%	67
		FFC+	1	N	1		
					—	A%	57
		FChia	1				
			—		7		
			7				

Apperceptive type: (W) –D; Experience balance: 0:½ EW: 0 (E)

The record is remarkable for its constricted formalism, which, although the subject allows himself abundant time, does not adhere to a higher form level such as would be typical of endogenous depression. After a first try, he does not venture upon whole responses. Though explicitly aware of colors, he avoids or denies non-formal determinants even where they are commonly employed and might be expected ("shape of –") except for achromatic color (white = lamp). The score given to "shape of a cloud" in Card I is determined by usage and might equally well read DF–. Caution, self-restriction or repression, anxiety and depression can be inferred from these signs. The pronounced red shock to Card II points to their neurotic origin and is corroborated in Card III, but compensated by fair interpretations of the red in both cards. The experience balance is constricted almost to the point of total coarctation. Finally, it is hard to deny the symbolic significance of the quite unusual "mouse and cat" to Card III, where the two smaller black parts indeed are frequently seen as animals, but almost always as two of a kind. Did the patient not feel himself as the mouse in the cat's claws?

We gained our first experience here with the massive migrainoid headaches of the Iranian women – no mere vapours or megrims, but severe illnesses that not seldom render their bearer unable to work for one to several days a week. Our "other" psychosomatic cases were one of eczema and one with truly polymorphous symptoms.

The six cases of clinical oligophrenia present no special features and were, as far as could be ascertained, cryptogenetic, except for one nine year old girl who had suffered an undiagnosed severe febrile disease in early childhood and remained backward thereafter. No case seemed to call for the diagnosis of psychopathy.

Turning from diagnoses to degree of severity, we find their distribution in Table B I 9. Herein we have treated the three villages separately. One having been subjected to a census study, the others to random sampling, their comparison is of interest. The sample sizes all lie between 150 and 200. Psychiatric morbidity of every degree appears to be highest in the smallest, most thoroughly investigated village (Qassemabad), which at the same time offers the largest sample (239). Easy though it would be to attribute this to the undoubted advantages of the census study per se, the attribution does not carry full conviction to the field worker. The colleagues of the public health

Table B I 9. Psychiatric Cases by Degrees of Severity

Village	Degree of severity 1	2	3	Sum of cases	Per 100 of 50 cases	Survey population	Per 1000 of survey pop.
Qassemabad	6	14	2	22	44	195	113
Zangiabad	4	7	3	14	28	159	88
Kenareh	4	9	1	14	28	146	96
	14	30	6	50	100	500	100
Sum of $P_2 + P_3$		36					
P_3 alone			6				
Per 100 of 50 cases	28	60	12				

Table B I 10. Neurological Cases by Degrees of Severity

Village	Degree of severity 1	2	3	Sum of cases	Public health survey population	Per 1000 of survey population
Qassemabad	2	3	1	6	321	19
Zangiabad	2	0	1	3	250	12
Kenareh	1	0	1	2	249	8
	5	3	3	11	820	13
Sum of $P_2 + P_3$		6				
P_3 alone			3			

survey agreed in judging the general health situation in Qassemabad to be the poorest. This village had been the longest without a school, had no home demonstration agent, had received the least developmental effort (itself abruptly interrupted), was remotest from the paved highway and considerably the most difficult of access. These may be regarded more or less as impressions, but the disproportionate share of cases belonging to the middle category of severity (P_2) rather than to the mild (P_1) despite more thorough coverage and, as appears in Table B I 10, the rather surprisingly large number of purely neurological cases (neuropsychiatric cases are included together with the purely psychiatric) tend to confirm them.

As we shall see later, the prevalence of all mild or P_1 cases in Marvdasht with only 28 per 1000 was much lower than in most of our other surveys and was in all likelihood an artefact due to insufficiently concentrated follow-up of suspects identified but not examined during the first intensive campaign of field work. On the other hand, the rates for the medium and severe categories P_2 and P_3 agreed well with those found in Khuzestan. Therefore we shall postpone discussion of the diagnostic distributions within the several categories of severity, as shown in Tables B I 5 to B I 8, until the findings from Khuzestan have been presented in Chap. B II and comparisons can be drawn.

4. Qassemabad 1963 and 1976[1]

The National Iranian Census of 1976 gave a fresh impulse to psychiatric epidemiology. The first author was called to Tehran for consultation in August 1976, discussed a number of projects aimed at an enumeration of the mentally ill, was forced to advise against many of them as impractical under the given conditions but agreed with his Iranian colleagues that a resurvey of an already surveyed area was likely to prove most informative. Since the survey had to be performed in the autumn of the same year and the Adviser could be absent from his university duties only for a limited holiday period, the choice fell upon Qassemabad as not too large, easily accessible from Shiraz with all

[1] A brief account was published in 1978 [32].

the supporting facilities of the city and the university, already covered by a census study and subject to substantial socio-economic changes since the first survey in 1963. Both authors therefore returned to Iran early in October, 1976, spent several days in Tehran for organization and short intensive training of field workers (15 young graduates of the University of Tehran with a Bachelor's degree in psychology and with some field experience already behind them) and were in the field with these from October 7 to 20, 1976.

Though methods were basically the same as before, we now employed a modification of the Block Design Test for Illiterates using platelets instead of true blocks and a new Arithmetic Test for Literates, both tested in Shiraz in 1969/70 and described in Part C.

Qassemabad in 1963 was an exclusively agricultural village gaining its livelihood both from field crops (mainly wheat) and animal husbandry (sheep and goats). Shortly after our first survey the fertilizer factory commenced operations and has been built up since into a small petrochemical complex. Close to it, some 5 km from Qassemabad, a new settlement called Kuh Sabz (Green Mountain) had come into being with better housing of brick and cement, a primary and secondary school and a community center. A number of former Qassemabadi had moved there and could be traced, but time did not permit a survey of the new town which we should have liked to carry out. An asphalted, much traveled road now led from the Shiraz-Persepolis-Isfahan highway to the factory, the settlement and on to Qassemabad, beyond this to a still newer factory for canned meat products and up to the construction site of the still unfinished Darius Dam. The two factories and the dam had attracted new residents to the region, and yet other workers were brought daily by bus from Marvdasht and the adjacent towns. The pattern of work and livelihood had changed radically. The great majority of the men now had jobs in the factories and either did a little farming on the side or left this to their families. The type of the worker-farmer (*Arbeiterbauer*) familiar from so many Swiss valleys with small industries, dominated the scene. Some men were engaged in trucking and light commerce. A few went to Marvdasht or even to Shiraz daily for work. Mobility had come to the formerly stagnant, almost isolated village. They were mostly light, all-purpose trucks that came and went, some motor bicycles, a few passenger cars. In nearly every house the women and girls were industriously knotting carpets of traditional design. Most boys were at school, five even attending the secondary school in Kuh Sabz, and more girls were going to classes than in 1963 (data below). There was, however, somewhat to our surprise no adult literacy class. We were told that one had been started, but the teacher came irregularly from Shiraz, attendance flagged, their double occupation claimed too much of the men's time, and the attempt was abandoned. On the other hand four teachers from Shiraz, no longer Literacy Corps members but employees of the Ministry of Education, now taught in the school. They obligingly placed its rooms at our disposal, pointed out their problem pupils and provided us with much helpful information.

In its physical aspect Qassemabad had altered little at first sight except for the poles and wires that struck us from afar and for the television antennae atop many of the houses. Electric current had been switched on only three days before we began our resurvey, nearly all houses were wired, and the rejoicing was great. There were even a few street lights. The six rows of hard construction houses outside the wall were completed and almost all the units were occupied. There had been hardly any new

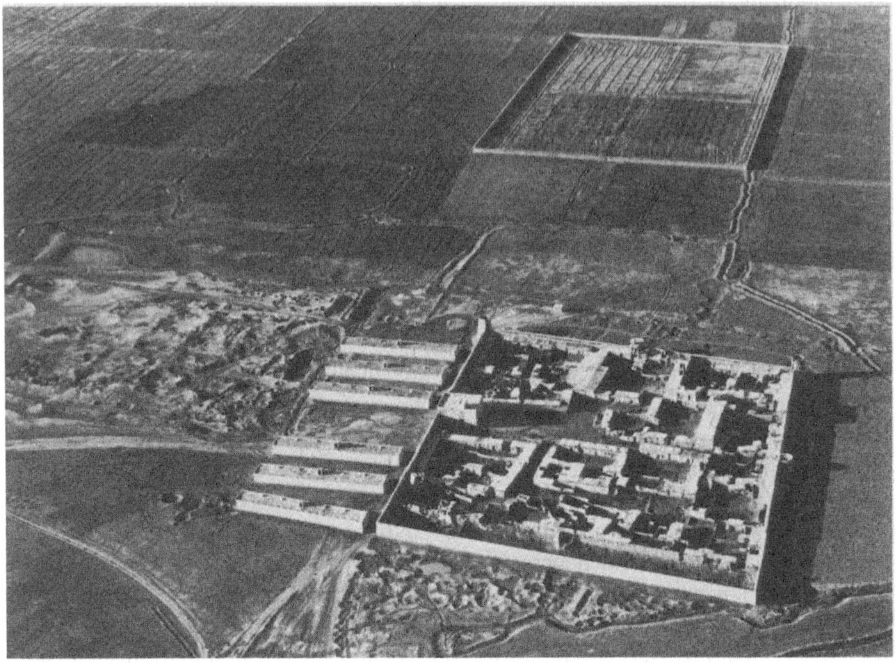

a

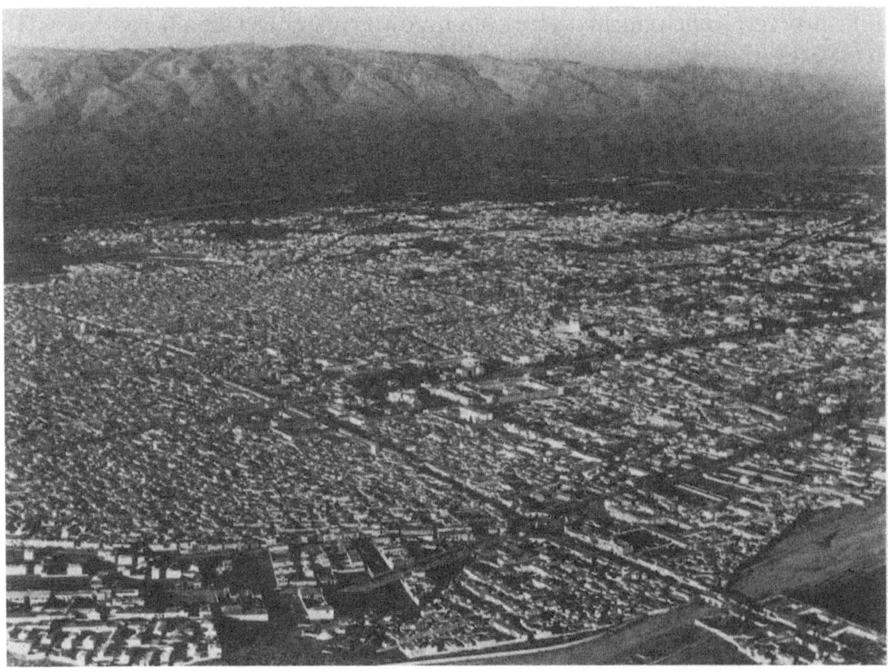

b

Plate B I. a Qassemabad **2** Shiraz (Aerial photographs by A. Jessup)

building inside the wall, but it quickly became noticeable that many rickety door and window frames had been replaced by iron ones with firm doors and glass panes and that at least some floors of beaten clay had been covered with cement. Not so, however, in the streets and alleys, where the dust and refuse accumulated as it had ever done. Most striking was the improvement in the household furnishings with cupboards taking the place of chests or the simple niche in the wall, refrigerators and electric fans (no luxury in the hot climate), television sets, appliances of all sorts, more pans and crockery. Tables, chairs and beds had not become utensils of life in Qassemabad as they had in some lower-class dwellings in the city. There was no telephone. Conditions of sanitation and hygiene had changed, so far as we could see, not at all. Vilely contaminated water for washing and for the household animals was drawn as before from shallow wells in the courtyards, drinking water fetched by the women in cannisters, jars and even yet in goatskins from the little river about one kilometer away. Neatly stacked along the road lay pipes that were to bring clean water from the Darius Dam to the villages below it: we can only hope that it is flowing now. A tiny general shop had set up in business. The dominant architectural feature of the village, the headman's two story house straddling the main gate, in which we had performed much of our testing in 1963, was crumbling and no longer inhabited after the headman had moved to Kuh Sabz, where we met him and his family. There was, in fact, no headman in Qassemabad in 1976, though there were several petty aspirants and pretenders without any real authority.

Public medical care, the inauguration of which had given the signal to the survey of 1963, had ceased, the official reason being that the petrochemical factory provided medical service for its employees and their families. This took care of a sizable share, but by no means the whole of the population. We heard many bitter complaints over this, encountered here and there some understandable reluctance to co-operate because the promise given by the government thirteen years ago had been broken and were enjoined again to intervene with the public health authorities to have a physician sent on periodic rounds. This we did to the best of our ability, but with what results we do not know. On the other hand, access to both public and private medical services in Marvdasht and Shiraz had become far more facile than before. We were not in a position to conduct a public health survey, but it seemed to us that many once conspicuous woeful pictures of malnutrition, chronic sores and infections had become noticeably less. No newer cases of poliomyelitis came to our attention. Smallpox and malaria evidently had remained under control.

The standard of clothing had become considerably better. Garments of mere rags were rare. People clearly had money in their pockets, were spending it and had gained a new self-confidence from this without losing their openness, hospitality (which greatly facilitated the survey) and courtesy. A new life had come into the village. A trip to nearby Marvdasht was commonplace, to Shiraz no longer a rare privilege and an adventure, and every now and then we encountered news of a husband or son who was away for weeks or months on business, usually dealing in agricultural products. There was no lack of complaints about working conditions particularly in the ill-smelling meat factory, but on the whole, we estimate, satisfaction over having a source of regular cash income prevailed. Obviously Qassemabad and its surroundings would have been a nearly ideal object for a sociological and economic study, but we had no persons with such training on our field force and could not even undertake amateurish investigations ourselves for sheer lack of time. As in all our field work we refrained from questions about income, but some people volunteered the information themselves, and it was always possible to discuss the price of the ubiquitous carpets. On the other hand, changes having been so numerous and in part so recent, in some cases almost certainly out of proportion to real income, we did not feel ourselves able to undertake such a classification by socio-economic levels on the basis of a summary glance as we had done in Shiraz. Neither did we have time to inquire more particularly into the only slightly differing levels of occupation of the factory workers. The technical and administrative staff of the two factories did not live, except for one technician, in Qassemabad, but either in factory-provided housing within the industrial area or in Shiraz. Though we had planned to do so, we also had to renounce our intention of inquiring in the petrochemical plant about workers' health, etc. No official health statistics for the village by itself existed.

Our sole attempt at gathering sociological information besides the standard questions of the Shiraz survey was inspired by our delayed realization in 1963 that a great numbers of the villagers had never in their lives been in the city only some 70 km away. We therefore included a routine question about how often the person interrogated had been or as a rule went to Shiraz. Furthermore we asked the number of rooms per household. As the statements about this varied astonishingly from one member of the family to the other depending, e.g., upon whether storerooms, stalls and the like were included or excluded, we reluctantly abandoned any attempt to evaluate the highly questionable and inconsistent findings. We first tried to have our field workers reconcile their divergencies, but this entailed long explanations and attempts at definition with which they seemed unable to comply. Checking every household ourselves would not have been intrinsically difficult but would have demanded a couple of additional days that we did not have at our disposal.

In the following we shall first present and discuss comparable data for the survey of 1963 and the resurvey of 1976 as far as such exist, thereafter data gained in the resurvey only. Already in the general characteristics and the population figures we encounter slight deviations from those stated in earlier publications [20, 29, 30] which were obtained by hand count. The present data have been punched and machine counted. The differences are trifling and alter no criteria of significance and no conclusions.

In Table B I 11 we note that the population had increased by 38 % over the thirteen years, while the proportion of children under six years had remained identical. Coverage in the resurvey was better, reaching 90 %, and could have been improved if we had had more time. The number of families had increased, but also the family size. A glance at Table B I 12 shows that the increase was mainly in the 6–14 and 15–19 age groups, whilst the percentage of young adults from 20 to 39 had decreased and the shares of the elder were practically unchanged, just as were those of the pre-school children. The mean number of live births per woman of ten years or over was 3.8 in 1976. When the 52 women who had never given birth to a living child were excluded, the mean became 6.2, identical with the mean given by Petrossian and Jessup [166] for 64 Qassemabadi women who had had at least one pregnancy in 1963. The mean number of living children per woman of ten or over was 2.6 in 1976 or, when again the women are excluded who had never given birth, 4.4. From the preliminary census figures for 1976 a crude fertility rate was estimated of 8.1 for the country and 4.6 for the city, placing Qassemabad neatly in between. Looking ahead to the Shiraz Survey figures of 1970, we find a mean of 4.4 births and 3.5 live children per woman, including

Table B I 11. General Characteristics, Subjects Scrutinized

	1963			1976		
General Characteristics						
Total population			321		478 +38 %	
Target population (≥ 6 years of age)			239 = 74 %		355 = 74 %	
Population actually scrutinized			195 = 82 %		320 = 90 %	
Number of families			57		74	
Mean family size			5.6		6.5	
General psychiatric morbidity per 1000			113		88 −22 % ns	
Subjects Scrutinized						
	m	f	m + f	m	f	m + f
1963 only	37	29	66	–	–	–
1963 and again 1976 in Qassemabad	52	44	96	52	44	96
1976 in Qassemabad	–	–	–	20	23	43
removed after 1963 but found and re-examined 1976 outside Qassemabad	13	11	24	–	–	–
died since 1963	4	5	9	–	–	–
other[a]	–	–	–	80	103	183
Sum	106	89	195	151	169	320

[a] Explanation in text.

women who had not borne. In the intervening six years the government had made strenous efforts to promulgate family planning. Although we do not know how many women were using contraceptives in Qassemabad in 1976 and refrained from asking because of the circumstances under which the survey had to be performed (short time, little privacy, partly male examiners), we know that some were, and it is difficult in view of the data not to surmise that family planning had exercised an effect. Had it not, one would expect a percentual rise in the number of pre-school children paralleling or exceeding that of the six to fifteen year-olds. That these increased, on the other hand, can be accounted for without difficulty on the reasonable assumption that during the thirteen years from 1963 to 1976 access to and employment of medical services had improved, as they unmistakably had, and that this had preserved a number of children and young people alive. This holds despite the circumstance that the local dispensary had been closed, partly because of the greatly increased mobility of the population, partly because a substantial part of this was covered by the medical service of the petrochemical factory. Regrettably indeed, we do not know and cannot ascertain how the equivalent rates may have changed in Shiraz between 1970 and 1976. The rise in family size goes naturally with the relative increase among those younger age classes most of whom are still living with their parents.

The rubrics in the lower half of Table B I 11, "Subjects Scrutinized", need some explanation. The class "1963 only" is smaller here than in reality, for it comprises only those subjects from the 1963 survey of whom we could be sure that they were not

Table B I 12. Populations by Age, Sex and Literacy

Age	1963 Male ill.	lit.	ill. + lit.	Female ill.	lit.	ill. + lit.	All	1976 Male ill.	lit.	ill. + lit.	Female ill.	lit.	ill. + lit.	All
	Absolute Numbers													
6–14	9	35	44	22	3	25	69	2	56	58	37	27	64	122
15–19	4	2	6	9	0	9	15	0	13	13	19	6	25	38
20–39	32	2	34	40	0	40	74	21	22	43	49	4	53	96
40–59	15	4	19	11	0	11	30	27	5	32	21	0	21	53
60 +	3	0	3	4	0	4	7	5	0	5	6	0	6	11
Sum	63	43	106	86	3	89	195	55	96	151	132	37	169	320
	Percent of Total Populations													
6–14	4.6	17.9	22.6	11.3	1.5	12.9	35.4	0.6	17.5	18.1	11.6	8.4	20.0	38.1
15–19	2.1	1.0	3.1	4.6	0	4.6	7.7	0	4.1	4.1	5.9	1.9	7.8	11.9
20–39	16.4	1.0	17.4	20.5	0	20.6	37.9	6.6	6.9	13.4	15.3	1.3	16.6	30.0
40–59	7.7	2.1	9.7	5.6	0	5.7	15.4	8.4	1.6	10.0	6.6	0	6.6	16.6
60 +	1.5	0	1.5	2.1	0	2.1	3.6	1.6	0	1.6	1.9	0	1.9	3.4
Sum	32.2	22.1	54.4	44.1	1.5	45.9	100	17.2	30.0	47.2	41.3	11.6	52.8	100
	Percent Literate by Age Class and Sex													
Children		79.5			12.0		55.1		96.6			42.2		68.0
Adult		12.9			0		6.3		43.0			9.5		25.3
All		40.6			3.4		23.6		63.6			21.9		41.6

embraced again by the resurvey. The second line carries the same qualification: it applies only to matched cases and thus only to subjects who in 1976 were at least 19 years old. The third line covers part, but only part of the population increment. The "removed" in the fourth were found mostly in nearby Kuh Sabz, but a few also in the town of Marvdasht, in Shiraz and in a couple of villages near Qassemabad. Time did not permit tracking down more. The last line "other" comprises, besides the rest of the increment, a substantial number of subjects concerning whom we could not be sure, for one reason or another, whether they had lived in Qassemabad in 1963 and had been scrutinized there or not. As our coverage in 1963 was only 82 %, it was altogether possible that some people then missed were caught in the resurvey, while others could be missed in both. Furthermore, though some subjects in 1976 said they had been living in Qassemabad in 1963 and were more than six years old then, their questionnaires and tests could not be matched convincingly with any previous ones. Age differences were unreliable; names became frequently altered in fact or in spelling, got new forenames attached to them (often simply a different one out of several), were or were not changed upon marriage, etc., etc. Subjects' own recollections of whether they had participated in the previous survey or not were partly misleading and sometimes flatly contradicted by the facts, as when, after a firm denial, a record with identical name and appropriate age was recovered from 1963. Patterns of consanguinity and marriage often clinched an identification, but as often failed. The quota of those who assuredly were scrutinized twice thus is equal to the sum of the second line in 1976 and of the fourth in 1963, i.e. 96 + 24 = 120 or 61 % of the population actually scrutinized in the initial survey.

The sex proportion in the survey population has become practically reversed from 54:46 in 1963 to 47:53 in 1976, which may be due to the fact that not a few adult men were "on the move", working outside, traveling or in military service. The pre-survey census of 1976 does not appear sufficiently reliable to warrant comparisons. The literacy rate had improved to an overall 42 %, but very unevenly – far more among the children than the adults, as might be expected, and percentually more among the girls than the boys, who had a better starting position and were already 80 % literate in 1963. In contrast thereto, only slightly more than half this percentage of girls was literate in 1976, and the women's literacy had increased from zero to nearly ten percent. The village school taught then as later up to the sixth grade. In 1963 only five persons, all male, had profited by any instruction beyond this level, of whom four were in the age class 40–59 and almost certainly had attended a Qoranic school. In 1976 on the other hand not less than 61 persons had received or were receiving some form of education beyond the sixth grade, and thirteen of these were female. The secondary schools in Marvdasht and more recently in Kuh Sabz accounted for the majority, technical and trade schools in Marvdasht and Shiraz for most of the rest. No one possessed an academic degree.

In order to understand the following tables of best and worse memories (B I 13 and B I 14) and of positive responses to items from the psychiatric questionnaire the reader will be forced to cast ahead to the relevant chapters (I and II) of Part C or to wait until he has read at least their introductory pages in which the constitution and purpose of the tables are explained. The data are nevertheless presented here for the sake of coherency rather than attaching them unorganically to general chapters in which more sweeping comparisons are made. The numbers at the left side of the Tables B I 13 and

B I 14 designate classes of memories which are described in Part C, Chap. II 1 a. They are given in parallel in absolute numbers and percentages for the two surveys, and the difference between these, where statistically significant, is indicated as described in the Table of Abbreviations and Signs. The procedure is similar for the psychiatric questionnaire except that absolute numbers and percentages could not be listed in parallel for reasons of space. Our interest concerns mainly the differences between rates, not numbers; therefore only such are given in Table B I 16 and then not numerically. The populations of 1963 and 1976 are treated as independent of each other in the computation of differences and their significance. In a sense, of course, they are not independent, as a number of individuals are common to both. The procedure is statistically debatable, though we believe it to be defensible. In hardly any more than a formal and legal sense are these common individuals the "same". They have retained their names, their gender, their bones and sets of engrams, but even most of the cells of the body outside the central nervous system have been renewed. The implications are very different from mixing experimental groups simultaneously or after short intervals. Employing semi-mixed groups such as these enabled us to take cross-sections of the village at widely separated points in time. Alternatively we should have been compelled to form three much smaller groups (1963 only, 1963 and 1976, 1976 only) and evaluate the middle group twice, once for each survey. Further subdivision by age and sex would have resulted in such miniscule classes that it is questionable whether any significant differences at all could have been ascertained, the more so as the large proportion of the "other", more than half the survey population of 1976, would have fallen by the wayside. We do not preclude such a detailed study later but did not find it feasible or justified under the circumstances.

We now turn to the tables as they stand and assume that the reader has acquainted himself with their intention, construction and meaning. Comparisons are drawn in Tables B I 13 and B I 14 (best and worst memories) for illiterate adults and literate boys only as there were not enough adult literates in 1963 to render them justifiable in case of the men or even possible in case of the women. Data for the literate men in 1976 are given as a matter of interest and can be compared with those for the literate in the same tables. Apart from mere tendencies, which may still be due to chance, significantly more women report in 1976 that their happiest memory is that of pregnancy and childbirth (No. 5). As we shall see in Part C, Chap. II 1, relatively few women in Marvdasht gave this as their best memory in 1963. One may speculate at least whether the change is not referrable to family planning with its resultant spacing of children and reduction of burdens and to more readily accessible medical facilities in the nearby towns and cities. The men recall significantly more often than before connubial life (No. 7) and weddings, festivals and feasts (No. 11) as their happiest memory. The most noteworthy findings, though, is that both sexes very significantly less than in 1963 assert that they have no pleasurable memory (No. 22). The amount and the very high statistical significance of the change speak for a distinct brightening of the prevailing mood in the village over the past thirteen years; something which we could feel ourselves, but can document here. Hope was dawning for most of the adult villagers in 1976 and had even fulfilled itself concretely for some. That the literate boys showed no significant changes in their best memories between the two surveys is hardly a matter for surprise, since effectively very little had changed for them. Attending school had been become already rather a matter of course rather than an exceptional opportunity (this is to be compared with Khuzestan later).

Table B I 13. Affirmations of Best Memories

	Illiterate Men 1963 N	Perc.	1976 N	Perc.	Illiterate Women 1963 N	Perc.	1976 N	Perc.	Literate Men 1976 N	Perc.	Literate Boys 1963 N	Perc.	1976 N	Perc.
1.	2	3.7 (‹)	6	11.3	2	3.1	2	2.1	2	5.1			2	3.7
2.							1	1.1	1	2.6	1	2.9	2	3.7
3.														
4.	2	3.7	5	9.4	7	10.9	10	10.5	5	12.8			1	1.8
5.	5	9.3 (‹)	10	18.9	2	3.1 ‹‹	17	17.9	2	5.1				
6.							1	1.1						
7.		‹	3	5.7	5	7.8	7	7.4	2	5.1				
8.							2	2.1					1	1.8
9.			1	1.9	1	1.6	1	1.1	1	2.6			1	1.8
10.	1	1.9			1	1.6	1	1.1	2	5.1				
11.	1	1.9 ‹	5	9.4	4	6.3	11	11.6	5	12.8	3	8.6	1	1.8
12.	2	3.7	1	1.9		(‹)	3	3.2	1	2.6				
13.									1	2.6				
14.	2	3.7	1	1.9			2	2.1	1	2.6			1	1.8
15.	1	1.9	1	1.9			1	1.1					1	1.8
16.									2	5.1				
17.	1	1.9												
18.									5	12.8	10	28.6	17	31.5
19.							1	1.1	1	2.6			2	3.7
20.			1	1.9	2	3.1	2	2.1						
21.	4	7.4 (›)	1	1.9	1	1.6	2	2.1			3	8.6	2	3.7
22.	28	51.9 ››	15	28.3	37	57.8 ›››	27	28.4	7	18.0	16	45.7	19	35.2
23.						(‹)	3	3.2	1	2.6	1	2.9	4	7.4
24.			1	1.9			1	1.1						
25.					2	3.1								
26.	5	9.3	2	3.8							1	2.9		
Sum	54		53		64		95		39		35		54	
% of pop.		27.7		16.6		32.8		20.0		12.2		17.9		16.9

Table B I 14. Affirmations of Worst Memories

	Illiterate Men 1963 N	Perc.	1976 N	Perc.	Illiterate Women 1963 N	Perc.	1976 N	Perc.	Literate Men 1976 N	Perc.	Literate Boys 1963 N	Perc.	1976 N	Perc.
1.			1	1.9	1	1.6	2	2.1						
2.	1	1.9	1	1.9			1	1.1					3	5.6
3.	1	1.9							1	2.6	1	2.9		
4.														
5.					1	1.6	1	1.1						
6.	5	9.3	12	23.1	9	14.1	14	14.7	7	18.0	2	5.7	4	7.4
7.	3	5.6			6	9.4	10	10.5	1	2.6				
8.	2	3.7	4	7.7	1	1.6	4	4.2	1	2.6				
9.	3	5.6	5	9.6	1	1.6	4	4.2	8	20.5			4	7.4
10.					1	1.6	3	3.2	1	2.6				
11.									1	2.6	1	2.9	1	1.8
12.	2	3.7												
13.	5	9.3	5	9.6	4	6.3	1	1.1	1	2.6				
14.	1	1.9												
15.													1	1.8
16.	1	1.9							2	5.7				
17.	4	7.4			3	4.7	2	2.1	1	2.6			1	1.8
18.							1	1.1	1	2.6			1	1.8
19.									2	5.7	1	2.9		
20.	1	1.9			1	1.6	2	2.1			1	2.9		
21.	4	7.4	1	1.9	5	7.8	4	4.2	5	12.8			3	5.6
22.	21	38.9	23	44.2	31	48.4	44	46.3	6	15.4	29	82.9	31	57.4
23.							2	2.1	1	2.6			4	7.4
24.													1	1.8
25.														
Sum	54		52		64		95		39		35		54	
% of pop.		27.7		16.6		32.8		20.0		12.2		17.9		16.9

Among the worst memories we see a compensatory, symmetric and confirmatory change in the men's recollection of connubial life (No. 7), it being now in 1976 significantly less often their worst memory just as it is also significantly more their best. The women, interestingly enough, have not changed either way! One would like to know why, but we have no basis for an answer. Among their worst memories the men in 1976 more often give bereavement other than loss of an own child (No. 6), which we suspect to be due to the general reduction of infant and child mortality. They recall less often (in fact not at all) overwork and exhaustion (No. 17), less often also "other ill memories" (No. 21) than those classified. The single significant change among the women is that they less often mention financial difficulties, poverty and debt (No. 13). The literate boys do furnish us with certain significant differences among their worst memories, though they did not among their best. They tend to recall more often in 1976 ill treatment at others' hands (No. 2). This rests on only three cases and reminds us how often a certain teacher with a propensity for beating the children was mentioned with anger and fear. He had happily departed when we arrived, and his replacement was a model of gentleness. Four boys recall their own illness or accident as their worst memory in 1976, none in 1963, and the difference, though statistically "significant", may well be fortuitous, having only four cases to support it. In No. 22 we encounter the converse of the adults' marked decrement of "no pleasurable memories" inasmuch as the literate boys in 1976 much less frequently affirm that they have no ill memories. More of them, too, give no response (No. 23). The percentual decrease is substantial, the numerical however not great and may be explained by the several small increases (Nos. 2, 9, 21, 23) mentioned above.

Taking these shifts in best and worst memories over the thirteen years together and considering their implications, we must conclude that they do furnish us with incontrovertible indications of a much less gloomy retrospection than prevailed in Qassemabad in 1963 and with a fund of more or less pleasurable experience which did not formerly exist. That elusive thing called "quality of life" becomes tangible in such responses and by them had changed for the better.

The alteration is even more apparent, and in part strikingly so, when we regard the affirmative responses to the psychiatric questionnaire in Tables B I 15 and B I 16. First, we have taken the mean number of affirmative responses per person (exclusive of Q 12: magic) as a crude "complaint score", even though this is not exactly true, since certain answers to Q 7: excitement could imply being beside oneself with joy. In the overwhelming majority, however, affirmations implied some degree of subjectively recognized affective disturbance. We note that the complaint rate has dropped sharply and significantly for all groups except the male children and recall that the literate boys (who were 97 % of the male children in 1976) also presented no shift in their best memories between 1963 and 1976 and not many in their worst. Their score has even risen numerically from 1.1 to 1.3, but the difference is far from statistical significance and may justly be neglected. Among the percents by column one is impressed by the significant and in many cases quite substantial decrease in the men's affirmations to eight of the ten questions. In regard to Q 6: depression there is only a tendency, though in the same direction. This is reversed in the case of headache (Q 3), where the rate more than doubles. One must remind oneself here that a great many of the men were working in 1976 in a petrochemical plant, exposed to the usual range of organic solvents etc., others in a meat canning factory, and that both were malodorous. However, there

Table B I 15. Affirmative Responses to Items from Psychiatric Questionnaire by Sex and Age Class

	Adults				Children			
	Male		Female		Male		Female	
	1963	1976	1963	1976	1963	1976	1963	1976
	Absolute Numbers							
Q 1 Paralysis	9	6	7	0	3	0	0	0
Q 2 Fits	7	4	4	6	2	4	1	2
Q 3 Headache	12	43	12	46	5	23	4	15
Q 6 Depression	39	48	40	59	8	12	6	8
Q 7 Excitement	20	11	16	25	14	16	9	8
Q 8 Anxiety	27	19	30	37	8	10	4	7
Q 9 Suspicion	17	5	17	10	1	6	3	3
Q 10 Estrangement	14	7	14	11	2	2	3	2
Q 11 Voices	10	7	11	10	5	4	6	3
Q 12 Magic	7	2	7	5	0	1	1	1
Subjects	62	93	64	105	44	58	25	64
Complaints per subject[a]	2.5›››	1.6	2.4›››	1.9	1.1	1.3	1.4›››	0.8
	Percent by Column							
Q 1 Paralysis	14.5›	6.5	10.9›››	0	6.8›	0	0	0
Q 2 Fits	11.3›	4.3	6.3	5.7	4.5	6.9	4.0	3.1
Q 3 Headache	19.4‹‹‹	46.2	18.8‹‹‹	43.8	11.4‹‹	39.7	16.0	23.4
Q 6 Depression	62.9(›)	51.6	62.5	56.2	18.2	20.7	24.0(›)	12.5
Q 7 Excitement	32.3››	11.8	25.0	23.8	31.8	27.6	36.0››	12.5
Q 8 Anxiety	43.6››	20.4	46.9(›)	35.2	18.2	17.2	16.0	10.9
Q 9 Suspicion	27.4›››	5.4	26.6››	9.5	2.3(‹)	10.3	12.0	4.7
Q 10 Estrangement	22.6››	7.5	21.9›	10.5	4.5	3.4	12.0(›)	3.1
Q 11 Voices	16.1›	7.5	17.2(›)	9.5	11.4	6.9	24.0››	4.7
Q 12 Magic	11.3››	2.2	10.9(›)	4.8	0	1.7	4.0	1.6
of population	31.8	29.1	32.8	32.8	22.6	18.1	18.5	20.0

[a] Excluding affirmations of Q 12.

Table B I 16. Significance of Differences in Frequency of Affirmative Responses to Items from Psychiatric Questionnaire by Sex and Age Class

	1963				1976			
	Male : Female		Adults : Children		Male : Female		Adults : Children	
	Adults	Children	Male	Female	Adults	Children	Male	Female
Q 1 Paralysis		(›)		›	››		›	
Q 2 Fits								
Q 3 Headache						›		››
Q 6 Depression			›››	›››			›››	›››
Q 7 Excitement					‹	›	‹‹	›
Q 8 Anxiety			››		‹			›››
Q 9 Suspicion		‹	›››	››				
Q 10 Estrangement			››					›
Q 11 Voices		(‹)						
Q 12 Magic			›					

is the same rise in Q 3 for the women, and they were not factory workers. Since they too recorded fewer open affective complaints, though their decrement was less regular, less marked and generally less highly statistically significant than the men's (this does not apply, be it noted, to the total complaint score), the hypothesis lies close at hand that, together with the decrease of overt complaints, there may have occurred an increase of covert ones, in other words of largely psychosomatic headache. This is not corroborated and even appears contradicted by our psychiatric prevalence tables, which show six psychosomatic cases in 1963 and only three in 1976, with four cases of female migrane in 1963 and none in 1976, but we have included in them only such cases as we have considered to be of "clinical" severity. These disabling cases had indeed vanished, as far as we could tell, but, as the table shows, over two fifths of the women instead of one newly complained of occasional headache of no crippling degree. The same complaint had increased among the male children significantly and among the female at least numerically. Closer environmental investigations would be needed, but in the absence of these we regard the hypothesis of a general trend toward mild somatization of residual affective disturbance as at least worthy of discussion. The drop in Q 1: paralysis is partly real thanks to energetic and successful immunization against poliomyelitis, though of course this does not account for all the subjects who registered such a symptom in 1963 and did not in 1976, they being much more numerous than the actual polio victims. The very real fear of this dread disease, thanks to which almost any mere transitory numbness of a limb could lead to interpretation as a symptom and to panic, was dying out also. Notably the women show no significant change in their rates of affirmative answers for depression (the men, to be sure, at most a tendency) and excitement (the men do), only a tendency toward less anxiety (the men a significant decrease), but join their spouses in a reassuring decline in suspicion. Rather surprisingly there is a tendency for this to rise, nevertheless, among the male children. The girls take an opposite course, though the difference does not attain statistical significance. We are frankly at loss for an explanation and can think of only one objective difference that might be invoked: the school, which practically all the boys, but less than half of the girls were attending and which few of their parents had attended. While it is far from our purpose to indict the schools as the root of all psychological evils, we have too many memories of complaints about ill treatment at teachers' hands, not seldom with subsequent withdrawal by the parents or refusal by the child to attend, to omit mention of this possibility. Western type schooling in the Iranian countryside was still very new then, and who can wonder if the mostly inexperienced teachers easily fell back into the tradition of corporal chastisement that had obtained for centuries in the homes?

It seems worth remarking that in certain respects significant alterations in the girl's and the men's complaints go together (Q 6, 7, 11) but find no counterpart among the women and the boys. Paradoxical though this appears, there is one circumstance which we think can account for it: the lives of both the former groups had undergone and were undergoing more profound socio-economic and cultural changes than those of the two latter. The transformation in the economy has been described: it was almost exclusively a men's affair. Women's rights existed on paper and were gradually coming into practice. The attitude toward female children, hitherto regarded at best as a burden and at worst as a curse, was changing – not everywhere, and in some families and circles not at all, but on the whole perceptibly and recognizably changing. If only 42 % of the girls were literate in 1976, that percentage was a mere 12 in 1963 and was constituted of three little girls in the first grades. Who can doubt that this was felt by the rest and came to be reflected even in our crude statistics? The women benefited by the general economic improvement, but their occupations and roles were not fundamentally altered; neither were those of the schoolboys.

Tables B I 16 compares the four sub-populations of each survey among themselves, i.e. not over time. In 1963 we observe no sex differences among adults and few among children, only one in fact being significant. Girls affirm suspicion more than boys. In 1976 they no longer do so, whereas it is the boys who have significantly higher rate of headache (Q 3) and excitement (Q 7). For 1976 there is a highly significant adult sex difference in regard to paralysis (Q 1), which six men, but no women report. This is not to be taken literally, but refers more to transitory complaints such as arthritic pains, etc., cf. above. Other adult sex differences are to be found in respect of excitement (where the gradient is opposite to that between the boys and girls) and anxiety, the women leading. This may be due to a cultural stereotype which, in Iran as in the West, permits and encourages women to express such feelings more than men, but leaves the question open why no such difference was demonstrable in 1963 when the stereotype certainly was no less operative. Referring to what was said above, we suspect that the finding reflects rather a decrease in excitement and anxiety among the men than an increase among the women and see this confirmed in Table B I 15.

In the age comparisons the adults lead wherever significant differences are to be found with one exception: excitement rates are higher in 1976 among the boys than the men. As very similar findings turn up elsewhere we shall not discuss them here, but postpone this until the results from the questionnaire are analysed both in general and with local reference in Part C, Chap. II 2. There the data for the Marvdasht Survey, of which the first Qassemabad Survey in 1963 was a constituent, are to be consulted. The parallel, as expected, is close except in one column: the comparison of the adult male and female populations. As mentioned, we find no significant differences in Qassemabad in 1963, but a number of them for Marvdasht as a whole. Any attempt to account for this would entail a detailed analysis of the other two Marvdasht villages, Kenareh and Zangiabad, separately – a task which we cannot undertake at present.

What is denominated here by the key word "magic" (Q 12) corresponds to an affirmation of the question "Have you ever been put under a spell?", by which formulation we aspired to obtain more concrete information than if we had inquired merely about an abstract belief. It is not in fact a psychiatric question, but is included here for convenience and will be treated separately in the larger context of Part C, Chap. II 1 d. Significantly less men in 1976 thought that they had ever been victims of magic in this sense, and there was a slight reduction in the number of the women also. In 1963 the men had believed more in spells than the boys, but this gradient had disappeared in 1976, as might be expected from the foregoing.

Other aspects of the survey and resurvey that invite comparison are intelligence and the Z Test. As we shall see later, mean intelligence quotients are moderately but significantly lower in all rural surveys than in the city, and this remains true when only the illiterate are compared. We have surmised that more intellectual stimulation and exigency may tend to raise the IQ in an urban environment. Qassemabad was by no means urban in 1976, but there had been a great opening, an enhancement of mobility, an increase of communication and commerce with Shiraz and with the secondary center of Marvdasht town, to say nothing of the number of men who took themselves and their trucks even farther afield. It would have constituted a confirmation of our hypothesis and surprised no one if a general rise in the IQ, independent of schooling, had occurred. The circumstances and structure of the survey and resurvey, however, restricted the possibilities for such a comparison drastically. It will be recalled that the Block Design Test employed in 1963 proved unsatisfactory and was replaced both in Shiraz and in the resurvey of Qassemabad. This left the Arithmetic Test, which remained the same for illiterates throughout (Arithmetic A), but for literates was replaced again in Shiraz and the Qassemabad Resurvey by a new Arithmetic Test B. In 1963 there were not enough literate men to justify a comparison, and there were no literate women. The only valid comparison that could be drawn therefore was that between the illiterates of both sexes in 1963 and 1976 on the Test of Mental Arithmetic (A). Since only one sub-test was involved, there was no need to convert the raw into weighted scores and these into IQs. We could and did compare the raw scores directly for both sexes, for the age groups 15–19, 20–39, 40–59, 60+ and all ages together and found no even remotely significant difference anywhere except for the men of 60 and over, whose mean raw point score on Arithmetic A had dropped conspicuously from 15.67 ± 3.21 in 1963 to only 10.00 ± 4.36 in 1976, the critical ratio being 2.63 and $p < 0.005$. The size of the difference was startling, but the means rested upon such very small numbers (3 men in 1963 and 5 in 1976) that we place little confidence in them despite their statistical "significance". In most other mean values there was, if anything, a very slight numerical tendency to decline. This may seem at first glance to controvert our hypothesis, but it does not necessarily do so. The comparison was drawn between the illiterate then and now, i.e. in 1976, and it seems a reasonable supposition that those who had remained illiterate in 1976 were on the whole the less enterprising and the less intelligent, those less open to the influence of intellectual stimulation, in other words a negative selection (though this certainly could not be affirmed of all cases). It seems further likely that the illiterate men beyond sixty had simply given up and turned over such arithmetical tasks as were inevitable to the more adaptable younger generation. It would be best, we opine, not to draw or force any far-reaching conclusions from such a small segment of our respective populations and to leave the question open for further study.

While we do possess comparable Z Tests from both Qassemabad surveys, evaluation of them remains a task for the future. We shall mention only one impression: that in the records of 1976 there were less indications of manifest pathology, but more of neurotoid structure and thus of potential or latent neurotic development, which must by no means necessarily grow into a neurosis. This would correspond quite well to the suspicion we expressed in connection with the conspicuous rise in the "headache" score, which nevertheless had no counterpart in the clinical cases of migraine or other forms of headache.

Before reaching the psychiatric findings we offer several short tables containing data gathered in 1976 only. We have no comparable figures from other rural surveys, but only from Shiraz. Fertility rates have been stated and discussed above. Orphanism (Table B I 17) is slightly higher in the city (where 62 % have both parents alive, in Qassemabad 69 %). In Shiraz there are somewhat more single than married men (Table B IV 4), in all likelihood due to an influx of job-seekers from the country, whereas in Qassemabad in 1976 62 % of the men ten years old or older were married

Table B I 17. Orphanism

	Absolute Numbers			Percent of Population		
	Ch.	Ad.	Ch. + Ad.	Ch.	Ad.	Ch. + Ad.
Both parents alive	111	109	220	34.8	34.2	69.0
One parent dead	8	39	47	2.5	12.2	14.7
Both parents dead	3	49	52	0.9	15.4	16.3
Subtotal	122	197	319	38.2	61.8	100.0
nc		1	1			
Total	122	198	320			

(Table B I 18) as compared to 58 % of the women. For these, the proportions of single and married are not greatly different between village and city. In 1970 about 73 % of the Shirazi residents had been born there (Table B IV 15), but in 1976 only 62 % of the Qassamabadi had been born in the village (Table B I 19). The great majority of the immigrants to the village had been born in other villages of Fars, together with a sprinkling of nomads. This appears contradicted by Table B I 20, where only 44 % claim to have lived in Qassemabad all their lives, but as a matter of fact not a few had resided in other places for a time and returned thence (this applies especially to widowed and divorced women, but there were also men who had tried their luck elsewhere and returned when the new factories afforded opportunities for employ-

Table B I 18. Marital Status (persons from 10 years upward)

	Absolute Numbers			Percent by Column		
	m	f	m + f	m	f	m + f
Single	44	46	90	37.3	33.6	35.3
Married	73	80	153	61.9	58.4	60.0
Deprived (widowed, divorced, separated)	1	11	12	0.8	8.0	4.7
Subtotal	118	137	255	100.0	100.0	100.0
nc		2	2			
Total	118	139	257			

Table B I 19. Place of Birth

	Absolute Numbers			Percent by Column		
	m	f	m + f	m	f	m + f
Qassemabad	97	97	194	65.5	59.5	62.4
Cities in Fars	2	5	7	1.4	3.1	2.3
Villages in Fars, nomads	42	57	99	28.4	35.0	31.8
Outside Fars	7	4	11	4.7	2.5	3.5
Subtotal	148	163	311	100.0	100.0	100.0
nc	3	6	9			
Total	151	169	320			

Table B I 20. Length of Residence in Qassemabad

	Absolute Numbers			Percent by Column		
	m	f	m + f	m	f	m + f
Lifelong	48	46	94	47.5	40.4	43.7
Ten years or more, but not lifelong	34	29	63	33.7	25.4	29.3
Five to nine years	3	6	9	3.0	5.3	4.2
One to four years	7	17	24	6.9	14.9	11.2
Less than one year	9	16	25	8.9	14.0	11.6
Subtotal	101	114	215	100.0	100.0	100.0
nc	50	55	105			
Total	151	169	320			

ment). Moreover, information on length of residence proved much more unreliable and difficult to collect, as the large number of nc in Table B I 20 shows. Statements tended to be vague and uncertain, while those about places of birth were not. The influence of the factories appears again in the 23 % who had lived in the village for less than five years, but there are also notably more female immigrants in this period: girls who had married into the village or in some cases daughters who had rejoined their families as carpet weaving began to flourish. Correspondingly there were less women who had lived there for ten years or longer but not always, and we may presume that they had mostly married outside.

We must take ourselves to task for having realized just too late in 1963 that we should have inquired systematically whether and how often each subject had been to the geographically near, but socio-economically and culturally remote city. A great many of the women and a substantial share of the men never had been or, if they had, only once or twice in their lives. In 1976 we did ask, with the results to be found in Table B I 21. The pattern is not unexpected, with the men registering more visits than the women and the adults more than the children. Certain items have impressed us and certainly could not have been encountered in even distantly comparable dimensions thirteen years before. Over forty percent of the men went to town oftener than once a month, and over ten percent of the women did. A small number of men were commuting daily to the city for work. Only six adult women had never been there at all,

Table B I 21. Frequency of Visits to Shiraz

	Absolute Numbers				Percent by Column			
	Male		Female		Male		Female	
	Ad.	Ch.	Ad.	Ch.	Ad.	Ch.	Ad.	Ch.
Never	0	13	6	19	0	23.6	6.0	31.7
Seldom ever	5	23	28	25	5.4	41.8	28.0	41.7
Seldom per year	28	12	45	11	30.4	21.8	45.0	18.3
Every couple of months	5	1	5	2	5.4	1.8	5.0	3.3
Monthly	9	1	5	0	9.8	1.8	5.0	0
Oftener than monthly	38	5	11	3	41.3	9.1	11.0	5.0
Daily	7	0	0	0	7.6	0	0	0
Unknown	1	3	5	4				
Sum	93	58	105	64	100	100	100	100

and none of the men. These figures are eloquent to those who knew Qassemabad in 1963. Other categories require no comment.

This table of visits rounds off a series of socio-psychological findings that document objectively deep and meaningful alterations in the habits, sentiments, feelings and propensities of the Qassemabadi population over thirteen years during which equally profound environmental changes had taken place. It would be folly to deny any connection between the two, even though not all the connecting threads can be traced singly. The socio-psychological alterations were consistently in the direction of more pleasurable, of fewer oppressive and gloomy memories, of fewer complaints about emotional disturbances within the normal range, especially of diminished excitation, anxiety and above all suspicion, whereas references to depression, not altogether as we had expected, had hardly declined. The reflection of all these we shall meet in the psychiatric findings, which the socio-psychological data help in part to understand and explain. Alterations of this kind affected the men more than the women and the girls more than the boys, the men and the girls being those whose form and presumably also content of life had changed or was changing more than the rest.

The psychiatric findings are given by diagnosis in Table B I 24, which may be compared with Table B I 23 for 1963. They are summarized again, by sex and degree of pathology only, in Table B I 22, in which both the total cases identified in 1976 and the new cases in the resurvey, either not of age, not present or not yet morbid in 1963, are shown separately.

The total psychiatric prevalence decreased numerically from 113 per thousand in 1963 to 88 per thousand in 1976, but the difference was far from statistical significance. Very significant however is the much larger share of female patients as against male in both survey and resurvey, very significant also ($p < 0.001$) the decrease in severity of pathology when P_2 and P_3 are combined and compared by fourfold X^2 table with P_1. P_3 is not even represented in 1976, and P_2 has receded from 14 cases to 3. A single new P_2 case was discovered. The rest are mild cases of degree P_1, and it is noticeable that in the new P_1 the sex ratio is coming nearer to a balance.

Where is this alteration diagnostically localized? Neither in the first survey nor in the resurvey did we find any case of functional psychosis. Since the expectation of such lies around 1:1000–2000 it is rather less than more likely that a case would occur in a population of only 200–300. Its absence tells us nothing. The constitutional anomalies too are represented by such small numbers that a case more or less may well be fortuitous and no conclusions can be drawn from their apparent decrease from 20 per thousand in 1963 to half that much in 1976.

The bulk of our cases, 86 % in the resurvey, are reactive, and among them changes of significant proportion and no little interest have occurred. Their overall increase

Table B I 22. Psychiatric Cases

	1963			1976			New in 1976		
	m	f	m + f	m	f	m + f	m	f	m + f
P_1	2	4	6	10	15	25	10	13	23
P_2	2	12	14	0	3	3	0	1	1
P_3	1	1	2	0	0	0	0	0	0
P	5	17	22	10	18	28	10	14	24

from 77 % in 1963 is not, however, statistically significant. The simple reactions and developments accounted for 36 % of the total morbidity in 1963, but only for 14 % in 1976, and similarly the psychosomatic cases have declined from 27 % to 11 %. The neuroses, on the contrary, have increased from 14 % to 61 %. A number of the simple reactions and developments contributed to the P_2 cases in 1963. If we now combine the neurotic and psychosomatic cases, in which by Binder's definition repression and dissociation are at work, and compare them with the simple reactions and developments with repression but without dissociation, we find the increase of the neurotic disorders in the extended sense (i.e. with psychosomatic included) over against the simple to be significant at the 5 % level of confidence. That is, we see a decline of the simple but in 1963 more severe, predominantly anxious-depressive reactions, but an increase of milder neurosis. Comparing now the strictly neurotic with the psychosomatic cases of the two surveys we find the difference to be significant at the 0.025 level of confidence. Theoretically this could be interpreted as meaning that heavier repression by itself (in the P_2 simple reactions and developments) had declined, while lighter repression combined with dissociation (the mostly P_1 neurotic and psychosomatic cases in 1976) had risen. If we accept Mitscherlich's illuminating hypothesis of double repression in psychosomatic illness [151] we can go a step further and conclude that the generally milder reactive disorders at the time of the resurvey were tending to meet on a common plane of relatively light repression and also light dissociation.

Table B I 22 enables the calculation of an incidence rate for total psychiatric morbidity. Twenty-four new cases had emerged in 13 years, i.e. 1.8 cases per year. The mean between the 195 subjects examined in 1963 and the 320 under scrutiny in 1976 is 258. Lacking exact year by year figures we are compelled to fall back on the almost certainly not wholly valid hypothesis that annual population growth was regular, though it is more likely that there were rather abrupt increases when the two factories began to recruit laborers. Under this hypothesis nonetheless we can arrive, with appropriate reservation, at an incidence rate of 24:(13x258)=7.2 per thousand per year.

A principal objective of the resurvey was to learn the fate, as far as practicable, of our former cases from 1963. The catamnestic data are shown numerically in Table B I 25. We succeeded in retrieving 16 of the 22 cases we had diagnosed in 1963 and re-examined most of them ourselves, while in a few instances we had to rely upon information from third parties that seemed adequate. Some were identified in Kuh Sabz or in neighboring villages and interviewed there. Some, as we were told, had removed to Shiraz, Marvdasht or more or less remote villages whither we could not trace them in the time at our disposal. A few had simply vanished. To these last belonged an epileptic with severe alteration of personality (P_3) from the first survey. The other P_3 case from it, an imbecile girl, had died. Thus no case of this severest degree remained, and no new ones were discovered. Ten out of 14 cases of medium degree diagnosed in 1963 could be found again in 1976. Eight of these had recovered, two were unaltered, none merely improved (that is from P_2 to P_1). This need occasion no surprise, as we have seen that the great majority were reactive disorders. Their tendency to spontaneous recovery over longer periods has been demonstrated and well documented by such authors as Ernst, Kind and Rotach [69] and Cremerius [59]. A number of severe migraine cases from 1963 belong here. One P_2 diagnosis had to be revised. The then ten year old girl of coarse appearance, backward in general and test performance, to all

Table B I 23. Psychiatric Diagnoses of All Cases in 1963

Diagnoses	Number of cases					p. 100 of 22 cases					p. 1000 of 195 subjects				
	m	f	m + f			m	f	m + f			m	f	m + f		
I. Funct. psychoses			0					0					0		
1. Schizophrenia															
2. Affect. psychoses															
II. Acute symptomatic psychoses															
III. Subchronic & chron. sympt. psychoses & residual states			1					4.5					5		
1. Epilepsy				1					4.5					5	
a. cryptogen.	1	0			1					4.5					
b. symptomatic															
2. Sen. & arterioscl.															
3. post-infectious															
4. post-traumatic															
5. endocrine															
6. addiction															
7. other															
IV. Reactive disorders			17					77.3					8.7		
1. Simple path. dev.				8					36.4					41	
a. anxious	0	2			2					9.1					
b. depressive	0	5			5					22.7					
c. irritable															
d. neurasthenic	1	0			1					4.5					
e. other															
2. Neuroses				3					13.6					15	
a. anxious	1	0			1					4.5					
b. phobic															
c. depressive	0	1			1					4.5					
d. hysterical															
e. hypochondriac	0	1			1					4.5					
f. neurasthenic															
g. self-insuff.															
h. negativistic															
i. other & polym.															
3. Psychosomatic				6					27.3					31	
a. headache															
1. migrainoid	0	4			4					18.2					
2. other															
b. gastro-intest.	1	0			1					4.5					
c. asthmatic															
d. other & polym.	0	1			1					4.5					
V. Constitutional disord.			4					18.2					21		
1. Clin. oligophrenia				4					18.2					21	
a. cryptogenetic	1	3			4					18.2					
b. genetic															
2. Psychopathy				0											
a. irritable															
b. anti-social															
c. schizoid															
d. other															
Total	5	17	22	22	22			100	100	100			113	113	

Table B I 24. Psychiatric Diagnoses of All Cases in 1976

Diagnoses	Number of cases					p. 100 of 28 cases					p. 1000 of 320 subjects				
	m	f	m + f			m	f	m + f			m	f	m + f		
I. Funct. psychoses			0					0					0		
1. Schizophrenia															
2. Affect. psychoses															
II. Acute symptomatic psychoses			0					0					0		
III. Subchronic & chron. sympt. psychoses & residual states			1					3.6					3		
1. Epilepsy															
a. cryptogen.															
b. symptomatic															
2. Sen. & arterioscl.															
3. post-infectious															
4. post-traumatic															
5. endocrine															
6. addiction	1	0		1	1				3.6	3.6				3	
7. other															
IV. Reactive disorders			24					85.7					76		
1. Simple path. dev.				4					14.3					13	
a. anxious	0	1			1					3.6					
b. depressive	0	3			3					10.7					
c. irritable															
d. neurasthenic															
e. other															
2. Neuroses				17					60.7					54	
a. anxious	1	4			5					17.9					
b. phobic															
c. depressive	2	2			4					14.2					
d. hysterical															
e. hypochondriac	0	1			1					3.7					
f. neurasthenic															
g. self-insuff.	1	4			5					17.9					
h. negativistic															
i. other & polym.	2	0			2					7.0					
3. Psychosomatic				3					10.7					9	
a. headache															
α. migrainoid															
β. other	0	1			1					3.6					
b. gastro-intest.	0	2			2					7.1					
c. asthmatic															
d. other & polym.															
V. Constitutional disord.			3					10.7					9		
1. Clin. oligophrenia				3					10.7					9	
a. cryptogenetic	3	0			3					10.7					
b. genetic															
2. Psychopathy				0											
a. irritable															
b. anti-social															
c. schizoid															
d. other															
Total	10	18	28	28	28			100	100	100			88	88	

Table B I 25. Catamneses

	1963			1976										
				Retrieved			Unchanged			Recovered			Died
	m	f	m+f	m	f	m+f	m	f	m+f	m	f	m+f	f
P_1	2	4	6	2	3	5	0	2	2	2	1	3	0
P_2	2	12	14	1	9	10	0	2	2	1	7	8	0
P_3	1	1	2	1	0	1	0	0	0	0	0	0	1
P	5	17	22	4	12	16	0	4	4	3	8	11	1

seeming dull and grossly unintelligent had grown into a still somewhat undifferentiated but otherwise unremarkable young woman who was living with her parents and working carpets. She had no complaints except some anxiety in the dark. Her intelligence quotient was 88, and the Z Test likewise indicated rather low intelligence, but not feeble-mindedness. A couple of other children who seemed extremely shy and inhibited in their performance in 1963 had undergone a gratifying development into inconspicuous normalcy.

Finally we should like to illustrate with four short histories the origin and dissolution of such disorders as we have discussed above.

1. The early orphaned patient, thirty years old when we first saw him, had grown up under the custody of his elder brothers, who by his own account plagued him more than they cared for him. He had married in 1957 and had two sons, one of whom uttered the same complaints as his father and one of the latter's brothers. These consisted above all in stomach aches with loss of appetite, in our patient's own case also insomnia, irritability and depression. He declined to designate the circumstances of his life as either good or bad and added that one must bear life as it came. He appeared tense, held his hands crampedly clasped and commanded the attention even of lay field workers. A gastric ulcer had been confirmed radiologically in a Shiraz hospital. We diagnosed a psychosomatic gastric disorder of degree P_2 on the basis of his early orphanism and unhappy youth. In 1976 he had eight children, but his economic position was fairly satisfactory notwithstanding. A nephrectomy of the right kidney had been performed seven years ago. The man had some back pains, but no more in the stomach. He mentioned understandable, unpathological worries about the remaining kidney and that his sleep was sometimes disturbed by pains in the head and back, but he was able to work at full capacity, was living to all appearances in good relations with his wife and the numerous children, seemed far less tense than formerly, behaved politely and considerately both towards his family and the investigators and gave no indication of depression. The intelligence quotient was 100. The ZTest remained slightly neurotic.

2. The second case serves to illustrate an urgent problem of the Iranian women. In 1963 we had come upon a thirteen year old girl whose father had died and who was living with her mother and her second husband, a brother and six year old sister from the mother's first marriage. There had been no issue from the second. The brother and the little sister were allowed to go to school, but not our patient. She seemed already physically and mentally mature beyond her age, self-controlled, keen witted, gave brief and clear answers to our questions and uttered no complaints. When we asked whether she would not like to attend school she replied with a simple affirmation, but added that at the normal time for entrance there had been no school in the village and that she herself was afraid that she could not catch up. The IQ of 86 fell below our expactation, but the ZTest disclosed a massive anxious-depressive pseudo-debility. The mother denied any tension between the stepfather and daughter, praised the latter as a quick and clever girl but had no ear for our pleas, supported by such Iranian officials as we could mobilize, that she should send her to school (education was "compulsory" by law). She needed her at home to work carpets! We took especial pains to find again the now twenty-six year old woman, whom

we had noted as a privileged candidate for a more severe neurosis, and did so with no difficulty in Kuh Sabz. She received us warmly, remembered well our former encounter, had married a year thereafter through the customary mediation of the parents and had never been to school, though she had borne three children who were all attending. She declared that she herself was content but was taking contraceptive pills regularly, did not want more than three children, but intended to see that all received a good education. Her marriage was not unhappy, and they had not financial worries. Sometimes she quarreled with her mother (whom we also saw again) and did not think much of the fact that the latter had recently become pregnant anew. Her manner was as before, only somewhat freer, the IQ 87, the Z Test no longer severely pathological but certainly neurotoid.

An elderly couple illustrates the genesis of new cases. Both partners were judged unremarkable in 1963.

3. The husband, turned 67, had the typical complaints of aging and could not get a job in the factory. As his happiest memory he recalled his youth with bodily mobility and with success in business and in the next instant denied having any happy recollection at all. His son had moved away, the neighbors wanted to put a bad spell on his house, and he was afraid of lightning. After losing his job four years ago he had begun to seek consolation in opium. The intelligence was normal with IQ 94. There were "spooks" in the Z Test and signs of a querulatory depression. We made the diagnosis of a paranoid-depressive development with opium habituation of degree P_1.

4. His fifty-five year old wife was worse off. Although they had enough to live on, she had developed a gastric ulcer when the husband lost his job and had to go about once a month to the doctor in the city. The ulcer was radiologically confirmed. She slept poorly, said herself she was nervous and irritable and added that if she became annoyed in the morning she would quarrel the whole day. Her IQ had dropped from 106 in 1963 to 93 in 1976 and the Z Test had altered even more than her husband's, had deteriorated in quality and was full of signs of neurotic anxiety and opposition. As she was constantly under medical care for her evidently psychosomatic illness we designated her as a medium case of degree P_2.

II. Khuzestan[1]

1. General

The Upper Khuzestan Plain is described by Gremliza [87] as "an area of almost 41 000 square kilometers . . . in the southwest of Iran. It is essentially a continuation east of the Iraqi border of the great Mesopotamian Plain", the breadbasket of the Middle East in Sassanian times. Long before that it was the center of the Empire of Elam (the modern Shush, where French archaeological teams have been excavating for decades), under the later Achaemenians the site of the city and University of Gundi Shahpour (near contemporary Dezful), whither the last of the Greek philosophers were expelled when Byzantium was christianized. After the Arab conquest the dams and irrigation canals, of which traces abound and a few have remained in use until the present, fell into disrepair and the plain into aridity (cf. Adams, [1]). North of Dezful it is bounded by the steep escarpments of the Zagros Range, through which the River Dez cuts its way by a deep and narrow gorge and flows to meet Iran's one navigable river (up to Ahwaz), the Karun, which at Khoramshahr combines with the already united Euphrates and Tigris to form the Shatt-el-Arab and empty itself into the Persian Gulf. Rainfall is minimal (300–400 mm per year), and after irrigation collapsed the work of dessication was completed by torrid winds that flattened the remaining vegetation and leveled the sandy, increasingly rootless and, from lack of drainage, saline soil.

After initial survey and on recommendation of the Development and Resources Corporation of New York to the Plan Organization of Iran, it was decided in 1957 to institute a Development Program for Khuzestan, the core of which was to be a large dam in the gorge of the Dez that would impound some 3300 million cubic meters of water to be used both for irrigation and for power and which in addition would control the floods that from time to time swept over the Upper Khuzestan Plain. It was completed in 1963. Irrigation canals and power lines were built at the same time, sugar cane cultivation was re-instituted after a lapse of centuries at Haft Tapeh (Seven Hills) between Dezful and Ahwaz, and electric current was supplied to Ahwaz, the capital of the province, and to the twin port cities of Khoramshahr and Abadan.

Parallel with the construction of the Dez Dam and the channels for its water and electricity the Khuzestan Water and Power Authority (KWPA), an agency of the Plan Organization of Iran, began a survey of the condition and resources of the future development area, taking as its object a central and presumably typical strip of land roughly 25 kilometers long and 10 kilometers wide comprising a population of over eleven thousand persons in 57 villages between Dezful and Haft Tapeh. This Dez

[1] A brief account has been published in 1969 [26].

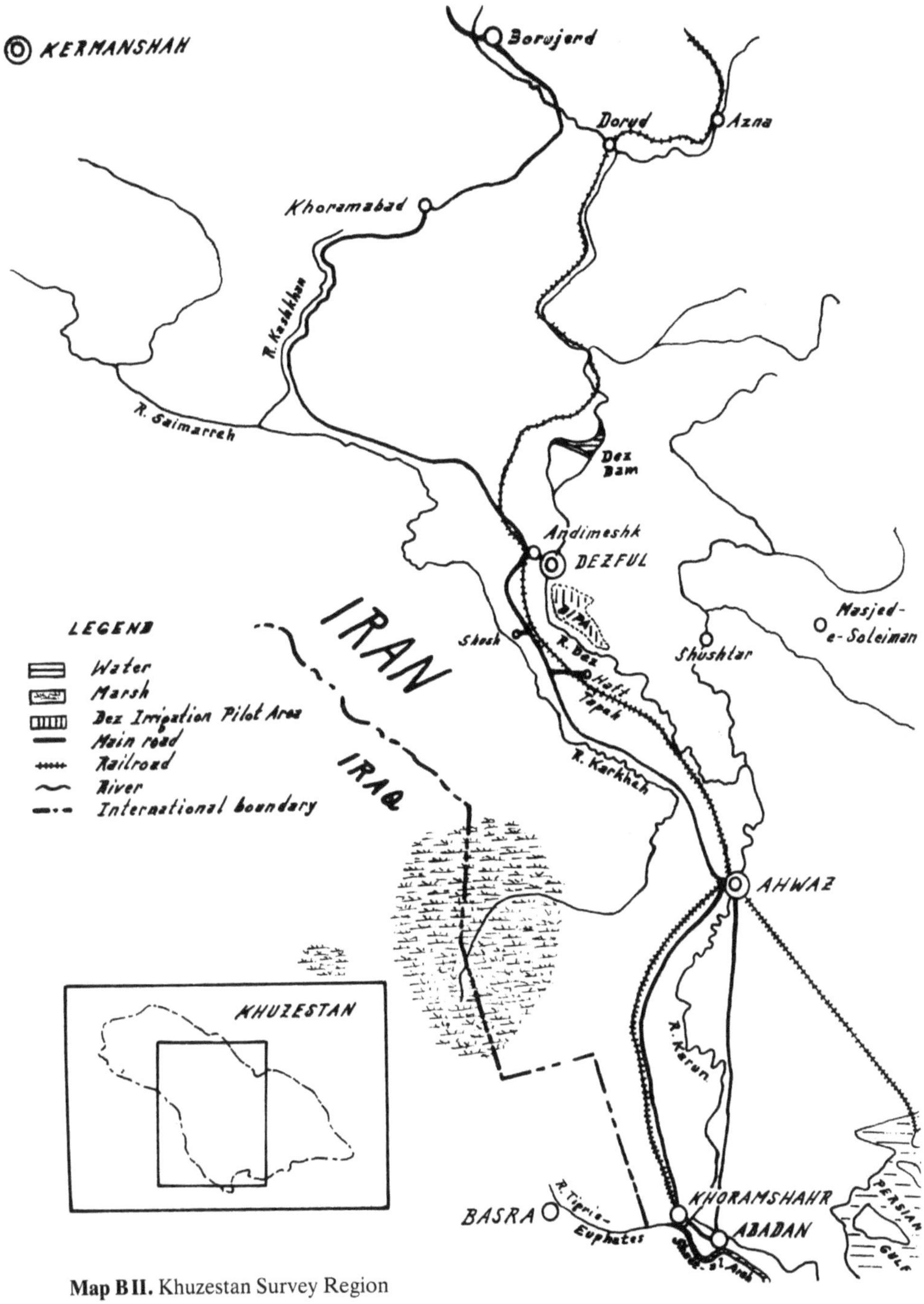

Map B II. Khuzestan Survey Region

Irrigation Pilot Area (DIPA) was not only to be studied, but was to be the prime recipient of water, power and the corresponding infrastructures – a laboratory for the subsequent development of the Greater Dez area that included most of the Upper Khuzestan Plain. An investigation of health conditions and needs formed part of the program and was intrusted to Dr. F. G. L. Gremliza. His public health survey, begun with a handful of Iranian technicians, whom he himself trained, in jeeps and tents in 1959, had been brought to a preliminary completion in 1960/61 and published in his compendious "Ecology of endemic diseases in the Dez Irrigation Pilot Area" in 1962 [87]. Periodic resurveys checked the original data and sought to measure change as the intended developments did in fact take place. Since the authors worked with Gremliza mainly in 1964 and 1965 during the phase of resurvey and consolidation, they had the immense advantage of a large body of carefully verified demographic and public health information, a mobile laboratory, a population accustomed to surveys and interviews and ready to bestow confidence upon strangers introduced by one whom they already knew as their benefactor and friend, technical help from Dr. Gremliza's staff and – not least – the day to day reliable, understanding and resourceful co-operation of an outstanding and very highly esteemed colleague to whom they gladly render their sincere thanks. Included therein is Dr. Gremliza's then counterpart and later successor, who ably abetted him and us.

Gremliza characterized the health situation of the DIPA as he first found it succinctly: The crude birth rate was 57.4 per thousand, the fertility rate in females between 16 and 40 years 288.6 per thousand per year, the crude death rate 24.9 per thousand, the infant mortality rate (below one year of age) 221.2 per thousand. Illiteracy in the age groups 11 to 50 years was 97.8 %. Diets were generally deficient in first class proteins, especially among the young and the aged. As regards these age groups, 46.7 % of the population was 15 years of age or under, while only 0.4 % was 61 or over. "Soil-transmitted intestinal worms constitute a major public health problem and are among the major causes of illness." The over-all sex ratio was 105 males to 100 females but varied substantially in different age groups, as we shall have occasion to observe below.

As remarked in Chapter A II, the then Adviser first met Gremliza on a duty trip to Ahwaz in 1960 and discussed with him during most of a long train trip back to Tehran the idea of a mental health survey. Gremliza was justly sceptical, but invited the Adviser to return, look over the field and experiment. He did so for a few days in 1961. Problems were beginning to arise concerning the selection of foremen, minor technicians and candidates for training for the multifarious public, agricultural, industrial and administrative services that the development program was introducing or about to introduce. Unsystematic trials convinced both Gremliza and the Adviser that the tests which the latter proposed to use, and to the choice of which Gremliza had contributed invaluable suggestions, did differentiate between aptitudes and abilities among the indigenous, then almost wholly illiterate population, and the conviction was carried to the Khuzestan Water and Power Authority. A mental health survey as part of Gremliza's resurveying was envisaged but, because of many complications connected with the completion of the Dez Dam, could not be executed until the spring of 1964. The Adviser's departure from Iran was already imminent, but in April of that year he did spend a week in the DIPA at the invitation of Gremliza and the Khuzestan Water and Power Authority and performed preliminary investigations with the understanding that they should be expanded into a systematic survey at a later date.

Since time did not suffice for any sizeable investigation and at the most two to three Iranian staff members of the KWPA could be spared for the field work, who also had to be introduced to the simplest techniques of psychological test administration and recording in a matter of hours, the Adviser decided to concentrate on persons whom Gremliza and his staff, familiar with every village and almost with every house and individual in the Pilot Area, could point out as to their knowledge pathological or suspect of pathology in a psychiatric and neurological sense. The compass had to be restricted, and as Gremliza's mobile laboratory and office and his staff's camp were at the time not far from a cluster of five small villages that had just been rendered accessible by a very newly built gravel road but otherwise barely touched by the on-going development program, and that Gremliza and the officials of the KWPA regarded as typical, the choice was easy. An irrigation canal also had recently reached them, a first school had been erected, a bath-house and a dispensary were planned for the near future. On Gremliza's rating scale for village public health status [88], which ran from +4 to –4, this cluster occupied the position –2. For five days the Adviser worked in a trailer or circulated in the villages and had brought to him by the experienced DIPA staff their psychiatric waifs and strays, who came almost without exception willingly and at the same time were given the routine medical laboratory tests that the resurvey required. A few supposedly "normal" relatives were also examined and interviewed. In this way the Adviser collected findings from 19 subjects whom he considered to exhibit significant psychiatric or neurological pathology, and the DIPA staff confirmed that these were all such as were known to them in that circumscribed area. In June 1964 the Adviser left Iran.

The KWPA was winding up its work in 1965 preparatory to handing over to the government, which had already set upon the Greater Dez Development Project vastly exceeding the scale of the DIPA. The government itself meanwhile had become interested and applied to the World Health Organization, Regional Office for the Eastern Mediterranean (WHO/EMRO), to bring the Adviser back for the mental health survey in Khuzestan. Gremliza happily was still there and in the field, putting the finishing touches on his work, when the two authors returned to Khuzestan in October, 1965, this time under the auspices of the Iranian Ministry of Health and the Department of Public Health of the Ostan of Khuzestan, though in closest personal association with Gremliza and his faithful crew. Some of these again lent a helping hand, as their chief did untiringly. It was clear that the same five villages in their entirety must be our target. Though registers of the whole DIPA population had been carried from the first counting, a fresh census of these villages was made just before our work began. The Director General of the Ostan Department of Public Health put at our disposal a land-rover with driver, a vaccinator and a public health educator from his staff. As a temporary employee, lent by the KWPA, a former assistant to the works physician during construction of the Pahlavi Dam collaborated with us. These young men, able, eager, accustomed to field work and familiar with the mentality and speech of the peasants, quickly comprehended what we were about, mastered the necessary techniques, took a lively interest and pride in the survey and proved to be both ideal collaborators and good comrades. No less so our driver, a bright, unfailingly good humored, skillful man who had been forced to leave school at an early age. After looking on at testing for a couple of days, his eyes sparkling with interest, he asked to be allowed to try it once himself, did so and soon was testing and interviewing along with and fully as well as the rest. Each of the two authors thus supervised a pair of testers, so that we were able to observe practically every test, take part in interviews, supplement questions, conduct not a few clinical examinations on the spot, make inquiries of relatives and neighbors and the like. For convenience we began our work in the tiny dispensary and bath-house but soon went into the villages, the courtyards and houses, the schools (of which there were now two) and out into the fields, where shepherds for instance could not leave their herds. Working in this way from mid-October to late December, 1965, we learned to know not only every person in the five villages, but also their likes and dislikes, habits, peculiarities and personal relationships and were able gradually to overcome the last barriers of withdrawal and mistrust that had rendered a handful of people reluctant to co-operate. Only three out of our target population of 485 persons finally could not be examined: a man who lay severely ill throughout in the Dezful hospital, an ancient, cachectic, moribund appearing woman who nevertheless managed to survive until the end of the survey and a younger woman who was staying the whole time with relatives in a remote place. A few others, gone for longer visits to villages in the vicinity, we sought out and examined there. A great many of our subjects were seen with or without intent several times over. Each evening the authors checked through the records of the day, determining which persons needed closer scrutiny, and performed this as soon thereafter as practicable. The partly blind evaluations of the Marvdasht and the later Shiraz survey thus were lost completely, so that we can draw no conclusions from the Khuzestan survey as to the relative efficiency of various indicators of pathology. Even the examiners' judgments were influenced unavoidably by their continual interchange of views with the two psychiatrists. If there was thus some methodological loss, it was more than compensated by the abundant opportunity for direct, immediate and often repeated observation and by the close personal contact that grew up over the two and a half months between villagers, testers and psychiatrists. For all these reasons the Khuzestan survey remains for the authors both the happiest and the most thorough, and they place most confidence in its results.

Gremliza had recorded the origins of all the peasants. In our five villages these were so homogeneous that the rare exceptions could be neglected, practically all being Dezfuli. There was a certain amount of inter-village migration, but little exchange of population between the villages and the town, i.e. Dezful, Shush or Shustar. One girl had married into a village, retained her chadour (not worn as a rule by the peasant women) and had some difficulties of assimilation. The DIPA included at its southern tip a handful of Arab villages, but these we excluded from the very beginning, as the Arab speaking minority is on the whole small. Our villages spoke Persian with an admixture of Bakhtiari and Lar dialect. They had neither mosque nor shop.

Trading was done in Dezful. At the Adviser's first visit to the area in 1961 one rutted road was the longitudinal artery of communication in the DIPA. To reach a village one turned off that road and jolted in a jeep or land-rover over barely discernible dirt tracks, crossing on a few sticks meandering ruts in which a trickle of water might carry some moisture to the parched fields. On these peasant women cut or rather tore scrawny stalks of grain with soft iron hooks in sickle form but with no sharp edge. In a few places the KWPA had begun to build schools and bath-houses, but in our five villages there were none yet. In 1964, one year after land reform, there were more of both, but the five villages were still waiting for their share. One school, as mentioned, had been built, but the Literacy Corps teacher had soon finished his term and to the intense disappointment of all had not been replaced. When the Adviser urged on the mother of a bright little girl the necessity of sending her to the school as soon as it should be re-opened he received the unforgettable answer:

ما نمیتنیم بخوانیم یا بنوسیم ، مثل حیوانی هستیم .
شما از ما انسان میخواهید بکنید

("We do not know how to read and write, we are like the kine. You want to make human beings of us.") Water in a properly constructed irrigation canal and a graveled road were present, and in the vicinity, though not in the immediate proximity of the villages, fields were beginning to show a fair yield of grain. Gremliza's trailer-laboratory was dispensing immunizations and first aid and collecting samples of urine, feces and blood, including intravenous blood, which had been impracticable in Marvdasht. A year and a half later when the survey proper was begun the graveled road had become good, and bicycles were beginning to circulate on it, though the peasants had neither cars, telephones nor electricity. A power line carried this from the Dam to Dezful and Ahwaz but had no feeders. The harvest of wheat was underway, water buffaloes thrashed it in endless rotation, and the villagers winnowed it into heaps. A second school had been built, and both were functioning. Also built was the bath-house, to which the villagers came in regular turns, getting first aid and medicines at the same time if needed. Clothes, shoes, bicycles, lamps and cheap "luxury" articles testified to improvement in the economy, which had begun to reorganize itself. The large landowners having been dispossessed, there remained a few small ones, share croppers, hired farm laborers, gardeners and shepherds (comprising altogether for the whole DIPA according to Gremliza 96 % of the active male labor force between 16 and 50 years of age, the remainder being 1 % laborers in Dezful or Haft Tapeh and 3 % permanently disabled) to constitute the adult male population. The adult female population consisted entirely of housewives, nearly all of whom also labored in the fields.

The five villages, with their characteristics as given by Gremliza in 1961 and their population as re-counted in 1965, were:

Table B II 1. Village Populations and Living Conditions

Village	Census 1960 (all ages)	Number of rooms	Persons per room	Condition 1960[a]	Census 1965 (age ≥ 6 y.)
Qaleh Now Askar	136	31	4.4	M	128
Jeibar	112	23	4.8	−1	90
Rob-e-Jeibar	63	15	4.2	M	59
Hadjiabad	108	20	5.4	−2	88
Chiti	114	20	5.7	−2	117
Total	533				482
				All ages	614

[a] Ratings run from + 4 to − 4, M = medium.

Superficially alike as they appeared, there were nevertheless differences, though not such as to render the pooling of results unsuitable. One village, earlier rated –2, had formed an active and apparently successful co-operative and seemed a shade better off than the rest. On the other hand, within its precincts one could usually hear an altercation going on around the person of the headman's shrewish wife, whom we diagnosed as an irritable psychopath with a gastric ulcer, for which she was ever demanding new and more medicine. Another village, also of –2 rating, had established no co-operative, lagged behind the rest, drowsed beside a stagnant pool into which tortoises would disappear from time to time with a mild splash and found itself in such a condition of insanitation that our Iranian staff spontaneously betitled it the deh-e-magaz or village of flies – a designation which we found no reason to contradict. It is difficult to attribute to mere chance the fact that we found a little group of imbecile cretins in this village and in it only.

The smallest and newest had been spawned off, as its name Rob-e-Jeibar (Quarter of Jeibar) indicated, from another, the population of which had outgrown its walls, and stood close to its parent with the newer of the two schools between. In the largest of the five, Qaleh Now Askar, a tendency to fission was already noticeable, there being two fairly distinct "quarters" with separate gates.

The DIPA like much more of Khuzestan was engulfed in 1979 by the Iraq-Iran War. When the first author revisited Iran in 1984 he was unable to travel to Khuzestan and was told in Tehran that the village inhabitants had been removed early in the war to larger centers for easier provisioning and better protection, then evacuated from Khuzestan altogether, mostly to cities of the Persian Gulf. The villages in question no longer existed.

2. Tests

Psychological test procedures and results are similar to those in Marvdasht. The unsatisfactory block design test with cubes was utilized once again in order to see whether its failure represented an isolated or fortuitous result. The composition of the test and survey population is shown in Table B II 2. For the uneven age distribution we have no explanation but note that it follows Gremliza's for the DIPA as a whole. This shows a marked deficit for the 11–15 year old group (409) as compared with the children from 6–10 (912). We can only suspect a catastrophe such as a famine or an epidemic. Inquiries remained fruitless.

The relatively large number of "literate males" in the age classes 9 and 10 raises the literacy rate from Gremliza's 2 % to 16 % but, despite real progress, creates a misleading impression, as it is made up mostly of boys who had attended school for the brief period of the first Literacy Corps teacher's residence, then dropped out for a year and resumed their schooling only recently when a new teacher arrived.

For comparisons by age, sex and literacy cf. Chap. C I 6. As in Marvdasht, the difference between males and females in all adult groups is large and statistically highly significant ($p < 0.001$) throughout. When compared with Marvdasht illiterates by means of the t test the adult male scores from Khuzestan do not anywhere show a significant difference. The female scores do, however, the Khuzestani 15–19 year old

Table B II 2. Distribution of Test Subjects by Age, Sex and Literacy

Age	lm	im	m	lf	if	f	m + f
6	1	9	10	0	4	4	14
7	3	9	12	2	8	10	22
8	7	5	12	1	8	9	21
9	17	5	22	3	11	14	36
10	10	0	10	0	3	3	13
11	5	1	6	0	8	8	14
12	3	4	7	0	9	9	16
13	8	3	11	0	10	10	21
14	4	7	11	0	3	3	14
Sub-total children	58	43	101	6	64	70	171
15–19	3	32	35	0	27	27	62
20–39	6	57	63	0	83	83	146
40–59	3	54	57	0	32	32	89
60 +	1	4	5	0	9	9	14
Sub-total adults	13	147	160	0	151	151	311
Total	71	190	261	6	215	221	482

girls being higher, the 40–59 year old women lower than in Marvdasht (in both cases $p < 0.05$). One might conjecture, though it would be difficult to prove, that the Khuzestani girls had been more stimulated by the atmosphere of change and development in the DIPA while their mothers had dropped behind. This effect does not show among the boys, but education had begun for them in some Marvdasht villages before it did in Khuzestan. The 15–19 year old illiterate youths from Marvdasht might thus on the whole constitute rather a negative selection. As the mean raw score for the entire illiterate adult population is the same in Marvdasht and Khuzestan even to the decimal point for the men and almost so for the women, too much should not be made of minor differences between groups.

3. The Remarkable and the Blind

In Khuzestan, but there only, we have undertaken the experiment of adding a marginal category to that of the frankly ill: a category of probands judged not to constitute "cases" according to our criteria, but to exhibit some mental trait, state, property or peculiarity that made them in any way remarkable in a negative sense among their non-pathological fellows – the so-called "normal". We have designated them, following Binder [36], as the "remarkable within the range of the normal" (*auffällig im Rahmen der Norm*) or, for brevity's sake, simply as the "remarkable", using this word rather in the neutral sense of the German *auffällig* than in the predominantly meliorative sense of the English words by which it is commonly rendered such as "exceptional", "outstanding", "striking" or "remarkable" itself, all which usually carry the connotation of superiority. Even then our use of it is not strictly neutral, but rather carries the opposite connotation to that of the unsatisfactory English equivalents – a connotation of negative deviation causing or apt to cause distress for its bearer. Such might correspond roughly to the Types III and IV of the Stirling County Survey ("probable psychiatric disorder" and "doubtful"), which covered together 63 % of the population, and to the categories of "mild" and "moderate symptom formation" of the Midtown Manhattan Study [186], which were applied to 58 %. We wanted to see whether the use of such a category in Iran would lead to comparably high rates such as those which startled the psychiatric community at their publication and have been the object of no little controversy since. The idea had suggested itself to us early in field work but was not put into execution for reasons given in Chap. A III. Here, where we had more time at our disposal and enjoyed a closer contact with most probands, came the opportunity to do so. A borderline category such as this had not been used in any European studies then know to us but has been employed very recently by Dilling and Weyerer in their investigation of a South German sample, where it is defined as "Degree 1: mild impairment not requiring medical intervention" (*leichte Beeinträchtigung, keine medizinische Intervention notwendig*) and is applied to 22 % of the adult population.

The Iranian members of this category were recruited mostly by personal observation during the census study. Many of them had appeared suspect of psychopathology by one or another indication, but on clinical examination had been rejected as candidates for P_1. Tables B II 3, 4 attempt to classify them empirically. Leaving aside for the moment the reactions to sensory defects, the headings hardly require comment and correspond in the main to attentuated forms of diagnostic

Table B II 3. "Remarkable" Adults

	m	f	m + f
1. Reaction to sensory impairment (mostly blindness) or physical illness	4	8	12
2. Reaction to other untoward circumstances or personal misfortune	1	8	9
3. Recovery after pathological psychic reaction with only minor trace	2	2	4
4. Abnormal personality traits, including under-accomplishment	10	5	15
5. Clinical underintelligence	1	3	4
6. Involution	3	5	8
Total	21	31	52

Table B II 4. "Remarkable" Children

	m	f	m + f
1. Mild environmental damage	2	0	2
2. Abnormal personality traits, including under-accomplishment	5	6	11
3. Clinical underintelligence	6	7	13
Total	13	13	26

pathological groups. In regard to "abnormal personality traits", the majority appeared neurotic and only three raised the question of psychopathy, but the distinction seemed too uncertain to justify a separate classification. "Under-accomplishment" in its pathological form becomes "pseudo-debility", a neurotic disorder, and is therefore listed here in the same category. "Clinical underintelligence" includes some, though not all, cases of borderline or moronic intelligence – those namely which manifested themselves as such by their lack of intellectual adaptability, their clumsiness, dullness, often coupled with a typically moronic appearance, and by their poor test performance – zero or near zero. On the other hand, the group does not include all poor test performers.

Table B II 6 shows again the "remarkable" by age (adults and children) and sex as do Tables B II 3 and 4, but now compares them with the entire Khuzestani collective and with its pathological constituents. It furthermore groups the remarkable with the pathological for comparison with the wholly unremarkable (in the sense here implied) remainder of the collective. (If sometimes hereinafter the epithet "normal" be applied to the remainder, this is solely for the sake of brevity and convenience. It is not meant to imply that the remainder is actually, unequivocally either the one or the other or both.) It first emerges that the numbers and proportions of the remarkable and the pathological are roughly equal, both being close to 15–16 %, together 31.1 %. Thus their sum still falls far short of the quotas of the "abnormal" or "impaired" given in some surveys, in which the "normal" are lucky to achieve the rank of 30 %! Secondly, when the proportions of the remarkable, of the pathological and of both together are compared by age and sex with the "normal", i.e. the unremarkable and unpathological, a female predominance appears in the adult groups that is moreover statistically significant (for the remarkable $X^2 = 4.087$, df = 1, $0.05 > p > 0.02$, for the remarkable and pathological adults together $X^2 = 7.763$, $0.01 > p > 0.001$). Not only does this disappear in the children's groups, but it even seems to be converted into a male predominance: the sex differences here, however, are not statistically significant. Observation of the sex ratios helps to explain this. We give them below in Table B II 5 for our Khuzestani sample along with Gremliza's for the DIPA as a whole for comparison (his age boundaries are slightly, but immaterially different).

Thus the excess of males in childhood, in our sample, causes the share of remarkable and remarkable plus pathological youths in the total population to increase without implying that a greater share of them is truly remarkable or pathological. Lest our sex ratio of 144:100 for boys and girls be regarded merely as a chance fluctuation in a small sample, it should be mentioned that no less imposing imbalances occur in the much larger DIPA sample, though not always in the same age ranges. Gremliza records

Table B II 5. Sex Ratios

	Khuzestan Sample (Bash)		DIPA (Gremliza)	
	Age boundaries	Ratio m : f	Ratio m : f	Age boundaries
Adults	≥ 15	106	103	≥ 16
Children	6–14	144	108	6–15
All ages	≥ 6	118	105	0–

Table B II 6. Unremarkable, Remarkable and Pathological Individuals: Adults and Children; Males, Females and Both Sexes

	Number Adult	Child	Ad. + Ch.	Per 100 of 482 Adult	Child	Ad. + Ch.
Unremarkable and non-pathological						
male	119	72	191	24.6	15.0	39.6
female	89	52	141	18.5	10.7	29.2
both sexes	208	124	332	43.1	25.7	68.8
Remarkable						
male	21	13	34	4.4	2.7	7.1
female	31	13	44	6.4	2.7	9.1
both sexes	52	26	78	10.8	5.4	16.2
Pathological						
male	20	16	36	4.1	3.3	7.4
female	31	5	36	6.4	1.0	7.4
both sexes	51	21	72	10.5	4.3	14.8
Remarkable and pathological						
male	41	29	70	8.5	6.0	14.5
female	62	18	80	12.9	3.7	16.6
both sexes	103	47	150	21.4	9.7	31.1

for his 31–40 year old class a ratio of 142, but in his neighboring classes between 16–20 years a ratio of only 83 and from 21–30 years a ratio of 94.

Among the so-called "remarkable" the blind were so by their very number. Trachoma, by far the leading cause of blindness in southern Iran, has been present for centuries in Khuzestan and has earned for Dezful and Shushtar the sorry epithet of "cities of the blind". With a general prevalence of 34.8 % in the DIPA, equally distributed between the sexes, it is hyperendemic, nor were our five villages favored, for their rates lay between 35–42 %. Early infection is the rule (according to Gremliza 58.4 % of children from 0 to 2 years), and its influence was counterbalanced until recently only by the equally catastrophic infant mortality rate. For us as psychiatrists the blind were as remarkable by the different ways and relative degrees of success they exhibited in dealing with their misfortune. We found opportunity to observe nearly every extreme and gradation between them. Some bore their blindness patiently, uncomplainingly and found cheer in other aspects of life, some with resignation more or less tinged by sorrow or embitterment, while for yet others, both literally and figuratively, light was gone out from their lives. Indifference to such a disability as blindness, one surmises, can occur only at the sublimest or most abysmal levels of spiritual development, in the sage or the idiot, and Khuzestan did not present us, among the blind, with either. There was food for reflection, however, in the wide range of attitudes and adjustments of mostly rather simple people to such an objective catastrophe. We denominate it objective in the sense that it is not inflicted by fellow men as violence, robbery and various forms of social injustice are and that the sufferers on the whole did

Table B II 7. Proportions of Adults and Children in Normal, Borderline and Pathological Groups

	Number Adult	Child.	Ad. + Ch.	Per 100 of group Adult	Child.
Unremarkable and non-pathological	208	124	332	62.6	37.4
Remarkable	52	26	78	66.7	33.3
Pathological	51	21	72	70.8	29.2
Remarkable and pathological	103	47	150	68.7	31.3
Psychiatric survey population (total)	311	171	482	64.5	35.5

Childhood as a whole would seem less liable to psychopathology or its borderline conditions, as the above table suggests. The differences, however, nowhere attain statistical significance, not even when we compare the strictly pathological children (29.2 %) with the unremarkable and non-pathological (37.4 %).

not apprehend society's capacity and responsibility for preventing the common forms of blindness. This can lead to further reflections upon the hardly less various reactions of mankind to social injustice that is apparent as such, so that a study of reactions to blindness may carry more implications than appear upon the surface.

In Table B II 3 our first category of adults remarkable by reason of their "reaction to sensory impairment . . . or physical illness" comprises twelve persons, all blind. One was moderately deaf as well, several others had somatic ailments or impediments. Yet the blind, by implication from above, were more numerous and were to be found also in the flanking groups: in the truly pathological and in those who, except for the very fact of their blindness, were unremarkable. Their total number in Khuzestan was 28 out of 482 = 5.8 %. By comparison we found in Marvdasht only 8 out of 505 = 1.6 %, though Läufer [119], working 1963/64, gives a rate of 4.6 % of "economic blindness" in twelve villages of the Shiraz District, one of which (Qassemabad) was identical with the village we had studied by the census method. In Shiraz the number was strikingly smaller: two out of 928. That all our blind patients were adults corresponds with Läufer's findings in as much as he does not tabulate any cases of economic blindness in the age groups below 25 years. The great majority of cases were due in all likelihood to trachoma, though the other usual causes of blindness such as trauma, cataract, etc. naturally exist. Their share in causing economic blindness is not apparent from Läufer's report, which is restricted to communicable eye diseases. It was not our purpose, nor were we qualified, to investigate them. It is necessary on the other hand to define what we mean by "blind". The term includes here 1. the truly sightless, 2. those whose vision was so reduced in both eyes that they were nearly sightless and by Swiss insurance standards would be compensated to the same extent as the totally blind, being able usually to distinguish only light and dark or at best large, obvious contrasting forms and hindrances, 3. impairment similar to 2 caused by amaurosis of one eye and substantial reduction of vision in the other, 4. partial amaurosis of both eyes resulting in marked impairment of everyday functions, though not so severe as under 1 to 3, and finally 5. half-blindness, i.e. total or nearly total lack of vision in one eye without grave impairment of the other. Though we did not test vision formally, observation of ordinary and particularly of test behavior permitted individuals who were blind in the senses just defined to be identified easily. For this very reason a number of block design and Z Tests could not be completed, or else the results, in cases of less than total blindness, had to be discarded as psychologically invalid. The wholly or almost wholly blind also could not identify the coins of the arithmetic test by sight, but a few did by touch. The half-blind, as a rule, could perform all tests, and one might question whether it was proper to include them here, since blindness of one eye hinders the bearer usually far less than partial amaurosis of both and permits daily life, particularly in a fairly simple village environment, to be carried on much as usual (in a technicized urban environment the consequences, e.g., for driving, may be greater). We have included them nevertheless because in several cases there was an obvious neurosis of insufficiency centered about the blindness of the one eye with corresponding over-valuation of the defect. Not included are the numerous cases of corneal opacities or scars, incipient cataracts, more or less severe but transient conjunctivitis and intermittent glaucoma, i.e., cases of partial and lasting but not grave, or else temporary though possibly grave impediments of vision.

A first glance at Table B II 8 showing the number of half-blind and the blind by sex and by psychic condition reveals a heavy over-representation of the female sex, which has twice as many half-blind and nearly thrice as many blind as the male.

The superficial expectation that all the nine half-blind would be psychically unremarkable or nearly so does not fulfill itself, but for varying reasons. Two men could be regarded as wholly unremarkable except for the fact of their sensory defect. Four women are listed as remarkable in normal range, but one in fact is simply unintelligent, though blind in one eye. Another reacts with a tinge of melancholy to her partial loss of sight. A third is involutional and also mildly melancholic, but it can hardly be said

Table B II 8. The Blind

	Male	Female	Both sexes	
Half-blind				
Unremarkable	2	0	2	
Remarkable in normal range	0	4	4	
Pathological	1	2	3	of whom 2 P_1, 1 P_3
	3	6	9	
Blind				
Unremarkable	0	4	4	
Remarkable in normal range	4	5	9	
Pathological	1	5	6	of whom 4 P_1, 1 P_2, 1 P_3
	5	14	19	
Total blind and half-blind	8	20	28	

whether her melancholia is due to the one or the other condition or to both. The fourth finally, 35 years old and for six years blind in one eye, has abundant family problems including the care of a likewise half-blind arteriosclerotic paternal aunt of her husband's (P_3) to be mentioned below, tends to react demonstratively if not hysterically and probably suffers from an undiagnosed somatic illness beside. It does not seem possible to extricate her reaction to her semi-blindness from the sum of the traits that cause her to be looked upon as remarkable, though not pathological. In the frankly pathological cases such a separation becomes even more difficult and in fact artificial, wherefore we do not even attempt it. One is a neurosis of insufficiency (female P_1) in which the connection is obvious. The second concerns a senile-arteriosclerotic psychosis with cataract of the left eye referred to above, and the third a psychically hardly remarkable posttraumatic epilepsy with infrequent attacks (male, classed as a neurological case of grade P_1). The same trauma, a kick from a mule, obliterated the eye and precipitated the epilepsy. In three at least of the half-blind, accordingly, including one of the four "remarkable" and one of the pathological, there is no evidence and not even much ground for suspicion that the sensory defect has led to any noteworthy distortion of personality.

Turning to those with total or nearly total amaurosis or with severely impaired vision of both eyes we observe that out of 19 such four women, but no men, can be classified as psychically unremarkable. They have achieved an adequate mental adjustment and a pragmatic adaptation to their misfortune – surely no small feat and doubly meaningful in the unsparing environment in which they dwell. Two of the "remarkable" men and three of the women are mildly depressive, two men and one woman exhibit other neurotic traits, and one woman is involutional. We have therefore among the "remarkable in normal range" in Table B II 8 actually one half-blind woman and three blind women whose peculiarity is not traceable to their blindness, while there remain three half-blind and five blind women whose peculiarity presumably is. These are the eight females who appear in Table B II 3 as remarkable for their reaction to sensory impairment whereas four blind or semi-blind women are psychically remarkable for reasons not connected with the defect or at least not directly referable to it. From this the seeming discrepancy between Table B II 8 and B II 3 arises.

Finally, the pathological cases among the blind are composed of three depressive developments or neuroses, all female and P_1, and of three senile-arteriosclerotic disorders: one of degree P_1 in a man and one each of degrees P_2 and P_3 in two women.

Regrouping again in an endeavor to analyze more particularly the effects of blindness on mental health, it emerges that two half-blind men and four blind women out of 28 altogether, about one fifth, are not noticeably affected by their sensory deficiency. Summing the remarkable and the pathological together, we can trace a clear and scarcely doubtful connection between amaurosis on the one hand and psychic peculiarity or psychopathology on the other in 10 of the remaining 22 and a probable one in six more. In yet another six the connection is doubtful or obscure, often inextricably complicated by other factors. As an approximation we can say that roughly are one fifth of the blind in our rural sample seem psychically unaffected, one fifth are problematic, while three fifths develop a perceptible and sometimes pathological reaction to their blindness. These three fifths make up 3.3 % of our total psychiatric survey population.

4. Psychiatry and Neurology

Psychiatric investigation in Khuzestan not only could be executed with more leisure and thoroughness than elsewhere, but it also afforded us the opportunity of observing a certain cohort of cases twice, with an interval of a year and a half between. In April 1964 the Adviser had identified nineteen cases with psychiatric or neuropsychiatric pathology of a significant degree in the five villages on the basis of information furnished by the medical staff of the DIPA, and the staff had confirmed that these were all the cases of such a nature known to them. Returning in October-December 1965 we found eighteen of these cases still present and re-examined them all. One had removed to an impracticable distance. Comparison of our findings in 1964 and 1965 may shed light on the usefulness of informants, here themselves informed, in epidemiology, on consistency in diagnosis and on changes to or loss from cohorts through recovery or improvement, especially when we apply the criterion of degree of severity. Since the survey in 1965 naturally was more comprehensive and more thorough, its disclosure of more cases tells us nothing about possible incidence in the interval.

Table B II 9. Psychiatric Cases Seen in Presurvey 1964

male	ICD-9	female	ICD-9
P_1		P_1	
2 conversion hysteric neuroses	300.1		
1 schizoid psychopathy (probably remitted schizophrenia)	301.2		
1 simple anxious development	309.2		
1 psychogenic headache (not migrainoid)	307.8		
1 moderate oligophrenia	318.0		
6		0	
P_2		P_2	
3 postcommotional states	310.2	1 neurotic pseudodebility with infantile hemiplegia	300.8
1 symptomatic psychosis with anemia	294.8		
1 symptomatic epilepsy of psychomotor type	345.4		
1 mild oligophrenia with congenital hemiparesis	317		
1 moderate oligophrenia from trauma in infancy	318.0		
7		1	
P_3		P_3	
		3 severe oligophrenias	318.1
		1 with infantile hemiplegia	
		1 mongoloid	+ 758.0
		1 cretin	+ 343
		1 senile-arteriosclerotic dementia	290.9
0		4	
Subtotal males: 13		Subtotal females: 5	
Total both sexes: 18			

The eighteen cases from 1964 are listed in Table B II 9 by sexes, degrees of severity and diagnoses. One would expect the severest cases to be as a rule the most noticeable if only by reason of their incapacitating character and therefore to be brought primarily to one's attention by informants not specifically trained in psychiatry, and to a large extent this was in fact what occurred. Four out of five cases classified in 1965 as P_3 (severe) were reported already in 1964. It is easily understandable why the fifth case was not, as it concerned a 51 year old woman with multiple and obvious somatic complaints (blindness from trachoma, deformity and pain from an old untreated fracture of the spinal column, cachexia) who was also quite clearly and prematurely organically demented, though it could not be ascertained with any reasonable reliability whether the dementia was due to the same accident (fall from the roof) that had broken the spinal column 15 years ago or to intercurrent diseases as the patient's replies were extremely sparse, while her son and daughter-in-law seemed to know little about her past (the same difficulty was to meet us over and over, as a great many of the simpler people in Iran, especially outside the towns, pay, so far as we have been able to observe, little regard to time and to the succession of inner or outer events. Happenings may be recalled vividly, but with small awareness of their temporal remove or order). Unable to stretch her body because of back pain, she huddled bent double throughout the nights and implored Allah and the people about her to let her die. Because of her resistance and distress we could not even perform a physical examination, but noted that the peripheral blood vessels were hard and sinuous as they might be in a woman of seventy or more. The patient could scarcely move her legs, but shuffled cowering along the ground. Her total infirmity made a classification of P_3 indisputable, though the amount of psychiatric disorder alone might not have justified it.

The reader will have noted that all the P_3 cases in Khuzestan in 1964 proved to be female, although in the final survey results the sexes exactly balanced each other, and that they included still another case of organic dementia. The picture changes abruptly to one of male dominance when we move to the regions of medium and slight severity. In P_2 we find seven males to only one female. Five of the seven involve trauma, to which males are more exposed, and which may explain in great part the much larger proportion of male cases. In nearly all the P_2 and P_3 cases there was an organic component, either causal or accessory (the single P_2 female showed a neurotic pseudodebility probably as a reaction to her infantile hemiplegia: a neurosis of insufficiency in the sense already described).

The mild cases (P_1) that were brought to our attention in 1964 were exclusively male – an interesting observation in itself since in 1965 we came upon no less females of like degree. The more value that is placed upon an object, the quicker as a rule will a defect in it be noted, and there is no question but that in rural Iran the man counts for more than does the woman. Objectively also in an agricultural economy where most labor is performed by manual strength, her well-being depends much on his. There might seem to be occasion for surprise in that almost as many P_1 cases were reported as P_2. The cases, however, were mostly such as would attract attention to themselves, this applying especially to the two hysterias, and they would nearly all seem graver to the non-psychiatric observer than they actually were. In one way or another they were functioning socially well enough that a classification of P_2 did not seem to us justified. The oligophrenia, for instance, we took to be more than slight and classified it by the ICD as 318, but the docile youth managed not badly in an undemanding, illiterate environment and in all likelihood would be able to earn his living in the future as a farm hand or laborer without unusual difficulty.

Two cases in the P_1 group demand special attention as they were the only ones in which a change in diagnosis or classification by severity was taken earnestly into consideration. The first concerned a 54 year old married share-cropper. He had five living children but had lost three, each within a few months of their birth. Fifteen years ago after having felled a tree he felt tired in the evening and awoke in the morning with a paralysis of the left side of the body that lasted for some twenty days and disappeared when he went on a pilgrimage to the Shrine of Imam Reza in Meshed. Previous to that he affirmed that he had no particular cares, worries or distresses, but later came fits of sadness that he dispelled with the help of purchased written charms, vague fears for which he could give no reason, and difficulties with his brother over money matters. A short time before he was seen in 1964 he had been to a physician complaining of stomach pains and a "wandering heart" and fearing that he would die, but had recovered after an injection of coffein. He was then feeling well, was talkative and superficially cheerful, showed no neurological abnormalities, no atrophy and no indication of former paralysis or paresis. In view of the protracted anamnesis the Adviser was inclined in 1964 to regard him as an hysterical personality or hysterical psychopath, but finding him in 1965 still well, with no history of relapse during the past year and a half and presenting the same personality picture as before, we diagnosed an hysterical neurosis, the manifestations of which had abated rather than increased. As he was supporting his family without any considerable impairment he was assigned to P_1.

A 44 year old married farmer, who was said by his step-daughter to quarrel a good deal with his wife, had no history of illnesses in childhood and youth. Fifteen years ago, by his own account in good physical and mental health, he several times heard a voice call his name loudly and clearly in the house, in the village street and in the fields, told others about his experience and finally referred it to his guardian angel. Thus far the account is almost commonplace, as not a few peasants have such an experience of hearing their names called – usually however when alone in the fields or the desert or else at night, seldom more than once and rarely with such distinctness as our patient described. Though the voices did not return, the man fell upon evil days, had trouble with his neighbors, moved temporarily to another village, was convinced that everyone was trying to harm him, though unable to say why or how. He recovered, but for about two years prior to 1964 had been feeling unhappy at times without a particular reason. At interview he appeared somewhat melancholy, but reacted with adequate intellectual and emotional adaptation, spoke clearly and in an orderly fashion and showed no signs of mental dissociation. Neighbors and the DIPA staff testified that he had been peculiar, distrustful, morose and withdrawn over several years, but was better now although he tended to preserve a distance from his fellows. In 1965 the picture had not changed. The Z Test showed signs of anxiety, self-uncertainty and a struggle to maintain external adjustment in a rather sensitive personality. It was noticeable that the initial response to Card I was "dive" (itself not too uncommon) and that the initial response to the chromatic Card II made inadequate use of a tiny white detail, interpreting it quite exceptionally as "white soup", i.e. white as a pure color response confined to a very small area. To the same card he gave three good chromatic form-color responses but terminated the test with a color-form answer to the medial red of

Card III. Human content was wholly lacking except for the anthropomorphic "spirit", and the form level was low, but three popular responses showed that he was not out of touch with conventional modes of apprehension. Direct findings thus were slight, but taken together with the evidence of the neighbors, the demeanor of the patient and the ZTest indicated enough abnormality to ascribe him to P_1 as a schizoid personality or, in the long view, a psychopath. From the history it seemed very probable that he had suffered at least one episode of paranoid-hallucinatory schizophrenia which had happily remitted to such a point that the diagnosis no longer could be sustained. We therefore placed him finally as a schizoid psychopath, but by some practices he might have been counted as a schizophrenic. The question is not indifferent as the total number of schizophrenias in our material is small and the inclusion or omission of a case or two influences prevalence rates. We shall return to this later when discussing this topic.

The survey of 1965 disclosed 72 cases, in which men and women participated in exactly equal numbers. In the population there were 261 men and 221 women, i.e. 54 % males and 46 % females or a sex ratio of 118:110. Thus a larger share of the females were classified as pathological (16.3 % as against 13.9 % for the males), but the apparent difference fell far short of statistical significance (X^2). This result is quite different from that in Marvdasht, where women outnumbered men almost two to one. We shall return to this question later, when larger figures are available. From the 72 one third had been identified with the help of informants in the presurvey. The proportion is again quite different from that in Marvdasht, where informants accounted for only ten per cent of the identifications, but the circumstances were also very different, our informants being better trained and professionally experienced. Nevertheless it must be noted that even with such expert and semi-expert help from workers long familiar with the field, their identification attained merely a third of that from the survey, was deficient not only at the level of low, but also at that of medium severity, and even at that of high severity missed one case from five.

The diagnostic distribution appears in Table B II 10–13. No manifest schizophrenia was encountered (but see above). The single affective psychosis was represented by a thirty year old married woman, less profoundly than persistently dysphoric and depressed without having, as she herself and her family assured us, any reason for it, though the death of her parents and a brother several years in the past seemed to have had some precipitating effect. Vaguely and unconvincingly she spoke of a "paralysis" after the birth of a child three years before, which had passed away. The present dysphoria had begun in Ramazan eleven months ago. She had carried on her work but felt constantly ill, voiced a number of depressive-hypochondric complaints, had no clear diurnal rhythm, but a noticeable habitus that did not alter during the weeks we observed and repeatedly talked to her, a resigned and unhappy tone and remarked time and again that she was glad life passed quickly. Physical and laboratory findings were unremarkable. Attitude and behavior were in no way hysterically demonstrative. Observation and interrogation of husband and children revealed no hint of conflict. Intellectual performance was modest as was the form level of the Z Test, but it was noticeable that here she avoided the bright colors, gave a single form-color response to the brown spots of Card II, but a movement response to Card I, the rest being simple animal answers. Though the symptoms were not pronounced, their persistence, consistency and duration tended to confirm us in the diagnosis.

Table B II 10. Psychiatric Diagnoses of Mild Cases (P_1)

Diagnoses	Number of cases					p. 100 of 72 cases					p. 1000 of 482 subjects				
	m	f	m + f			m	f	m + f			m	f	m + f		
I. Funct. psychoses		1	1				1.4	1.4				2.1	2.1		
1. Schizophrenia															
2. Affect. psychoses		1		1			1.4		1.4			2.1		2.1	
II. Acute symptomatic psychoses			0					0					0		
III. Subchronic & chron. sympt. psychoses & residual states	1	1	2			1.4	1.4	2.8			2.1	2.1	4.1		
1. Epilepsy															
a. cryptogen.															
b. symptomatic															
2. Sen. & arterioscl.	1			1		1.4			1.4		2.1			2.1	
3. post-infectious															
4. post-traumatic															
5. endocrine		1		1			1.4		1.4			2.1		2.1	
6. addiction															
7. other															
IV. Reactive disorders	18	12	30			25.0	16.7	41.7			37.3	24.9	62.2		
1. Simple path. dev.	6	7		13		8.3	9.7		18.0		12.4	14.5		27.0	
a. anxious	2	1			3	2.8	1.4			4.2	4.1	2.1			6.2
b. depressive	3	4			7	4.2	5.5			9.7	6.2	8.3			14.5
c. irritable		1			1		1.4			1.4		2.1			2.1
d. neurasthenic															
e. other	1	1			2	1.4	1.4			2.8	2.1	2.1			4.1
2. Neuroses	11	4		15		15.3	5.5		20.8		22.8	8.3		31.1	
a. anxious	5	1			6	6.9	1.4			8.3	10.4	2.1			12.4
b. phobic	1				1	1.4				1.4	2.1				2.1
c. depressive	2	1			3	2.8	1.4			4.2	4.1	2.1			6.2
d. hysterical	2				2	2.8				2.8	4.1				4.1
e. hypochondriac															
f. neurasthenic		1			1		1.4			1.4		2.1			2.1
g. self-insuff.		1			1		1.4			1.4		2.1			2.1
h. negativistic	1				1	1.4				1.4	2.1				2.1
i. other & polym.															
3. Psychosomatic	1	1		2		1.4	1.4		2.8		2.1	2.1		4.1	
a. headache					2					2.8					4.1
١. migrainoid		1					1.4					2.1			
ب. other	1					1.4					2.1				
b. gastro-intest.															
c. asthmatic															
d. other & polym.															
V. Constitutional disord.	3	1	4			4.2	1.4	5.6			6.2	2.1	8.3		
1. Clin. oligophrenia	2	1		3		2.8	1.4		4.2		4.1	2.1		6.2	
a. cryptogenetic	2	1			3	2.8	1.4			4.2	4.1	2.1			6.2
b. genetic															
2. Psychopathy	1			1		1.4			1.4		2.1			2.1	
a. irritable															
b. anti-social															
c. schizoid	1				1	1.4				1.4	2.1				2.1
d. other															
Total	22	15	37	37		30.5	20.8	51.4	51.4		45.6	31.1	76.8	76.8	

Table B II 11. Psychiatric Diagnoses of Medium Cases (P_2)

Diagnoses	Number of cases					p. 100 of 72 cases					p. 1000 of 482 subjects				
	m	f	m+f			m	f	m+f			m	f	m+f		
I. Funct. psychoses			0					0					0		
1. Schizophrenia															
2. Affect. psychoses															
II. Acute symptomatic psychoses			0					0					0		
III. Subchronic & chron. sympt. psychoses & residual states	6	5	11			8.3	6.9	15.3			12.4	10.4	22.8		
1. Epilepsy				1					1.4					2.1	
a. cryptogen.															
b. symptomatic	1				1	1.4				1.4	2.1				2.1
2. Sen. & arterioscl.		3		3			4.2		4.2			6.2		6.2	
3. post-infectious	1	1		2		1.4	1.4		2.8		2.1	2.1		4.1	
4. post-traumatic	3			3		4.2			4.2		6.2			6.2	
5. endocrine															
6. addiction															
7. other	1	1		2		1.4	1.4		2.8		2.1	2.1		4.1	
IV. Reactive disorders	3	9	12			4.2	12.5	16.7			6.2	18.7	24.9		
1. Simple path. dev.				0					0					0	
a. anxious															
b. depressive															
c. irritable															
d. neurasthenic															
e. other															
2. Neuroses	2	4		6		2.8	5.5		8.3		4.1	8.3		12.4	
a. anxious															
b. phobic		1			1		1.4			1.4		2.1			2.1
c. depressive															
d. hysterical															
e. hypochondriac		1			1		1.4			1.4		2.1			2.1
f. neurasthenic															
g. self-insuff.		1			1		1.4			1.4		2.1			2.1
h. negativistic	1				1	1.4				1.4	2.1				2.1
i. other & polym.	1	1			2	1.4	1.4			2.8	2.1	2.1			4.1
3. Psychosomatic	1	5		6		1.4	6.9		8.3		2.1	10.4		12.4	
a. headache					5					6.9					10.4
α. migrainoid		4					5.5					8.3			
β. other	1					1.4					2.1				
b. gastro-intest.															
c. asthmatic		1			1		1.4			1.4		2.1			2.1
d. other & polym.															
V. Constitutional disord.	5	2	7			6.9	2.8	9.7			10.4	4.1	14.5		
1. Clin. oligophrenia	3	1		4		4.2	1.4		5.5		6.2	2.1		8.3	
a. cryptogenetic	3	1			4	4.2	1.4			5.5	6.2	2.1			8.3
b. genetic															
2. Psychopathy	2	1		3		2.8	1.4		4.2		4.1	2.1		6.2	
a. irritable	1	1			2	1.4	1.4			2.8	2.1	2.1			4.1
b. anti-social															
c. schizoid															
d. other	1				1	1.4				1.4	2.1				2.1
Total	14	16	30	30		19.4	22.2	41.7	41.7		29.0	33.2	62.2	62.2	

Table B II 12. Psychiatric Diagnoses of Severe Cases (P_3)

Diagnoses	Number of cases					p. 100 of 72 cases					p. 1000 of 482 subjects				
	m	f	m + f			m	f	m + f			m	f	m + f		
I. Funct. psychoses			0					0					0		
1. Schizophrenia															
2. Affect. psychoses															
II. Acute symptomatic psychoses			0					0					0		
III. Subchronic & chron. sympt. psychoses & residual states		2	2				2.8	2.8				4.1	4.1		
1. Epilepsy															
a. cryptogen.															
b. symptomatic															
2. Sen. & arterioscl.		1		1			1.4		1.4			2.1		2.1	
3. post-infectious															
4. post-traumatic															
5. endocrine															
6. addiction															
7. other		1		1			1.4		1.4			2.1		2.1	
IV. Reactive disorders			0					0					0		
1. Simple path. dev.															
a. anxious															
b. depressive															
c. irritable															
d. neurasthenic															
e. other															
2. Neuroses															
a. anxious															
b. phobic															
c. depressive															
d. hysterical															
e. hypochondriac															
f. neurasthenic															
g. self-insuff.															
h. negativistic															
i. other & polym.															
3. Psychosomatic															
a. headache															
١. migrainoid															
ب. other															
b. gastro-intest.															
c. asthmatic															
d. other & polym.															
V. Constitutional disord.		3	3				4.2	4.2				6.2	6.2		
1. Clin. oligophrenia		3		3			4.2		4.2			6.2		6.2	
a. cryptogenetic		2			2		2.8			2.8		4.1			4.1
b. genetic		1			1		1.4			1.4		2.1			2.1
2. Psychopathy				0					0					0	
a. irritable															
b. anti-social															
c. schizoid															
d. other															
Total	0	5	5	5		0	6.9	6.9	6.9		0	10.4	10.4	10.4	

Table B II 13. Psychiatric Diagnoses of All Cases

Diagnoses	Number of cases					p. 100 of 72 cases					p. 1000 of 482 subjects				
	m	f	m + f			m	f	m + f			m	f	m + f		
I. Funct. psychoses		1	1				1.4	1.4				2.1	2.1		
1. Schizophrenia															
2. Affect. psychoses		1		1			1.4		1.4			2.1		2.1	
II. Acute symptomatic psychoses			0					0					0		
III. Subchronic & chron. sympt. psychoses & residual states	7	8	15			9.7	11.1	20.8			14.5	16.6	31.1		
1. Epilepsy				1					1.4					2.1	
a. cryptogen.															
b. symptomatic	1				1	1.4				1.4	2.1				2.1
2. Sen. & arterioscl.	1	4		5		1.4	5.5		6.9		2.1	8.3		10.4	
3. post-infectious	1	1		2		1.4	1.4		2.8		2.1	2.1		4.1	
4. post-traumatic	3			3		4.2			4.2		6.2			6.2	
5. endocrine		1		1			1.4		1.4			2.1		2.1	
6. addiction															
7. other	1	2		3		1.4	2.8		4.2		2.1	4.1		6.2	
IV. Reactive disorders	21	21	42			29.2	29.2	58.3			43.6	43.6	87.1		
1. Simple path. dev.	6	7		13		8.3	9.7		18.0		12.4	14.5		27.0	
a. anxious	2	1			3	2.8	1.4			4.2	4.1	2.1			6.2
b. depressive	3	4			7	4.2	5.5			9.7	6.2	8.3			14.5
c. irritable		1			1		1.4			1.4		2.1			2.1
d. neurasthenic															
e. other	1	1			2	1.4	1.4			2.8	2.1	2.1			4.1
2. Neuroses	13	8		21		18.0	11.1		29.2		27.0	16.6		43.6	
a. anxious	5	1			6	6.9	1.4			8.3	10.4	2.1			12.4
b. phobic	1	1			2	1.4	1.4			2.8	2.1	2.1			4.1
c. depressive	2	1			3	2.8	1.4			4.2	4.1	2.1			6.2
d. hysterical	2				2	2.8				2.8	4.1				4.1
e. hypochondriac		1			1		1.4			1.4		2.1			2.1
f. neurasthenic		1			1		1.4			1.4		2.1			2.1
g. self-insuff.		2			2		2.8			2.8		4.1			4.1
h. negativistic	2				2	2.8				2.8	4.1				4.1
i. other & polym.	1	1			2	1.4	1.4			2.8	2.1	2.1			4.1
3. Psychosomatic	2	6		8		2.8	8.3		11.1		4.1	12.4		16.6	
a. headache					7					9.7					14.5
١. migrainoid		5					6.9					10.4			
ب. other	2					2.8					4.1				4.1
b. gastro-intest.															
c. asthmatic		1			1		1.4			1.4		2.1			2.1
d. other & polym.															
V. Constitutional disord.	8	6	14			11.1	8.3	19.4			16.6	12.4	29.0		
1. Clin. oligophrenia	5	5		10		6.9	6.9		13.9		10.4	10.4		20.7	
a. cryptogenetic	5	4			9	6.9	5.5			12.5	10.4	8.3			18.7
b. genetic		1			1		1.4			1.4		2.1			2.1
2. Psychopathy	3	1		4		4.2	1.4		5.5		6.2	2.1		8.3	
a. irritable	1	1			2	1.4	1.4			2.8	2.1	2.1			4.1
b. anti-social															
c. schizoid	1				1	1.4				1.4	2.1				2.1
d. other	1				1	1.4				1.4	2.1				2.1
Total	36	36	72	72		50	50	100	100		74.7	74.7	149.4	149.4	

Acute symptomatic psychoses did not occur during the period of observation. A single case of epilepsy showed relevant psychiatric disturbance, was of psychomotor type and probably post-infectious. Cases of organic dementia without ascertainable exogenous cause, such as, to our mild surprise, we had not encountered in Marvdasht, made their appearance in Khuzestan: eight in all, of which six were female. Five, including one male, presented fairly typical pictures of simple dementia, probably compounded with arteriosclerosis, and were classed accordingly under III.2. As their mean age was 61 and the eldest 65 (if the statements can be trusted), it might be more appropriate to speak of pre-senile than of senile dementia. Among the three "other" (III.7) there was a 50 year old man with an anemia (Hb 40 %) of unknown origin, for which he was receiving liver extract and vitamin C. He had suffered repeated syncope. Psychiatrically he was bradyphrenic, depressed, perseverated dully in his responses, ever and again lost the thread, but managed an IQ of 94 on arithmetic test A when given time. Typically, he could do nothing at all with the block design. His responses to the Z Test were few and undifferentiated. He was diagnosed as a chronic symptomatic psychosis presumably due to anemia of unknown cause, P_2. The second was a woman of 51 years with typical incipient organic character alteration, but hardly demented: P_2, while the third was also a woman of only 51 years, but already far gone in organic cachexia, suffering from an unset fracture of the vertebral column and from trachoma: P_3. The single endocrine case was that of a hypothyreotic female with marked neurotic overlay.

The reactive disorders will be discussed in a more general context, as they did not exhibit any features peculiar to this site.

Like organic dementias, clinical oligophrenias proved to be more frequent in Khuzestan (10 cases) than in Marvdasht (6 cases, the populations being of nearly equal size), though this apparently had no influence on the mean arithmetic test performance (see above and Part C, Chap. I 6). We found a mongoloid case with struma and two cretins without mongoloid features, but both with extensive struma diffusa, among them. Their siblings were unremarkable. One was said to have had a quadriplegia at the age of six years and to have been treated successfully for this by being tied into a jackal's skin! An earlier cerebral affection therefore might have caused the evident mental retardation, but the pendulous cheeks, thick lips and deep bridge of the nose beside the struma itself spoke for the endocrine origin.

Of the two irritable psychopaths the village shrew has been mentioned. Her male counterpart was a typical "sociopath", a feckless ne'er-do-well who could stick to no job and carry no task to its conclusion. Both had long histories reaching back to childhood but, so far as we could discover, no somatic or reactive antecedents that would have justified a diagnosis of pseudo-psychopathy or of neurosis. The schizoid case also has been described. The "other" was that of a fifty year old man who initially claimed to be seventy without looking it. He referred numberless complaints and fears about his objectively unimpaired physical health to a snake bite many years ago and pleaded incapacity to work because of anesthesia in the bitten foot, but on neurological examination revealed no trace of sensory deficiency. Any kind of injection tended to relieve his ills for a few days. His persistent hypochondria had impaired him socially and economically to such an extent that we had to class him as P_2. The Z Test accorded well with the diagnosis and was not of a hysterical character, as his complaints also were too fleeting and superficial, too overlaid by general anxiety about his health to deserve the term "hysteric" in the sense of conversion symptoms.

Table B II 14. Psychiatric Cases (67) and Neuropsychiatric Cases (5) by Degrees of Severity

Degree	Number of cases	Per 1000 of 72 cases	Per 1000 of 482 Survey Pop.
P_1 mild	37	51	77
P_2 medium	30	42	61
P_3 severe	5	7	11
Total	72	100	149
$P_2 + P_3$	35	49	72

As all villages were subjected to census studies by identical techniques, and as the number of inhabitants in each was small, favoring fortuitous differences, we do not give separate prevalence figures as for the three Marvdasht villages. The total prevalence rate in the Khuzestani cluster of five ranged from 12 to 18 per 100. It may or may not be due to chance that the lowest rate was found in the town that had a thriving farmers' co-operative and a slightly better socio-economic situation. Table B II 14 shows the distribution by grades of severity for psychiatric and neuropsychiatric cases together.

Their number is now large enough that a comparison of diagnostic distributions by degrees of severity becomes meaningful. It is provided byTables B II 10–12.The single functional psychosis is encountered, somewhat contrary to expectation, under P_1, illustrating again that "psychosis" cannot be equated with "grave" or "severe". It constitutes a different kind, not a degree of psychiatric disorder. The symptomatic psychoses and residual states are sparingly represented in P_1, are mostly to be found in P_2 and contribute, as would be expected, a proportionally large share to the small absolute number of P_3. In Khuzestan no reactive disorders fall into this disabling category, about 12 % of all psychiatric cases into P_2 and 51 % into P_1 (percentages here and hereafter are referred to the total of 72 cases of all kinds and degrees unless otherwise stated). Within the mild group men and women share about equally in the simple pathological developments. Among the neuroses we find 11 males (5 with anxiety neuroses) to only 4 females. The two psychosomatic cases are almost too few for comment, but even this pair exhibits the typical allocation of migrainoid headache to the woman and of non-migrainoid to the man. If we now compare the reactive disorders of medium degree (P_2, Table B II 11), we note that the simple pathological developments are missing, that the females outnumber the males in regard to neurosis by two to one and in regard to the more plentiful psychosomatic disorders by a much greater proportion, due again mainly to migrainoid headaches. Under the constitutional disorders the mild and severe degrees are about equally represented with 4–5 %, the medium degree with double the rate, i.e. about 10 %. In this last figure the oligophrenias and psychopathies participate about equally, while among both the lighter and graver cases the psychopathies are few or absent. The numbers are too small to be conclusive.

Only six purely neurological cases were found here, including two cryptogenetic epilepsies and one posttraumatic, all without episodic psychiatric disturbances, alteration of character or organic psychosyndrome of more than trifling degree (a fourth case of epilepsy characterized by fugues, psychomotor attacks and occasional auditory hallucinations, but with no major fits since the illness began after the patient was kicked by a mule and lost the sight of one eye two years before, was classified as psychiatric). The other three were the single case of neural muscular atrophy encountered in all our work in Iran – a man who bore his ill fate with almost cheerful fortitude, a postcommotional syndrome confined to neuro-vegetative complaints, and a hemiparesis of unclear origin that had set in only half a year ago after the 41 year old man had slept a night in the field and awoken with pains in the head and back that had not ceased since. Besides this his subjective complaints were weakness in the entire left side, vertigo, a heavy tongue and some difficulty in speaking, which later could be confirmed objectively. There was slight anisocoria (left pupil and lid aperture somewhat wider than the right), but the pupillary reactions were normal. The left temple, supraorbital point, neck and shoulder were sensitive to pressure. All tendinal reflexes of the left side were greatly heightened as compared to the right, and sensibility for touch was reduced in the left hand and arm, but not in the lower extremity. In the finger-nose test there was some deviation and a light spastic tremor, but in the position experiment the hands did not sink on either side, and the grip appeared to be equal. The reflexogenic zone for the patellar tendon reflex was extended upward on both sides, not only on the left. The Babinsky group was negative. Tentatively and in the absence of any clinical resources for further neurological examination we considered the diagnosis of a multiple sclerosis, though, aware that this disease is rare in Iran, we would by no means advance this diagnosis as definite.

Because of their small numbers the neurological and neuropsychiatric cases are listed together in Table B II 15 (neurological diagnoses, with psychiatric complications, which also have their place in Table B II 13, mentioned in parentheses) and in Table B II 16 (distribution by degrees of severity). Since both categories are combined in Table B II 16 and are referred to the psychiatric survey pupulation only (children under 6 years excluded, whereas in Marvdasht they were included in the calculation of the neurological prevalence rate) the prevalence emerges almost twice as high as in Marvdasht. If we correct for this by omitting the one neurological patient younger than six years in Marvdasht and taking the psychiatric survey population of 500 there too as our basis for reference, we obtain a neurological prevalence rate of 10:500 = 20 per thousand, or very near to what we have found in Khuzestan (23 per thousand).

Table B II 15. Neurological Diagnoses

Diagnosis	m	f	m+f
Infantile or juvenile hemiplegia or hemiparesis (of which 2 neurotic, 1 moron, 1 imbecile)	2	2	4
Traumatic hemiparesis (in moron)	1		1
Epilepsy (with little or no mental alteration)			3
a. cryptogenic	2		
b. symptomatic	1		
Sclerosis multiplex (probable)	1		1
Neural muscular atrophy	1		1
Postcommotional syndrome (only vegetative, without significant psychiatric symptoms)	1	–	1
Total	9	2	11

Table B II 16. Neurological and Neuropsychiatric Cases by Degrees of Severity

Degree	Number of Cases	Per 1000 of 482 Survey Pop.
P_1 mild	3	6.3
P_2 medium	6	12.4
P_3 severe	2	4.1
Total	11	22.8

III. The Qashqai

1. The Nomadic Qashqai

The total tribal population of Iran was estimated in 1963 at between three and four million, that of the Fars of Ostan at something less than half a million. Even the best figures from the later census can only be rough, partly because of the almost insuperable difficulties of counting a so widely dispersed and mobile population, partly because the very definition of "tribal" or "nomad" presents great problems when extensively applied, even though members of a tribe will unhesitatingly declare whether a given person belongs to it or does not. The tribal structure is closely knit. Barth's [14] careful description of the relatively small Basseri tribe (ca. 20000 people) holds in its major features for the much larger Qashqai tribe also, which constitutes about half the tribal population of Fars and which Barth calls a confederacy rather than a single tribe. Unlike the Basseri and the Khamseh Confederacy to which they belong, the Qashqai are Turkish, not Persian-speaking. Oberling has written their history.

Some tribal people are nomadic, some not, and there is a good deal of spontaneous alternation between the two modes of life. The word "nomad" is likely to conjure up false ideas when applied to the non-sedentary tribal members. Their pattern of life and movement is altogether different from that of the nomads of, e.g., the Arabian deserts and is circumscribed within the relatively close limits of long strips of territory which may extend for several hundred kilometers from north to south but only some twenty to fifty from east to west. Within these the several tribes or sub-tribes move free of interference with each other on mostly well defined though unmarked paths with rights of transit and freeway hardly less precise than those of an English countryside. They are migratory rather than nomadic and follow with their flocks of sheep and goats the seasonal pastures from the plains of the south in winter to the lusher slopes of the Zagros in summer and back in annual cycle, the duration of stay at any camp site being determined first of all by the grazing conditions, then by weather, water and the like. The cycle is familiar in Alpine countries, where the horizontal distances are less and the harsher winter is passed under firm shelter. The Persian tribesmen are not raisers of cattle like the Alpine peasants. Sheeps and goats are their livelihood, donkeys and sometimes camels their transportation, the jackals of the stony desert and an occasional leopard (besides man) their threat, fierce dogs their protection. Their existence depends on their flocks. For supplementary income some weave the well-known carpets and blankets, raise a little wheat, vegetables or poultry, but these more for their own consumption.

Reza Shah Pahlavi I had attempted with some success forcefully to settle the tribes, but after his abdication the majority returned to their migratory way of life. Over years they were left more or less alone but regarded by the central government with suspicion, their loyalties being to their own chiefs and leaders. Pressure upon them to settle again had begun to rise in the early sixties, was increased by the land reform of 1963 and led to revolts against the government in southern Fars that were put down *manu militari*. This action had been completed by the time our survey began, leaving thousands none the less on their traditional migratory paths and ways of life. The year before had brought a disastrous drought, as already mentioned in connection with the Marvdasht Survey; over half the animals had died of starvation, the economy was precarious and the population depressed. It was a matter of wonder that a tribal survey could be carried out, however incompletely, at all.

That it could be was due largely to the good offices of the Tribal Education Division of the Ministry of Education. This prepared teachers, who were themselves tribesmen, after their general education in a one year pedagogical course at a special seminary in Shiraz, after which they returned to their own tribes and, moving with them, held classes wherever the tribe went. The white school tent topped by the tiny green, white and red flag stood out among the black ones, and the children trooped eagerly to it. At the urging of this Division the Khan in question consented to a public and mental health survey of his sub-tribe along the same lines as in Marvdasht when it would be encamped at a reasonably accessible site in the vicinity of Shiraz in the autumn of 1963. With a tremendous organizational effort on the Iranian side, complicated by the fact that the University had begun its term and therefore a number of participants could get away only with difficulty, almost the whole staff of the Marvdasht Survey was mobilized once more. These circumstances limited strictly the time available for the survey, as did the tribe's movement, dictated by the scrawny pasture, on the other. It camped in the stony dry river beds of Syach and Darengoon southwest of Shiraz. Even reaching the encampment was more consuming of time than it had been in Marvdasht and required first nearly an hour's drive over the newly paved Shiraz-Kazerun road, then another half hour or more as the jeeps threaded their way between boulders and jolted over rocks up to the camp or rather the camps. A main group had set up their tents around the Khan's big one and the school tents (there were two of these), but there were other clusters of tents scattered about at considerable distances and reachable only by foot, as Map B III shows. After census taking the survey was conducted on three consecutive days in October, 1963, after which the staff had to be disbanded and the tribe moved on.

This tribal group had been visited before by malaria teams and their tents sprayed (of 144 thick smears taken, none were positive for malaria). The Khan welcomed us personally, recommended us to his people and came forward himself with his family as the first to be examined. Naturally the principal group of tents about his own and the school tents, to which children came trudging from all the rest, were both the headquarters of the survey and the main center of attention, an especial endeavor being made to examine all the school children as far as possible. This latter succeeded to a high degree. The sub-tribe counted 499 souls. Though these were not more than in Marvdasht, it became apparent in the first day's work that, due to the dispersion and occasional reluctance of the justly wary subjects, it would not be possible in the remaining two to examine them all either physically or mentally. Neither was strict randomization by tent numbers practicable in that time as it would have necessitated hour long expeditions on foot to outlying tent clusters with the not inconsiderable likelihood of finding no one there except a grandmother and a couple of small children,

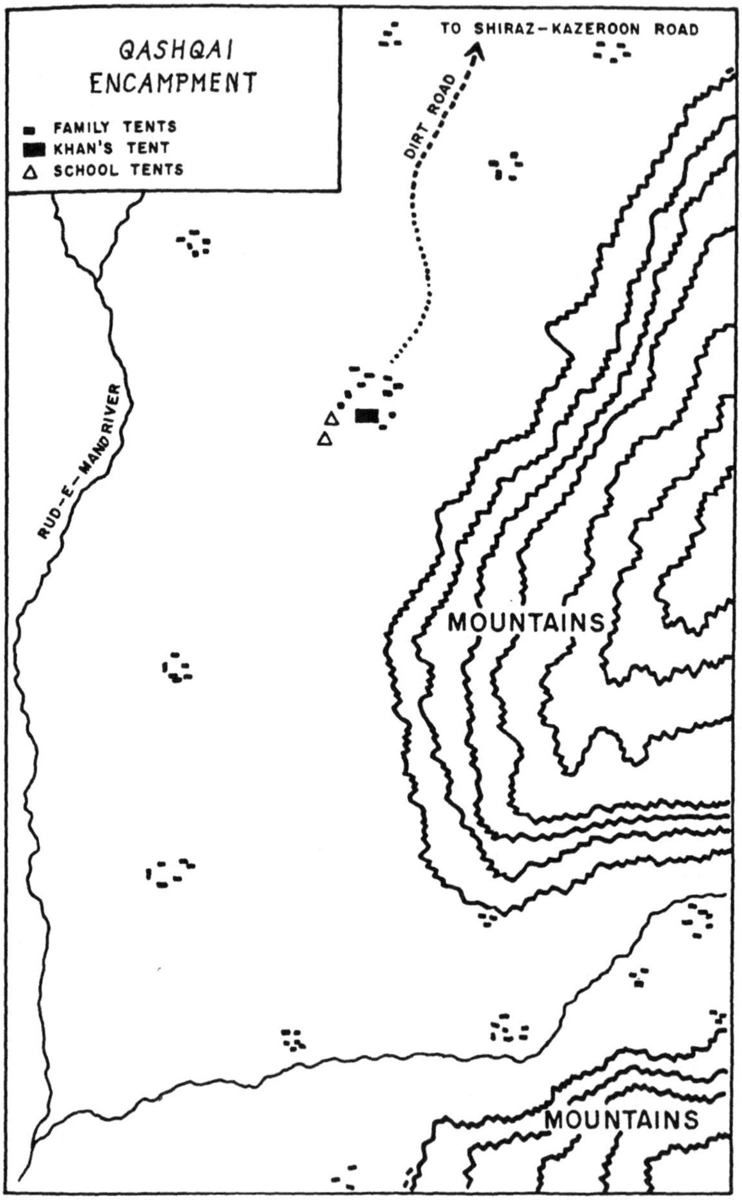

Map B III. Qashqai Encampment

the rest of the family being out grazing the goats and sheep beyond calling distance. The Adviser did take several such walks when returning examiners reported suspicions of a case but was not rewarded by coming thus upon a positive one. Our subjects therefore were nearly all the dwellers in the central tent cluster, all or nearly all the school children, adults and children from the outlying tents drawn to the central group by chance, curiosity or persuasion and such others from these peripheral tents as we could reach. When an intended subject showed unwillingness we spent little time urging him, as not all individuals could be examined in any case, and this circumstance is likely to have caused a certain psychiatric selection. The Khan and the two teachers willingly pointed out the few persons whom they believed to have any kind of neuropsychiatric disorder. For the rest, our selection was "random" in the sense frowned upon by statistics but here enjoined by necessity.

This held for the public health as for the mental health survey, and in fact somewhat more individuals on the whole were tested psychologically (189) than were given the full set of physical and laboratory examinations (148). The total population, as already stated, was 499, of which 52.9 % were male and 47.1 % female, and lived in 72 tents. The average family size was 6.7 persons. Fifty-six percent of the population was below 15 years of age. The birth rate was 55.6 per thousand, the crude death rate 11.1 per thousand, the death rate for children under five years 142 per thousand live births. The median age at the time of marriage for the tribal women was 15 years. In five of the 67 tribal families there were two wives, in 17 (25 %) the husband and wife were blood relatives. Each family lived in a black, home-woven, goat-hair tent provided with carpets. The tent sides are kept up in summer for ventilation, down in winter for warmth. Cooking is done in front of the tents on an open fire using wood or more often brush for fuel. River water was carried over three kilometers in goatskins. Five people at the time of the survey were recovering from typhoid fever. The camp has no sewage disposal facilities, the place of which is taken by the ample desert, abetted by the scorching sun. Smallpox vaccination had been performed, but 175 children were newly vaccinated during the survey. Of 97 people given the Snellen vision test, eight had a demonstrable visual defect of one eye and six of both eyes. Conjunctivitis and respiratory infections were common.

Psychological test procedures and results are similar to those in Marvdasht and Khuzestan. The composition of the population on which they are based is shown in Table B III 1. The relatively large number of "literate males", who even outnumber the illiterate, is deceptive as it was in Khuzestan and for the same reason: it is composed for the greater part of schoolboys. The tent school had 35 boys and 4 girls enrolled and taught six classes, i.e., up to the age of 12–13 years. Among the literate males we observe a sharp drop after this period. Only seven literate males are to be found in the higher age classes. Neither is it certain that all the ten literate 12 and 13 year olds were still attending school, though it is highly probable that they had attended it. Disappointingly few girls did, and none of their mothers had attained literacy. The age distribution is uneven as it was in Khuzestan but is more likely here than there to be caused by an artefact of sampling, especially as we concentrated on the school or school-age children.

Arithmetic test scores are given as in Marvdasht and Khuzestan only for the illiterate adults of both sexes, and for the same reasons, the other groups being too small (Table C I 1–2). The sex differences again are marked and are very highly

Table B III 1. Distribution of Test Subjects by Age, Sex and Literacy

Age	lm	im	m	lf	if	f	m + f
6	4	1	5	1	1	2	1
7	8	1	9	1	4	5	14
8	12	0	12	0	3	3	15
9	2	0	2	0	2	2	4
10	9	0	9	0	2	2	11
11	1	0	1	0	0	0	1
12	8	0	8	1	6	7	15
13	2	1	3	0	1	1	4
14	0	1	1	0	4	4	5
Sub-total children	46	4	50	3	23	26	76
15–19	1	1	2	0	13	13	15
20–39	4	20	24	0	35	35	59
40–59	2	8	10	0	11	11	21
60 +	0	11	11	0	7	7	18
Sub-total adults	7	40	47	0	66	66	113
Total	53	44	97	3	89	92	189

significant throughout. For the men we find a significant difference only in the age group 40–59 ($p < 0.05$) between the Qashqai (mean arithmetic test score 10.5) and the Khuzestani (13.4), which does not hold for the Marvdashti although their mean score too is higher (11.7). When all male groups are pooled, however, a difference is suggested ($0.05 > p > 0.1$) between the Qashqai (10.6) and the Marvdashti (11.9). The scores of the Qashqai women are nowhere significantly different from those of the village women. It is not easy to account for the single significant difference between the nomads and the peasants, the more so as it appears in one age group only. Comparing mean scores, however, we observe that the Qashqai males generally tend to score lower than those in the villages, although the differences with the exception mentioned are not significant. As this again holds only for the males, one could ask oneself whether their relative isolation from interchange with others, from commerce and trade, did show its effects in a tendency to lower arithmetic test performance and whether this effect was not stronger upon the elder generation whose life had been more isolated and traditional than that of the younger. If correct, this hypothesis could also explain why no differences, either statistically significant or in the form of trends, were discovered between the female groups, as they take less part in trade and bartering in any case and have departed less from tradition than the younger men have done.

The block design test was carried out among the Qashqai as it had been in Marvdasht a few months before, but with similarly unsatisfactory results, which therefore are not tabulated.

Coming now to our main theme, neither inquiry from the Khan and the two teachers, the tests and our examiners' judgments, nor the observations of the numerous medical staff busied in all kinds of ways at the survey revealed any case of significant psychiatric disorder among the 189 persons under scrutiny. A number of factors already mentioned may be invoked to account for this surprising result. Nevertheless, while the Adviser would hesitate to present on the basis of this experience a wholly clean bill of mental health, as it were, to the tribal or any other group, he is not inclined, on the basis of other field experience, to consider the failure to meet with even a single case in the course of three days intensive field work as wholly fortuitous or due altogether to the adverse circumstances just referred to. A comparison can be drawn in the next chapter. Easy though it is to miss mild cases (P_1) or even those of medium severity (P_2), it seems hardly likely that severer or grave cases (P_2–P_3) would be overlooked completely if they were actually present – cases for example such as idiocies, dementias or other severe brain damage. Not one came, or was brought, to our attention. One not improbable explanation is that more or less incapacitated persons are left behind in villages, towns or other tribal settlements, of which we shall come to speak presently, or that, if they are taken upon the perennial migrations, they do not survive this harsh mode of existence. But this type of natural selection would not explain the absence of medium cases, nor does anything suggest that all such are left in the towns. The Adviser's impression remains that the tribal group, as far as he came into contact with it, showed a better level of general mental health than the peasants did, whereas a comparison with the urban group was not yet possible.

Some indication may be afforded by the examiners' judgments made, it will be remembered, by the same examiners who had worked in Marvdasht and therefore comparable as a whole, though the examiners' eyes may have been sharpened by their accumulated experience. They affirmed that psychiatric investigation was required in 19 cases out of 178 subjects (189 less 11 for whom no unequivocal judgment was ascertainable) or 10.7 % and had done so in Marvdasht in 50 cases out of 500 – 16 = 484 subjects or 10.3 %. Remarkable in the tribal group was that the affirmative judgments were rendered 13 times for females and only 6 times for males, although the numbers of both sexes (89) were exactly equal. If we assume that about half of the examiners' judgments would be confirmed on clinical investigation as in Marvdasht (54 %; cf. Part D, Chap. II), then about 9–10 of the 19 cases would be positive, corresponding to some 5 % of the population, and the prevalence would be distinctly lower than in Marvdasht with its 10 %. There the examiners' judgments were the principal means of identification for 46 % of the positive cases, again about one half. If we double this, we arrive afresh at roughly 10 %, i.e. about the same as in Marvdasht, but less than in Khuzestan – this under the unflattering but nevertheless conceivable assumption that the authors had failed to recognize all the cases with which they were confronted! The value of such extrapolation remains questionable, however, especially in view of the remarkable bias toward the female sex such as we have encountered nowhere else, including Marvdasht itself with its majority of female cases. Looking over the protocols so designated we observe that several indeed were described as unhappy and depressed, more however as simply unco-operative and withdrawing because of language difficulties. We did not have enough Turkish-speaking helpers to handle them. Several women also had lost sons or husbands in the recent fights with the government forces, and we have no satisfactory basis for estimating whether their normal mourning would lead over into a pathological depression or not. The scanty evidence we can glean from these figures tends to suggest that mental health is rather better in the nomadic tribal group than in other populations heretofore studied.

What our colleagues did find and our informants did point out were, in contrast to the city, several neurological and other cases, which we shall summarize singly.

1. A25 year old man has been subject to major epileptic siezures, which always occur during sleep, for about seven years. They take place at irregular intervals varying roughly from a day to a month without prodromes, are accompanied by tongue biting and urinary incontinence and leave the patient feeling prostrated. The family history was negative, there was no history of precipitating illness or accident, and the patient was psychiatrically unremarkable. He had never received treatment: we left him anti-convulsant medication and urged him to replenish it when the group was in the vicinity of a town. P_2.

2. A35 year old woman, married to a somewhat older husband, was pregnant at the time of interview. Since early childhood she had been suffering from predominantly nocturnal epileptic seizures that occurred once or twice a week. They tended to be heralded by prodromes of yawning, gastric and esophagal spasm and nausea. She asserted, and her husband confirmed, that she did not have tonic-clonic spasms, but would lose consciousness for about one hour. She had no subjective feeling of mental abnormality or weakness of memory but was rather uncommunicative, less open than most of the Qashqai women, and the not inexperienced husband, whose fourth wife the patient was, said he found her rather difficult and ill-tempered. The description of the symptoms suggested a psychomotor epilepsy with typical gastric aura. This is the one case that might also have been rubricated as neuropsychiatric, but the psychiatric symptoms did not seem to be very pronounced nor to exceed greatly the ordinary range of variation. P_2.

3. A five year old girl, youngest of a sibship of five, had been subject according to her mother for the last two years to attacks of loss of consciousness in which she turned pale, clenched her teeth and had convulsions affecting all the limbs. They were said to last two or three minutes with rapid recovery and without either tongue biting or incontinence and always to be provoked by some external factor such as a "nervous upset" or punishment. The family and personal antecedents were unremarkable. No sure diagnosis could be made, but epilepsy was regarded as probable. P_1.

4. A two year old girl was apparently well during her first year of life, then showed a weakness in her legs and difficulty in learning to walk. No history of febrile or other associated conditions could be obtained. The child was restless and difficult to examine. Contractures affected the joints of both lower limbs, with obvious weakness of the left, where the foot was flaccid and the reflexes more sluggish than on the right. A poliomyelitis residue P_2 seemed probable.

5. Three children (two boys aged 14 and 6, and one girl aged 12) totally unable to sweat were discovered in one family. The father and mother were first cousins. The father died, the mother remarried, and the one child by the second father was normal. The three affected children were brought to Nemazee Hospital in Shiraz and studied there. Biopsy confirmed the complete absence of sweat glands in the skin, demonstrating an anhidrotic ectodermal dysplasia. All three children were intelligent, suffered from absence of temperature regulation particularly in the hot summers and were accustomed to drink large quantities of water with little relief, but adapted well to the circumstances and showed no personality disorder. Neither were there any complicating somatic malformations. They have been described in [32].

Time did not suffice for the psychological examination of the two adult cases of epilepsy, both of whom were discovered toward the very end of our field work in the Qashqai encampment. Therefore they do not fall into our sample of 189 persons and are not included among the epileptics listed in Table D IV 8. Two children (Nos. 3 and 4 above) were below our age limit, and the three anhidrotic children are neither neurological nor psychiatric cases, but are mentioned for the sake of interest.

Both adult epilepsies were of medium severity with frequent attacks, and the two year old girl was damaged not a little when we saw her, with further recovery unlikely and rehabilitating measures unavailable. In the light of these cases the hypothesis that invalids are left behind or die loses some of its probability. If psychiatric cases of similar degree existed, then why, must we ask, did they not come to sight? The answer remains open.

2. The Settled Qashqai in Qalandari

a. General. The investigation here to be described was not foreseen as part of the Shiraz Survey, but came as a postscript to it through good fortune and the help of a colleague and friend. While working in Shiraz we learned that he had undertaken several village health studies [133] since our previous co-operation on the Marvdasht Survey, one with more than usually good co-operation and satisfying results in the village of Qalandari, about 70 km west of Shiraz by the Kazerun road, after turning off which several kilometers had to be traversed by a dirt road in fair condition. The word "qalandar" (قلندر) denotes a wandering dervish, "qalandariyeh" (قلندریه) the order of such dervishes, but we did not succeed in establishing a connection with the indigenous name of the village. This was more commonly called "deh-e-nou" or the "new village". The appellation had more significance for us as it stemmed from the fact that the village had been newly founded only eight years previously by Qashqai tribesmen who had determined to settle down. It thus presented an ideal object for comparison with the migratory Qashqai group described above, the more so as it possessed a well-established school which most of the children were attending. The Qashqai Khan under whose jurisdiction the village fell was well disposed to the undertaking. Together we called on him in the late spring and received his promise of assistance and co-operation as well as that of the teachers. As the more intensive phase of the Shiraz Survey gave way to the pursuit of stragglers and the verification of findings, setting free some examiners and cars and relaxing somewhat the pressure on the authors, we undertook on June 21st and 23rd, 1970, the survey of Qalandari, returning on July 15 with only a few assistants to see certain individuals who had been away on our previous visits and to check some information.

On both principal working days we were happy to have the company and advice of a colleague from the Department of Psychology of the University of Shiraz, who made interesting proposals for supplementing our testing program (see below) and also, being of Turkish mother tongue, could carry out interviews with the few residents who still had acquired little or no command of Persian.

A census had been prepared before we arrived on the scene. There were 193 habitants, of whom 153 or 79.2 % were six or older, living in 27 houses, one family to a house, i.e. 7.2 persons on the average to a family. Seventy-nine were male, 65 female, yielding a sex ratio of 122:100. Our headquarters were the school house, not in session then. The teachers gave us understanding, valuable co-operation. Procedure was as elsewhere except that tests and the questionnaire were given immediately after the family sheet had been filled out. Most of the men were present and were tested first, as the Khan had asked them to remain at home until we had seen them. The examiners immediately reported anyone who seemed suspect of pathology to the authors, who then went to examine the suspect person. When not engaged thus we circulated through the village from house to house, saw all the inhabitants (with the exceptions to be noted below), could observe testing and intervene much as we had done in Khuzestan. None refused, but a problem arose because of the interchange between sedentary and migratory Qashqai mentioned in connection with the first tribal group. During the summer some of the residents of Qalandari joined the migrants for shorter or longer periods, visited relatives or went on business or in search of work to cities. Thus one young man had gone to Tehran, and another was said to be in Shiraz but could not be traced. Seven others, mostly young, were off with the tribes for the summer and could not be followed. For a time we were threatened with even more drop outs until by dint of much questioning and after several false starts we learned that a half a dozen people from two families were encamped at a not excessive remove and got one of the village residents to go with us in the land-rover and show the way. There had been a vague talk of half an hour's drive, which extended itself to an hour and a half over first dirt roads, then a rutted and barely visible track twisting, diving and climbing over bush covered foothills and leading into a wild but beautiful, uninhabited country quite different from the rolling open ground sparsely dotted with scrub and grass, in sight of other villages, where Qalandari lay. In this remoteness we came upon three black tents beside a clear brook where our villagers were spending the summer with their relatives and their flocks in surroundings of rugged beauty and splendid isolation. The afternoon just sufficed for the testing and interviewing. The following afternoon, the last one planned with the full force, was curtailed by a pressing call to an emergency case nearby. We found an acute abdomen, suspected cholecystitis or hepatitis, sent the women in a station wagon ahead to the hospital in Shiraz with a nursing aide, then crowded our examiners and ourselves into the remaining two larger and one small car to return to the city. The final visit in July served to conclude that day's tasks as well as to interview a few previous absentees and supplement some incomplete information.

b. Tests. Psychological test procedures in Qalandari were the same as in Shiraz, with additions to be mentioned, the survey of this village having been undertaken at the very end of our work in the city and after corresponding test modifications as against Marvdasht, the nomadic Qashqai and Khuzestan had been put into effect. Only the raw scores on the arithmetic test A for illiterates, therefore, are directly comparable with raw scores from other villages, and there are too few such from Qalandari to warrant statistical comparison. In individual cases comparison should be made only after conversion into weighted scores and intelligence quotients.

Table B III 2. Distribution of Test Subjects by Age, Sex and Literacy

Age	lm	im	m	lf	if	f	m + f
6	0	4	4	0	1	1	5
7	2	3	5	1	2	3	8
8	7	1	8	0	1	1	9
9	0	0	0	5	0	5	5
10	4	0	4	0	0	0	4
11	2	0	2	2	0	2	4
12	5	0	5	5	1	6	11
13	4	0	4	0	0	0	4
14	3	0	3	3	1	4	7
Sub-total children	27	8	35	16	6	22	57
15–19	6	2	8	2	7	9	17
20–39	7	13	20	0	25	25	45
40–59	3	5	8	0	6	6	14
60 +	1	7	8	0	3	3	11
Sub-total adults	17	27	44	2	41	43	87
Total	44	35	79	18	47	65	144

The composition of the test and psychiatric survey population appears in Table B III 2. From this it can be seen that most of the boys of school age are in fact attending school: we find no illiterate males between 8 and 15. A respectable number of their fathers, too, have learned their letters, whether in their own youth or in adult literacy classes. A fair number of girls are to be found in school, but after the age group 15–19 all women are illiterate. The age distribution is not as strikingly uneven as e.g. in Marvdasht, but the sharp drop in numbers after 40 is noticeable and probably must be referred to the quite recent founding of the village.

Following a suggestion of a colleague who had worked with both tests in Shiraz, we applied in addition to our standard battery the Goodenough-Harris Draw-a-Man-Test [91] to children from 6 to 14 and the Short Form of the Maudsley Personality Inventory to the adults. The Goodenough-Harris Test demands that each subject make two full drawings of human figures, one of a man, the other of a woman. The village population counted 57 children aged 6 to 14, of whom 45 made scoreable drawings. Some of the youngest scribbled, shied or balked, as did a few of the older. A few drawings were not of a full figure, and one was an all too obvious copy. Several of the pairs were not completed: 36 were, of which 22 were done by boys and 16 by girls. All drawings were evaluated by Goodenough and Harris's rules. The point scores were converted by their tables into standard scores, which in this case are equivalent to intelligence quotients. The number of drawings of each sex by each sex, the mean standard scores for each of the four groups and for the two sexes are given in Table B III 3.

As on all other intelligence tests we have applied in Iran, the girls score lower than the boys, though the difference in this case is not great and relatively much less than on the arithmetic and block design tests. Harris writes [91, p. 103) that "there is a slight but quite consistent tendency for girls to score higher than boys on the Man scale," and (p. 106) that "the advantage held by the girls increases appreciably in drawing their own sex." Neither the one nor the other appears to be confirmed for Iran. Because of the small numbers involved it seemed unrewarding to compute statistical measures of significance etc. and not only unrewarding but meaningless to draw age-progress curves when some age and sex classes were represented only by a couple of members. We content ourselves with presenting these rough mean values as a stimulus to further investigation. The tendency that they show corresponds to what we have found in more extensive studies (cf. Chap. C I). We must add that in this as in other cases foreign scoring norms cannot be applied without restandardization to Iranian test subjects, who would all appear by these standard scores to be feeble-minded. The mean combined IQ on the arithmetic and block design tests for this entire population of

Table B III 3. Mean Standard Scores on Draw-a-Man Test

28 drawings of men by boys	71
22 drawings of women by boys	72
All boys' drawings	71
16 drawings of men by girls	67
17 drawings of women by girls	63
All girls' drawings	65

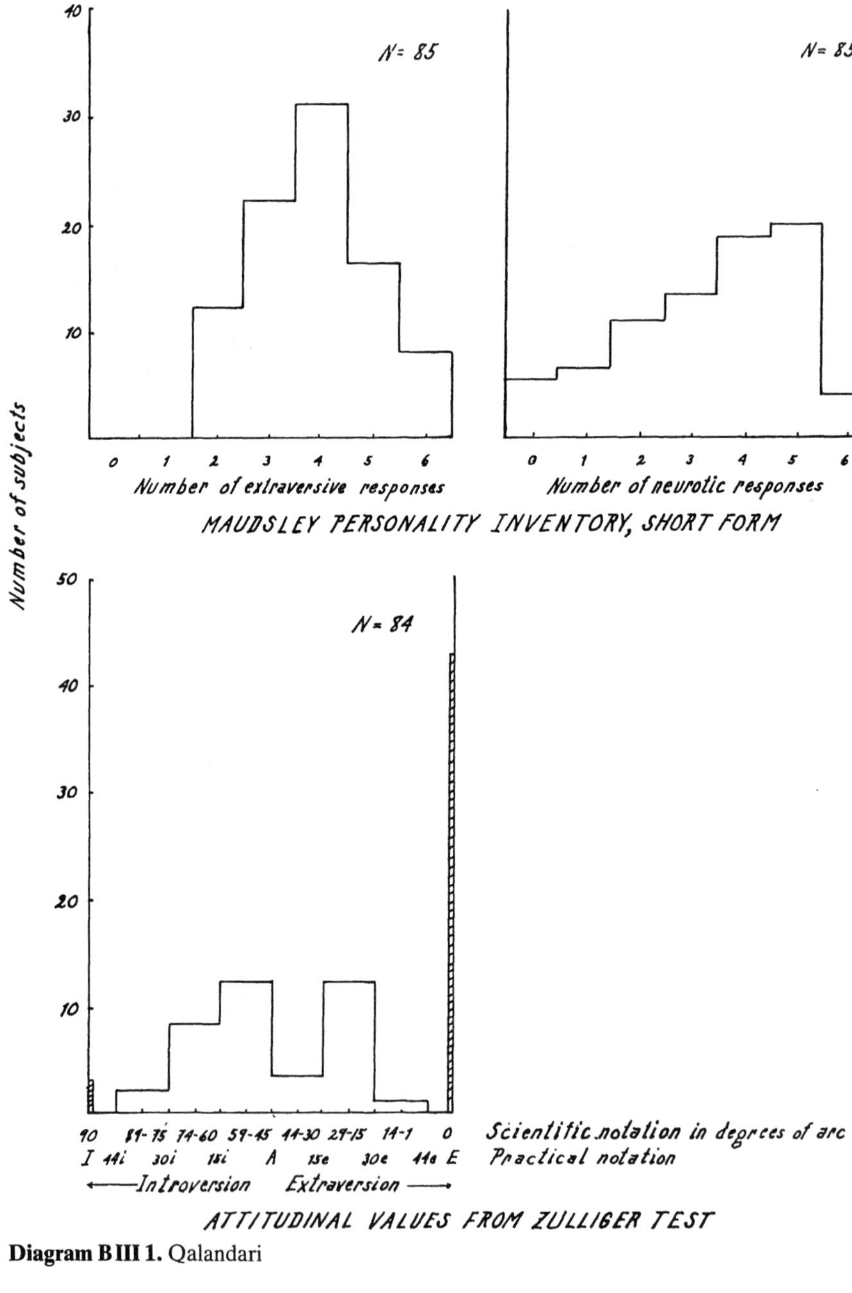

Diagram B III 1. Qalandari

children who completed at least one scoreable drawing, omitting the six and seven year olds as explained in Chap. C I 3, was 106, however, proving indubitably that Qalandari ranked well on the Iranian scale. The product-moment correlation for 37 children who produced both scoreable drawings and combined intelligence quotients on the arithmetic and block design tests was only 0.35.

The Short Form of the Maudsley Personality Inventory [MPI; 73] consists of twelve questions, six of which are supposedly relevant to extraversion (really to the dimension introversion-extraversion, but Eysenck speaks only of the latter) and six to neuroticism. The two scales are practically independent of and hardly correlate with each other. The score on each ranges from 0 to 6, every affirmative answer to a question counting one point. There is no lie scale as there is in the full form of the MPI. Eighty-five adults gave useable records. The distribution of their scores can be seen in the upper half of Diagram B III 1. The extraversion scores distribute normally, with the expected peak at 4 in mid-range. The neuroticism scores do not, but pile up progressively to their mode at 5. If neuroticism is a pathological characteristic or one bordering upon the pathological, the opposite kind of skewing must be expected. This short "neuroticism scale" therefore measures in this Iranian village, if anything, a trait or tendency that has nothing in common with the psychiatric diagnosis of neurosis. Because it attains its mode just short of the maximal scalar value, it seems doubtful whether it measures anything at all.

Another measure of introversion-extraversion was available since all the subjects had been given the Z Test and their attitudinal values (AV)[1] could be calculated from the experience balance, except in one case with the indeterminate balance 0:0. In order to obtain a distribution with the same number of classes as Eysenck's Short Extraversion Scale the range of attitudinal values from 0 to 90 was divided as follows: 0 (= introversionless), 1–14, 15–29, 30–44, 45–59, 60–74, 75–89, and 90 (= extraversionless). The number of subjects in each class was counted and their scatter histogram (lower half of Diagram B III 1) compared with that of the Eysenck extraversion scores. Be it noted that the attitudinal values in "scientific notation" run along the abscissa in the opposite direction to the Eysenck scores, namely from right to left, as a low attitudinal value and a high Inventory score correspond to extraversion and vice versa. One is impressed first by the large number (43 out of 84) of introversionless, i.e. one-sidedly extraverted subjects with an experience balance of 0:X and therefore an AV = 0. They have only three extraversionless counterparts at the opposite extreme with experience balance X:0 and AV = 90. In between we find not a normal, but a bimodal distribution. The fact of this bimodal distribution need not occasion surprise. It is found regularly when groups of subjects are tested with the Rorschach Test and their experience balances are converted into linearly distributed attitudinal values [15, 16]. Distributions of introversion and extraversion obtained from questionnaires are sometimes unimodal, sometimes slightly bimodal, as is Eysenck's own published curve [74] from his Maudsley Personality Inventory, and sometimes do not show any clear modality, while distributions from projective tests such as the Rorschach and the Zulliger are usually bi- and occasionally trimodal. This lends confirmation to C. G. Jung's typological concept and substantiates it for Iran also.

---

[1] For explanation cf. Part C, Chap. II 3 d.

The distributions of the attitudinal values of the two sexes in Qalandari did not show any noteworthy difference. The mean attitudinal values were 23 e for men and 21 e for women, i.e. practically equal and also nearly the same as the values we have found for the sexes combined among the related, still migratory Qashqai nomads (19 e) and in Khuzestan (21 e). The mean E values were 3.8 for the men and 3.9 for the women. On the other hand, both Mehryar and Baraheni, working independently, using the full scale of 24 items and Iranian undergraduate students of both sexes as subjects, have found a normal distribution of the extraversion and neuroticism scores and practically no correlation between the two. In this respect we can confirm their and Eysenck's original findings. The Pearson product-moment correlation of the two short scales in

Table B III 4. Psychiatric Cases by Sex and Degrees of Severity

	male	ICD-9		female	ICD-9
P_1			P_1		
				20 y., illiterate, married. Repeated miscarriages, one surviving child. Migrainoid headache.	346
				35 y., illiterate, unhappily married at 12 y. Migrainoid headache (with occasional hysteriform seizures).	346 (300.1)
				45 y., illiterate, intelligent, married. Anxiety neurosis (with migrainoid headache).	300.0 (346)
	0			3	
P_2			P_2		
	8 y. Febrile disease with transient hemiparalysis at 5 y., since then abnormally excitable and irritable, dispensed from first school year. Status postencephaliticus.	310.8		30 y., illiterate, married. Typhoid fever at 25 y. Grands maux with considerable alteration of character.	345.1
	32 y., literate, twice married. Manifold, principally cardiovascular psychosomatic complaints (with neurotic depression).	306.2 (300.4)			
	38 y., illiterate lowgrade imbecile, able to perform simple menial tasks.	318.1			
	3			1	
P_3			P_3		
	0			0	
	3			4	

Qalandari was only 0.28, and V by Cramer's method was 0.25.[1] Baraheni emphasizes that neither his nor Mehryar's group can "be regarded as a representative or random sample of the normal Iranian student population." Qalandari too had its special characteristics, but the sample did encompass nearly all adults residing there.

c. Psychiatry and Neurology. The relatively small population was of the same order of magnitude as the migratory Qashqai group so far as this was actually scrutinized, but thanks to its compactness could be studied in the same time much more thoroughly. Nevertheless and in spite of close observation by both authors throughout, the sample of 144 persons yielded only 7 psychiatric cases = 49 per 1000. Exceptionally we have added to this short table a minimum of personal data and (in parentheses) such accessory diagnoses as seemed called for. These are not included in the main tables and are given here for the sake of interest only.

The advantages of almost ubiquitous presence and direct observation proved themselves in Qalandari through a harvest of four neurological cases, whereas in the much larger city of Shiraz only two were found (plus six neuropsychiatric), rendering it practically certain that the rate for Shiraz is much too low. These four cases were:

1. A 7 year old boy with a flaccid paresis of the left foot, in all probability a polio residue. ICD 044, P_1.
2. An 85 year old man, in excellent mental condition, with a Parkinsonian tremor, which he smilingly shrugged off as a minor accompaniment of advanced years. ICD 342, P_1.
3. A 43 year old man with a probable discopathy and a paresis of both lower limbs. ICD 725.1, P_2.
4. A 23 year old woman with flaccid paralysis of the right lower limb and foot after poliomyelitis, using a crutch. ICD 044, P_2.

The neurological prevalence rate comes out at 28 per 1000 or practically the same as found everywhere else but in Shiraz.

---

[1] We thank Prof. J. Gadourek, Groningen and formerly NIAS, for the calculations.

IV. Shiraz

1. The City and Its Survey

After two rural and one nomad survey had established a foundation for reference and had confirmed our methodology, an urban sample was needed. Though the Adviser was urged to attempt this in Tehran he was reluctant for various reasons. The metropolis with its now several million inhabitants, its manifold stratification and steep socio-economic gradients, its wider exposure to foreign influences and its higher level of industrialization and commercialization could not and cannot be regarded, though it is the capital of the country, as typical of Iran as a whole. Even if it could have been, the resources available were far from adequate for so complex a task. Our methods and tests had not yet been tried out in an urban setting, and we did not know what the response of an urban population, to which we could offer no form of direct or indirect assistance as we had in Marvdasht and Khuzestan, would be. It seemed unwise to undertake our first experiment in the largest and most problematical city of all Iran. As on the other hand a minor city could provide us, at least in the early and middle 'sixties, with hardly any of the essential supporting facilities, the choice of a site was essentially restricted to one of the provincial capitals.

Shiraz was the obvious choice. Historically, geographically and culturally it has always belonged to the heartland of Persia. These aspects have been well and lovingly described by Arberry in his *Shiraz: Persian City of Saints and Poets* [9]. The ancient Achaeminian capitals of Pasargadae and Persepolis are within easy driving distance today, the latter being a principal tourist attraction (cf. Dutz, W.: *Das Gebet des Königs* [65]). By diplomatic submission Shiraz at first escaped the devastation visited by the Mongols upon most of the rest of Iran in the thirteenth century, though Timur harrowed it later out of displeasure over the real or imagined misdeeds of its administration. Precisely in those perilous times, mayhap because of them, poetry and Sufi mysticism, the one almost inseparable from the other, burgeoned there to an unparalleled flowering. Two of the towering pillars of Iran's and the world's literature, the poets Saadi and Hafez were its sons, and their tombs are places of literary pilgrimage to this day, while their verses live on in the hearts and upon the lips of Iranians whether literate or illiterate. The mystic Ruzbehan was their townsman and near contemporary. In the eighteenth century, after the Afghans had extinguished the brilliance of the Safavids, the great Regent Karim Khan Zand restored light briefly to Central Iran, furnished Fars with a model administration and laid straight through his capital Shiraz the broad avenue that still carries his name. Even under the renewed darkness of later dynasties Shiraz with its port of Busher retained importance as a center of trade, distribution and administration for much of South Persia – a function it still fulfills in part. From this and from its reawakened cultural mission derives the significance of Shiraz today, to which has been added its importance as a military base since the outbreak of the Iraq-Iran War. Though industry (principally textiles, cement, sugar refining and manufacture of telephone apparatus) exists and is increasing, Shiraz has been far less subject to the intensive process of industrialization than Isfahan and Tabriz, not to mention Tehran. While there may be no such thing as a typically Persian city, Shiraz could probably lay a better claim to the title than any other. Its citizens almost without exception speak Persian, eliminating language problems such as would have rendered a survey difficult in predominantly Turkish speaking Tabriz or in Ahwaz with its substantial Arab population. Its University was flourishing, had already shown a lively and active interest in our work and declared its willingness to participate in a new survey of the city itself and to assist therein as far as possible. We had worked out of Shiraz before in the Marvdasht Survey and knew places and people on whose aid we could count whether officially or unofficially. A survey of considerably larger compass than hitherto could only be executed by a corresponding staff. This could be assembled better in Shiraz than anywhere else in Iran and also could be kept together over the year that we estimated would be required, since most of it, including our immediate professional colleagues, was resident – a factor of crucial importance in Iran, where most technically trained people tend to congregate in a few cities that they are reluctant to leave even for brief periods.

After preliminary conversations in Tehran the authors arrived in Shiraz early in October, 1969, passing Pasargadae and Persepolis, recrossing the familiar and in the intervening years partly reforested Marvdasht, traversing the rocky outcrops that separate it from Shiraz, emerging through the classic defile of the Ruknabad and joining their breaths with those of the ancient travellers, who, after long leagues in the desert, at the sight of the fair city in its verdant plane were wont to exclaim in delight "Allahu Akbar! God is Great!". Shiraz lies at a height of about 1500 m in a well watered, wide and fruitful valley of the southeast slope of the Zagros Range and is connected by a paved highway (a dirt road when the Adviser first visited it in 1960) and by frequent air services with Isfahan and Tehran, nearly five hundred and a thousand kilometers respectively distant. At the national census in 1966 the population totaled around 270000. We were fortunate in that the Department of Public Health in the very fall of 1969, while our preparations were under way, conducted a fresh census of all households with a view to a campaign of oral immunization against poliomyelitis, in the train of which we followed. As only children of fourteen and below were to be immunized, these alone were enumerated personally, but great care was taken to search out and number every household in the city. The municipality had been divided rather arbitrarily into eighteen districts, not coinciding with the administrative or police districts, using the main thoroughfares as boundaries. The households of each district were numbered consecutively by a pair of workers who began at a convenient point of access and threaded their way through the maze of streets, painting numbers in red, one for each household, on walls or at doors and gates after ascertaining how many families lived behind them and describing their route by local landmarks, squares and street names in a notebook. Since only the houses on certain principal avenues have regular numbers and no generally available large scale city map existed (the administration and police possessed wall-size maps of their own) these numbers and notes were to be our whole reliance. We set as our target a random one per cent sample of all households, excluding for technical reasons as before individuals below the age of six years. For each district we drew a two-place number by chance from a table of random numbers, then examined as far as possible every hundredth household the number of which ended with the randomly chosen number. In the few instances in which this was not possible because e.g. the house in question had been abandoned or demolished we took the next house in which people were living.

For the more detailed registration of the census and of demographic data, psychological testing, administering the psychiatric questionnaire and following up answers the Department of Public Health placed at our disposal fifteen female members of the Health Corps – girls mostly of 18–19 years who had all completed twelve years of school and been drafted as auxiliaries into military service. It should be emphasized that they were not nurses or nurse aides and had received no medical training whatsoever. Some had participated in the polio census and immunization campaign already mentioned. Similar in age and schooling, they were in other respects a heterogeneous group that displayed all degrees of willingness or unwillingness, application and skill. An undoubted advantage was that they could obtain access to nearly all homes, particularly to those from which the men were absent during the day and to which the housewives or their daughters probably would not have admitted a male interviewer. By this time too the national services such as the Health Corps had achieved a respected status. Seldom was any door closed to the mostly cheerful girls in their trim uniforms, in whom not even the most sceptical imagined a threat of the tax collector or the police. Balancing disadvantages were their relative immaturity and their great differences in motivation. In contrast to the professional or semi-professional Iranian co-workers on the rural surveys, they had been ordered, not asked to take part. Some did so gladly and developed into indefatigable, resourceful staff members; some simply got through the job; two were caught inventing their "results".

In a two week course the future examiners received short talks on the background and purpose of the survey, followed by detailed instructions about recording demographic data and administering the tests and questionnaire. They practiced first on each other, then on non-psychiatric out-patients, on school pupils and on miscellaneous relatives and friends, while the authors and the assisting supervisory staff – a nurse, a nursing aide, a technician and a social worker – continually checked their performance, skills and records. Every examiner was given a mimeographed book of instructions in Persian, and every two received a set of testing material. It was agreed at the outset that it would be more prudent and even necessary for them to work in pairs to counteract both their own feelings of insecurity and also any disapproval that might be visited, at least in the more traditional and conservative quarters of the city, upon a girl roaming the streets, as it were, alone. Less than two decades ago this would have been unthinkable. The few professionals were accustomed to working alone and did so from the beginning, as several of our more skillful, interested and self-reliant girls later did also. The common procedure was for a car to take out a group to a strategic point from which they dispersed and from which they were later collected. Usually one girl of a pair talked or tested while the other recorded. Several trips to a house might be necessary until all members had been reached. Men were sought out at their places of work, children, if attending, at school. Employers made hardly any difficulties, teachers and principals none. It quickly became apparent that the most favorable time for interviewing and, if indicated, subsequent psychiatric examination usually was in the evening, when the whole family was likely to be assembled. The majority of the girls were reluctant to perform evening visits and were not obligated to do so, though some were willing to go with one of the authors or the supervisory staff, and our best after a time began making evening home visits alone. As it became more and more urgently necessary to increase the night work above all in order to interview our male probands we received most welcome succour from the Training School for Male Nursing Aides. Four young aides in training joined our nocturnal excursions, worked diligently and ably far into the nights and thus reached a considerable number of subjects whom otherwise we should have missed. The necessity for such work after hours jeopardized the Survey for a time when the drivers' overtime pay was slow in coming, for not only was the city much to extensive to cover on foot, but also our late visits were often scattered over wide areas, serving to fill in gaps that could not be closed during the day. Frequently this implied tramping the streets from eight p.m. to near midnight, searching around dark corners and in dim, dusty or muddy alleys with flashlights for numbers scrawled on walls, persuasions at hesitant doors and the like more. The reader will have asked himself more than once by this time how such unsolicited, especially nightly, intruding visits were received, and we must answer: well, far beyond our expectation. For this a number of reasons suggest themselves.

Our young, unformidable examiners in uniform with a certain recognized public status but with no threatening power, nearly all well mannered and often personable, gained easier entry than a more professional, experienced group might have obtained. The sex of the majority was no doubt an asset. Nevertheless we observed that our young men also had little difficulty. It must be recalled, however, that they were in a sense "professionals" or on their way to becoming so, had already enjoyed at least a year of training in hospital and public health work and had entered this field voluntarily, besides which the Directress of the School obligingly picked out for us her four best. After much discussion of the matter with our Iranian colleagues no preparatory action by local radio or newspaper was undertaken, though the public health officials did "spread the word" in the policlinics and through their field staff. We commenced operations in the most densely populated, poorest and most conservative section of the city immediately adjacent to the Department of Public Health, in which this Department had been most active and in which its workers enjoyed a great deal of confidence. The inhabitants were not unused to surveys and campaigns of immunization of various kinds nor to visiting the policlinics of the Department. The Maternal and Child Health Section particularly had organized a well-functioning system of ongoing supervision and care for pregnant women, young mothers and their children up to two years of age, and as the majority of younger women in that district were having babies every year or two they were almost permanently in the care of the MCH Section over several years at a time. Not seldom when introducing ourselves to a young housewife or making inquiries about her we were smilingly told: بهداشت است یک مادر ("she's a Public Health Department mother"). A number of such willingly came to the Department themselves, combining their routine check-up with our examination, and brought their children, occasionally even their husbands. The news spread with the characteristic rapidity of neighborhood gossip, exonerated our crew of ill intentions and in many cases wakened such a friendly curiosity about the two foreigners who would actually come to talk with people and did not remain seated behind official or academic desks that we found many a house waiting for "its" visit or disappointed when the random number had excluded it. Thence we became heralded in other districts of the city. We had no Iranian physician working regularly with us, the Department being too short staffed, but for special cases one might be detached, and we could and did refer freely both psychiatric and somatic cases to the appropriate outpatient services. Though we naturally had no legitimation to practice in Iran and neither tried nor wished to transgress this, there were ways in which a modest extra help might be obtained for the needy such as a quicker acceptance by over-busied colleagues, a physician's sample, a reassurance about a child's or relative's health, a simple piece of advice and the ancient panacea of the psychiatrist: patient listening. An examination could resolve itself to a council on family problems or on family planning. A great aid unquestionably was the Iranian tradition of hospitality, especially to the stranger. Xenophobia does not exist in Iran. Time after time the authors and their collaborators were invited in, or back, for a chat, were regularly plied with tea, often with refreshments, to refuse which would have been crass rudeness, even asked to a meal. The question of "motivation" that had disquieted us not a little before the urban survey began resolved itself effortlessly. Neither did the inevitable evening visits constitute any major problem. First visits to a household we made in the daytime wherever possible, then arranged an appointment in the evening when required and have spent many an evening interviewing all the members of a family in their own room huddled around the cylindrical naphtha stove that is the usual provider of heat, laying blocks, presenting Z cards to puzzled eyes or scribbling notes by an oil lamp while the doorway and corners of the room in the half dark gradually filled with the faces of the curious neighbors whose attempts to supply the answers had to be restrained. Even when we sometimes inadvertently woke someone from sleep the victim nearly always remained courteous. A grocer might be tested at eleven at night among his greens where he had been waiting hopefully for a last customer before rolling up to sleep on a scrap of rug in the rear of the shop. Overborne by zeal we penetrated once late at night to a minute courtyard and, knocking, awoke an elderly man who had long settled down for the sleep of the just. He wondered, listened politely to our apologetic explanations, kindled the lamp and without remonstrance applied himself to the mental arithmetic exercises, failed one, solved another, failed, yawned, rubbed the sleep out of his eyes and then, instead of giving us the round cursing that we deserved, apologized and asked us if we could not come another evening a little earlier, as he usually did not get home from work until nine and for sheer weariness could not think of the replies to our questions. We came again, and he answered well.

If the poor, and particularly the very poor for whom we had nothing, accepted us so graciously, what, we wondered, would be our lot among the rich and the more sophisticated? We encountered no essential difference, though in a couple of cases, when a well known family possessed of property and power fell into our sample and the indicative number was painted on the gate of its walled estate, we realized just in time that our examiners had interviewed the gatekeeper's family and had shied off the owner. Going back ourselves we managed to see him and his relatives and have been received with elaborate courtesy upon priceless carpets or refreshed in one of the shady, luxuriant gardens that are the pride of Shiraz. Of course there were exceptions, which with a little persistance, a dose of persuasion and humor almost always were surmountable. Where resistance proved entrenched, one particularly of our Health Corps collaborators developed an astonishing ingenuity and a sporting joy in overcoming it and with a bare handful of exceptions succeeded. Once she had won the recalcitrant family, tested and questioned them and sometimes conversed with them by the hour she usually could persuade them to accept and even feel honored by our visit. In other quarters a physician whose benefactions to the city were well known and who enjoyed the full confidence of even the most conservative could and did intervene, as did other colleagues and friends.

Simple as the enumeration and random choice of households had been made for us, there remained problems to be solved that had not presented themselves in the villages. Shiraz like most other cities has a floating population of job-seekers, visiting relatives and friends, business people, military (as headquarters of an army corps), patients in hospitals and institutions, students and foreigners, a few of whom are connected with the university, while the majority come from the Persian Gulf States. We determined at the beginning not to include visitors and transients (whether guests in families, hotels or hospitals), the military except for the more or less permanent staff of instructors, technical and maintenance personnel settled in Shiraz and living outside of military quarters, into which we did not enter, students except those from Shiraz families and living with these outside the student residences, hospital patients with the same exceptions. We were prepared to include resident foreigners but were spared any quandaries over these as no such households fell into our sample. As mentioned in Chap. A IV, temporarily absent household members were sought out as far as possible, especially those reported to be in hospitals or institutions (including a private psychiatric hospital, general hospitals, a home for delinquent boys and the jail), while those absent and unreachable for the whole period from the completion of the lists until the end of the survey were dropped and not counted. Refusals were not substituted.

Such testing equipment as could not be procured in Iran had been duly ordered by the WHO at our request early in the summer of 1969, but when we arrived in October only a small part of it was at hand and much, including the indispensable stop watches, did not reach us until December or even later. Preparation, translation and offset printing of the numerous forms and instruction booklets proved a more formidable task than anticipated, mainly because the relatively few technically competent persons on whom we had perforce to rely, including the Nemazee Hospital printing office, were so besieged by their routine work that exacting extra tasks nearly overtaxed them. We are the more grateful to our colleagues who gave of their scant spare time. It was early in January 1970 before we could commence training our Health Corps staff and mid-January before field work actually could begin. Within a month or two it became clear that with persistence, the extension of the Adviser's ten month appointment for another month (to which the WHO/EMRO promptly agreed) and a modicum of luck it might still be possible to complete the first phase (demographic data, testing and questionnaire) for the whole one per cent sample (as in fact was done), but by no means the second, though we began with the clinical examination of suspect cases very soon after a fair number had been collected and the first technical difficulties had been more or less overcome. Soon the absence of a full-time Iranian counterpart and of an administrator, who could not be spared from the Health Department staff, made itself direly felt. As there was a constant coming and going in our policlinic headquarters with pairs and teams departing and returning, material to be distributed, new assignments to be improvised if the intended househoulds could not be reached, above all completed forms to be checked immediately and if necessary complemented, only one of the authors could go out at a time for direct supervision in the field and for clinical investigations. For supervision we had some assistance as described above, but the effectiveness of one or the other author's unforeseen appearance at the test sites or unannounced decision to accompany one of the teams for some hours was unmistakable. A limited number of cases could be invited or brought to the policlinic, but they remained a minority, and it was clear almost at once that the only way to secure anything approaching a satisfactory coverage was by persistent home visits. Examining all the suspect cases in this way would have carried us far beyond both the Adviser's assignment and his leave from his regular position. There were other administrative snags besides, so that we became forced most reluctantly to abandon our original aim of exploring psychiatrically in a second phase of the survey all subjects designated by whatever criterion as suspect of significant psychiatric disorder in the first.

It seemed preferable not to relax our criteria, as this would have invalidated comparison with our earlier surveys, this being precisely one of our principal objectives. Neither did we wish to confine ourselves to one stratum of urban society, e.g. the poorest, which would have been most readily comparable with our rural samples, while taking a smaller random sample from the whole city, say one-half of one per cent or rather less than one per cent, easily could have left us with such small strata or sub-groups that comparisons between them would have been statistically insignificant. Reflecting that the influence, if any, of socio-economic contrasts and of cultural transition, both of them strikingly apparent in Iran, upon psychiatric morbidity is one of the major questions of psychiatric epidemiology and social psychiatry, we decided to concentrate upon these contrasts and rather to study more carefully their extremes as far they were to be found in Shiraz than to attenuate a general sample to the point where they or their possible effects might disappear. That such contrasts existed in Shiraz was abundantly evident to the naked eye, as was also that cultural transition from the more traditional oriental to a style of life that for brevity's sake may be called "Western", and that at any rate in the Middle East is untrammeled by tradition, tended, with exceptions, to go with them. Rise on the socio-economic, especially on the economic scale in Iran as, in our experience, nearly throughout the Near and Middle East, brings with it as a rule at least outward "Westernization" whatever the professed opinion of the better-off person about the "West", however deficient or distorted his knowledge of it may be. Furthermore, the outward "Westernization" fairly regularly, inevitably and often unconsciously tends to penetrate the skin, with effects that are extremely various in various persons. It is not our purpose nor our province to describe, evaluate or philosophize about these here, but as psychiatrists simply to record the unchallengeable fact that Iran, like so many other "developing" countries or in this case as a redeveloping one, being the heir of an ancient and lofty civilization, was undergoing at a very rapid pace a profound cultural transition in the direction indicated, a transition that for many was unsettling and therefore might, but must not necessarily, lead to a change in the amount or pattern of psychiatric morbidity or in both. We do not undertake to define what is meant by "Westernization", but take the word at its current value in – so to speak – the bazar.

Shiraz possesses several smaller bazars and one large one, solidly built of brick vaults by the Karim Khan Zand mentioned at the beginning of the chapter and since known as the Bazar-e-Vakil or Regent's Bazar. It marks the very transition of which we have spoken, lying between the old town and the new. To the south and west of it is the densely clustered elder city with its mosques and shrines, their spacious courtyards, a few squares and wider or very recently widened streets and with innumerable angular narrow alleys, impassable for motor cars, between mud brick walls, from which wooden gates admit to miniature gardens, almost every one of which nevertheless, as in all Iran, has its frequently tiny pool. On two sides the old quarter, though not in itself walled, cuts off as sharply as a knife, on the others it merges into the newer. It is the center of religion, history, tradition, but also of poverty. Any casual walk through it conveys this last impression, which our systematic exploration of it confirmed. It corresponded to a great extent with the largest district drawn for the household census of the polio immunization campaign (District 4) and comprised about 61000 persons in 12224 households. It was also immediately adjacent to the Department of Public Health. We determined to take it as a sample or stratum representative of the more traditional style of life and of the lower socio-economic extreme for the second or clinical phase of the mental health survey.

From the Bazar-e-Vakil the pleasantly gardened Avenue Karim Khan Zand traverses the modern shopping and commercial center of the city and leads straight on to the Medical Faculty of the University, the Nemazee Hospital and the green, well-watered newer residential section. Parallel thereto comfortable to rich villas line the wide and shady Avenue Qasrodasht. The mud brick walls have vanished except for remnants around an abandoned garden waiting for its price. Big American cars bump over the pitted asphalt, some with conspicuous license plates on them of Emirates down the Gulf, the leaders of which keep a villa in Shiraz as a summer residence against the blasting heat of their own oil-rich sands. The style of life is eminently "Western", and a large proportion of the inhabitants have been educated abroad. Here if anywhere the other extreme was to be sought. The area had been cut up into several not very populous districts (Nos. 9, 10, 12, 13, 18) and contained about 39000 persons in 7779 households. Our final sample drawn from it consisted of 364 persons, that drawn from the poor district of 576 persons, both together of 940 persons or roughly one third of the one per cent sample that had been our goal. For convenience' sake we shall speak of the large, generally poor district of the old city as the "lower" district and of the cluster of the generally better-off districts in the newer, university and residential area of the city as the "upper", avoiding designations such as "poor" and "rich" or "well-to-do" for reasons that will soon become apparent. It may be emphasized again that in all districts exactly the same sampling technique was used, the same size of sample proportionate to the population was drawn and the same indications for following up suspect cases by clinical examination were employed. In the lower and upper districts the second phase of the survey was carried out as thoroughly as possible, the aim being stratification based on topography, while in the remaining districts we were forced to limit ourselves to the first phase. As this phase delivered the indispensable data for standardization of the tests as well as a body of representative demographic information it was by no means fruitless.

When it became apparent towards the spring that we might not be able unassisted to complete the second phase even with the limitations just described, urgent representations made to the Ministry of Health resulted in sending two psychologists and a psychiatric Head Nurse to Shiraz for the ensuing months. These excellent collaborators assisted us with supervision, administration, testing and interviewing, lent a hand wherever it was needed and truly made it possible to bring the survey within its limited bounds to a satisfactory completion. Adding several new workers increased our need for transportation, the Health Department's car and driver pool was exhausted, and here we were helped out most generously by the WHO Nursing Education Project and by the Faculty of Arts and Sciences. We had checked forms, scored intelligence tests, inspected and roughly judged Z Tests as we went along besides performing and writing up our clinical examinations, but the time that had been allotted initially for evaluation toward the end of the project had been consumed by the delayed start and the lack of supporting staff, so that we were occupied with collection of data from the field literally until the last days spent in Shiraz. We departed on August 6, 1970, leaving copies of all records in the Psychiatric Policlinic of the Department of Public Health. The originals were shipped first to Tehran, then to our home in Bern, Switzerland. Since we had to take up our professional duties and practice immediately upon returning there and have been able to pursue the evaluation of our findings only in our spare time until the year at the Netherlands Institute for Advanced Study presented us with a priceless opportunity, it will be understood why the results are late in appearing.

Numerical data for total, sample and actual survey populations are presented together with similar data from other sites in Table D III 1 and in more detail in Tables B IV 1–2.

Long deferred though definitive publication has been, we endeavored soon after returning to Switzerland to evaluate, diagnose finally and categorize our pathological cases, reviewing once more all those which seemed to lie athwart the borderline and settling upon our ultimate decision how these were to be rubricated, with a view to preliminary communication. Comparison of prevalence rates in the lower and upper districts, our intended basis of stratification, led to the remarkable and statistically significant ($p < 0.01$) result that morbidity was higher in the upper districts (21.0 %) than in the lower (14.0 %). Though remarkable indeed, the conclusion came to us not altogether as a surprise, for field work had disclosed to us what the casual visitor, being driven mayhap to a host's comfortable home in Qasrodasht, does not see and not only we ourselves, but also our Shirazi friends had not fully realized when the stratified survey was planned: that the upper districts did in fact include a substantial portion of the financial means, the more prominent social positions and the higher education of Shiraz, all of them conspicuous to the eye, but also in back streets often just behind the villas with their park-like grounds and largely concealed by them a by no means inconsiderable number of poor houses, even wretched huts and hovels with a high population density. On the fringe of these upper districts and included in them were also two not particularly well-to-do villages that had lately been incorporated into the municipality and that presented a picture similar to that of its poorer central areas or even in part to that of our rustic villages of earlier surveys. On the ultimate fringe we discovered to our surprise, beside the bed of Shiraz's usually dry river and only a few minutes from the professorial villas of the Nemazee Hospital, a settlement of true gypsies (not nomads, with whom they are not to be confused) in huts of straw, cardboard and tin. It did not count as transient, had been included in the poliomyelitis campaign and had its huts numbered, so we duly sampled it, regretting that time did not allow us to give it the more thorough study it deserved. A counterpart was a shanty town of a kind that had sprung up in empty lots within the city. Its motley, non-gypsy population regarded any kind of intrusion with disfavor, but here too we succeeded in testing the household that the random number had allotted to us. It did not come within the psychiatric survey sample. It was evident that topographical stratification had played us a prank and that no reliable conclusions could be drawn from it. The conclusion that seemed to present itself was at variance with nearly all the findings of social psychiatry hitherto. This was not a reason to reject it, but there were plentiful grounds for regarding it with skepsis and examining its validity.

We had been in the habit of making brief, though unsystematic, notes about the socio-economic conditions of the households we visited in Shiraz and of recording many comments of our examiners, had visited ourselves not all, but a major share of all those who fell into the psychiatric survey sample (to exclude negative cases besides identifying and examining positive ones), still retained distinct recollections of most and were able to draw fairly probable conclusions as to socio-economic status from the data and comments available on the rest. We set ourselves therefore, regrettably remote from the field, to classify the households on the basis of our composite impression gathered from all the above indicators and any others we could summon socio-economically into three groups: the poor, the middle class and the comfortable or well-to-do. We found ourselves able to do this for all the households in the psychiatric survey sample and for the great majority of the rest. Separation between social and economic status seemed to us under the given conditions impossible, as it probably would have been even if we had had trained sociologists and economists to perform it. An Iranian family's means and income are closely guarded secrets, are said to be mirrored not without distortion in the equally secret tax lists, are hidden the more jealously for this very reason from inquiring persons, in or behind whom the tax collector is suspected and are certainly not to be uncovered by direct questioning, any attempt at which would have utterly destroyed the confidence on which our survey was based. We made judgments by appearances, well aware how delusive these can be, but also with eyes sharpened for signs that an investigator unfamiliar with Iranian society and manners of living might miss or evaluate differently. Those who are convinced without having explored the ground themselves that such subjective appraisals are worthless are at liberty to disregard them and will find everywhere data for the psychiatric survey population as a whole that are independent thereof. The dissatisfaction of the sociologists shares the company of our own. As will be shown in detail below, restratification by individual household status rather than by district boundaries reversed the former conclusion, again to a statistically significant degree.

The statuses that we tried to distinguish were, like the degrees of severity in illness, three in number. An attempt to differentiate more levels in either case, we felt, would have plunged us disproportionately deep into subjectivity. Medical realities seemed to call for three in regard to severity of illness if any attempt was to be made, as we had determined from the beginning to make it, to identify and enumerate more than the gravest, essentially incapacitating cases corresponding to our P_3. This can be done reasonably in very extensive, but less intensive surveys, the target of which is the major psychoses and the ruinous constitutional disorders. In occupations we have used the five-fold classification that has become internationally accepted. Theoretically we might have rested socio-economic grading upon the occupational level of the principal breadwinner, but meanwhile unexpected difficulties (to be discussed below) in the determination of this level had revealed themselves, while to our personal observation all too frequently the two levels failed to match. It was the extremes which it seemed possible to differentiate by the slender, unsystematic and subjective information we possessed: the poor on the one hand and the well-to-do or rich on the other (despite its awkwardness we retain generally the expression "well-to-do" since inclusion only of the "rich" would have made the class numerically very small and carried connotations that we wished to avoid. The German *vermögend* would convey much better our intentions, while all the English equivalents that suggest themselves such as "comfortably situated", "upper middle class" and the like are still more cumbersome than "well-to-do" or "well off". "Upper class" by itself again carries other, societal and traditional implications that would have been misleading.) "Poor" we took to mean that the household was at, below or very little above the subsistence level and, if above it, had not much assurance of being able to remain so. The wolf, if not at the door, was on the prowl nearby. Our "well-to-do" showed indications of being able without jeopardizing themselves to indulge in some comforts and even luxuries over and above the ordinary desires and needs of an Iranian who is not considered as poor by his fellow Iranians. There were some rich, a few very rich among them, but the majority of this group might have been reckoned elsewhere to the upper half of the middle class. This implies, of course, that most of our so called "medium" or "middle" group would have been assigned to the lower half of the middle class or even in some cases to the poor in an Anglo-European economy. It should not be forgotten that a middle class in every sense of that vague and encompassing word is for the most part new in Iran and still relatively small, though rapidly increasing and surely by the time of this book's publication larger than it was when the survey was performed.

2. Demography and Social Psychiatry

The first Iranian National Census was carried out in 1956. Others have followed at ten year intervals. The figures stated in the decennial census for the population of the City of Shiraz, the number of households comprising it and the mean number of persons per household are:

Census year	Population	Number of households	Mean persons per household
1956	170 659	no information	
1966	269 865	52 548	5.14
1976	425,813	86 769	4.91

Immediately the question presents itself how far our survey population, encompassing about one per cent of the total population six or more years old (cf. Table B IV 1a, b), was representative of this, and the same question arises for the Psychiatric Survey Population (PP) drawn from the Survey Population (SP) according to the considerations described in the preceding chapter. The answer cannot be derived from a comparison with the official census figures. In the relatively short period of about three years from the national census-taking to the enumeration of households for poliomyelitis immunization, on which our sampling was based, Shiraz, like most other Iranian cities, had undergone much growth and change. The household enumeration did not suffice to define them, for its goal, after identifying and counting as far as possible every household within the city limits, was merely to list all children of fourteen years or below, who would then be given the immunizing drops. Individual adults were not counted. At first query we were told that there were 64386 households, which, multiplied by the approximate factor of 5, would afford an estimate of 321930 persons.

Later the official figure was revised downwards to 62723 households. As we found in our Survey Population a mean of 5.75 persons of all ages per household, we can now multiply by this factor to obtain a new estimate of some 361000 total population in the city of Shiraz in the fall of 1969. This would correspond to a population increase of about 91000 persons in three years, which can be ascribed to several factors: natural growth, incorporation of some suburbs into the city and, as we then suspected more strongly than we do now, the migratory trend from the rural to the urban areas that prevails in most of Iran, though probably more to Tehran and Isfahan than to other cities. The increase of population by one third within a few years proves in any case that census figures from 1966 cannot be matched against sampling results from 1969. Neither is there any reason to assume that the composition of the population will have remained essentially the same, whereas there are several grounds such as the incorporation of suburbs already mentioned, generally increased mobility, the spread of literacy and education, the restructuring of rural economics through land reform, increase of industrialization, etc., to suspect that it has not. We shall see them reflected in our demographic data and must address ourselves anew to the question: how far are these representative for the city as a whole?

The reply to this depends largely on the thoroughness of the household enumeration performed by the Department of Public Health, on which we had two controls. The first was direct observation of the enumerators' and immunizers' work. We could accompany them several times in different parts of the city during the fall of 1969 and convinced ourselves that it was not superficial. Those who executed the actual registration were all public health staff members with years of experience, devotion to their job and understanding of its significance, as most of them had participated in such campaigns before and had witnessed their effectiveness in practically wiping out, within the city at least, such scourges as smallpox and trachoma. The immunizing drops were administered partly by the same young Health Corps members who were subsequently transferred to our survey. Their supervision, as we could see for ourselves, was thorough. Even so they were not responsible in the main for ferreting out the households and enumerating these and the children belonging to them. Secondly, since we had determined upon a strictly random sampling, we could again observe several months later that the search for the designated household numbers took us into every nook and corner of the city, from its wealthiest villas to its shanty-town slums, from the mountain side by the Qoran Gate down to the central bazars and across the valley in which Shiraz lies. From these observations we are little inclined to doubt the representativeness of our demographic findings even when they are at variance with the census of 1966 and with certain expectations.

A first overview of these findings is offered in Table B IV 1a, b. It shows the age and sex distributions of our Shiraz Survey Population (SP), representing a very nearly complete one per cent random sample of the entire municipal population aged six or more, of the Psychiatric Survey Population (PP), which is contained in the SP and constitutes about one-third of it, and finally of the pathological cases identified within the PP and abbreviated simply P. We list these three populations, each one to the right

Table B IV 1a. Population by Age and Sex

	Survey Population (SP)			Psychiatric Survey Population (PP)			Pathological cases (P)		
	m	f	m+f	m	f	m+f	m	f	m+f
	Absolute Numbers								
Age									
6	48	51	99	12	17	29	1	0	1
7	55	61	116	17	16	33	3	1	4
8	67	43	110	23	11	34	6	1	7
9	58	59	117	11	14	25	2	0	2
10	63	63	126	17	18	35	1	1	2
11	47	51	98	16	19	35	4	1	5
12	69	72	141	21	24	45	1	1	2
13	56	44	100	19	11	30	6	4	10
14	56	63	119	17	23	40	1	4	5
Sub-total children	519	507	1026	153	153	306	25	13	38
15–19	228	198	426	78	75	153	7	12	19
20–29	163	236	399	56	62	118	14	8	22
30–39	205	214	419	54	69	123	8	20	28
40–49	171	136	307	54	45	99	8	12	20
50–59	77	76	153	32	26	58	2	8	10
60–69	73	51	124	29	23	52	6	5	11
70+	29	31	60	11	8	19	2	4	6
Sub-total adults	946	942	1888	314	308	622	47	69	116
Total	1465	1449	2914	467	461	928	72	82	154

being contained in the foregoing one to the left, parallel to each other for easier comparison, with the percentages by age groups per column below them. Regarding the age groups in this table, some additional comment besides what has been offered in Chap. A IV is required. As the population is relatively large and single errors in the determination of age tend to cancel each other out, we present data here for single years from 6 to 14 and sum them together as "children". The five-year class 15–19 covers adolescence and corresponds to the culmination of the age-growth curve for test intelligence. Thereafter we have usually employed intervals of twenty years, wide though they are, for practical reasons as explained in the introductory chapters. In Tables B IV 1a, b age classes are constituted by decades from 20 on for the convenience of those who may wish to make their own calculations to different boundaries than ours. For brevity we shall recur in most subsequent tables to the larger intervals or simply compare "children" with "adults", it being understood that the former refers to ages 6–14 and the latter to all ages from 15 upward.

Though the PP is comprised in the SP, it is not necessarily a representative sample of this and was not designed to be one, but rather to accentuate its socio-economic extremes. It does not follow from this that the age and sex distribution must be the same or nearly so. Actually, though, the share of the sexes turns out to be identical in the SP and PP even to the decimal place for the two populations as wholes, and the variations between corresponding age groups are nowhere large.

Table B IV 1b. Population by Age and Sex

	Survey Population (SP)			Psychiatric Survey Population (PP)			Pathological cases (P)		
	m	f	m + f	m	f	m + f	m	f	m + f
	Percent by Column								
Age									
6	1.6	1.8	3.4	1.3	1.7	3.1	0.6	0	0.6
7	1.9	2.1	4.0	1.8	1.7	3.6	1.9	0.6	2.6
8	2.3	1.5	3.8	2.5	1.2	3.7	3.9	0.6	4.5
9	2.0	2.0	4.0	1.2	1.5	2.7	1.3	0	1.3
10	2.2	2.2	4.3	1.8	1.9	3.8	0.6	0.6	1.3
11	1.6	1.8	3.4	1.7	2.0	3.8	2.6	0.6	3.2
12	2.4	2.5	2.8	2.3	2.6	4.8	0.6	0.6	1.3
13	1.9	1.5	3.4	2.0	1.2	3.2	3.9	2.6	6.5
14	1.9	2.2	4.1	1.8	2.5	4.3	0.6	2.6	3.2
Sub-total children	17.8	17.4	35.2	16.5	16.5	33.0	16.2	8.4	24.7
15–19	7.8	6.8	14.6	8.4	8.1	16.5	4.5	7.8	12.3
20–29	5.6	8.1	13.7	6.0	6.7	12.7	9.1	5.2	14.3
30–39	7.1	7.3	14.4	5.8	7.4	13.2	5.2	13.0	18.2
40–49	5.9	4.7	10.6	5.8	4.8	10.7	5.2	7.8	13.0
50–59	2.6	2.6	5.2	3.4	2.8	6.2	1.3	5.2	6.5
60–69	2.5	1.7	4.3	3.1	2.5	5.6	3.9	3.2	7.1
70 +	1.0	1.1	2.1	1.2	0.8	2.0	1.3	2.6	3.9
Sub-total adults	32.5	32.3	64.8	33.8	49.7	67.0	30.5	44.8	75.3
Total	50.3	49.7	100.0	50.3	49.7	100.0	46.8	53.2	100.0

The distribution of the sexes in the City of Shiraz according to various criteria is as follows:

	m	f	m+f
Census 1966	142846	127019	269865
Census 1976	227757	198055	425812
Shiraz Survey	1465	1449	2914

The proportions of the sexes by age classes are shown in Table B IV 2 for the census of 1966 and the Shiraz Survey, but not for the census of 1976 because this does not present age-stratified data for the City of Shiraz alone, but only for urban and rural populations within the Ostan of Fars. As the "urban" comprise a number of secondary cities from which people were emigrating to Shiraz in the 1970's a direct comparison is not admissible.

The census figures show a male surplus almost throughout, which increases steadily up to the third decade and does so again in the fifth. The preponderance of females in the sixth seems to reflect Western experience that women on the whole live longer but is contradicted by a resurgence of male preponderance after 60. This is even more marked in the Shiraz Survey Population, and we have no ready explanation for it. For the steady male increase up to adulthood a grim explanation suggests itself that cannot

Table B IV 2. Proportions of the Sexes

Age	National Census of 1966 % m	% f	m:f	Shiraz Survey Population of 1970 % m	% f	m:f
< 5	50.3	49.7	101:100			
5–14	52.4	47.6	110:100	50.6[a]	49.4[a]	102:100[a]
15–19	53.7	46.3	116:100	53.5	46.5	115:100
20–29	55.0	45.0	122:100	40.8	59.2	69:100
30–39	53.0	47.0	113:100	49.9	51.1	96:100
40–49	57.5	42.5	135:100	55.7	44.3	126:100
50–59	46.8	53.2	88:100	50.3	49.7	101:100
60 +	51.4	48.6	106:100	55.4	44.6	124:100
All listed ages	59.9	47.1	112:100	50.3	49.7	101:100
	National Census of 1976					
All ages	53.5	46.5	115:100			

[a] The lower age limit of the Shiraz Survey Population is 6, not 5 years.

be rejected out of hand: girl children are less desired and, as repeated personal observations tend to confirm, often receive less care.

The figures from the Shiraz Survey agree with those from the census of 1966 roughly within the usual range. How large this can be we have seen in Khuzestan, and in districts of Shiraz that all fell into the Survey it could extend from 142:100 to 70:100. Nevertheless, they do not show a general male surplus, but on the contrary a rather striking female surplus in the decades of most active occupation from 20–29 and 30–39 such as hardly can be attributed to chance. At the time of our survey the tourist or casual visitor to Shiraz would rarely, but the resident inevitably notice that no few men, not all young, were to be encountered and at night literally stumbled over, curled up upon a scrap of carpet in a sheltering doorway, under counters, behind bales or quite simply on the curb, whose home for the time was nowhere, who neither constituted nor belonged to a household and therefore dropped through the meshes of the household census. This is not to imply that all watchmen, doorkeepers, assistants who sleep in a shop and the like belong to this partly amorphous category, but a number do. Neither does it include squatters, shantytown residents and inhabitants of the little gypsy settlement, all which were duly included in the polio immunization census and were visited personally by the authors. The young men we mean are, at least for the time, adrift, footloose, houseless and, as far as the city is concerned, homeless, though they may have a house and relations somewhere in the countryside. It is conceivable, though very difficult to prove, that just such men may constitute a large part of the apparently "missing", and that their being missed was an artefact of the method of enumeration. Be that as it may, we must draw upon the data we possess.

In the fifth decade the proportion of females drops sharply both in the census and the SP. One can hypothesize that the toll taken by childbirth in the past among the generation of women now entering that stage of life might play a part.

Agreement between the SP and PP in regard to sex ratios is gratifyingly close and enables us to take the latter, in this respect at least, as representative of the former.

Turning finally to the 154 pathological cases (P), 72 = 47 % were male and 82 = 53 % were female, the sex ratio being 88:100. The difference, when compared to the PP, is not remotely significant ($X^2 = 0.78$). This ratio lies close to that prevailing in all our Iranian surveys taken collectively, in which we find 46 % male and 54 % female cases with a sex ratio of 84:100 (cf. Chap. D III). The age distribution of the psychiatrically ill as compared to that of the larger samples is shifted to the advantage of the younger classes up to about age 30 and to the disadvantage of the elder.

Having established the similarity of the SP and PP in regard to such fundamental biological characteristics as sex and age, we direct our attention to a socially characteristic constituent of the PP: socio-economic status or SES. The PP was intended to embrace and emphasize its two extremes. For better statistical analysis of relations between SES and psychopathology, we no longer present figures for the PP as a whole, but for its unpathological and pathological members separately in Table B IV 3. (Figures for the whole PP can be obtained by simple addition. For the tables at least we have adopted the rather cumbersome headings "unpathological" and "pathological" in order to avoid the sometimes excessive implications of words like "healthy" and "sick" or "well" and "ill", though we shall have recourse to these simpler terms from time to time in the text and, where necessary, to keep table headings short. "Well" or "healthy" is then not intended to imply more than the absence of demonstrable psychopathology under the conditions of field study and by the methods described, while "ill" or "sick" implies no more than its presence.) Since both are contained in the SP, only limited comparisons can be drawn with it.

The first of these is a comparison between the unpathological of the PP and the SP with regard to SES. In the former both the poor and the well-to-do are more, the middle class less represented than in the SP. Far from falsifying the comparison, this confirms that our original, unsatisfactory attempt at topographical stratification did

Table B IV 3. Distribution of Populations by Socio-Economic Status, Sex and Pathology

	Shiraz Survey Population (SP)			Psychiatric Survey Population (PP)					
				Unpathological			Pathological		
	m	f	m+f	m	f	m+f	m	f	m+f
	Absolute Numbers								
Poor	616	609	1225	179	165	344	33	52	85
Middle	710	701	1411	161	161	322	27	24	51
Well-to-do	123	117	240	55	53	108	12	6	18
nc	16	22	38	0	0	0	0	0	0
Total	1465	1449	2914	395	379	774	72	82	154
	Percent by Column								
Poor	42.0	42.0	42.0	45.3	43.5	44.4	45.8	63.4	55.2
Middle	48.5	48.4	48.4	40.8	42.5	41.6	37.5	29.3	33.1
Well-to-do	8.4	8.1	8.2	13.9	14.0	14.0	16.7	7.3	11.7
nc	1.1	1.5	1.3	0	0	0	0	0	0
Percent of sex	50.3	49.7		51.0	49.0		46.8	53.2	

achieve one desired result: the accentuation of the socio-economic extremes referred to above. With this we are in a better position to investigate the relation between SES and psychiatric morbidity. The accentuation is increased among the pathological cases. There, for the sexes taken together, the middle class dwindles and the poor multiply. For a 3 x 2 table with 2 df X^2 =6.16 and $p < 0.05$. The difference becomes much more striking when we regard the sexes separately. The percentage of poor men is only a trifle higher among the pathological than among the unpathological, but the percentage of poor women soars: $X^2 = 4.24$ and $p < 0.05$. While sensible percentage sex differences do appear, with the share of the pathological middle class and well-to-do women dropping compensatorily to the increase of the poor females, the same fourfold X^2 comparison by sex and pathology or lack of it for the two better-off socio-economic classes yields no significance. Nevertheless, the fact that by percent of their sex only about half as many well-to-do females become pathological as remain free from pathology hardly can be disregarded and seems more likely to represent an artefact of the small numbers.

What is the marital status of these men and women? Table B IV 4 states this for the members of the Shiraz Survey Population who are 10 or more years old, i.e. of nubile age. The annual age classes from 10 to 14 are summed. Marriage below 15 is not infrequent in the country, but in the Shiraz Survey no male below 15 was recorded as married and only two females, one of 12 and another of 14 years. The table

Table B IV 4. Marital Status in the Shiraz Survey Population. Men and Women ≥ 10 years only

Age	Men Single	Marr.	Depr.	nc	Sum	Women Single	Marr.	Depr.	nc	Sum
	Absolute Numbers									
10–14	291	0	0	0	291	291	2	0	0	293
15–19	228	0	0	0	228	129	63	6	0	198
20–39	105	258	4	1	368	46	390	14	0	450
40–59	4	240	3	1	248	4	149	56	3	212
60 +	1	94	5	2	102	0	15	67	0	82
Total	629	592	12	4	1237	470	619	143	3	1235
	Percent by Column									
10–14	46.3	0	0		23.5	62.0	0.4	0		23.7
15–19	36.2	0	0		18.4	27.4	10.2	4.2		16.0
20–39	16.7	43.6	33.3		29.7	9.8	63.0	9.8		36.4
40–59	0.6	40.5	25.0		20.0	0.8	24.1	39.2		17.2
60 +	0.2	15.9	41.7		8.2	0.0	2.4	46.8		6.6
	Percent by Row									
15–19	100.0	0	0		53.5	65.2	31.8	3.0	0	46.5
20–39	28.5	70.1	1.1	0.3	45.0	10.2	86.7	3.1	0	55.0
40–59	1.6	96.8	1.2	0.4	53.9	1.9	70.3	26.4	1.4	46.1
60 +	1.0	92.1	4.9	2.0	55.4	0.0	18.3	81.7	0	44.6
Total	50.8	47.9	1.0	0.3		38.1	50.1	11.6		

Key: Marr. = married; Depr. = maritally deprived, i. e. widowed, divorced, separated; nc = not classified or not known.

demonstrates with all clarity the tendency of the young women to marry much earlier than their husbands. At 19 years of age 32 % of the girls, but (at least officially) none of the youths are espoused. By forty, more than 70 % of the men are married, but 86.7 % of the women, and for these deprivation from the husband by separation, divorce or widowhood already has appreciably begun. By the time they are sixty, over a quarter of them are so deprived, whereas the percentage for the men is only 1.2. The age disparity, with consequent early widowhood for the wife, accounts for this in large part, but not wholly. Though divorce is not rare, it is not fully reflected in our data, for many divorced as well as widowed men remarry, while divorced women find it harder to do so.

In Table B IV 5 such data from Table B IV 4 as bear upon the Psychiatric Survey Population are extracted, divided into the unpathological and pathological and classified by socio-economic status rather than by age, for the sexes separately. Turning to the men first, we observe that the distribution of marital status for all SES together is practically the same in the SP and the unpathological PP. Everywhere the number of the deprived is so small as to render it unsuitable for statistical treatment, and the like holds in mitigated degree for the well-to-do. In the PP we are reduced mainly to comparing the single and married poor and middle-class males. It strikes the eye that the single poor and the married middle-class seem relatively more numerous among the pathological, whereas the married poor and the single middle-class seem relatively more frequent among the unpathological. By X^2 tests, however, the differences are not significant. Among the women, the shares of the single and married unpathological again agree well with those in the SP, and the share of the deprived becomes substantial. The percentages of both single and married pathological women among the poor are higher, among the middle class lower than among the unpathological, confirming the female excess among the pathological poor already demonstrated in Table B IV 3. The finding is not new, but leads to the question as to what role marital deprivation, to which women in Iranian culture are far more subject than men, may play in the prevalence of psychiatric disorder among females. A comparison of the deprivation rates in pathological males (5.0 %) and pathological females (20.0 %) sustains 2.56 times its standard deviation and is thus highly significant ($p < 0.013$). When unpathological and pathological married and maritally deprived females are compared alone, X^2 comes to 4.083 and $p < 0.05$. Marital deprivation among women thus does appear to play a significant part. What are its causes? Reference is made frequently to divorce, but this appears seldom in our statistics. Taking pathological and unpathological subjects together, we find that out of 8 maritally deprived men 2 are widowed, 3 divorced and 3 separated. Widowhood among women thus far overshadows all other causes, as may be expected from the data on age and marital status in Table B IV 4.

Table B IV 6 describes numerically the issue of the marriages with which we have just been concerned. It is limited to the PP for reasons that will be elaborated in connection with the next table regarding family size, and it is also limited, as are the preceding tables regarding marital status, to females ten or more years old. Any girl of ten or above was taken for statistical purposes as a potential mother without heed to whether she had menstruated or not, because information on menstruation, as we shall see, proved exceedingly difficult to procure under the circumstances and unreliable when it was recorded. Furthermore, a girl who has already menstruated at ten is

Table B IV 5. Marital and Socio-Economic Status of Marriageable Persons (from 10 Years Upward) in the Shiraz Psychiatric Survey Population

	Unpathological					Pathological			
	Single	Marr.	Depr.	nc	Sum	Single	Marr.	Depr.	Sum
MEN	*Absolute Numbers*								
Poor	67	80	4	0	151	16	10	2	28
Middle	72	68	1	2	143	9	12	1	22
Well-to-do	29	21	0	0	50	4	6	0	10
Total	168	169	5	2	344	29	28	3	60
	Percent by Column								
Poor	39.9	47.3	80.0		43.9	55.2	35.7	66.7	47.7
Middle	42.9	40.2	20.0		41.6	31.0	42.9	33.3	36.7
Well-to-do	17.2	12.5	0		14.5	13.8	21.4	0	16.6
	Percent by Row								
Poor	44.4	53.0	2.6	0	100.0	57.2	35.7	7.1	100.0
Middle	50.3	47.6	0.6	1.3	100.0	41.0	54.5	4.5	100.0
Well-to-do	58.0	42.0	0	0	100.0	40.0	60.0	0	100.0
Total	48.8	49.1	1.5	0.6	100.0	48.3	46.7	5.0	100.0
WOMEN	*Absolute Numbers*								
Poor	51	71	17	1	142	12	29	9	50
Middle	49	77	8	0	134	5	12	7	24
Well-to-do	21	23	3	0	47	2	4	0	6
Total	123	171	28	1	323	19	45	16	80
	Percent by Column								
Poor	43.1	41.5	60.7		44.0	63.2	64.4	56.2	62.5
Middle	39.8	45.0	28.6		41.5	26.3	26.7	43.8	30.0
Well-to-do	17.1	13.5	10.7		14.5	10.5	8.9	0	7.5
	Percent by Row								
Poor	37.3	50.0	12.0	0.7	100.0	24.0	58.0	18.0	100.0
Middle	36.6	57.5	5.9	0	100.0	20.8	50.0	29.2	100.0
Well-to-do	44.7	48.9	6.4	0	100.0	33.3	66.7	0	100.0
Total	38.1	52.9	8.7	0.3	100.0	23.8	56.2	20.0	100.0

Key: Marr. = married; Depr. = maritally deprived, i. e. widowed, divorced, separated; nc = not classified or not known.

unlikely to give birth before she has become eleven, but for the reason mentioned it was practically impossible to take statistical account of this natural circumstance. We have perpetrated a conscious simplification, therefore, by placing all females over nine into one class as candidates for immediate maternity. The division into unpathological and pathological has been retained, and for convenience the combined data are also presented for the over nine year old females of the PP as a whole.

In many cases the desired information could not be obtained, as is evident from the number rubricated "not known". The principal reason was not objection or reluctance,

Table B IV 6. Marital and Socio-Economic Status of Marriageable Women in the Psychiatric Survey Population (Females from 10 Years Upward)

	Unpathological Single	Marr.	Depr.	nc	Sum	Pathological Single	Marr.	Depr.	Sum
	Absolute Numbers								
Poor	53	71	17	1	142	12	29	9	50
Middle	49	77	8	0	134	5	12	7	24
Well-to-do	21	23	3	0	47	2	4	0	6
Total	123	171	28	1	323	19	45	16	80
	Percent by Column								
Poor	43.1	41.5	60.7		44.0	63.2	64.4	56.2	62.5
Middle	39.8	45.0	28.6		41.5	26.3	26.7	43.8	30.0
Well-to-do	17.1	13.5	10.7		14.5	10.5	8.9	0	7.5
	Percent by Row								
Poor	37.3	50.0	12.0	0.7		24.0	58.0	18.0	
Middle	36.6	57.5	5.9	0		20.8	50.0	29.2	
Well-to-do	44.7	48.9	6.4	0		33.3	66.7	0	
Total	38.1	52.9	8.7	0.3		23.8	56.2	20.0	

Key: Marr. = married; Depr. = maritally deprived (widowed, divorced, separated); nc = not classified or not known.

but the circumstance of the survey that such information not seldom had to be requested from informants other than the woman herself. When the informant was a male relative or e.g. an aunt, niece or the like, the information was frequently faulty or wanting. Unless there was ground to suspect pathology in the woman she was not pursued further, as the collection of such data was not the main purpose of the survey and would have entailed an expenditure of time and resources that we could not afford. Elder women in particular usually had experienced a number of abortions and still-births and had trouble in remembering the number of children actually born alive. First attempts to gather information about the number of miscarriages were abandoned for these very reasons. That confusion with miscarriage etc. was a minor factor, however, may be concluded from the fact that the number of living children is unknown in only slightly fewer cases than the number of live-born.

The results as reported in Table B IV 7, strike one at first as almost disappointing in their uniformity. Of the differential fertility usually reported in Western studies there is hardly a trace, whether the difference be sought in the SES or in the presence or absence of psychopathology. The mean number of live births lies in nearly all groups between 4.3 and 4.6. The two where it does not are so small and so subject to the influence of chance that the apparent deviations are meaningless. In the middle-class group of pathological females two sets of more than ten live births drove the rate up. The well-to-do pathological group counted only six mothers. The like holds for the number of living children, which lies between 3.4 and 3.7 with the same two exceptions. Thus in Shiraz, as far as our findings go, neither the poor nor the pathological, and especially not the pathological poor, are more fertile or lose more children, as is

Table B IV 7. Number of Live-Born and Still Living Children per Woman: Psychiatric Survey Population (Females from 10 Upward Only)

SES	No. of women	Live-born children	Births per woman	No. of women	Living children	Living child. per woman
Unpathological Females						
Poor	86	384	4.47	86	301	3.50
Middle	77	331	4.30	83	288	3.47
Well-to-do	22	101	4.59	27	100	3.70
Subtotal	185	816	4.42	196	689	3.52
Not kown	138			127		
Total	323			323		
Pathological Females						
Poor	36	155	4.31	38	134	3.53
Middle	18	95	5.28	18	87	4.83
Well-to-do	6	17	2.83	6	14	2.33
Subtotal	60	267	4.45	62	235	3.79
Not kown	20			18		
Total	80[a]			80[a]		
Unpathological and Pathological Females						
Poor	122	539	4.42	124	419	3.38
Middle	95	426	4.48	101	375	3.71
Well-to-do	28	118	4.21	33	114	3.45
Subtotal	245	1083	4.42	258	908	3.52
Not kown	158			145		
Total	403			403		

[a] Not identical with the number of female cases from the total PP (82) because two cases were below the age of ten years.

commonly reported in surveys from Western countries. There is some indication nevertheless that this situation may have been changing at the very time of the survey. While we gave up inquiring about abortions and still-births and about menstrual status generally because the youth, inexperience and sometimes shyness of our female Health Corps examiners all too often warped or left gaps in the information, we did inquire about pregnancy and lactation. Here, too, many cases had to be designated "unknown", but from the rest emerged a remarkably consistent pattern: a negative correlation between the proportions of women involved at the time in gestational processes and the SES of these same women, as can be read from the condensed Table B IV 8.

Table B IV 8. Gestating Women ≥ 10 Years by SES

	Poor	Middle	Well-to-do	Total (= 1128)
Pregnant	4.3 %	2.1 %	1.1 %	3.0 %
Lactating	4.8	2.7	3.2	3.5

The actual size of families and their distribution by numbers of members are shown in Table B IV 9 for the PP only, here subdivided into families without pathological members and families with such. A comparison with the SP was intended but proved unfeasible. Our coding system was based on the enumeration of households, but there could be several families in one household. Attempts to distinguish between households and families by mechanical sorting turned out so unsatisfactorily that we were forced to resort to a hand count, the execution of which for the entire SP we felt to be excessively time-consuming. It has been performed and repeatedly checked for internal and external consistency for families, numbers of live-born children and of living children in the PP. Such a count of children was unavoidable, as there might be and sometimes were two or more mothers in one household. Mechanical count led to 613 households in the SP against our 629 family dossiers, and to 198 households in the PP against our 205. The discrepancy, though not large, was far from negligible. We were interested first in any relations that might be discovered between family size, SES, and pathology, then in the calculation of the true size of the PP and its pathological sector. This could be performed by multiplying the number of families of a given size by the number of members of all ages from the newborn upward and summing the products, as has been done in Table B IV 9. Here discrepancies by a few, especially large families (the largest was 14) could affect the sum greatly. The total of 1178 persons given for the PP in Table B IV 9 is naturally larger than the total of 928 persons under psychiatric

Table B IV 9. Sizes of Families of Psychiatric Survey Population (Members of All Ages Included)

No. of members	All Families		Families without pathological members		Families with pathological memb.	
	No. of fam.	per 100 families	No. of fam.	per 100 families	No. of fam.	per 100 families
1	4	1.9	3	2.7	1	1.1
2	17	8.3	13	11.8	4	4.2
3	25	12.2	11	10.0	14	14.7
4	23	11.2	14	12.7	9	9.5
5	29	14.1	19	17.3	10	10.5
6	37	18.0	22	20.0	15	15.8
7	20	9.7	7	6.4	13	13.7
8	18	8.8	9	8.2	9	9.5
9	15	7.3	6	5.4	9	9.5
10	10	4.9	4	3.6	6	6.3
11	3	1.5	1	0.9	2	2.1
12	1	0.5	0	0	1	1.1
13	0	0	0	0	0	0
14	3	1.5	1	0.9	2	2.1
Total fam.	205	100	110	100	95	100
Total memb.	1178		585		593	
Mean memb. per fam.	5.75 ± 2.62		5.32 ± 2.51		6.24 ± 2.71	
			D = 0.92			
			$SD_D = 0.369$			
			$D/SD_D = 2.49$			

Table B IV 10. Shiraz Survey Population: Relation of Family Members to Head of Household

	Number	per 100
Self	617	21.2
Spouse	562	19.2
Child	1480	50.8
Subtotal	2659	91.3
Parent	81	2.8
Parent-in-law	19	0.7
Sibling	50	1.7
Servant	28	1.0
Other	75	2.6
Subtotal	253	8.7
nc	2	0.1
Total	2914	100

scrutiny given in other tables because it includes children below six. They constitute 18 % of the total population corresponding to the PP (cf. Table D III 1, Chap. D III).

Families with pathological members are larger than those without, the median for the latter being 5, for the former 6 persons. The difference between the means is 0.92 and is statistically significant ($D/SD_D = 2.49$, $p < 0.01$). In good agreement with this is the finding that the 154 pathological persons identified in the PP are distributed over only 95 families, or 1.6 to a family. The tendency to cluster that we remarked in the field is confirmed by numerical analysis. Certain families seem to breed pathology, whether we regard this breeding as a genetic or environmental process or a combination of both [175]. It is perhaps worthy of note also that of 17 families in the PP with 10 or more members each, 11 contain pathological members and only 6 do not, although the total number of members in both groups of families is roughly equal.

The rather large mean of 5.75 members per family contrasts with the mean of 5.13 calculated from the census of 1966 but harmonizes well with the mean number of living children per woman, 3.52, when the two parents are added to this number on the presumption that they are both alive, giving a sum of 5.52. The remaining difference is accounted for easily by other family members, servants, etc., the share of whom can be read from Table B IV 10. It amounts to about 9 %, which when added to 5.52 gives just over 6 persons per household. The difference between the estimated figure of 6.02 and the empirical one of 5.75 can be explained by the fact that not always both parents are alive or are actually members of the household and by the occasional doubling of families in households, to which reference has been made above. The amount of parent loss appears in Table B IV 11. It does not vary substantially by SES, and the number of full orphans among the children is happily lower than might be anticipated.

Returning to the families and their SES as shown now in Table B IV 12, it is reassuring to observe in the upper half of the table, which takes account of residence, confirmation that our attempt at topographical stratification was not in vain. The share of poor families in poor districts is definitely higher than in the non-poor districts, as is that of the well-to-do families in the non-poor districts, while the percentage of middle class families is about equal in both. Of more immediate interest to us is the relation

Table B IV 11. Orphanism in Shiraz Survey Population

SES	Children: Both parents alive	Children: One parent dead	Children: Both parents dead	Adults: One parent dead	Adults: Both parents dead	nc	Total
	Absolute Numbers						
Poor	689	13	0	178	197	148	1225
Middle	731	24	4	242	190	220	1411
Well-to-do	131	3	0	36	36	34	240
Not class.	15	1	0	10	4	8	38
Total	1566	41	4	466	427	410	2914
	Percent by Row						
Poor	56.2	1.1	0.0	14.5	16.1	12.1	100
Middle	51.8	1.7	0.3	17.2	13.5	15.6	100
Well-to-do	54.6	1.2	0.0	15.0	15.0	14.2	100
Total	53.7	1.4	0.1	16.0	14.7	14.1	100

between families with pathological members and poverty. Of families with pathological members 57 % are poor, of those without such members "only" 42 %. Compensation occurs almost wholly in the middle class, the difference in percentages of well-to-do families being trifling. Adding the middle class to the well-to-do as before to form a class of the non-poor permits the construction of a convenient four-fold table, from which a $X^2 = 4.02$ is calculated. Thus the association between poverty and families with pathological members proves to be significant with $p < 0.05$.

Data so far suggest that the poor are more afflicted by psychiatric illness than the better-off, and it now becomes necessary to ascertain the prevalence rates for the PP as a whole and for the three SES constituting it. In order to avoid duplication of tables we introduce here also the degrees of severity of disorder as defined in Chap. A III and already applied to other surveys. The results are given in Table B IV 13, where the prevalence rates appear under "Percent by Row". Quoting now by rates per thousand rather than per hundred in order to eliminate the inconvenient decimal, we note a total psychiatric prevalence rate for the Shiraz Psychiatric Survey Population of 166 per 1000. This appears higher than the rate of 149 per 1000 in Khuzestan, but the difference

Table B IV 12. Socio-Economic Status of Families in Psychiatric Survey Population

	Absolute Numbers: Poor	Mid.	WTD	Tot.	Percent by Row: Poor	Mid.	WTD	Tot.
In poor districts	71	49	2	122	58	40	2	100
In non-poor districts	29	31	23	83	35	37	28	100
Total	100	80	25	205	49	39	12	100
Without path. members	46	50	14	110	42	45	13	100
With pathol. members	54	30	11	95	57	32	11	100
Total	100	80	25	205	49	39	12	100

Key: Mid. = middle class; WTD = well-to-do.

Table B IV 13. Distribution of Psychiatric Cases by Socio-Economic Status and by Degrees of Severity

SES	Psych. Survey Pop. (PP)	Unpath.	P_1	P_2	P_3	All path. (P)
	Absolute Numbers					
Poor	429	344	42	37	6	85
Middle	373	322	30	19	2	51
Well-to-do	126	108	8	7	3	18
Total	928	774	80	63	11	154
	Percent by Column					
Poor	46.2	44.4	52.5	58.7	54.5	55.2
Middle	40.2	41.6	37.5	30.2	18.2	33.1
Well-to-do	13.6	14.0	10.0	11.1	27.3	11.7
Total	100	100	100	100	100	100
	Percent by Row					
Poor	100	80.2	9.8	8.6	1.4	19.8
Middle	100	86.3	8.0	5.1	0.5	13.6
Well-to-do	100	85.7	6.3	5.6	2.4	14.3
Total	100	83.4	8.6	6.8	1.2	16.6
Sum of $P_2 + P_3$ = 74 cases = 8.0 % of 928						
	Percent by Row of Pathological Cases Only					
Poor			49.4	43.5	7.0	100
Middle			58.8	37.3	3.9	100
Well-to-do			44.4	38.9	16.7	100
Total			52.0	40.9	7.1	100

is not statistically significant by the X^2 test. The rate of 80 per 1000 for the middle and severe degrees of psychiatric illness taken together lies very near to that found in Khuzestan (72 per 1000) and in Marvdasht (71 per 1000). As the number of milder cases diagnosed in Marvdasht is certainly too low and reflects itself in the total prevalence rate, we do not compare either with the corresponding rates for Shiraz.

The higher morbidity of the poor as compared to both the middle class and the well-to-do strikes the eye immediately. Using the X^2 test and fourfold tables, it proves to be statistically significant as compared both with the middle class alone ($p < 0.05$) and the sum of the non-poor (middle and well-to-do: $p < 0.02$), all three degrees of severity being taken together. So does the striking difference in P_2 ($p < 0.05$), the cases of medium severity. The difference in the mild cases (P_1) alone is not significant. Measures of significance were not calculated for the severe cases (P_3) by themselves because of the small numbers, apparent differences being due in all likelihood to chance. No significant differences emerge between the middle class and the well-to-do, nor do they between the poor and well-to-do, presumably because of the small numbers in the latter group (for total morbidity significance is suggested with $p < 0.2$). We can conclude thus that *total psychiatric morbidity* and morbidity of medium (in all likelihood including severe) degree is *significantly higher among the poor* in the Shiraz Psychiatric Survey Population, whereas a significant difference between the middle class and the well-to-do cannot be demonstrated.

One would then like to know whether the poor are not only more afflicted in number, but also in degree. Disregarding again the rates for P_3 based on too small numbers, it would appear from the percentages by column that a larger share of the P_2 cases falls to the poor than to the non-poor, and the like manifests itself in the percentages by row, where 8.6 % of the poor belong to P_2, but only 5.1 % of the middle class and 5.6 % of the well-to-do. We have therefore calculated the percentages by row of the pathological cases only and find confirmed afresh that the poor have the largest proportion per 100 (43.5) of P_2. Nevertheless, these differences do not stand any test of statistical significance and indeed are remote from such, so that no conclusive answer can be given to the question raised.

These conclusions take no regard to the subjects' residence and environment, i.e. to the topographical stratification with which we had begun and which led to paradoxical conclusions, but none the less to interesting results. The "poor" district was in fact predominantly, though not exclusively poor, as the fact indicates that 305 out of 429 poor subjects and 71 out of 100 poor families resided in it. The other, supposedly upper class districts were far more mixed, did include a large proportion of the more comfortable and wealthier houses in Shiraz, but also hovels and mean alleys behind them, middle class and small business areas and also some truly poor ones, these being mostly on the periphery of the city and corresponding to two villages of predominantly rural character recently incorporated into it. Since our psychiatric survey population had now become stratified in two ways, by only partially representative topography and by what we hoped was an approximation to real socio-economic status, it became a point of interest to inquire whether the type of surroundings had any relation to prevalence of psychiatric disorder within a given socio-economic class[1], the expectation being that it might have, especially for such of the poor as were directly confronted with a more prosperous environment in which they had no share. We therefore classified our poor, middle class and well-to-do subjects in Table B IV 14 according to whether they lived in a poor district or in one of those that we had assumed at the outset to be better off, although, as pointed out, these latter were not actually homogeneous.

The members of each of the three socio-economic classes were further classified within each type of residential district according to absence or presence and, if present, according to severity of psychopathology. As the last classification led to excessively small sub-groups, prevalence rates were finally calculated by class of subject and district for total pathology only. From Table B IV 14 we see that the poor, contrary to expectation, have practically identical prevalence rates whether they live in poor or generally more prosperous surroundings. On the other hand the prevalence among middle class subjects in middle class and well-to-do districts turns out to be three times as high as that among middle class subjects in poor districts ($p < 0.001$) and higher than any other prevalence rate to be found in the table. Being in doubt as to what the situation among the truly well-to-do might be, we kept this smaller group separate instead of combining it with the middle class as our first results had suggested and found a difference in the same direction, but one that could not be verified statistically because of the small numbers, particularly of the well-to-do in poor districts. Not

[1] Following a suggestion of Prof. A. Stinchcombe of NIAS and the University of California, for which we thank him.

Table B IV 14. Prevalence of Psychopathology by Residence and Socio-Economic Status

Residence	Well	P_1	P_2	Ill P_3	P	Well + Ill	χ^2 well : ill	
Poor Subjects								
Poor districts	245	31	24	5	60 = 19.7 % of	305	0.0	ns
Non-poor districts	99	11	13	1	25 = 20.2 % of	124		
Middle Class Subjects								
Poor districts	227	11	7	1	19 = 7.7 % of	246	20.21	$p < 0.001$
Non-poor districts	95	19	12	1	32 = 25.2 % of	127		
Well-to-do Subjects								
Poor districts	14	1	0	0	1 = 6.7 % of	15	0.26	ns
Non-poor districts	94	7	7	3	17 = 15.3 % of	111		
All Subjects								
Poor	344	42	37	6	85 = 19.8 % of	429	4.92	$p < 0.05$
Middle Class	322	30	19	2	51 = 13.7 % of	373	0.0	ns
Well-to-do	108	8	7	3	18 = 14.3 % of	126		
All SES	774	80	63	11	154 = 16.6 % of	928		

χ^2 for all subjects poor: well-to-do : : well:ill = 1.62 ns

significant was the difference between the middle class in non-poor districts and the poor in either kind of environment.

It is commonly suspected that psychiatric morbidity is greater where socio-economic statuses clash, where wealth so to speak is flaunted in the face of poverty, but the present findings do not appear so far to support this for Shiraz. The poor do suffer more psychiatric disorder than the non-poor, but they suffer it, so far as our results go, wherever they live – among themselves or at the foot of the tables of the rich. It is difficult here not to invoke the age-old and not yet wholly dissipated Islamic view of poverty as fate or the Will of Allah, before which man must bow. Also, in Islamic countries no stigma or disgrace attaches to poverty. Modern Western welfare states would vehemently protest that it no more does there either, but the times when it did are not long gone, and one may be permitted to ask whether, in bitterly competitive economies, they are really gone at all. On the other hand whole living generations in Iran have grown up with no other thought than that poverty had to be endured like drought, locusts, malaria and other "natural" ills and have felt themselves separated from the better-off by such an unbridgeable gap that it was inconsequential whether this yawned up the street or at their door. It is hardly necessary to add that this attitude is changing swiftly.

Somerset Maugham, who knew the poor of London, for a time shared their poverty himself by dour necessity and told of them as few since Dickens have done, wrote pertinently in *Of Human Bondage* [136, p. 866]: "Philip learned how little there was in common between the poor and the classes above them. They did not envy their betters, for the life was too different, and they had an ideal of ease which made the existence of the middle classes seem formal and stiff; moreover, they had a certain contempt for them because they were soft and did not work with their hands. The proud merely wished to be let alone, but the majority looked upon the well-to-do as people to be exploited; they knew what to say in order to get such advantage as the charitable put at their disposal, and they accepted benefits as a right which came to them from the folly of their superiors and their own astuteness."

What, then, of the middle class? Among the poor they are the non-poor, even the favored. Living in the better districts, they are constrained to measure themselves against their social and economic peers and against the really well-to-do, even the rich. The fatalistic attitude that yet may reign among a number of the poor cannot be theirs. They are moving up on the whole, and they wish presumably to move higher and faster. Especially in rapidly changing societies such as the contemporary Iranian there is no longer any conventional upper limit for the ordinary man's striving, no level at which he may tacitly come to rest and feel that he and his family have attained their place. To a certain degree this is of course true for all open societies, but it would seem to be both more marked and more perilous in such as are undergoing a swift economic expansion. We can suspect, but only suspect, that for this reason mainly the middle class, where set voluntarily or involuntarily in competition with their equals, rivals and superiors, are more subject to psychiatric disturbances (which, be it noted, does not hold for the middle class as a whole).

We have striven to delve deeper into this question by inquiring whether the middle class display a different pattern of disorder according to the type of their environment. They might, for example, show more reactive disorders in general, more depressions in particular, in surroundings that forced them into competition or conflict rather than in surroundings over which they had demonstrated their ascendency. This does not prove to be the case. Neither the distribution of the main categories of psychiatric illness (symptomatic psychoses and residual states, reactive disorders and constitutional disorders, the functional psychoses being omitted here because they are so sparingly represented in comparison to the rest and afford contents of cells that are zero or close to zero) nor that of the three principal sub-groups of reactive disorders (simple, neurotic and psychosomatic) shows a statistically significant difference between the middle class in the poor and the non-poor areas according to X^2 tables with 3 x 2 cells and 2 df. Nevertheless, as we have observed above, the middle class in a concordant, middle to upper class environment exhibit a very significantly higher over-all psychiatric morbidity rate than in a discordant (poor) environment, while the poor show no such difference. This would accord well with the hypothesis that the poor had either given up or never taken up the fight, while the middle class among themselves were tenaciously engaged in it.

Instead of calculating expectancies in the standard manner by X^2 tables of n x 2 dimensions, in which both columns to be compared enter proportionally to their sums, one can take as the "normal" case a group living in its concordant environment and calculate therefrom the expectation for a corresponding group in a discordant environment. When we do so for the poor we observe that those in a better environment exhibit a rather striking surplus of symptomatic disorders (9 observed against 4 expected), only slightly less reactive and constitutional disturbances than expected, and no functional psychoses (3 observed in the concordant environment with an expectation of 1 in the discordant). Expectancies for the middle class estimated by the same priciple turn out to be rather similar inasmuch as there are more symptomatic cases in discordant environments (7 observed, 4 expected), the difference being made up by somewhat fewer reactive cases (10 observed, 14 expected), while observation and expectation agree in regard to the constitutional disorders (2 cases in discordant, 3 in concordant environments). Turning to the three types of reactive disorder we find no noteworthy discrepancies among the middle class. Among the poor living in a non-poor environment the number of simple developments corresponds to expectation (3 cases). There are less neurotic disturbances (5 observed, 8 expected), but more psychosomatic cases (4 observed, 1 expected). Though the differences are numerically not great and ill suited for calculations of significance, they give food for thought. Upon superficial consideration one might anticipate a surplus of simple, probably depressive developments in the poor dwelling among the better off, but this resolves itself into an excess of psychosomatic cases instead. Assuming again that psychosomatic illness rests essentially upon a mechanism of double repression, this agrees as above with the hypothesis that the poor were either not engaged in the struggle (hence few simple developments) or sternly repressed it.

Harder to explain is why, in more prosperous surroundings, both the poor and the middle class exhibit more and not less symptomatic disorders. As bad hygiene usually goes with poverty and in Shiraz certainly does so, one would expect rather the reverse. The answer cannot be reached by statistical manipulation or conjecture. When we compare the frequencies of seven single diagnoses (not groups of diagnoses, cf. Table B IV 31) under the heading of symptomatic psychoses and residual states according to socio-economic status (two-fold) and environment (also two-fold), only one of the resulting 28 cells contains more than 3 subjects. Its column is that of the poor in non-poor districts, its row is that of the post-infectious cerebral disorders, and the number of subjects in it is six. To this can be added one further post-infectious case: a middle class subject in a concordant environment. When we look at these cases individually, it turns out that every one of the six, though resident in a better-class district, actually lives under very poor to outright slum conditions, several in the newly incorporated peripheral area of the city already mentioned, and that two of them even belong to the same poverty-stricken family in a most unsanitary hut. In the seventh case, though the family was not badly situated and lived in a middle class neighborhood, the house was memorable for its dirt and disorder. In sum: topography has again played us a trick, and the six poor post-infectious cases found in supposedly better areas were one and all living in a familial environment that had to be classed as poor to wretched, as was the one middle class case also. A four-fold table comprising only the poor in Shiraz and comparing them by their residential environment on the one hand, by the presence of a symptomatic, residual psychiatric disorder or of any other psychiatric disorder on the other, gives a X^2 value of 2.77, so that the level of confidence lies between 10 % and 5 %. The circumstances just described, however, atone for any numerical deficit in confidence. This leaves us with a final question: why did we not find any cases of post-infectious residue among the residents of the poor district, whether the residents themselves were poor or not? Since we encountered them in other districts, we can hardly suppose we were blind to them there, and it is equally difficult to imagine that they simply did not occur. It is well to look now to the village populations, which were generally poor and lived almost without exception under very unsanitary circumstances. In Marvdasht we found no post-infectious case, in Khuzestan only two, i.e. roughly 2 per 1000 among a poor population living in a poor environment in which infectious diseases of every kind were or at least had been rife.

The rate is remarkably low, as it is among the correspondingly situated group in Shiraz. Mere chance becomes an improbable explanation when we consider the agreement between the three surveys, and we find ourselves forced back upon the suspicion that had already arisen in the nomad camp: that the victims did not survive. In the relatively more favored districts of the city there may be more opportunity for the poor and also more social pressure upon them to seek aid, receive treatment and, e.g., keep a childhood victim of meningo-encephalitis alive. This is not to belittle the free medical care that the Department of Public Health provides to the truly poor areas of Shiraz, to which it is immediately adjacent, but it is meant to suggest that the motivation to seek and take advantage of such help may not be the same in sociologically diverse areas and that in such a category of cases influence of the wider may even prevail over that of the narrower, familial environment by such a simple circumstance as a more understanding neighbor adjuring: "Get your child to a doctor!" The post-infectious cases were mostly residues from childhood. Where the poor flock together there is an observable tendency, however bitterly a child's illness may be bewailed, to accept it as an unavoidable stroke of fate – a tendency that diminishes as the congregation of poverty thins and different attidudes, ideas and examples begin to infiltrate. We can scarcely bring a final proof of the above hypothesis from this material, but it does seem to agree with the available findings and to be contradicted by none of them.

Where do the patients come from, and is there any relation between their origins and their socio-economic status? Table B IV 15 offers the relevant iformation. Its categories of origin are somewhat simplified from the original seven to four. Only eight persons in the SP were of nomadic birth: they have been classified with the villagers of Fars Province. Three further categories, villages outside Fars, cities outside Fars and Tehran, have been condensed into a single one ("outside Fars") because of the small numbers in each.

When we compare the unpathological by column, we see that the percentage of born Shirazis hardly varies from one socio-economic class to another. It is lower among the pathological poor, whereas in this same group the share of those born within the province, but outside its capital city is higher. For the middle class and the well-to-do it is rather lower than among the unpathological. Comparison by row renders this even more apparent. The difference for the poor born in Shiraz and in villages of the same province or as nomads is significant ($X^2 = 6.94$, $p < 0.01$), while the difference for the middle class or for all non-poor together is not. Neither is the seeming difference, based on small numbers, between the middle class and the poor born in cities of Fars outside Shiraz. Other differences of appreciable magnitude do not appear. We can conclude at most that born villagers from Fars make up a disproportionately large share of the pathological poor found in the city. As we have seen in Table B IV 3, the poor in the city have a significantly higher prevalence rate for psychiatric morbidity than the non-poor. If we calculate the expected prevalence among the 429 poor according to the observed rate of 13.8 % found among the 499 non-poor, it comes to 59.2 or approximately 59 persons. Actually we find among the poor 85 pathological persons, i.e. 26 more than the expectancy. The pathological poor of village or nomadic birth from Fars number 24 persons and are thus practically equal in number to the excess – a finding that gives rise to reflections. The total morbidity rates, as we have seen, do not differ significantly between city and country, but the rates for the poor and non-poor within the city do. We now compare the rate for the urban poor, which is 19.8 %, with that for Khuzestan

Table B IV 15. Place of Birth and Socio-Economic Status

	Shiraz Survey Population					Psychiatric Survey Population Unpathological				Pathological			
	Poor	Mid.	WTD	nc	Sum	Poor	Mid.	WTD	Sum	Poor	Mid.	WTD	Sum
	Absolute Numbers												
Shiraz	856	1017	194	30	2097	263	239	84	586	52	37	13	102
Other cities in Fars	120	128	7	5	260	25	16	3	44	8	2	3	13
Villages in Fars, nomads	178	105	8	2	293	55	19	5	79	24	5	0	29
Outside Fars	62	141	29	1	233	0	40	14	54	0	5	2	7
nc	9	20	2	0	31	1	8	2	11	1	2	0	3
Total	1225	1411	240	38	2914	344	322	108	774	85	51	18	154
	Percent by Column												
Shiraz	69.9	72.1	80.8	78.9	72.0	76.5	74.2	77.8	75.7	61.2	72.5	72.2	66.2
Other cities in Fars	9.8	9.1	2.9	13.2	8.9	7.3	5.0	2.8	5.7	9.4	3.9	16.7	8.4
Villages in Fars, nomads	14.6	7.5	3.3	5.3	10.0	16.0	5.9	4.6	10.2	28.2	9.8	0.0	18.8
Outside Fars	5.1	10.0	12.1	2.6	8.0	0.0	12.4	13.0	7.0	0.0	9.8	11.1	4.6
nc	0.7	1.4	0.8	0.0	1.1	0.3	2.5	1.9	1.4	1.2	3.9	0.0	1.9
Total	100	100	100	100	100	100	100	100	100	100	100	100	100
	Percent by Row												
Shiraz	40.8	48.5	9.3	1.4	100	44.9	40.8	14.3	100	51.0	36.3	12.7	100
Other cities in Fars	46.2	49.2	2.7	1.9	100	56.8	36.4	6.8	100	61.5	15.4	23.1	100
Villages in Fars, nomads	60.7	35.8	2.8	0.7	100	69.6	24.0	6.3	100	82.8	17.2	0.0	100
Outside Fars	26.6	60.5	12.4	0.5	100	0.0	74.0	26.0	100	0.0	71.4	28.6	100
Total	42.0	48.4	8.2	1.3	100	44.4	41.6	14.0	100	55.2	33.1	11.7	100

Key: Mid. = middle class; WTD = well-to-do; nc = not classified or not known.

(= 14.9 %) where the whole population was regarded as poor, and obtain a X^2 value of 3.45, nearly equal to the critical value of 3.84 for $p < 0.05$ and 1 df. Very probably there are more pathological poor in the city, and very probably also the excess comes from the country. Why? The perennial problem raises its head: do the poor pathological migrants to the city migrate because they are psychiatrically ill, or do they become ill as a consequence of their migration?

In a first endeavor to reach an answer to this question we have examined the case histories of all the 52 pathological immigrants among the Shiraz PP regardless of their origin. In three instances their present socio-economic status could not be determined. These were dropped, leaving 49. In all these cases we tried to ascertain whether the psychiatric disorder that had led us to judge the person in question as pathological had begun before or after migration to the city. The results appear in Table B IV 16. In most cases we could decide whether the incidence of the disorder preceded or followed migration with a fairly high degree of probability, though not always with certainty, whereas in 7 we could not. Of the remaining 42, 28 or exactly two-thirds were certainly or probably disordered before they moved to Shiraz. Of the poor alone, approximately three-fourths, or 20 out of 27, were, and this holds whether they migrated to Shiraz from the countryside or from other cities. Among the non-poor the relation of incidence to migration is ambiguous. Their numbers are small, but they remain roughly equal for incidence before and after migration regardless of origin and regardless of whether they belong to the middle class or the well-to-do. Case analysis confirms what numerical analysis suggested: that the pathological poor constitute a group unto themselves.

It now becomes necessary to inquire into the types of disorders from which the pathological immigrants suffered before and after migration. In Table B IV 17 we distinguish between the 27 poor and the 15 non-poor, 42 altogether. The constitutional disorders existed by definition before migration. All the six cases lie among the poor.

Table B IV 16. Pathological Immigrants to Shiraz: Sites of Emigration and Relation of Incidence of Psychiatric Disorder to Migration

	Incidence of Psychiatric Disorder in Relation to Migration			
	Before	After	Unknown	Sum
	Pathological Immigrants from Villages			
Poor	14	5	5	24
Middle	3	2	0	5
Well-to-do	0	0	1	1
Total	17	7	6	30
	Pathological Immigrants from Cities			
Poor	6	2	0	8
Middle	3	3	0	6
Well-to-do	2	2	1	5
Total	11	7	1	19
	All Pathological Immigrants to Shiraz			
Poor	20	7	5	32
Middle	6	5	0	11
Well-to-do	2	2	2	6
Total	28	14	7	49

Table B IV 17. Pathological Immigrants to Shiraz: Incidence and Type of Psychiatric Disorder According to Socio-Economic Status

	Poor before migration	Poor after migration	Non-poor before migration	Non-poor after migration	Altogether before migration	Altogether after migration
Symptomatic	3	1	1	2	4	3
Reactive						
Simple	1	3	1	1	2	4
Neurotic	7	3	4	1	11	4
Psychosomatic	3	0	2	3	5	3
Constitutional	6	0	0	0	6	0
Subtotal	20	7	8	7	28	14
Total	27		15		42	
Not classifiable					10	

Five were psychopathies, one an oligophrenia. At the head of the table are the symptomatic disorders. It is not surprising that two dementias manifested themselves after long residence in the city; no connection need be postulated in these between migration and pathology. Two more patients were victims of cerebral traumas in Shiraz. Of the remaining three, two epilepsies had originated in villages before migration, and the third patient undoubtedly had brought from there the warped personality that misled him into opium addiction and dementia.

Turning to the reactive cases, the simple developments of such severity that they must classed as pathological are few. So far as the small numbers permit any conclusion, it appears, again unsurprisingly, that they tend to arise after migration (4 cases) rather than before (2 cases). It is otherwise in the neuroses, the most numerous category. Among the poor we meet with 7 cases before and 3 after, among the non-poor 4 to 1. The psychosomatic diseases are not so consistent. All three among the poor were manifest before migration, among the non-poor 2 before and 3 after. In respect to sex, all 4 female cases (3 of hemicrania) and one male case had been manifest before migration, whereas the three cases subsequent to migration were all male.

Of the 32 pathological poor immigrants to Shiraz, 21 were female. Out of the villages came 15 women to 9 men, and out of the cities 6 women to 2 men. Among the pathological immigrants of the upper and middle classes, the small numbers were roughly balanced for the sexes whether they emigrated from village or city. In the entire group of 49 who could be classified by SES there were 30 women to 19 men, but among the 27 poor who could be so classified 18, i.e. two thirds, were female. From the seven poor who indubitably became ill after migration all but one were women. Notable among the poor pathological immigrants were four families with 1 x 4 and 3 x 2 ill members. The four patients in a single family were a mother with three neurotic and five apparently undisturbed children. Her husband, a baker, was not abnormal. His wife was rather unintelligent, emotionally unstable, in her own words "worried and sad from life", forced to care for her 75 year old father-in-law besides the eight children, unable to cope with a city life in poverty, harking back mournfully to her youth as an unmarried country girl. With marriage and the first pregnancy, before removing to Shiraz, the anxiety and ever-increasing self-uncertainty had begun.

This case affords a clue to the preponderance of females among the pathological poor immigrants. In western countries they might be sought among rustic girls who had set out to make their way in the city and failed, but such a career is rare indeed in Iran. As we have seen, girls marry, or are married, young, and when the husband emigrates to the city they must follow if he demands (some do not, but leave wife and child in the village). Not only are family ties strong, but replies to inquiries about happiest and unhappiest memories show clearly that their maintenance, restoration or breakage mean more to the female sex in Iran than to the male. It will be recalled that M. Bleuler [39, p. 536] in his exhaustive investigation of the role of peristatic factors in schizophrenia could demonstrate beyond doubt, and with full statistical significance, that "personal relations – in childhood to the parents, later to other persons close to oneself – plays a significant part in the origin and course of schizophrenic psychoses in women."[1] Bleuler surmises that they do for men also, but was unable to bring the same stringent proof and concludes that their importance for men is probably somewhat less. Our findings suggest strongly that impairment or rupture of personal relations plays a greater part for women than for men in the origin and course of psychiatric disorder in general, and not for schizophrenia alone.

Reverting to the larger question of the relationship between migration and mental disorder, it now seems clear that no single, simple answer fits the reality. Both, disorder following migration and migration following disorder, occur, and they do so in the middle and well-to-do classes in about equal proportions. The temporal sequence does not always imply a causal one, as the case of the arteriosclerotic woman who had resided for three decades in Shiraz illustrates. In the majority of cases, though, there seems to be ground to suspect, at least, a relationship of partial causality. If this be accepted, then the evidence speaks for the preponderant role among the poor of psychiatric morbidity as an instigator rather than as a consequence of migration from the country to the city. The very close agreement between the excess of pathological poor in the city and the number of poor immigrants thereto who are found to be pathological offers confirmation. Life in Shiraz in the third quarter of the twentieth century by Gregorian calender or in the second quarter of the fourteenth by Iranian chronology does not seem to exercise by itself any very substantial pathogenic influence as compared with life in the country. To generalize from this to other countries and epochs would be fraught with risks.

Does the length of the immigrants' residence in Shiraz affect their morbidity? Several hypotheses are conceivable. Morbidity might diminish with acclimatization, it might increase under the sustained presumptive stress of an unaccustomed environment, or there might be no change. If there were none, this might be because the factors just named either did not operate or canceled each other out. It might also be because the migrants were impelled to migrate by their own latent or manifest pathology which was hardly influenced by a change of environment, as we have found reason to suspect. We had hoped to obtain some light upon these questions when we asked each subject how long he or she had been residing in Shiraz and, for those who had not lived there always, subdivided the period of residence into a number of intervals (less than one year, 1 to 4 years, 5 to 10 years, over 10 years but not always).

[1] Translated by the present authors.

Table B IV 18. Duration of Residence in Shiraz and Socio-Economic Status

	Shiraz Survey Population					Psychiatric Survey Population Unpathological				Pathological			
	Poor	Mid.	WTD	nc	Sum	Poor	Mid.	WTD	Sum	Poor	Mid.	WTD	Sum
	Absolute Numbers												
Lifelong	856	1014[a]	193[a]	30	2093[a]	263	239	83[a]	585[a]	51[a]	37	13	101[a]
10 years	131	90	11	2	234	28	25	5	58	12	5	3	20
10 years	147	190	7	5	349	39	39	1	79	13	3	0	16
nc	91	117	29	1	238	14	19	19	52	9	6	2	17
Total	1225	1411	240	38	2914	344	322	108	774	85	51	18	154
	Percent by Column												
Lifelong	69.9	71.9	80.4	78.9	71.8	76.5	74.2	76.9	75.6	60.0	72.5	72.2	65.6
10 years	10.7	6.4	4.6	5.3	8.0	8.1	7.8	4.6	7.5	14.1	9.8	16.7	13.0
10 years	12.0	13.5	2.9	13.2	12.0	11.3	12.1	0.9	10.2	15.3	5.9	0.0	10.4
nc	7.4	8.3	12.1	2.6	8.2	4.1	5.9	17.6	6.7	10.6	11.8	11.1	11.0
Total	100	100	100	100	100	100	100	100	100	100	100	100	100
	Percent by Row												
Lifelong	40.9	48.4	9.2	1.4	100	45.0	40.9	14.2	100	50.5	36.6	12.9	100
10 years	56.0	38.5	4.7	0.9	100	48.3	43.1	8.6	100	60.0	25.0	15.0	100
10 years	42.1	54.4	2.0	1.4	100	49.4	49.4	1.3	100	81.2	18.8	0.0	100
nc	38.2	49.2	12.2	0.4	100	27.0	36.5	36.5	100	52.9	35.3	11.8	100
Total	42.0	48.4	8.2	1.3	100	44.4	41.6	14.0	100	55.2	33.1	11.7	100

[a] The discrepancies between these and the corresponding cells of Table are explained by a small number of persons who were born in Shiraz, moved away and returned.

Key: Mid. = middle class; WTD = well-to-do; nc = not classified or not known.

Again, the numbers in the subdivisions within the PP turned out to be so small that the table was condensed into three periods of residence: always, more than 10 but not always, and less than 10 years. Even this brought us no closer to a solution. The immigrant groups to the city remained so small in comparison to those who had lived their lives there that no even suggestively significant differences in their psychiatric morbidity could be discovered. Among the poor the percentage differences between the permanent residents and the immigrants seemed conspicuous but failed to meet any statistical test, whether we took the shorter and longer term immigrants separately or together. This does not contradict what was said above in connection with Table B IV 16 about the relatively large share of poor immigrants to the city among the pathological there, since in Table B IV 16 comparison was made between pathological sub-groups, whereas it is made here in Table B IV 18 between a pathological sub-group on the one hand and the whole group of the unpathological poor on the other.

Turning now to factors that are even more distinctly social, the first that occurs in quasi-biographical order is that of literacy in its relation to socio-economic class and to pathology. In the Survey Population we encounter the expected positive correlation between literacy and SES. Tables B IV 19 and B IV 20 are again condensed. The first category "illiterate" comprises both the truly illiterate of all ages (above five and a half) and a few children who had not yet entered school. The second, "elementary eduction", comprises those who either were attending the first six school grades or had ceased their formal education at latest after completing the sixth grade, this being the recognized limit of elementary education in Iran. We also put into this category those who had acquired their literacy by the "old" means of education, i.e. with the help of relatives, tutoring, their own efforts or – most commonly – the traditional religious type of school (and are aware that by so classifying them we have done grave injustice to a handful of learned scholars, to whom we tender our apologies). The third category of "higher education" comprises all formal education beyond the elementary up to and including the university. In gathering data we had distinguished between not less than twelve categories, but again found the higher all so sparingly represented that their separation would have confused rather than clarified the relationships.

The basic information of Table B IV 19 requires little comment. Comparing the sexes by column, female illiteracy on the whole far outweighs male. Up to 19 years, however, both sexes take approximately equal advantage of elementary education. In subsequent years the share of the girls and women in both elementary and superior education falls off sharply. That the younger generation of women is faring better educationally than their mothers is suggested again by comparison by row. Here the percentages of males and females between 20–39 who are enjoying a more than elementary education are equal, whereas by column less girls of this age group go on to a higher school. The proportion by column is nearly equalized for both sexes in the 6–14 year class, however.

Before condensing the data for these tables we could ascertain that among persons 20 or more years old 32 out of 717 males or 4.5 % and 11 out of 744 females or 1.5 % were attending elementary or secondary, but not higher classes. This may afford some indication of the number participating in adult education, i. e., for the most part, literacy programs.

Table B IV 20 is more instructive with regard to social psychiatry. From it we see that the majority (60 %) of the illiterate are poor, but only 42 % of the poor are

Table B IV 19. Age and Degree of Education in Shiraz Survey Population

	Males						Females					
	Absolute Numbers											
	6–14	15–19	20–39	40–59	60 +	Sum	6–14	15–19	20–39	40–59	60 +	Sum
Ill.	56	11	89	104	60	320	67	35	206	160	71	539
Elem.	398	68	163	108	37	774	380	59	162	34	8	643
Sup.	65	149	114	36	5	369	60	104	82	18	3	267
nc	0	0	2	0	0	2	0	0	0	0	0	0
Total	519	228	368	248	102	1465	507	198	450	212	82	1449
	Percent by Column											
Ill.	10.8	4.8	24.2	41.9	58.8	21.8	13.2	17.7	45.8	75.5	86.6	37.2
Elem.	76.7	29.8	44.3	43.5	36.3	52.8	74.9	29.8	36.0	16.0	9.8	44.4
Sup.	12.5	65.3	31.0	14.5	4.9	25.2	11.8	52.5	18.2	8.5	3.6	18.4
nc	0.0	0.0	0.5	0.0	0.0	0	0	0	0	0	0	0
Total	100	100	100	100	100	100	100	100	100	100	100	100
	Percent by Row											
Ill.	17.5	3.4	27.8	32.5	18.7	100	12.4	6.5	38.2	29.7	13.2	100
Elem.	51.4	8.8	21.1	14.0	4.8	100	59.1	9.2	25.2	5.3	1.2	100
Sup.	17.6	40.4	30.9	9.8	1.4	100	22.5	38.9	30.7	6.7	1.1	100
Total	35.4	15.6	25.1	16.9	7.0	100	35.0	13.7	31.1	14.6	5.7	100

Key: Ill. = illiterate; Elem. = elementary schooling; Sup. = higher schooling, beyond elementary; nc = not classified or not known.

Table B IV 20. Literacy and Socio-Economic Status

	Shiraz Survey Population					Psychiatric Survey Population Unpathological				Pathological			
	Poor	Mid.	WTD	nc	Sum	Poor	Mid.	WTD	Sum	Poor	Mid.	WTD	Sum
	Absolute Numbers												
Ill.	515	311	20	13	859	143	77	4	224	48	13	3	64
Elem.	593	709	92	23	1417	165	160	39	364	33	24	7	64
Sup.	116	390	128	2	636	36	85	65	186	4	14	8	26
nc	1	1	0	0	2	0	0	0	0	0	0	0	0
Total	1225	1411	240	38	2914	344	322	108	774	85	51	18	154
	Percent by Column												
Ill.	42.0	22.0	8.3	34.2	29.5	41.6	23.9	3.7	29.0	56.5	25.5	16.7	41.6
Elem.	48.4	50.2	38.3	60.5	48.6	48.0	49.7	36.1	47.0	38.8	47.0	38.9	41.6
Sup.	9.5	27.6	53.3	5.3	21.8	10.5	26.4	60.2	24.0	4.7	27.4	44.4	16.8
nc	0.1	0.1	0.0	0.0	0.1	0	0	0	0	0	0	0	0
Total	100	100	100	100	100	100	100	100	100	100	100	100	100
	Percent by Row												
Ill.	59.9	36.2	2.3	1.5	100	63.8	34.4	1.8	100	75.0	20.3	4.7	100
Elem.	41.8	50.0	6.5	1.6	100	45.3	43.9	10.7	100	51.6	37.5	10.9	100
Sup.	18.2	61.3	20.1	0.3	100	19.3	45.7	34.9	100	15.4	53.8	30.8	100
nc													
Total	42.0	48.4	8.2	1.3	100	44.4	41.6	14.0	100	55.2	33.1	11.7	100

Key: as for Table B IV 19.

illiterate. Nearly half of the urban poor proceed to elementary school and nearly one-tenth beyond. Half of the middle class too go or have gone to elementary school, but more than a quarter beyond, while less than a quarter is illiterate. Somewhat more than half the well-to-do enjoy a better than elementary education, and only 8 % remain illiterate or have not yet begun school. In the unpathological sector of the Psychiatric Survey Population the relationships are basically similar but are accentuated, as we should expect from the nature of the sample, for the well-to-do and the poor when we regard the percentages by row. By column, i.e. SES, they are practically the same as in the SP for the poor and the middle class, while the share of the well-educated well-to-do is more conspicuous. Among the pathological prevalent illiteracy is noticeable both by row and column for the poor. The proportions among the middle class are not greatly different from those in the healthy members of that class. The pathological well-to-do seem to exhibit less higher education and more illiteracy, but the numbers are too small to be conclusive. Statistically the representation of the illiterate poor among the pathological (31.2 %) is quite significantly larger than among the unpathological (18.5 %; the difference is 3.58 times its SD, $p < 0.001$). Because the middle class relationships remain practically unaffected by pathology, we can infer that those among the well-to-do are actually, though not statistically significant. Since the great majority of the immigrant villagers are both poor and illiterate, as our rural surveys confirm, and since we have established already that these contribute a disproportionately large share of the pathological poor in the city, it becomes probable that the excess of the illiterate among the pathological poor is made up in no small part of just such immigrants. Of the 48 illiterate pathological poor in fact 24 or 50 % have come from outside Shiraz. Seven of these were male, 17 female.

Table B IV 21 makes clearer the relations between place of birth or origin, sex and educational opportunity and hardly requires comment. The city dwellers are favored, and in the city the men before the women, but this holds only for Shiraz itself. The "other cities in Fars" show a pattern of education and (il-)literacy that is practically identical with that of the villages, and this for both sexes. For those from "outside Fars" the picture is brighter. They came for the most part from major cities of other provinces, including Tehran, and were again for the most part people in business or administration who had moved to Shiraz for reasons connected with their work. One feature to be remarked is that, while there are many more illiterate Shirazi women than men, the percentage of women who pass beyond the elementary school into some form of higher education is only slightly less than that of the men, as seen already in Table B IV 19. Most of them are to be found among the girls who go on to complete the ninth grade of school instead of stopping at the sixth. Little is gained by applying these classifications to the Psychiatric Survey Population, so we give figures for the SP only.

Intimately connected with birth and origin is religion. The religious affiliation of our sample can be shown quite simply (cf. Table B IV 22).

After education usually follows occupation. We address ourselves to this interesting and important chapter not without reluctance. In regard to hardly any other question, simple though it may seem, did the inadequacies of our young and inexperienced examiners become more apparent or were they more difficult to counter. All too often their statements of subjects' occupations were vague, inaccurate or even irrelevant. The commonest example of the last was the frequent designation of a subject as an "employee" (karmand کارمند) without any indication of the employer or the position

Table B IV 21. Place of Birth and Degree of Education in Shiraz Survey Population

	Absolute Numbers					Percent by Row				
	Ill.	Elem.	Sup.	nc	Sum	Ill.	Elem.	Sup.	nc	Sum
Males										
Shiraz	192	577	265	2	1036	18.5	55.7	25.6	0.1	100
Other cities in Fars	51	60	24	0	135	37.8	44.4	17.8	0.0	100
Villages in Fars, nomads	55	67	25	0	147	37.4	45.6	17.0	0.0	100
Outside Fars	17	60	51	0	128	13.3	46.9	39.8	0.0	100
nc	5	10	4	0	19					
Total	320	774	369	2	1465	21.8	52.8	25.2	0.1	100
Females										
Shiraz	317	517	227	0	1061	29.9	48.7	21.4	0.0	100
Other cities in Fars	87	28	10	0	125	69.6	22.4	8.0	0.0	100
Villages in Fars, nomads	102	35	6	0	143	71.3	24.5	4.2	0.0	100
Outside Fars	28	59	21	0	108	25.9	54.6	19.4	0.0	100
nc	5	4	3	0	12					
Total	539	643	267	0	1449	37.2	44.4	18.4	0.0	100

Key: as for Table B IV 19.

Table B IV 22. Religious Affiliation of the Shiraz Survey Population

Moslem	97.2 per 100
Jewish	2.1 per 100
Christian	0.2 per 100
Zoroastrian	0.0 per 100
Other or not recorded	0.5 per 100

in which he was employed. The Persian term, like the English, refers to anyone receiving a regular salary, though not necessarily under contract, i.e. to someone whose position could be regarded as relatively stable and moderately assured. Most of the girls came from such families. In a labile economy with a good deal of unemployment and poverty the attainment of such a status understandably seemed crucial. As elsewhere, a regular employee was likely to possess somewhat better qualifications than a worker or hired hand, but this is far from being necessarily so or from indicating the level of skill at which the employee might be working. Even the place of employment, upon which we soon began to insist, told little. A "government employee" might mean anything from a municipal streetsweeper to a high-ranking official; a "university employee" might mean anything from a maid in the student dormitories (and in one case did!) to a professor, just as "gardener" served for anyone from the owner of a large and profitable truck garden down to the boys who weeded the patches and toted the endless cans of water. Numberless, repeated explanations of what we wanted in this respect and why we wanted it seemed to make little impression on the majority of the girls, whose scanty experience in life had not equipped them to comprehend the meaning and importance of such distinctions as we sought, whereas our elder and generally more experienced collaborators understood at once. Coming upon such designations, we strove to clarify them and render them more precise wherever possible, but all too often the essential information was not to be had without revisiting the household in question. For this time could not always be spared. The quality and exactitude of our occupational data therefore leave much to be desired. They are most reliable where they relate to simply and easily identifiable categories such as housewife or pupil, least where they concern the skilled and professional. The number of such was relatively few at best, but lack of precision here was especially regrettable because it was exactly these upper categories that were absent in our rural surveys.

We had adopted as a basis the fivefold classification of occupations commonly used for such work, e.g. by Shepherd and Strotzka, this being:

I. Professional, highly specialized or academic
II. Lower grade professional or academic (below doctorate or licentiate)
III. Skilled
IV. Semi-skilled
V. Unskilled

Equally commonly, housewives and dependent children are assigned to the grade of their husbands or fathers. This seemed inappropriate in a swiftly changing, mobile society such as Iran's had become. Too often we could observe marked disparities – most often naturally where the children were exceeding the father's level not only in literacy, but also in vocational or professional training. In a number of cases the husband had some education, the wife none, and in a few more we came upon the converse. We therefore decided to put all housewives not gainfully employed into one category. The same was done for all pupils and students including the handful of the latter who were working besides their studies. At first treated separately, they remained too few to justify either a category to themselves or a splitting of categories with all the difficulties in computation this would have incurred. In the final classification our Iranian colleagues helped us greatly. Even so, a regrettably large number of subjects had to remain without occupational classification – nearly one-fifth in all.

What emerges, then, from Tables B IV 23–24 corresponds to expectation. Regardless of SES, the housewives make up a significantly larger share of the pathological (34.4 %) than of the unpathological (23.8 %) in the Psychiatric Survey Population (Table B IV 24, Percent by Column; $X^2 = 7.10$, $p < 0.01$). Taking their percentages by row, that of the housewives among the poor mounts sharply from 43.5 % among the unpathological to 60.4 % among the pathological, corresponding to the excess of the poor and mostly illiterate women already ascertained among the pathological cases. The relation is reversed, again according to expectation, among the pupils and students, who constitute (by column, without regard to SES) 42.1 % of the

Table B IV 23. Occupation and Socio-Economic Status: Shiraz Survey Population

	Poor	Middle	Well-to-do	nc	Sum
	Absolute Numbers				
Skilled	4	115	45	0	164
Semi-skilled	118	248	20	0	386
Unskilled	221	36	2	0	259
Housewife	298	381	54	12	745
Pupil	473	563	107	14	1157
nc	111	68	12	12	203
Total	1225	1411	240	38	2914
	Percent by Column				
Skilled	0.3	8.1	18.7	0.0	5.7
Semi-skilled	9.6	17.6	8.3	0.0	13.2
Unskilled	18.0	2.6	0.8	0.0	8.9
Housewife	24.3	27.0	22.5	31.6	25.6
Pupil	38.6	39.9	44.6	36.8	39.7
nc	9.1	4.8	5.0	31.6	7.0
Total	100	100	100	100	100
	Percent by Row				
Skilled	2.4	70.1	27.4	0.0	100
Semi-skilled	30.6	64.2	5.2	0.0	100
Unskilled	85.3	13.9	0.8	0.0	100
Housewife	40.0	51.1	7.2	1.6	100
Pupil	40.9	48.7	9.2	1.2	100
nc	54.7	33.5	5.9	5.9	100
Total	42.0	48.5	8.2	1.3	100

"normal", but only 27.9 % of the pathological cases ($X^2 = 10.22$, $p < 0.01$ and very nearly reaches the value of 10.83 required for $p < 0.001$). Attempts to find other statistically significant differences do not succeed unequivocally, but for the semi-skilled against all others X^2 is 3.66 and thus near to the critical value of 3.84 for the 5 % level.

Finally, a question was included as to the habit of clay eating, which is encountered not too rarely in rural Iran, more among children than adults. It does not seem to be a food substitute to which resort is taken in poverty or famine but rather to correspond roughly to Western gum chewing. It has been brought into relation speculatively with the zinc deficiency that some authors claim to have demonstrated and this again with some cases of mental deficiency [8, 186]. As a good deal of work on this debated subject has been centered in Shiraz and interest in it was lively, we inquired about it routinely. From 2914 subjects only 17 = 0.6 % said that they habitually ate clay. 2329 = 79.9 % denied doing so, and from 568 = 19.5 % no reply to this question was recorded.

Table B IV 24. Occupation and Socio-Economic Status: Psychiatric Survey Population

	Unpathological				Pathological			
	Poor	Middle	Well-to-do	Sum	Poor	Middle	Well-to-do	Sum
	Absolute Numbers							
Skilled	2	27	25	54	1	9	5	15
Semi-skilled	45	59	3	107	6	5	1	12
Unskilled	66	3	1	70	15	2	1	18
Housewife	80	80	24	184	32	17	4	53
Pupil	131	141	54	326	23	16	4	43
nc	20	12	1	33	8	2	3	13
Total	344	322	108	774	85	51	18	154
	Percent by Column							
Skilled	0.6	8.4	23.1	7.0	1.2	17.6	27.8	9.7
Semi-skilled	13.1	18.3	2.8	13.8	7.1	9.8	5.6	7.8
Unskilled	19.2	0.9	0.9	9.0	17.6	3.9	5.6	11.7
Housewife	23.2	24.8	22.2	23.8	37.6	33.3	22.2	34.4
Pupil	38.1	43.8	50.0	42.1	27.1	31.4	22.2	27.9
nc	5.8	3.7	0.9	4.3	9.4	3.9	16.6	8.4
Total	100	100	100	100	100	100	100	100
	Percent by Row							
Skilled	3.7	50.0	46.3	100	6.7	60.0	33.3	100
Semi-skilled	42.1	55.1	2.8	100	50.0	41.7	8.3	100
Unskilled	94.3	4.3	1.4	100	83.3	11.1	5.6	100
Housewife	43.5	43.5	13.0	100	60.4	32.1	7.5	100
Pupil	40.2	43.3	16.6	100	53.5	37.2	9.3	100
nc	60.6	36.4	3.0	100	61.5	15.4	23.1	100
Total	44.4	41.6	14.0	100	55.2	33.1	11.7	100

Table B IV 25. Psychiatric Diagnoses of Mild Cases (P_1)

Diagnoses	Number of cases					p. 100 of 154 cases					p. 1000 of 928 subjects				
	m	f	m+f			m	f	m+f			m	f	m+f		
I. Funct. psychoses		1	1				0.6	0.6				1.1	1.1		
1. Schizophrenia															
2. Affect. psychoses		1		1			0.6		0.6			1.1		1.1	
II. Acute symptomatic psychoses			0					0					0		
III. Subchronic & chron. sympt. psychoses & residual states	7	5	12			4.5	3.2	7.8			7.5	5.4	12.9		
1. Epilepsy				4					2.6					4.3	
a. cryptogen.	2	2			4	1.3	1.3			2.6	2.1	2.1			4.3
b. symptomatic															
2. Sen. & arterioscl.	2	2		4		1.3	1.3		2.6		2.1	2.1		4.3	
3. post-infectious		1		1			0.6		0.6			1.1		1.1	
4. post-traumatic	1			1		0.6			0.6		1.1			1.1	
5. endocrine															
6. addiction	1			1		0.6			0.6		1.1			1.1	
7. other	1			1		0.6			0.6		1.1			1.1	
IV. Reactive disorders	22	37	59			14.3	24.0	38.3			23.7	39.9	63.6		
1. Simple path. dev.	2	9		11		1.3	5.8		7.1		2.1	9.7		11.8	
a. anxious		1			1		0.6			0.6		1.1			1.1
b. depressive	2	8			10	1.3	5.2			6.5	2.1	8.6			10.8
c. irritable															
d. neurasthenic															
e. other															
2. Neuroses	10	23		33		6.5	14.9		21.4		10.8	24.8		35.6	
a. anxious		2			2		1.3			1.3		2.1			2.1
b. phobic		1			1		0.6			0.6		1.1			1.1
c. depressive	1	3			4	0.6	1.9			2.6	1.1	3.2			4.3
d. hysterical	2	4			6	1.3	2.6			3.9	2.1	4.3			6.5
e. hypochondriac	1	5			6	0.6	3.2			3.9	1.1	5.4			6.5
f. neurasthenic															
g. self-insuff.		1			1		0.6			0.6		1.1			1.1
h. negativistic															
i. other & polym.	6	7			13	3.9	4.5			8.4	6.5	7.5			14.0
3. Psychosomatic	10	5		15		6.5	3.2		9.7		10.8	5.4		16.2	
a. headache					10					6.5					10.8
ا. migrainoid	3	3				1.9	1.9				3.2	3.2			
ب. other	3	1				1.9	0.6				3.2	1.1			
b. gastro-intest.	3	1			4	1.9	0.6			2.6	3.2	1.1			4.3
c. asthmatic															
d. other & polym.	1				1	0.6				0.6	1.1				1.1
V. Constitutional disord.	5	3	8			3.2	1.9	5.2			5.4	3.2	8.6		
1. Clin. oligophrenia	3	2		5		1.9	1.3		3.2		3.2	2.1		5.4	
a. cryptogenetic	3	2			5	1.9	1.3			3.2	3.2	2.1			5.4
b. genetic															
2. Psychopathy	2	1		3		1.3	0.6		1.9		2.1	1.1		3.2	
a. irritable	1				1	0.6				0.6	1.1				1.1
b. anti-social															
c. schizoid	1				1	0.6				0.6	1.1				1.1
d. other		1			1		0.6			0.6		1.1			1.1
Total	34	46	80	80		22.1	29.9	51.9	51.9		36.6	49.6	86.2	86.2	

Table B IV 26. Psychiatric Diagnoses of Medium Cases (P_2)

Diagnoses	Number of cases					p. 100 of 154 cases					p. 1000 of 928 subjects				
	m	f	m + f			m	f	m + f			m	f	m + f		
I. Funct. psychoses		2	2				1.3	1.3				2.1	2.1		
1. Schizophrenia		1		1			0.6		0.6			1.1		1.1	
2. Affect. psychoses		1		1			0.6		0.6			1.1		1.1	
II. Acute symptomatic psychoses			0					0					0		
III. Subchronic & chron. sympt. psychoses & residual states	12	6	18			7.8	3.9	11.7			12.9	6.5	19.4		
1. Epilepsy				2					1.3					2.1	
a. cryptogen.	1				1	0.6				0.6	1.1				1.1
b. symptomatic	1				1	0.6				0.6	1.1				1.1
2. Sen. & arterioscl.	2	4		6		1.3	2.6		3.9		2.1	4.3		6.5	
3. post-infectious	5	1		6		3.2	0.6		3.9		5.4	1.1		6.5	
4. post-traumatic	1	1		2		0.6	0.6		1.3		1.1	1.1		2.1	
5. endocrine															
6. addiction	2			2		1.3			1.3		2.1			2.1	
7. other															
IV. Reactive disorders	10	22	32			6.5	14.3	20.8			10.8	23.7	34.5		
1. Simple path. dev.		5		5			3.2		3.2			5.4		5.4	
a. anxious		1			1		0.6			0.6		1.1			1.1
b. depressive		3			3		1.9			1.9		3.2			3.2
c. irritable		1			1		0.6			0.6		1.1			1.1
d. neurasthenic															
e. other															
2. Neuroses	9	12		21		5.8	7.8		13.6		9.7	12.9		22.6	
a. anxious		1			1		0.6			0.6		1.1			1.1
b. phobic															
c. depressive	2	2			4	1.3	1.3			2.6	2.1	2.1			4.3
d. hysterical	1	6			7	0.6	3.9			4.5	1.1	6.5			7.5
e. hypochondriac		1			1		0.6			0.6		1.1			1.1
f. neurasthenic															
g. self-insuff.	2				2	1.3				1.3					
h. negativistic															
i. other & polym.	4	2			6	2.6	1.3			3.9	6.5	2.1			8.6
3. Psychosomatic	1	5		6		0.6	3.2		3.9		1.1	5.4		6.5	
a. headache					3					1.9					3.2
α. migrainoid		3					1.9					3.2			
β. other															
b. gastro-intest.		1			1		0.6			0.6		1.1			1.1
c. asthmatic		1			1		0.6			0.6		1.1			1.1
d. other & polym.	1				1	0.6				0.6	1.1				1.1
V. Constitutional disord.	6	5	11			3.9	3.2	7.1			6.5	5.4	11.8		
1. Clin. oligophrenia	1	2		3		0.6	1.3		1.9		1.1	2.1		3.2	
a. cryptogenetic	1				1	0.6				0.6	1.1				1.1
b. genetic		2			2		1.3			1.3		2.1			2.1
2. Psychopathy	5	3		8		3.2	1.9		5.2		5.4	3.2		8.6	
a. irritable	3	1			4	1.9	0.6			2.6	3.2	1.1			4.3
b. anti-social	2				2	1.3				1.3	2.1				2.1
c. schizoid															
d. other		2			2		1.3			1.3		2.1			2.1
Total	28	35	63	63		18.2	22.7	40.9	40.9		30.2	37.7	67.9	67.9	

Table B IV 27. Psychiatric Diagnoses of Severe Cases (P_3)

Diagnoses	Number of cases					p. 100 of 154 cases					p. 1000 of 928 subjects				
	m	f	m + f			m	f	m + f			m	f	m + f		
I. Funct. psychoses	1		1			0.6		0.6			1.1		1.1		
1. Schizophrenia	1			1		0.6			0.6		1.1			1.1	
2. Affect. psychoses															
II. Acute symptomatic psychoses			0					0					0		
III. Subchronic & chron. sympt. psychoses & residual states	5	1	6			3.2	0.6	3.9			5.4	1.1	6.5		
1. Epilepsy															
a. cryptogen.															
b. symptomatic															
2. Sen. & arterioscl.		1		1			0.6		0.6			1.1		1.1	
3. post-infectious															
4. post-traumatic	1			1		0.6			0.6		1.1			1.1	
5. endocrine															
6. addiction	4			4		2.6			2.6		4.3			4.3	
7. other															
IV. Reactive disorders			0					0					0		
1. Simple path. dev.															
a. anxious															
b. depressive															
c. irritable															
d. neurasthenic															
e. other															
2. Neuroses															
a. anxious															
b. phobic															
c. depressive															
d. hysterical															
e. hypochondriac															
f. neurasthenic															
g. self-insuff.															
h. negativistic															
i. other & polym.															
3. Psychosomatic															
a. headache															
ا. migrainoid															
ب. other															
b. gastro-intest.															
c. asthmatic															
d. other & polym.															
V. Constitutional disord.	4		4			2.6		2.6			4.3		4.3		
1. Clin. oligophrenia	4			4		2.6			2.6		4.3			4.3	
a. cryptogenetic	3				3	1.9				1.9	3.2				3.2
b. genetic	1				1	0.6				0.6	1.1				1.1
2. Psychopathy			0					0					0		
a. irritable															
b. anti-social															
c. schizoid															
d. other															
Total	10	1	11	11		6.5	0.6	7.1	7.1		10.8	1.1	11.9	11.9	

Table B IV 28. Severe Cases (P_3)

No.	Sex	Age	SES	ICD	Clinical Characteristics
1	m	20	p	318.0 774.6 389.7	Imbecility after icterus neonatorum, deafmute
2	m	35	p	304.0	Opium addict
3	m	45	p	304.0 301.3	Opium addict, irritable psychopath
4	m	48	p	295.1	Hebephrenia (Case No. 3 of Table D IV 1)
5	m	65	p	304.0 294.1	Opium addict, demented, possibly also arteriosclerotic
6	f	80	p	290.0	Senile dementia
7	m	13	m	318.1 767.9	Imbecility, probably from perinatal trauma
8	m	30	m	294.8 854	Chronic symptomatic psychosis, probably after cerebral trauma
9	m	9	w	758.0	Mongoloid idiot
10	m	29	w	318.2	Congenital idiot
11	m	65	w	304.0 303 294.1	Opium and alcohol addict, demented

3. Special Psychiatry and Neurology

A summary of the Shiraz psychiatric findings has been presented in [31]. They are tabulated in more detail in the following Tables B IV 25–29. We met here two cases of schizophrenia, one in a man of 48, the other in a woman of 31 years. In both cases the circumstances and the accumulation of pathology in the households justify a brief description.

In the former one the examining team was received on their first visit by the patient's sister, a voluble woman of 45, married to a recurrently unemployed baker, in a cheaply built, sparsely furnished relatively new house in an area in which some renovation of the old district had been attempted. Not at all averse to voicing her complaints about the family's poverty and the burden of caring for her old mother and her "mad" brother, she nevertheless did not allow the girls to see him. When the first author accompanied them another time, he was first presented with the mother – a shrivelled little eighty year old lady with a cackling voice, huddled on the ground, disorientated in every respect and so far gone in senile dementia that she was classed unhesitatingly as P_3. The daughter had served up to our rather too guileless examiners a story of a tumor in the head, after the operation of which two physicians known personally to us had said she would never be well again. There was no sign of any operation. Our colleagues confirmed that they had seen the patient and made the same diagnosis as ourselves. We mention this as an illustration of the pitfalls laid for epidemiologists and still more for non-professional examiners by informants uninhibitedly exaggerating, mayhap not even intentionally, to create sensations, gain pity or calumniate physicians. On a little insistence from the author the informant led her brother in from a room in which she had been hiding him. Clad in trousers, shirt and a blanket over his shoulders he kept smiling blandly at nothing, hardly appeared to regard us, replied briefly and inattentively if at all, smoked a good many cheap cigarets and otherwise let his jaw hang open. He had no complaints, no enemies, was not bored from having no work and nothing whatever to do and, to our question whether he would not like to undertake some kind of

Table B IV 29. Psychiatric Diagnoses of All Cases

Diagnoses	Number of cases					p. 100 of 154 cases					p. 1000 of 928 subjects				
	m	f	m + f			m	f	m + f			m	f	m + f		
I. Funct. psychoses	1	3	4			0.6	1.9	2.6			1.1	3.2	4.3		
1. Schizophrenia	1	1		2		0.6	0.6		1.3		1.1	1.1		2.1	
2. Affect. psychoses		2		2			1.3		1.3			2.1		2.1	
II. Acute symptomatic psychoses			0					0					0		
III. Subchronic & chron. sympt. psychoses & residual states	24	12	36			15.6	7.8	23.4			25.9	12.9	38.8		
1. Epilepsy				6					3.9					6.5	
a. cryptogen.	3	2			5	1.9	1.3			3.2	3.2	2.1			5.4
b. symptomatic	1				1	0.6				0.6	1.1				1.1
2. Sen. & arterioscl.	4	7		11		2.6	4.5		7.1		4.3	7.5		11.8	
3. post-infectious	5	2		7		3.2	1.3		4.5		5.4	2.1		7.5	
4. post-traumatic	3	1		4		1.9	0.6		2.6		3.2	1.1		4.3	
5. endocrine															
6. addiction	7			7		4.5			4.5		7.5			7.5	
7. other	1			1		0.6			0.6		1.1			1.1	
IV. Reactive disorders	32	59	91			20.8	38.3	59.1			34.5	63.6	98.1		
1. Simple path. dev.	2	14		16		1.3	9.1		10.4		2.1	15.1		17.2	
a. anxious		2			2		1.3			1.3		2.1			2.1
b. depressive	2	11			13	1.3	7.1			8.4	2.1	11.8			14.0
c. irritable		1			1		0.6			0.6		1.1			1.1
d. neurasthenic															
e. other															
2. Neuroses	19	35		54		12.3	22.7		35.1		20.5	37.7		58.2	
a. anxious		3			3		1.9			1.9		3.2			3.2
b. phobic		1			1		0.6			0.6		1.1			1.1
c. depressive	3	5			8	1.9	3.2			5.2	3.2	5.4			8.6
d. hysterical	3	10			13	1.9	6.5			8.4	3.2	10.8			14.0
e. hypochondriac	1	6			7	0.6	3.9			4.5	1.1	6.5			7.5
f. neurasthenic															
g. self-insuff.	2	1			3	1.3	0.6			1.9	2.1	1.1			3.2
h. negativistic															
i. other & polym.	10	9			19	6.5	5.8			12.3	10.8	9.7			20.5
3. Psychosomatic	11	10		21		7.1	6.5		13.6		11.8	10.8		22.6	
a. headache					13					8.4					14.0
١. migrainoid	3	6				1.9	3.9				3.2	6.5			
ب. other	3	1				1.9	0.6				3.2	1.1			
b. gastro-intest.	3	2			5	1.9	1.3			3.2	3.2	2.1			5.4
c. asthmatic		1			1		0.6			0.6		1.1			1.1
d. other & polym.	2				2	1.3				1.3	2.1				2.1
V. Constitutional disord.	15	8	23			9.7	5.2	14.9			16.2	8.6	24.8		
1. Clin. oligophrenia	8	4		12		5.2	2.6		7.8		8.6	4.3		12.9	
a. cryptogenetic	7	2			9	4.5	1.3			5.8	7.5	2.1			9.7
b. genetic	1	2			3	0.6	1.3			1.9	1.1	2.1			3.2
2. Psychopathy	7	4		11		4.5	2.6		7.1		7.5	4.3		11.8	
a. irritable	4	1			5	2.6	0.6			3.2	4.3	1.1			5.4
b. anti-social	2				2	1.3				1.3	2.1				2.1
c. schizoid	1				1	0.6				0.6	1.1				1.1
d. other		3			3		1.9			1.9		3.2			3.2
Total	72	82	154	154		46.7	53.2	100.0	100.0		77.6	88.4	165.9	165.9	

activity, replied that other people did not need his help. In contrast to his ancient mother he was fully orientated even to the day and date, could read newspaper print and spoke, if he did speak, in an entirely orderly way, though often no answer was forthcoming and the affective rapport remained extremely superficial. We could gain no knowledge of his thoughts. While we turned to his sister for more information he aimlessly wandered in and out. According to her he had attended the sixth grade, but was taken mentally ill at about twelve years, ceased school and never worked. At the time he stopped school he masturbated a great deal and was severely reproached and beaten by his father, who thereupon procured him a temporary wife by the still sanctioned but seldom practised Shi'ite institution of the mut'a (marriage for a contractually stipulated term) for three months. The marriage was never consumated, and the patient after the age of fifteen showed no interest in women. In times past he was often deeply depressed and even wanted to throw himself into a well, but he later turned to laughing and talking to himself, though his sister could not repeat to us anything that he had said. Very religious in his youth, he was said to have become less so. He preferred to be alone, as his sister explained, wandered about the house, had no occupation or interests, no anxiety or enmity, no ideas of persecution and was completely harmless. He cared for his own bodily needs and appeared reasonably clean under the circumstances but otherwise was wholly dependent upon his sister, with whom he had been living for the past 25 years. He had been treated some 20 years ago in a Tehran mental hospital and had been to the Salami Hospital in Shiraz several times as an out-patient. There was no history of somatic illness. Though his father had died only four years ago and despite his proven orientation in time, he would affirm to his relatives that he quit school because of his father's death. It was instructive to note that, while two members of the household had severe mental illnesses of P_3 degree, the informant unhesitatingly presented to us her senile mother, but not her schizophrenic brother. Our diagnosis was chronic hebephrenia with severe affective alteration. The four children of the family and the informant's husband were unremarkable.

In the second schizophrenic case the family constellation was even more exceptional and confronted us with some diagnostic problems.

The patient's 65 year old husband, who initially claimed to be 50, was a superficially rather more than well-to-do businessman dealing in agricultural machines and parts but admitted to business difficulties because, as he asserted, his customers did not pay up. The couple lived in an opulent house with servants and a charming garden. The husband had sustained a "heart attack" ten years ago and had lain three weeks in hospital, a thrombophlebitis six months ago and a spell of dizziness while driving two months ago as well as (according to the description given by his wife) a transient hemianopsia. By his own complaint he was suffering from fatigue and an impairment of recent memory that caused him difficulty in the conduct of his business and had consulted a specialist in nervous diseases. From this colleague we received confirmation that the patient was not only hypertonic with a BP around 180 mm Hg, but was known to him and to the whole city as a high liver who was out every evening until far into the night, frequented different mistresses and was addicted to both opium and alcohol. Besides this he complained to his physician that his wife was making his life an inferno, that she was subject to attacks of blind rage in which she lost every control over herself and was even insensible to pain and that these occurred over the merest trifles or for no apparent reason at all, that she distrusted family, friends and neighbors, was constantly on the search for hidden motives, believed that everybody was plotting against her and even heard and saw things that did not exist.

The key patient in this case, less than half as old as her husband and the mother of two children by him, declared at once that she had only married him for his money after a first unhappy marriage that had ended in divorce and that her second marriage had been wretched from the beginning. She confirmed the account of her present husband that he himself and his physician had given us, her distrust of her neighbors and a real fear of her husband's first wife and son from that marriage, her own nervousness, excitability and attacks of depression. Once in such a condition she had thrown herself out of a window and cut her wrist badly. She denied phobic fears, but a little questioning brought out a terror of "microbes" such that she felt compelled to boil for a long time every dish and cup out of which visitors had eaten or drunk, besides a number of other compulsions. The abundant trials and provocations of the patient's life could have served to account for her psychopathological symptoms, but the second author was impressed besides by the patient's flickering glance, her ceaseless motor unrest and generally inappropriate, though not rejecting, behavior including crude attempts to flirt with the accompanying male psychologist in the psychiatrist's presence. The second author returned, experienced again the patient's abrupt oscillation between refusal and uninhibited revelation of intimate personal matters leading up to a description of how she "heard" the neighbors influencing the maid against her. Being asked *what* they said, she replied that she had not exactly heard them but knew it beyond doubt and hinted at yet other "knowledge" that she was not prepared to disclose. Although in common with former physicians we had considered the diagnosis of a grave reactive disorder and had been inclined to assume this after the first interview, the patient's characteristic manner and her unshakeable conviction of the plots against her together with her typically affirmed then attenuated acoustic hallucinations confirmed us in the diagnostis of a paranoid schizophrenia. Both the patient and her husband were adjudged to be of grade P_2. As the organic dementia from mixed causes including hypertonia and cerebrovascular insults dominated the picture and the man was already 65, he was diagnosed as an arteriosclerotic, and the important secondary diagnoses of addiction and neuroticism unfortunately were statistically lost. The 14 year old son was clever, spoiled, nervous and excitable, but since he was at puberty we left him the benefit of the doubt and did not class him as pathological although grounds for this were not entirely lacking. The 12 year old daughter appeared remarkably well equilibrated in spite of all. The husband's 16 year old daughter from his first marriage, who was attending school in Tehran, happened to be at home, and it was interesting to observe how the stepmother insisted that we also examine her, which we did without special result.

If our two schizophrenias were highly disparate cases nearly at opposite social extremes and with major familial complications, our two affective psychoses were very similar dim pictures in dark grey.

Both were female, the one 50, the other 55, and both had lived for several years in a state of chronic involutional depression without any previous history of either depressive or manic episodes. Both lived in poverty, had suffered sickness and bereavement and had ills and cares enough to make a diagnosis of reactive depression by itself plausible. The once divorced, then widowed 50 year old patient (the age is uncertain) became depressed before her husband died some eight years ago and left her a minute pension. Though she lives with her 15 year old son she feels lonely, neglected and hardly ever goes out of the tiny house. A change of outward circumstances would not help her, she said. She had consulted several out-patient clinics, including the psychiatric, without benefit. Her melancholy is strongest in the mornings and becomes better towards noon, is worse in summer. Formerly, she affirmed, she was able to work hard and well. To us she described such a series of bodily complaints that we thought a somatic examination necessary, suspecting hepatic disease and chronic bronchitis. Nemazee Hospital could not confirm any somatic illness. The patient was put on Tofranil and classed as involutional depression, P_2. The elder woman, 55, had lost her son-in-law and was looking after his six children as well as her husband and daughter-in-law, who was working in the woman's dormitories at the University. A pycnica with mournful cast of countenance, she replied to questions slowly but carefully. She awoke unrested, felt worst in the morning, complained of headache and failing eyesight, worried incessantly and had fears about everything, tried at first to refer her depression to the death of the son-in-law but let slip that it had set in a year before. We found again an involutional depression, but of lighter degree, as the patient in spite of all was still fulfilling important familial responsibilities and was not dependent upon medical help. She was correspondingly classed as P_1.

The epilepsies are predominantly cryptogenic, in contrast to the rural cases. Two boys of beginning school age were among them. A third male case concerned a 26 year old student of theology – a true morbus sacer! – whose mostly nocturnal fits had ceased five years ago but left him with a pronounced diffuse organic psychosyndrome and an impairment of memory that rendered the pursuit of his studies difficult. He had been subject to postictal acoustic hallucinations, but was so no longer. He and his wife subsisted in poverty on the daily allowance of a prominent mullah. In both of our females attacks had begun post partum. The single symptomatic case was referable to an undiagnosed severe febrile illness in early childhood. The patient was a 21 year old greengrocer with few seizures, but with such an alteration of character in the direction of irritable moodiness that he drove his relatives to despair and must be considered as a pseudo-psychopath. In only two of the six cases could any relation to diurnal rhythms be made out: both were nocturnal.

The 11 cases of senile and arteriosclerotic dementia ranged in age from a presenile 57 to a patriarchal 82, the mean ages of the whole group and of the male and female sub-groups separately being alike 68 and thus over a decade higher than in Khuzestan. All degrees were represented. For diagnosis of the "mild" cases we demanded more than the slight forgetfulness or irritability that not infrequently supervenes in the sixth or seventh decade and were convinced of the "more" in the instance of the 57 year old leader of a minor sect whose poor performance on the arithmetic and mediocre performance on the block design test contrasted with the more than minor official position he had occupied. The Z Test with a single answer per card (1 WF-, 1 DWF- of absurdly poor quality and 1 WF+ of "statues" where a WM would have been expected) was in keeping, and the clinical interview disclosed a sufficiently pronounced circumstantiality, egocentricity and unclearness of thought to confirm our suspicions. Two of our cases were opium addicts, one being the rich dealer in agricultural machines described above in connection with his schizophrenic wife, the other a post-apoplectic 60 year old woman servant. In both the obvious arteriosclerosis was regarded as weighing heavier than the addiction that had probably furthered it. Four cases were classified as P_1, 6 as P_2, 1 as P_3.

Six of the seven post-infectious cases were due surely or probably to a meningitis or encephalitis and were classed P_2. One was distinctly unintelligent, one showed a eunuchoid habitus and one woman had a residual paralysis of the right side. A seventh case, of milder grade (P_1) represented a malarial residue. These are the seven cases mentioned in the preceding chapter.

The four post-traumatic cases (three of them children of 11, 13 and 14 years respectively) require little comment beyond that three showed a typical focal syndrome with no great intellectual or memory impairment, the fourth case, a 30 year old man, having deteriorated in this respect also to P_3. We can mention in this connection our single "other" case, that of an 8 year old weak, shy and neurasthenic boy prematurely born at 7 months, whose intellectual performance was also below the norm and was rated with some skepticism as P_1 since he just contrived to carry on in school, though P_2 might have been appropriate.

More extended discussion is required and has been given in part elsewhere [23] of the seven cases, all male, in which addiction constituted the leading diagnosis. As we have seen already they are far from representing the sum of addicts to be found in the psychiatric survey sample even when the word "addiction" is used in a narrower sense than in the ICD and is taken to imply somatic dependance. Though at the time of the Shiraz Survey the former strict law against opium cultivation and the illegal use of drugs had been much relaxed so that addicts over 60 on a doctor's certificate could get a regular ration of government opium of good quality at a much lower price than had prevailed on the black market and opiates also could be prescribed regularly to patients under 60 under rather liberal conditions, there was still illicit traffic, and particularly younger users did not feel free to talk about the subject. In the larger interests of the survey we refrained from inquiring except in obvious cases or when offered a lead. Correspondingly 4 cases were rated P_3 (out of 11 P_3 in the whole sample), 2 as P_2 and only one – the sole alcoholic, a listless and unsteady psychopath with a gastritis alcoholica as well – as P_1.

The 91 cases of reactive disorders are much too numerous for individual discussion. Instead we shall give a few examples of the more frequent types or of those that present differential diagnostic problems. We see that as in the country the anxious and depressive cases with 26 patients led all the rest, and that the female sex with 21 out of the 26 dominated. Needless to say, a great many other reactive disorders were colored by depression where this did not constitute the sole or principal diagnosis. Let us regard two illustrative cases that will help to demonstrate the difference between simple and neurotic depression.

The scavenger's wife in the stinking courtyard of a neglected dwelling was 47 both by her own statement and her identity card but far gone in pregnancy. From poverty and general ill health she was sorrowful already before her marriage five years ago but found some consolation in memories of a not unhappy childhood and in hope for a better future. Into this marriage her 49 year old husband brought one eye, another wife and four children by her; the first wife and one of the children live apart from our proband, but three half-grown, noisy children inhabit another room of her house, take party with the husband against her and intrude themselves over and over into our conversation in the courtyard, intimidating the step-mother, from whom we get little information about her spouse except the unconvincing affirmation that he is "not angry". She has borne him one child already. The pregnancy was difficult, the partus apparently normal, but she had not enough milk and was gravely ill even to hospitalization for some time thereafter (no case history could be found, the description suggested mastitis). Avoiding direct accusations of her husband and the unruly step-children, she reiterated that she was always unhappy, indifferent and did not wish to live longer. While talking about her childhood she brightened perceptibly for a moment, then sank into renewed depression at the sudden realization that it was irrevocably gone. There were no diurnal mood swings and no evidences of concrete physical illness, though the patient seemed well-nigh exhausted. She was listless, apathetic, totally discouraged and despairing and heedless of the modest offers of help that we could make through a social aid society. We revisited her a month and a half later. She had given birth to a daughter, looked a shade better, but conveyed the same feeling of exhausted resignation and despair as before. The husband had been tested, had performed rather weakly on the intelligence tests and had given some evidence of insecurity on the Z Test. The examiners had described him as quiet and shy but did not feel that further investigation was necessary. We ourselves made several appointments to see him, which he broke. There was no doubt of a chronic severe depression, the main causes of which were evident to us and well known to the patient also, although she was endeavoring with slight success to dissimulate them both to herself and to us. Thus some dissociation, but no true repression was present. Somatic factors could not be excluded but were certainly not the only and probably not the main cause. We diagnosed a simple depressive development of grade P_2.

A thirty-five year old housewife of low intelligence, but not oligophrenic, was hopelessly overburdened by poverty, a 75 year old grandfather approaching infirmity and eight children, two of whom were confirmed bed-wetters. She took it out less in depression than in constant snapping, querulous ineffective scolding and was diagnosed as a simple irritable development, P_2.

Also opressed by poverty was the 16 year old daughter of an hysteric mother (glomus hystericus, P_1) and an unassuming, short-sighted greengrocer who had been compelled to leave school against her will by shortage of funds, as she asserted, but was merely helping a bit around the little house, was doing no remunerative work although at the time it was not difficult for girls to find domestic jobs, had worked for a short time as a seamstress and quit. She blamed her recurring fits of melancholia on her frustration but managed to smile, played a good deal with her hands and hair at interview, shook herself and conspicuously overbreathed, complained more or less jokingly of fears, particularly of going into the courtyard in the dark and even mentioned she sometimes thought someone was "calling" from there, though with so little conviction that we could exclude hallucinations. She was uneasy, aimless, moodily sad, then pleased to converse and even to jest a little about her plight. The Z Test gave evidence of neurotic depression with black as color, diffuse shading responses and sinister contents such as skeletons and scorpions and, to confirm her intelligence complex, showed four anatomy responses to Card II. The intellectual level of the Z Test was somewhat better than the mediocre performance on the two intelligence tests, which hardly would have qualified her for the profession of teaching that she had wished to embrace. Diagnosis: neurotic depression, P_1.

That not all depressive developments and neuroses stem from poverty becomes clear from the case, a pendent in many ways, of the 21 year old daughter of a comfortable or even well-to-do house that had achieved her aim of becoming a teacher as the preceding patient had not.

After high school she was undecided what she should do and took a one year training course that qualified her to teach in rural or small town schools, but not in Shiraz. She taught in a minor center but found no satisfaction in it, suffered from continual homesickness and had disciplinary difficulties with her classes. A second year there passed more unhappily than the first. She lost interest in everything, could envisage no goal ahead of her, slept poorly and could hardly bring herself to eat. Finally she quit her job some three months before we saw her and came home, expecting improvement to follow. It did not, and she consulted a psychiatrist, whose tablets yielded her little benefit beyond sleep. She was morosely killing time at her parents' house, tense, unhappy and at first little inclined to communicate, though after a while she began to talk more freely about herself. Under any physical or mental stress she was subject to headaches, felt continually unsure of herself, described herself as sensitive but reticent, whereas her sister would fly out at whatever provoked her. She had phobic fears of mice and cockroaches and was also afraid of the dark and of ghosts, but liked ghost stories! She looked much younger than her years, and her mother confirmed that the school inspectress had inquired several times if the age she stated was the true one. With no very concrete aim in life at all, she was vaguely considering taking up the study of psychology or journalism at the University but was reluctant to work for and present herself at the entrance examination. Diagnosis: depressive neurosis in infantile personality, P_2. A sister, two years older, presented a quite similar, more diffusely infantile and neurotic picture, was taking teacher training and herself teaching school, both part time and half-heartedly, was excitable, tense, moody, plagued by all manner of anxieties and dissatisfied with herself and with everyone else. As her symptoms were so manifold, while she was still barely able to function in a superficially "normal" manner and had not given up as her sister had, we diagnosed a polymorphic neurosis of grade P_1, also in an infantile personality. In regard to home background we may add that the father, chief accountant in a government office, was an open, cheerful and easy going man with no indication of personality disorder. The mother, 45, confessed that she had been rather excitable in her youth like her two daughters but had learned to keep herself in hand. She talked to us willingly and to all appearances openly, felt adequate to her responsibilities with a large house and six children and beyond a slight fear and dislike of the dark presented no neurotic symptoms. In the Z Test there was a mild initial stupor with only one response ("crab") to the first card, thereafter an unremarkable record.

The hysterical neuroses, of which we had seen few in the countryside, presented themselves in the city in numbers among rich and poor alike. One sketch of the familiar picture may suffice.

The 25 year old housewife had spent an agreeable childhood in comfortable circumstances, then married a driver and had been forced to live in more straitened ones. She had borne him moreover five daughters but no sons, about which he was unhappy. Things had gone passably until she was alone in the house with her third baby and was awakened by one of the elder children's returning, upon which she jumped up startled, fainted, awoke with people around her and could not speak for days afterwards. Over the past nine years such fits had followed not infrequently. She described vividly how she would become angry at one of the children, would like to scream but could not and then knew for certain that a fit was coming. She would fall but never injure herself, clench her teeth, thrash about and later come to herself. The husband would tell any bystanders to leave her alone! She had been to a neurologist and got tablets. Her mother had been subject to attacks of the same sort. One of the daughters was in hospital under treatment for rheumatic heart fever at the time, the rest of the family was unremarkable. The diagnosis was self-evident. Considering the frequence of the hysterical attacks, their severity and the general disruption of the household that they caused, we assigned the patient to P_2.

Along with the hysterical the not unrelated hypochondric neuroses also increased in the city far over what we had observed in the country (7 cases in Shiraz as against one each in Marvdasht and Khuzestan, the combined populations of the latter two being roughly equal) and were all female with a single exception. On the other hand we did not meet with diffuse neurasthenic neuroses in the urban environment.

The three self-insufficient neuroses in Shiraz deserve a brief depiction to explain the term.

The 13 year old son of a factory worker and a housewife afflicted with vicious attacks of migraine and anxious-depressive neurotic symptoms (P_2), both illiterate, was two years behind in school, as was his 10 year old sister. The boy's intelligence test performance, though not high, was not consonant with such retardation, but the Z Test exhibited marked neurotic traits, especially a repetition of supressed kinesthesias in the form of sculpture answers and an unchildlike avoidance of color, resulting in complete coarctation. His more excitable sister attained only 3 points on the arithmetic test and on the block design test none at all, delivered an equally neurotic Z Test with compensated color shock and animal stereotypy and was full of worries, fears and sorrow over the separation from her married elder sister. The influence of the neurotic, ever ailing mother and of the total lack of any intellectual stimulation in the environment were hardly to be doubted. In both instances we diagnosed a neurotic pseudo-debility from lack of intellectual stimulation and of emotional reassurance and classified the children in view of their pronounced failure at school as P_2. Their 14 year old sister was even further back (3 years), but showed both more adolescent complications and more indications of latent possibilities for compensation. As there was an admixture of demonstrative, irritable and even transient hysterical traits the diagnosis was made of a polymorphic neurosis or crisis of adolescence, and she was classified as P_1. The remaining case, a 10 year old boy who had struggled into the second grade, came from a similar intellectually and financially impoverished environment. He was as apathetic as his family appeared unconcerned. Examinations for parasitic infestation and for anemia were negative. The Z Test pointed to neurotic regression. P_2.

The "other and polymorphous" constitute the largest single subclassification. As the "polymorphous" far outweighed the "other", the nigh upon twenty cases cannot be described individually, but enough have been sketched already so that the reader can form an impression of this group. No purpose would be served by attaching pseudo-descriptive labels to them that could be nothing but arbitrary.

Among the psychosomatic cases there are a number of migranoid headaches as in the country, with the females in the majority, but perhaps the most striking feature is that the general female predominance among the reactive disorders (21 males to 49 females when reactive developments and neuroses are combined) here disappears. Eleven males as compared to ten females were found to be psychosomatically ill in the city. Of the two "other and polymorphous" male cases one concerned a cholecystopathy, one an incredibly fat twelve-year-old, neither intellectually very dull (he had repeated the second grade in school and just finished the fifth) nor sexually undeveloped. There was gynecomastia. The Nemazee Hospital could confirm neither a myxedema nor a morbus Froehlich, but observed that the youngster consumed enormous quantities of food, which his parents more or less surreptitiously provided even in the hospital. Even if his wants were not entirely fulfilled he remained placid and cheerful. Intelligence test performance was modest, but the Z Test was extremely stereotyped, poor in content and completed slowly while the boy from time to time laughed. His ten-year-old brother too was fat but intellectually and affectively far more lively. Two male children had died early, one at 1, the other at 3 years, and both had been unusually bulky, as we were told. The rather simple parents could make few useful statements about the brothers' childhoods or about the family situation and did not themselves impress us as pathological in any way. Though it was difficult not to persuade ourselves of an organic, presumably endocrine disorder the hospital findings made the diagnosis of an alimentary obesity with probably neurotic regression unavoidable. P_2.

The sex ratio among the clinically manifest oligophrenics was the reverse of that which had obtained among the reactive disorders: 8 males to 4 females, whereas in the villages the proportions had been equal. As sampling and examination were carried out in the same way throughout we have no explanation of this. By the usual clinical classification seven cases of the twelve could be counted as more or less gravely moronic, three as imbeciles, two as idiots. A male case of mongolism fell into this last, genetic category. There was one clinically typical case of Turner's syndrome and another probable one, in which the parents unfortunately would hear nothing of gynecological examination. No instance of Klinefelter's syndrome has occurred in our several samples.

Among the psychopaths the irritable and anti-social, mostly male, held the stage. Proceeding to the three female "other" cases we encounter one hysterical, one affectively labile and one anxious and self-unreliant. The 30-year-old man whom we finally, though not without lingering doubt, diagnosed as a schizoid psychopath perplexed us not a little and demands closer description.

After our examiners had recorded some of his striking responses to the questionnaire and had judged positively his need of special psychiatric examination we called one afternoon at the bakery where he worked, having learned already from his wife that he often stayed there throughout the night. Out of the sooty dark with a gleam of the inferno's flame that characterizes an open streetside bakery in the poorer quarters of an Iranian city appeared first the snowy flour-powdered head, then the short lithe figure of the unreluctant man, who politely explained that he could spend only a few minutes with us because of his work. During the interview a number of customers and gradually also of the curious did arrive and had to be served or fended off. The baker managed both calmly and without signs of annoyance.

Until about a year ago, he said, he had known no troubles beyond those of want (he was a low paid employee of the bakery). Then he was taken suddenly and violently ill with vomiting and diarrhea, was prostrated, thought at once that certain relatives of his wife's were trying to poison him and later saw with his own eyes how one of them put poison in his food. He had been occupying his brother's house but was ordered out of this as it needed repairs, took to sleeping in the bakery (in itself not at all uncommon in Iran) and was visited there by visions of animals, angels and devils, mostly inimical black figures, first during his sleep, later also when awake. These were neither ideas nor dreams, he affirmed, but a simple fact. They bothered him somewhat, and since their appearance had been connected with his "poisoning" he was not unwilling to visit the policlinic, made an appointment and accepted the card we gave him. His speech and gestures were orderly, even rather measured, without a trace of confusion. As his glance seemed slightly occluded we inquired cautiously about opium, the use of which he quietly denied.

We were scarcely surprised when the patient did not keep the appointment, but went to his home and found neither himself nor his wife there, but his sister-in-law. The rather dull young woman in the poverty-stricken and ill-kept dwelling could not state many precise details but even without prompting supplied illuminating general information such as that her brother-in-law was "always thinking" and that his thoughts were peculiar, although she could not explain why nor define them in any closer way. He had married her sister, a good wife, three years ago and to her knowledge had always been the same – a serious, very hard working man, liable to attacks of diarrhea and general weakness, easily but quickly calmed and incapable of doing harm to anyone. He had suffered no accident and never had epileptic seizures. His visions in the bakery had been well known to her for at least 3 years, i.e. since his marriage and had not altered (thus contradicting the patient's own assertion of a sudden commencement after a somatic illness only a year ago). They did not seem to excite her wonder in the least. He made trouble for nobody, not even for his brother who had more or less turned him out, although he was convinced that everyone was trying to make trouble for him. Further questions about ideas that might seem out of the way or bizarre were met with blank incomprehension. We left an invitation for the absent wife and were mildly surprised this time when she did in fact appear at the policlinic.

She too was apparently a dull woman, ground down by depression (classed as simple, P_1), poverty and care and, like her sister, able to answer only in the most general way. During four (!) years of marriage she had observed no abnormal or extraordinary behavior in her husband, who was to be sure taciturn, reclusive, but also hard-working and a good provider within his means. From time to time he got a headache and had to stay at home. He had said nothing whatever to his wife about the strange sights in the bakery.

In this quandary Dr. Moharreri managed to see the patient himself and talk to him more familiarly than we could. He was convinced that the "sights" were dreams, not hallucinations, and of a kind not extremely uncommon in the patient's environment. The next step clearly would have been a thorough physical and neurological examination to exclude as far as possible somatic disorders, but the subject had had enough and was not inclined to submit to this.

The man was illiterate and achieved merely four points on the arithmetic test and two on the block design, but did not strike one as unintelligent. Neither did the Z Test record reflect lack of intelligence. The protocol follows:

Z Test Protocol
Subject 04/02122/01, Shiraz, male, 30 years old, tested January 27, 1970

Beginning 11:04 o'clock

Card I Initial time 10 sec.

1. Eyes (two tiny white spots in upper central black)	DdSF+	Hd
2. Leaf of a tree (lateral grey detail with outstanding process)	DF–	Pl
3. A person with coat and trousers (entire central part, with middle black as coat)	DF+	H
4. Like wood (lower slender processes obliquely projecting downward and inward)	DdF+	Obj

Card II 11:08 o'clock, initial time 16 sec.

5.	The two brown parts are lions	DFFc+	AP
6.	The two green parts are flies	DF–	A
7.	The two red parts in the middle are like the leafs of a flower (entire red)	DFcF	Pl

Card III 11:12 o'clock, initial time 10 sec.

8.	The two lower black parts are mice ("legs" of mannekin)	DF+	A
9.	The two middle black parts are a cat (bodies and extended arms of mannekin, both sides)	DF–	AO–
10.	Both the red sides are a wolf (lateral red)	DF–	A

End 11:16 o'clock.

Total time 12 min., total responses 10, mean reaction time 72 sec.

W	0	F+	8		H	1	Space	1
D	8	F+		4	Hd	1	P	1
Dd	2	F–		4	A	5	Orig.	1
	—							
	10	FFc+	1		Obj	1	f%	85
		FcF	1		Pl	2	F+%	50
			—			—		
			10			10	A%	50

Apperceptive type: D – Dd
Experience balance: 0:1½ EW: O (E)

The opening tiny white space detail as "eyes" reflects anxiety in front of the heavy black mass and raises unavoidably the suspicion of something paranoic. The field is enlarged to the embracing upper dark area, which becomes the banal but formally unsuitable "leaf of a tree", and thence to the central black, which is seen not inappropriately as "a person with coat and trousers", a relatively well differentiated response. As if afraid of his own courage the subject "edges" and interprets the two small straight lower processes again banally as "like wood", i.e. sticks.

A variety of diagnoses seemed possible. Schizophrenia of the paranoid-hallucinatory type had been very much in our thoughts but did not convince our experienced colleague who had explored the subject longer than anyone else and in his own tongue, without intermediaries or the hindrance of a limited vocabulary. There were numerous references to somatic illnesses and complaints both on the part of the patient himself and on that of his relatives, but except the regular mention of recurring diarrhea (common enough in the poor districts anyhow and mostly of small moment) they were not consistent. The patient's visions and the mention of his headaches by his wife set our thoughts going in the direction of an organic cerebral disorder, e.g. temporal lobe epilepsy, but we could not confirm this and did not have grounds for more than a suspicion. The one point that seemed beyond doubt and on which all could agree was that the man was schizoid and, so far as we could ascertain, had been so for some years at least. There were few if any clinical or anamnestic indications of neurosis, and the Z Test definitely was not neurotic, leaving room to speak of a schizoid personality or a schizoid psychopathy. The condition seemed persistent and almost unchanging so far as we could learn, though the history of the remoter past was unsatisfactory. To assert that the patient "suffered" under his condition might have been to use too large a word, but his own initial readiness to accept medical advice indicated an awareness that not all was as it should be, and his relatives confirmed that they felt him

Table B IV 30. Diagnosis and Socio-Economic Status

Diagnoses	Poor					Middle					Well-to-do				
	m	f	m + f			m	f	m + f			m	f	m + f		
I. Funct. psychoses			3					0					1		
1. Schizophrenia	1			1								1		1	
2. Affect. psychoses		2		2											
II. Acute symptomatic psychoses															
III. Subchronic & chron. sympt. psychoses & residual states	11	8	19			9	4	13			4	0	4		
1. Epilepsy				4					2						
a. cryptogen.	2	1			3	1	1								
b. symptomatic	1				1										
2. Sen. & arterioscl.		4		4		2	3		5		2			2	
3. post-infectious	4	2		6		1			1						
4. post-traumatic		1		1		3			3						
5. endocrine															
6. addiction	4			4		1			1		2			2	
7. other						1			1						
IV. Reactive disorders	11	36	47			16	17	33			6	5	11		
1. Simple path. dev.	2	9		11			5		5					0	
a. anxious		2			2										
b. depressive	2	7			9		4			4					
c. irritable							1			1					
d. neurasthenic															
e. other															
2. Neuroses	6	22		28		10	7		17		4	5		9	
a. anxious		1			1	1	1			2					
b. phobic												1			1
c. depressive		2			2	3	2			5		1			1
d. hysterical	1	8			9		2			2	2				2
e. hypochondriac		5			5	1				1		1			1
f. neurasthenic															
g. self-insuff.	2	1			3										
h. negativistic															
i. other & polym.	3	5			8	5	2			7	2	2			4
3. Psychosomatic	3	5		8		6	5		11		2	0		2	
a. headache					5					7					1
α. migrainoid	1	3				2	3								
β. other	1					1	1				1				
b. gastro-intest.		1			1	3	1			4	1				1
c. asthmatic		1			1										
d. other & polym.	1				1										
V. Constitutional disord.	10	6	16			3	2	5			2	0	2		
1. Clin. oligophrenia	4	3		7		2	1		3		2			2	
a. cryptogenetic	4	2			6	2				2					
b. genetic		1			1		1			1	1				1
2. Psychopathy	6	3		9		1	1		2		0	0		0	
a. irritable	3	1			4	1				1					
b. anti-social	2				2										
c. schizoid	1				1										
d. other		2			2		1			1					
Total	33	52	85			28	23	51			12	6	18		

inarticulately to be a man somehow apart. We came therefore to a diagnosis of schizoid psychopathy, but only of grade P_1, since the patient was holding his own in the society of which he was a part as well as in his narrower family circle and even accepted with suspicious calmness the remarkable subjective experiences by which he was visited. His own utterances left no doubt as to the paranoid trends that the first response to the Z Test suggested. The question must remain open whether they are to be regarded as a manifestation of the schizoid character, possibly aggravated by physical illness, or of a paranoid schizophrenia. Certain it is that in the illiterate, impoverished and superstitious environment from which our patient came the readiness to take dreams and illusions that are congruent with popular imagery at their face value is enhanced, and the flame of the bakery fire under the sooty vault might play upon a disturbed imagination, oscillating between waking and dreaming, as the fires of the alchemist's oven have done upon brooding souls in times past. We leave the case with this diagnosis but shall return to it in connection with the schizophrenias and epilepsies in Part D.

Tables B IV 25–27 show how diagnoses are distributed according to degrees of severity in Shiraz, but we postpone a discussion until Part D, where comparisons can be drawn to other surveys as well. The relation of diagnosis to socio-economic status appears in Table B IV 30 and has been indicated for severe cases only in Table B IV 28 already. Discussion again shall be postponed. The total figures reveal no statistically significant higher morbidity rate for either sex, but those for the poor do. Females here constitute 61 % of the cases. Comparison by fourfold table between the poor and non-poor of both sexes gives $X^2 = 4.86$ and $p < 0.05$, confirming manifold implications of the same kind that we have met before. Comparison of single diagnoses by SES nowhere has led to statistically significant findings, while comparisons of categories of disease by sex and SES shall be reserved for Part D, where they can be extended in certain cases to other surveys.

Somewhat to our surprise only two exclusively neurological cases were identified, both presenting residual symptoms after poliomyelitis. In Table B IV 31 the neurological and neuropsychiatric cases are tabulated together, this time by their neurological diagnoses, with the psychiatric complications indicated in parentheses.

Four each of the above cases could be classed as mild and medium, i.e. 4.3 ‰ each, none as severe. The total neurologic plus neuropsychiatric morbidity rate of 8.6 per

Table B IV 31. Diagnostic Distribution of Neurologic and Neuropsychiatric Cases

	m	f	Sum m + f
Residues after poliomyelitis (2 psychiatrically unremarkable, 1 depressive neurosis)	2	1	3
Status after meningo-encephalitis (3 cases of affective disturbance, of which 1 eunuchoid, 1 with paresis, 1 with occipital headache)	2	1	3
Posttraumatic amblyopia (with affective disturbance following cerebral trauma)	1		1
Juvenile hemiparesis (with affective disturbance following subsequent cerebral trauma)		1	1
	–	–	–
Total	5	3	8

1000 is thus lower than in Marvdasht (20 ‰, children below six not included) and in Khuzestan (23 ‰), and for this difference $0.05 > p > 0.02$. The difference is "significant" but very probably deceptive. A smaller part of the survey sample in Shiraz was seen by physicians either Iranian or foreign, and the examiners whose obligation it was to report neurologically as well as psychiatrically suspicious cases had no medical training at all. Examiners in the two rural surveys, on the contrary, almost without exception possessed some medical background even if they were not physicians themselves. In their course of instruction our Shirazi examiners naturally were told something about neurological illnesses and asked to look for them, but their information could not be anything but extremely sketchy, nor had they any practice in recognizing what was meant. Our own regular attendance at the weekly neuropsychiatric case presentations at the Medical Faculty of the Pahlavi University did not afford us any reason to believe that neurological cases were more rare in the city than in the country. We strongly suspect that their seeming scarcity in our sample was an artefact of the method of case finding.

Part C Psychological Studies

I. Intelligence

1. Previous Studies with Intelligence Tests in Iran

So far as the authors' knowledge goes, it was Max Valentine, commissioned by the British Government as Visiting Professor of Psychiatry at the University of Shiraz from 1956 to 1958, who first attempted systematically to apply intelligence tests on a wide scale in Fars and perhaps in all Iran [195]. He was set the task of making a selection among the very numerous candidates for admission to the various collegiate and academic institutions there. For this purpose he used the Raven Matrices. Young men from the villages had applied for a one to two year course at the agricultural school; their number unfortunately is not stated. According to British norms the test results were very low; almost a third would have fallen into the group of the "feeble minded". Valentine refers this to anxiety and to basic unfamiliarity with such tasks and remarks justly that it would be ridiculous to interpret the results uncritically according to Western norms. A further group was formed of 120 from 340 candidates for the Faculty of Medicine after 210 applicants had been eliminated by previous academic tests. The distribution of the results was roughly normal, but the performance was merely average by Western norms although the group had passed through several processes of selection. For such a select group, it comprised an extraordinary number of poor performances. This "tail" was smaller in the third group of candidates for the Agricultural Faculty of the same university and the number of above-average performances was greater, as one would expect from a selected group. An entirely satisfactory explanation for this could not be given. Probably though, as Valentine suspects, a practice effect played some part since not a few candidates who were not accepted for the Faculty of Medicine thereupon applied to the Faculty of Agriculture, took the tests again and thus acquired some familiarity with them.

Valentine furthermore tested 627 secondary school pupils in the city of Shiraz, aged between 14 and 20 years, with the Raven Matrices. According to the British norms the age differences are particularly small in this range. The Iranian results lagged behind the British throughout, especially in the higher age groups, and those of the girls behind those of the young men. According to a personal communication of Raven's to Valentine, Raven had encountered the same peculiarity in other Oriental and African populations and referred them to unfamiliarity with Western ways of thought.

When the first author took up work in Iran in 1960, he sought contact not only with psychiatric, but also with educational and particularly with counseling institutions and found that practically all Western trained psychologists were indeed using the tests with which they had become familiar, but in translation, more or less free adaptation and with subjective, comparative evaluation. Rumors were rife then and many years after that this or that test was being, or already had been, standardized and was about to be, or already had been, published with due sets of Persian norms. Diligent inquiry up to mid-1978, when regular communication ceased, has not led to the discovery of even a single such test. If we have missed them, we regret this and apologize to their authors. This does not mean, on the other hand, that no research on psychological, particularly intelligence testing, has taken place. It has indeed, mostly at the instigation of A. Mehryar and with the co-operation of his group at Pahlavi University, Shiraz. A series of publications begins there about 1970 and shall be reviewed here rather briefly because the basic population remained largely the same and different intelligence tests when applied to it yielded rather similar results.

Mehryar and Shapurian [146, 147] began with Persian adaptations of Heim's AH4 and AH5 group tests [95, 96], the former being essentially a speed test "widely used for research and practical purposes in Britain" [147, p. 169], the latter "a high-grade group test which relies heavily on facts and skills associated with middle and higher education" [147]. The large basic population was formed first of 1008 pupils of secondary schools in Shiraz and soon enlarged to 3120 of both sexes, that "could be regarded as fairly representative of the socio-economic composition of the secondary school population of the city of Shiraz" [147, p. 168]. In the secondary schools specialization in the three branches of mathematics, natural sciences and literature had already begun. The first two were socially and economically more prestigious. The authors remark that "although no objective study of the relative standing of the three branches in terms of intelligence is available, it would seem to be generally assumed that the most intelligent and serious students go to the mathematics and natural science branches, and that a sizeable portion of those entering the literary branch do so not because of any particular talent or interest in arts and humanities, but because they were not able to find any other outlet for their wish to finish secondary education and enter university" [147, p. 168]. Results on both tests were basically similar to each other, to Valentine's, to those of preliminary unpublished research performed with adapted Western tests in Iran and, so far as comparison is possible, with our own to be reported below, showing on the whole a roughly normal distribution of scores, a rise in average performance with increasing age, discrimination between the three branches of specialization in the expected directions, average performances even among highly selected groups that were much lower than the British and consistently lower averages from female subjects than from male, although the smaller female groups at the higher educational levels were probably even more selected and almost certainly more motivated than their male counterparts. Girls following the mathematics and natural science branches of the upper grades did, however, score better than their male counterparts in the first, verbal part of the AH4, though not on the second, perceptual and remained behind them on both parts of the AH5. The authors, reflecting that "for the overwhelming majority of subjects . . . this experiment provided the first opportunity to take a Western type intelligence test under strictly controlled conditions" [147, p. 177], retested 107 subjects of both sexes with the AH4 after an interval of three months and found a very marked rise in average performance amounting to just over one standard deviation unit of the subjects' respective original scores, equivalent to a rise of over two years in mental age. Because of "the easy nature of the AH4 test and its obvious dependence on information and skills common to formal schooling" the authors did not attribute the poor performance of the Iranian students to the cultural content of the test, but discussed lack of test sophistication, the unaccustomed use of a separate answer sheet, the time restriction (contrary to Iranian custom and education style) and relative deprivation of cultural stimulation of Western type as possible reasons for it.

Analyzing the same collective tested with the AH5, Mehryar studied the influence of sociodemographic correlates on the results [139, 140]. He found a marked positive correlation between them and parental education (especially the father's) and a less marked negative correlation with family size, whereas small families seemed even more closely related with general academic success as indicated by passed and failed examinations than was the education of the parents. He quotes an unpublished study by Haghighi using almost ten thousand Persian university applicants and a Persian adaptation of Thurstone's PMA which showed a correlation of −0.258 between intelligence and family size. The girls came from an "obviously superior socio-economic background", scored consistently lower than the boys on the AH5 test and nevertheless recorded smaller ratios of past academic failure. Commenting on this, Mehryar remarks [139, p. 51] "that the apparent superiority of Iranian boys is most probably due to certain subtle differences in the early handling of boys and girls in this country. Perhaps a similar subtle difference in their early interactions with parents and the grown-ups underlies the observed differences between subjects coming from large and small families".

In an effort to find "Some Personality Correlates of Intelligence and Educational Attainment in Iran", Mehryar, Kahjavi, Razavieh and Hosseini [143] applied no less than six tests of intelligence and academic attainment, the Eysenck Personality Inventory and Eysenck's Psychoticism Scale to 878 students who had just left secondary school and were taking the annual university entrance examination. Unsurprisingly, there was an unequivocal negative relation between psychoticism and intelligence scores, but "an almost total lack of correlation between the neuroticism scale and measures of intellectual performance" – even less surprising in the light of our own experience with Eysenck's short form of his neuroticism scale reported in Chap. B II 2. The differences in relation to introversion and extraversion, as measured by Eysenck's scales, were neither very marked nor consistent. Extraversion seemed to go with superior achievement in boys, but with the contrary in girls. The authors comment on the "psychometric inadequacy" of the tests, and the present writers as psychiatrists cannot but indicate their doubts about the meaningfulness or usefulnes of a "psychoticism scale" for the general population at all.

In an investigation more closely related to some of ours than the preceding Mehryar [142] used the Tool Matching Scale of the General Aptitude Test Battery, Form B-1002B, developed by the U.S. Department of Labor [194], on 320 hitherto totally illiterate male workers at the lowest socio-economic level employed by the then very new National Iranian Steel Corporation in Isfahan and attending literacy classes run by the experimental Work-Oriented Adult Literacy Project organized jointly by the Government of Iran and the UNESCO. General findings were again distressingly below the American standards, but improved substantially when the Iranian subjects were allowed more time. The test was found to be significantly correlated with four of six measures of literacy achievement. The influence of age is of especial interest in connection with our own findings. The mean performance of Iranian subjects reached its peak at about age 18, declined somewhat toward age 23, remained more or less stable nevertheless over the decade from 21 to 30, declined again toward forty and sharply thereafter, whereas we found only a very moderate decline between 20 and 60.

2. Intelligence Tests Newly Standardized in Iran and Employed in the Present Studies

A detailed description of psychological tests, their administration and standardization, their respective merits and demerits, holds little interest as a rule for the epidemiologist. We therefore propose to keep this chapter brief. Directions for administration and the necessary tables for converting raw into standard scores and these into intelligence quotients (IQs) are meaningless except for those who are actually using the tests, so it is planned to bring such information together in a Test Manual in Persian, which will also include a description of the standardization and its criteria.[1]

As the time expendable for each subject was short and the intelligence test was intended more as a screening and research instrument than as one for individual diagnosis we confined it to two subtests, one of more theoretical, the other of more practical intelligence, anticipating that in the far from homogenous socio-cultural situation substantial differences between these aspects of general intelligence might be encountered. For the first we chose, not without a good deal of initial scepticism and hesitation, a set of straightforward exercises in mental arithmetic, in all four basic operations and including at the end a few fractions, familiar to us over years and then still employed in a large number of Central European psychiatric institutions. There was good reason to question whether it was suitable for use in a largely illiterate population that had not been formally trained in this last of the three R's. Nevertheless, all were living in a monetary economy and had a vital interest in mastering at least the simple operations demanded of them. Moreover, the test could be extended easily from a very low range (identification of current coins and addition of them to a prescribed sum, thereafter only mental arithmetic) up to a fairly high one ("How much is $^1/_2$ and $^1/_3$?"). Preliminary trials showed that the scores scattered widely and differentiated even better than we had expected. This we called Arithmetic Test A. Another one was required for school children and literates, mainly in Shiraz. For this we translated and adapted the Arithmetic Test of the Wechsler-Bellevue Scale, Form II and have retained it since then unchanged in spite of Wechsler's new versions for the sake of comparability and uniformity. It is known as Arithmetic Test B.

As a test of practical intelligence we first tried Wechsler's adaptation of the Kohs Block Design Test because this is generally considered to be one of the best of his subtests, correlating highly with the total score of the scale, often is used as an independent test of intelligence as by Kohs and also possesses diagnostic value as an indicator of diffuse brain damage. In the illiterate village and nomad populations it worked very poorly, differentiating hardly at all. The main reason seemed to be that the subjects were distracted by the sides of the cubes, could not abstract from them to concentrate on the two-dimensional design and kept on trying to build the colored sides into this. Following the wise suggestion of a Persian colleague we resorted to a device employed by Ord in New Guinea and described by Vernon in his book on *Intelligence and Cultural Environment* [198, pp. 101–102] and substituted flat pieces of the same dimensions for the blocks. The designs, time limits, etc. remained the same. This

[1] The Manual has in fact been written in English but not yet translated.

worked out quite well, so we used the platelets as Block Design Test A for the illiterates and the cubes as Block Design Test B for the literates. In the Marvdasht and Khuzestan Surveys we had still been using cubes for all. The results for the Block Design Test proved useless and were discarded. IQs for these surveys are based on the Arithmetic Test alone. The change was made with the Shiraz Survey, in which the proportion of the literates was much larger, and was retained of course in Qalandari and in the Qassemabad resurvey.

During field work we had recorded raw scores and judged intelligence by experience with these and by observation. When, after the surveys of Shiraz and Qalandari, facilities for data processing became available through the WHO, standardization was undertaken. As the tests for the literates and illiterates were not the same, these populations had to be standardized separately. The literate populations were those of Shiraz and Qalandari because the number of literates in the previously investigated villages and tribes was practically negligible and nearly confined to a handful of primary school children. This does not imply that the literates comprise an excessive number of somewhat better-off urban residents, for because of our strictly random sampling of the Shiraz Survey Population the less well-off and the poor were represented in exactly those proportions in which they occurred. It does imply, however, that both Block Design Tests A and B were standardized on the populations of Shiraz and Qalandari only. For Arithmetic A we drew on the adult populations of villages and nomads earlier studied as well, but not for Arithmetic B for the reasons given above. When it became apparent that the age progression from 6 to 7 and 7 to 8 was unsatisfactory we eliminated the age classes 6 and 7 from the standardization population and were left with the numbers in Table C I 1:

Table C I 1. Literacy of Men and Women in Iran

	Illiterate	Literate	Ill. + Lit.
Males	660	1186	1846
Females	1038	934	1962
	1698	2120	3808

Finally, account had to be taken of the very marked and obvious differences in test behavior and performance between the sexes in Iran. The sex discrepancies among the illiterates were great and statistically highly significant, tended to decrease with literacy, urbanization and higher education, but even in the higher SES did not become small enough to be neglected, let alone vanish. When, as an experiment, intelligence quotients for literate city women were calculated by the weighted scores for men they turned out to be about 5 IQ points lower. The reasons for this are hardly psychobiological, but much rather socio-cultural. We believe that they stem, at least in the far larger part, from an ingrained pattern of social behavior that was obvious even to the most casual observer in the villages but did not stop at the city boundaries. Akin to this may be the fact that, although most occupations and professions were open to women even in the 1960s and a number of women did occupy leading places among them, their number was relatively small. Outside of a thin upper layer of well-situated and educated families there was little insistence upon the female members to acquire genuine skills and to exercise them, to bear up under pressure and prove themselves by performance. Though every year increasing numbers of girls flocked to secondary and higher schools they tended to cling to the shelter of the home and the goal of marriage. This observation detracts in no way from the work done by many excellent and devoted female teachers, nurses, administrators, technicians and professional persons, but we are persuaded that it holds for a substantial majority. Statistical findings are a reflection of the majority. Typical test behavior especially of uneducated Iranian girls was to solve at most a couple of the easiest problems, risk a wild guess or two, giggle and resign. After consulting with several experienced test psychologists, both Iranian and foreign, we decided to standardize all tests separately for the two sexes.

This was done by following exactly Wechsler's procedure as described in [201]. The scores therefore are standardized or z scores, and the "intelligence quotients" are not true quotients but standard scores for the respective age class (the classes, n.b., are not identical with Wechsler's). The range of weighted scores per test was set arbitrarily at 20, the mean at 10 and the standard deviation at 3. One probable error (PE) above or below the mean corresponds to an IQ of 90 or 110. Age classes were by single years from 8 to 14, then 15–19, 20–39, 40–60 and 60+. The IQ distribution as shown in Diagram C I 1 turned out to be quite satisfactorily Gaussian except for a "hump" around IQ 85–90 for the illiterate males. Correlations between the Arithmetic and Block Design Tests are stated in Table C I 2 (numbers of subjects are lower than stated above for a variety of technical reasons, to account for which would require excessive space here):

Table C I 2. Correlations between Arithmetic and Block Design Test

	Males	Females	Males and Females
Illiterate subjects (Arith. A x Block A)			
Number of subjects	332	570	902
Correlation (r)	0.41	0.37	0.39
Standard error	0.05	0.04	0.03
Literate subjects (Arith. B x Block B)			
Number of subjects	1183	920	2103
Correlation (r)	0.54	0.50	0.52
Standard error	0.02	0.02	0.02

Further technical information must be reserved for another place.

Differentiation around the age of 8–10 years and for IQs below 80 or above 120 at all ages is not as good as we should wish it to be. We recommend employing the tests cautiously at these extreme ranges and regarding very low or very high IQ scores as indications for further investigation. Caution is likewise indicated in interpreting all results at ages 8 and 9, whereas at 10 and above they satisfy usual criteria of short test reliability and validity.

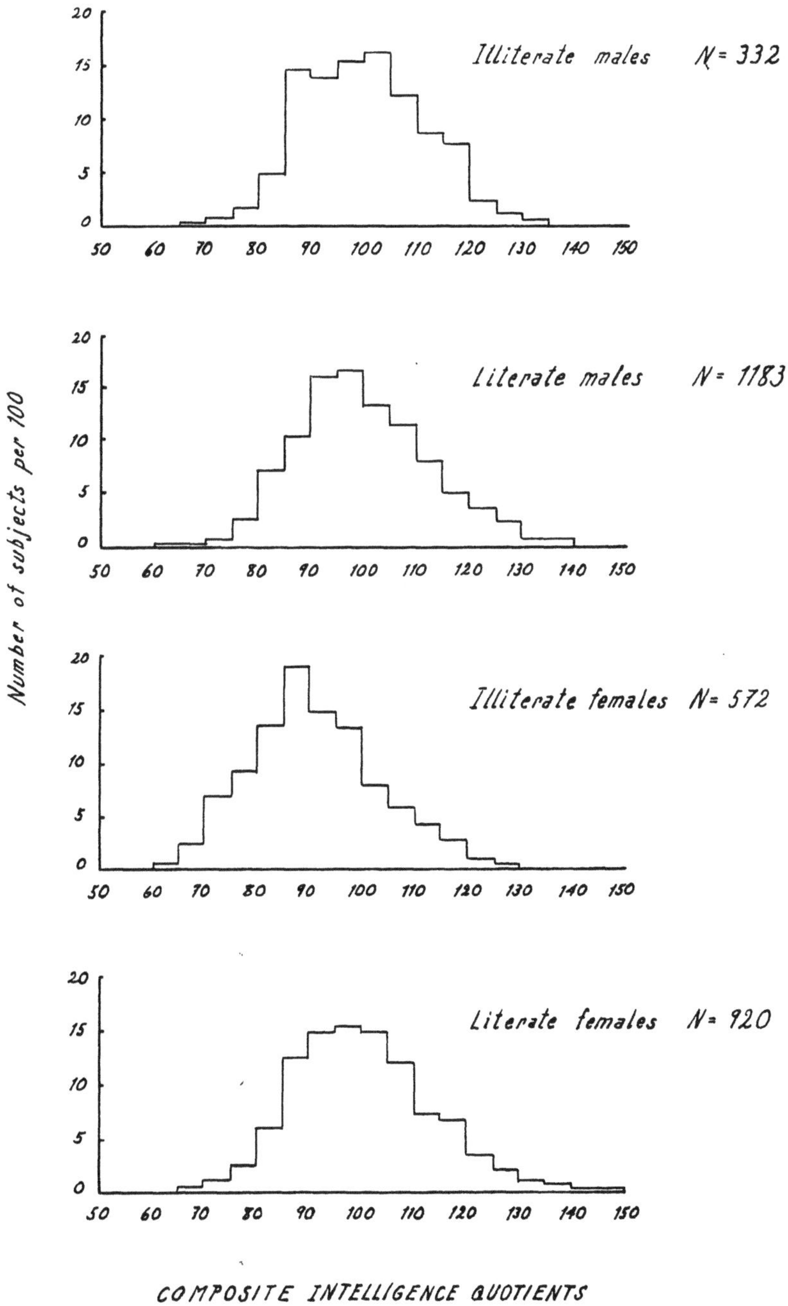

Diagram CI 1. Distribution of Composite Intelligence Quotients

3. Comparative Results of Intelligence Testing

Since Table C I 3 shows that the empirical means of the intelligence tests do in fact cluster very closely around the theoretical mean of 100, it becomes possible to compare the means of socio-economic, unpathological and pathological sectors of the Shiraz Psychiatric Survey Population on the one hand and the means of geographically and to some extent ethnically different populations on the other, bearing in mind that comparisons between the illiterate and the literate as between the sexes cannot be made directly because of the separate standardizations of the tests.

We begin with such comparisons as lie within the compass of Shiraz and Qalandari. The basic findings are set out in Tables C I 4–6. Table C I 4 covers the entire Shiraz Survey Population (SP) including Qalandari. Its first seven lines compare the mean IQs of subpopulations by socio-economic status, literacy and sex, although the two sexes are not compared with each other. A glance shows that with monotonous regularity, high to very high statistical significance and by IQ margins that, varying between 4.0 and 6.8 points, are factually and not only statistically significant, the poor do less well whether they are literate or illiterate, male or female. The results are familiar from many investigations in different countries and continents and lead always to the question whether poverty on the whole suppresses intellectual unfolding and performance (as in some cases it undoubtedly does) or whether relatively inferior intellectual endowment engenders poverty. Since there is some positive correlation between socio-economic status and educational opportunity and a higher one probably in developing countries such as Iran than in Western countries with nearly universal systems of compulsory free education up at least to primary level and often with many opportunities for scholarships after that, it is important to look at the literate and illiterate poor and non-poor separately. When we do so, we find no basic difference. Literacy per se does not, as far as these findings go, equalize or counterbalance the stultifying effect of poverty, nor can it be said that the poor are poor simply because of illiteracy. Otherwise we should not observe a nearly equal gradient (though a little steeper in the literate) between higher and lower socio-economic status in the literate and illiterate alike. The argument that illiteracy is one thing, but literacy many, from the first grade to the university and beyond, is irrelevant because it simply helps to explain on the one hand the already observed superior intellectual performance of the non-poor with their generally better educational opportunities but on the other does not in any way explain why the illiterate non-poor attain a substantially higher mean IQ than the economically less fortunate but equally illiterate.

The intellectual gradient between the non-poor and the poor does not appear to be related in any way to sex, as it is found in both sexes, whether literate or illiterate, alike.

The eighth line provides more food for thought. It compares the illiterate with the literate in seeming contradiction to what was said at the beginning of the chapter, but it does not do so directly. It compares the standing of the poor in each educational group against the mean of their fellows in the same group, which is approximately 100. The literate poor fall farther than the illiterate poor below this mean by 2.6 IQ points, and the difference, though not large, is statistically quite significant. The circumstance may cause surprise at first glance. At second it seems inevitable. The already mentioned correlation between socio-economic status, intelligence and educational opportunity is

Table C I 3. Mean Composite Intelligence Quotients for Arithmetic and Block Design Tests Combined

	Illiterate						Literate					
	Males			Females			Males			Females		
Age	N	Mean	SD	N	Mean	SD	N	Mean	SD	N	Mean	SD
8							71	99.07	11.95	42	99.76	12.86
9							56	100.04	12.88	59	99.58	12.71
10							65	99.80	12.78	62	99.63	12.06
11							49	99.67	12.13	52	99.08	11.80
12							74	99.76	13.41	72	99.76	12.39
13							58	99.72	13.34	41	99.59	13.58
14							58	99.79	12.68	61	99.74	13.48
15–19	12	100.42	14.19	43	99.84	12.18	223	99.75	13.16	164	99.67	13.17
20–39	100	99.58	13.01	229	99.56	12.60	285	99.61	13.18	243	99.68	12.64
40–59	107	99.94	11.47	160	99.86	11.87	145	99.90	12.74	51	100.22	12.63
60 +	59	100.12	11.40	69	100.01	11.40	42	100.02	12.79	10	99.60	13.19
All	278			501			1126			857		

Table C I 4. Survey Population from Shiraz (SP) and Qalandari: Mean Intelligence Quotients by Socio-Economic Class, Literacy and Sex

Classes compared	N	$\overline{IQ}$	SD/$\overline{IQ}$	N	$\overline{IQ}$	SD/$\overline{IQ}$	$\overline{\Delta IQ}$	Sign. t
	Non-poor			*Poor*				
all : all	1638	102.4	13.0	1329	97.3	11.6	5.1	›››
ill. : ill.	325	103.4	12.5	564	98.8	11.7	4.6	›››
lit. : lit.	1313	102.1	13.1	765	96.2	11.3	5.9	›››
m ill. : m ill.	95	105.0	11.7	234	98.8	12.1	6.2	››
f ill. : f ill.	230	102.8	12.8	330	98.8	11.5	4.0	››
m lit. : m lit.	737	102.5	13.2	433	95.7	11.3	6.8	›››
f lit. : f lit.	576	101.7	12.6	332	96.8	11.5	4.9	›››
	Poor			*Poor*				
ill. : lit.	564	98.8	11.7	765	96.2	11.3	2.6	››
	Non-poor			*Non-poor*				
ill. : lit.	325	103.4	12.5	1313	102.1	13.1	1.3	(›)
Tested	3005							
SES unidentified	38							
Effective pop.	2967							

Table C I 5. Psychiatric Survey Population from Shiraz (PP) and Qalandari: Mean Intelligence Quotients by Socio-Economic Status, Literacy and Sex

Classes compared	N	$\overline{IQ}$	SD/$\overline{IQ}$	N	$\overline{IQ}$	SD/$\overline{IQ}$	$\overline{\triangle IQ}$	Sign. t
all : all	505	102.5	13.7	555	95.7	11.7	6.8	›››
ill. : ill.	98	104.9	13.2	259	97.2	11.9	7.7	›››
lit. : lit.	407	102.0	13.8	296	94.4	11.3	7.6	›››
m ill. : m ill.	33	106.1	11.0	107	96.8	11.3	9.3	››
f ill. : f ill.	65	104.2	14.2	152	97.5	11.3	6.7	›››
m lit. : m lit.	227	102.7	13.9	169	94.7	11.0	8.0	›››
f lit. : f lit.	180	101.1	13.6	127	94.1	11.8	7.0	››
	Poor			*Poor*				
ill. : lit.	259	97.2	11.7	296	94.4	11.3	2.8	›
	Non-poor			*Non-poor*				
ill. : lit.	98	104.9	13.2	407	102.0	13.8	2.9	(›)

Tested 1060 = effective population

Table C I 6. Psychiatric Survey Population from Shiraz (PP) and Qalandari: Mean Intelligence Quotients by Pathology, Literacy and Sex

Classes compared	N	$\overline{IQ}$	SD/$\overline{IQ}$	N	$\overline{IQ}$	SD/$\overline{IQ}$	$\overline{\Delta IQ}$	Sign. t
	Unpathological			*Pathological*				
all : all	891	99.8	12.8	161	94.9	13.9	4.9	›››
ill. : ill.	285	100.2	12.1	69	96.1	13.9	4.1	›
lit. : lit.	606	99.6	13.0	92	94.0	14.4	5.6	››
m ill. : m ill.	118	100.3	12.1	21	92.9	15.0	7.4	›
f ill. : f ill.	167	100.1	12.6	48	97.6	12.5	2.5	(›)
m lit. : m lit.	339	100.3	12.9	54	93.4	14.2	6.9	››
f lit. : f lit.	267	98.7	13.1	38	94.8	14.7	3.9	(›)
	Pathological			*Pathological*				
ill. : lit.	69	96.1	13.4	92	94.0	14.4	2.1	
	Unpathological			*Unpathological*				
ill. : lit.	285	100.2	12.1	606	99.6	13.0	0.6	
Tested	1060							
Clinical examination refused	8							
Effective population	1052							

far from perfect. Every school has its dunces. Of 13 patients in the Shiraz Survey diagnosed as oligophrenic, 7 were by definition "literate". Unable to profit by what education they have received, they are naturally more apt than their classmates to swell the ranks of the poor and therefore to depress the mean measured intellectual performance of these. If this were not true, one must expect that the non-poor literates would do better than the non-poor illiterates. The ninth line shows that they do not and even indicates a not quite statistically assured tendency for them, by a small margin, to do worse. The comparison of these findings seems to offer a fairly conclusive answer to the question raised at the outset. In statistical terms, and with numerous painfully familiar exceptions, it cannot be said that poverty per se depresses intelligence, but that poorer intellectual equipment – weaker arms in the struggle for existence – increases the risk of poverty.

Table C I 5 based only on the Psychiatric Survey Population practically duplicated its predecessor and does not require separate discussion. Its value lies in the demonstration that the intellectual composition of the SP and PP are nearly identical, i.e. that the PP in this respect (though not in others) is an entirely representative sample of the SP. This becomes of importance when we now set out, within the PP, to compare the intelligence test performance of the unpathological and the pathological, as we can be confident that the results hold also for the larger collective.

We discover at first, in Table C I 6, a general confirmation for the obvious expectation that intelligence test performance sinks with psychopathology. In almost every case the degrees of significance are quite satisfactory even though slightly less than in the preceding tables because of the smaller numbers. Where they are not, and only approach significance, it is notable that they apply both times to female groups. We could not find any explanation for this in general, social, cultural or economic terms, but the explanation became obvious when we turned to the distribution of diagnoses in the two sexes. It becomes necessary here to anticipate results that will be discussed in Part D, Chap. III. From the table of all diagnoses in Shiraz (No. B IV 29) it will be seen readily that the men have double the rate of the women for subchronic and chronic symptomatic psychoses and residual states (25.9 as against 12.9 per thousand) and also for clinical oligophrenia (8.6 as against 4.3 per thousand). These are precisely the disease groups most apt to depress intellectual performance – the latter by definition. The women make up for this by a rate for reactive disorders: 63.6 per thousand, that is nearly twice as high as the men's: 34.5. Such disorders may influence intellectual performance unfavorably in some cases and at some times, but by no means to the same degree and never with a comparable regularity. The remaining cases are too few to affect the mean IQ in more than a slight degree.

The eighth line reflects only numerically, but without statistical significance, the difference between the illiterate and literate that we had seen in the foregoing tables. Pathology pulls down the schooled and the unschooled nearly alike. Apart from oligophrenia, it seems reasonable that acquired psychopathology should affect test performance even more in those who have had some training in this direction, i.e. in formal schooling. Those who have attained more have more to lose.

The ninth line does nothing more than to confirm the expectations of our test standardization.

It may be asked whether the inclusion of oligophrenics does not unduly depress the mean IQs of the pathological subjects and thus mask whatever influence psychiatric

Table C I 7. Mean Intelligence Quotients of Pathological Subjects with and without Oligophrenia

Class	of which oligophrenic with valid comp. IQ	Mean IQ Oligophrenia included	excluded
Male illiterate	4[a]	92.9	95.8
Male literate	3	93.4	94.4
Female illiterate	0		
Female literate	4	94.8	96.8

[a] Two members of this class had to be omitted from the calculation because they could not be tested. The total of cases is thus 13, not 11 as appears here.

disorders with process character may exert. We have therefore recalculated some mean IQs omitting the oligophrenics with the results shown in Table C I 7.

The mean IQs of pathological subgroups do rise as expected when the oligophrenics are excluded, but still remain substantially below the means of the unpathological.

We examine now the geographical differences, which in the case of the Qashqai are ethnic also. A more suitable instrument for doing this than the mean IQ is the raw point score on the mental arithmetic test for illiterates (Arithmetic Test A) for a number of reasons. The principal one is that it is the only test of the four which has been used unchanged in all surveys and has been applied with fair success to almost wholly illiterate village populations (the unrevised Block Design Test, it will be remembered, proved unsatisfactory there). Raw scores on the arithmetic test can now be converted into weighted scores and IQs, but little is gained and probably even some accuracy is lost thereby. Mean raw scores have to be rounded off to integers, and this rounding off by a few decimals upwards or downwards may lead to a displacement by one or more weighted score points and by several IQ points. We give the IQ values, without decimals, nevertheless for the sake of easier comparability with other tables, though in certain cases, as we shall see, they are probably misleading. This is due to the nature of the tests themselves and of the conversion tables with their rather gross steps, not to a fault in the general norms. These have been derived in fact from a standardizing population in which the illiterate villagers were generously represented, and if these sometimes fall short of the expected standard, it is not because they did not participate adequately in its composition. The differences may be taken to be real.

We treat the two sexes separately as throughout, omit age classes below 15, as many of them when distributed geographically would yield far too small numbers, and even thereafter do not calculate means etc. for classes or groups with less than 10 members. Inspection of the material showed that it was expedient to take as our basis of comparison the population of Shiraz and Qalandari and to compare against this, for each age group, the three rural or nomad populations of Marvdasht (closest to Shiraz, in the Province of Fars), Khuzestan and the Qashqai subtribe. A separate comparison of the nomadic Qashqai with the settled Qashqai of Qalandari might have seemed desirable, but is in fact hardly feasible in respect to Arithmetic Test A because too many of the already small population of Qalandari had been or were going to school. The age groups of the illiterate rest would have been again too small. Since, however, the Qalandari have been included in the Shiraz norms, a comparison of the Qashqai with these furnishes indirect information about Qalandari also. When we come later to the Z Test, this difficulty of the small subgroups disappears. It may be stated explicitly again that the norms under "Shiraz" in Table C I 8 include those for Qalandari, but no more. They are *not* the norms for the total standardizing population, to which Shiraz contributed extensively.

From the tables themselves we see that there are few significant differences between the Shirazi and the rural or nomad groups of corresponding age, although the mean scores of these tend almost throughout to be numerically lower. Even where this difference appears to be quite large, as in the age class 15–19 between the city on the one hand and Marvdasht and Khuzestan on the other, it is not significant against Marvdasht, presumably because of the small number there and of the large SDs, and merely suggestive of significance against Khuzestan ($0.10 > p > 0.05$). Significance is reached only in the age class 20–39 between the Shirazi and the Qashqai and in the age class 40–59 between the Shirazi and the Marvdashti, while the Qashqai here are too few for valid comparison. The interpretation is hardly clear. It would seem not amiss to attribute a certain intellectual stimulation, a sharpening of wits, to life in the city

Table C I 8. Ethno-geographical Comparison of Mean Raw Scores on Arithmetic Test A (Illiterates) and of Intelligence Quotients Derived from Them

Age group	Place	N	Mean score and SD	IQ	Place	N	Mean score and SD	IQ	Sign. of diff.
Males									
15–19	Shiraz	12	12.1 ± 5.33	101	Marv.	12	9.6 ± 2.64	95	ns[a]
					Khuz.	32	8.9 ± 5.04	90	(›)
					Qash.	1			
20–39	Shiraz	101	12.7 ± 4.23	99	Marv.	72	12.0 ± 4.87	99	ns
					Khuz.	57	12.0 ± 4.80	99	ns
					Qash.	20	9.9 ± 3.93	92	››
40–59	Shiraz	109	14.0 ± 3.86	101	Marv.	31	11.7 ± 4.77	94	››
					Khuz.	54	13.4 ± 4.89	94	ns
					Qash.	8			
60 +	Shiraz	65	12.6 ± 4.14	99	Marv.	16	13.8 ± 4.78	106	ns
					Khuz.	4			
					Qash.	11	11.9 ± 3.62	99	ns
Females									
15–19	Shiraz	43	8.8 ± 2.53	103	Marv.	29	5.3 ± 2.89	80	›››
					Khuz.	27	6.6 ± 3.79	87	›[a]
					Qash.	13	5.8 ± 5.04	80	›[a]
20–39	Shiraz	231	9.6 ± 3.41	99	Marv.	95	6.3 ± 3.48	81	›››
					Khuz.	83	6.6 ± 3.49	87	›››
					Qash.	35	6.0 ± 2.89	81	›››
40–59	Shiraz	166	10.3 ± 2.99	96	Marv.	31	6.9 ± 4.09	82	›››[a]
					Khuz.	32	5.7 ± 3.10	75	›››
					Qash.	11	6.6 ± 3.98	82	›[a]
60 +	Shiraz	73	9.1 ± 3.34	101	Marv.	12	6.3 ± 4.48	83	›
					Khuz.	9			
					Qash.	7			

[a] Calculated by Welch-Aspin Test, variances being unequal, otherwise by t test. Abbreviations: Marv. = Marvdasht, Khuz. = Khuzestan, Qash. = Qashqai.

whether one attended school or not, especially since there is or was probably more dealing with money, more practical exercise of arithmetic in the city, and this could affect especially the nomads who spend long times remote from monetary and similar transactions. The same might apply to the middle-aged Marvdashti, many of whom at that time had never been to the city at all and had left most of their affairs to the village proprietor, the head man and the money lender, but it does not altogether explain why there is no significant difference at the same age level between Shiraz and Khuzestan. We recall, though, that the villages studied in Khuzestan were just then at the edge of the Dez Development Project and enjoyed a degree of communication with the "outside" that was to reach Marvdasht only several years later. The suggested explanations, however, cannot be other than tentative.

The women's half of the table presents an unrelievedly depressing picture. In every age group and in every place, the rural or nomad women fall far behind the urban, who, be it remembered, are no more schooled than they. The significances, moreover, are almost uniformly high, and where they are merely modest, this seems clearly due to the small numbers in the classes. The vastly superior performance of the city women may even be exaggerated by the IQ. Differences in mean IQs are sometimes over 20, and the means of the rural women range around values that are ordinarily equated with feeble-mindedness (most striking in the case of the Khuzestani women between 40 and 59, whose test performance is only a little more than half that of the city and whose corresponding IQ as a group is 75!). Yet these women perform their part in daily life, and nobody would be so stupid as to assert they were so stupid as the test results make them. Is this a ground to discard the intelligence test or tests? In the light of the other data we have been able to present we think not, but it is certainly a warning to apply them only critically and with due regard to the social context.

Comparisons hitherto have been only urban-rural. Already in 1970 we have published comparisons of the three rural/nomad groups among themselves [28]. Since there were very few differences of moment, which moreover occurred sporadically rather than in a recognizable relation to populations or age classes and whose explanations were largely speculative, we mention them only and do not repeat the tabulation.

II. Personality

1. Best and Worst Memories; Magic

a. Method. It was Mr. Hushang Ordoobadi, Lecturer in Psychology at the University of Shiraz, who proposed including inquiries about the subject's best or happiest, worst or unhappiest memory (Q 4 and 5) in our questionnaire, so that this chapter in a real sense is his even though written by the present authors. He is, of course, not responsible for mistakes. The purpose was to gain information about our subjects' affective valuation of actual life events they had enjoyed, endured or suffered and to investigate whether these valuations differed significantly according to such major biosocial factors as age, sex and literacy as well as from one locality to another in which were reflected predominantly rural, urban or nomadic types of culture and society. The number of variables being large already, we confined ourselves to two age groups in the sense they have been used throughout: children (including youths and maidens) up to the age of 14 and adults from 15 onwards. By asking for memories only we hoped to keep closer to tangible facts, concrete and countable realities, whereas questions about wishes, ambitions and desires would have opened the sluices to an unmanageable flood of vague, variegated and often unrealistic fantasies. It proved no easy task either to hold our subjects to the concrete recollections that were our goal. Often they could be brought back only by some insistence from flights of imagination or invective and then sometimes shirked the point by saying they had neither good nor bad recollections – a circumstance to which we shall return.

The widely scattered replies had to be classified in some way if they were to be treated numerically at all. This was done purely empirically. A number of clusters were obvious at first glance. We looked then for others of roughly comparable magnitude and coherence, trying to balance the positive and negative, but finally included some with substantially smaller numerical and percentual representation because of what we judged to be their psychological significance (for example among the "best" memories Nos. 3, 13, 16, 17, 26; among the "worst" Nos. 10, 11, 16, 17). The classification upon which we finally settled, with the "best" and "worst" paired against each other where intrinsically possible, is as follows:

Best or Good Memories	*Worst or Bad Memories*
1. Childhood, youth, life with parents. Implied is a period before marriage and before assumption of adult responsibilities.	1. Family conflict, whether with parents and siblings or with spouse and parents-in-law (with whom a young bride often lives).

2. Getting playthings or presents; other kind treatment beyond ordinary care and affection.	2. Ill treatment at other's hands. More than its corresponding item to the left, this applies to adults as well.
3. Good fortune, achievement or success of a relative or friend. Excludes No. 8 below.	3. Personal mischance or misfortune, catastrophe (not strictly polar to No. 3 left, but empirically justified because replies of a polar character were scarce. Excludes Nos. 4, 5, 6, 7, 9, 13, 14, 15, 16, 18, 19 below).
4. Engagement and marriage.	4. Divorce.
5. Pregnancy and childbirth (not restricted to females, since many men affirmed that their happiest memory was the birth of a child, usually the first son).	5. Unwanted pregnancy or childbirth (in Iran practically, though not necessarily, confined to females).
6. Birth of siblings.	6. Bereavement other than loss of own child.
7. Connubial life.	7. Loss of own child or children. The distinction from No. 6 above is called for by the high infant mortality.
8. Good health or recovery of near relatives or friends (to be distinguished from No. 3 above).	8. Illness or accident in family or among close friends.
9. Own good health or recovery.	9. Own illness or accident (i.e. directly affecting one's own health and therefore to be distinguished from No. 3 above).
10. Reunion with relatives or friends.	10. Separation from relatives or friends.
11. Family weddings, festivals, feasts.	11. Fear of animals or situations, phobia.
12. Activity, achievement, success in work.	12. Dissatisfaction with employment or occupation.
13. Joy in accomplishment outside of work (skill, hobby, social acknowledgement not bound to educational promotion or gainful occupation).	13. Financial difficulties, poverty, debt, etc.
14. Travel, excursion, holiday, repose.	14. Material loss, bankruptcy (concrete and irredeemable loss as opposed to the threats and difficulties implied in No. 13).
15. Religious experience including pilgrimage (the latter overlaps often with No. 14 but is to be distinguished by its specifically religious intent).	15. Unemployment.
16. Military service; cf. below.	16. Military service.
17. Completion of or liberation from military service.	17. Overwork, exhaustion.
18. Attending school.	18. Interruption of or cessation of school.

19. Success in school or related examinations.	19. Failure in school or other examinations
20. "Always" or "very much" (i.e. happy).	20. "Always" or "very much" (i.e. unhappy).
21. Other pleasurable memories.	21. Other ill memories.
22. No pleasurable memories.	22. No ill memories.
23. No response.	23. No response.
24. Unspecific, unclassifiable response.	24. Unspecific, unclassifiable response.
25. Good harvest, etc.	25. Ill harvest, etc.
26. Land reform.	

Though we have striven to find brief headings, designations by a single word or at most two, for each class of answers, which could be employed in tables and would make referral to them easier, the task has proved insurmountable. "Good health" for example does not carry the same valence whether it applies to others or to oneself; "joy in accomplishment outside work" is hardly to be compressed; "bereavement" includes in Western usage the loss of children that is so much more frequent in Iran, and so on. Therefore in what follows we shall occasionally use short captions when the meaning and implications can be made clear, but in the main, and in the tables throughout, the abbreviations BM for best memory and WM for worst memory with the relevant number will be used.

Returning to the list of response classes, we observe that there are few precise opposites, but a number of more or less polar pairs, while certain good and bad memories with the same number are not polar at all. Thus "divorce" WM 4 is the opposite of "marriage" BM 4, and the same holds for BM and WM 5, but not for BM and WM 6, though the last pair are related. "Connubial life" BM 7 would have had to be paired against either "divorce" or "loss of husband": the first was pre-empted and the second numerically of much less weight than the far more frequent "loss of child". Pairs of strict opposites would have made it easier to read and compare the tables and to bear in mind their captions, but the wryness of the classification and the violence done to the material would have more than overweighed the formal advantage. Neither is there any real opposite to BM 11 "family weddings, feasts, etc." unless one take "burials" maybe, which are hardly ever mentioned, are in themselves short and simple ceremonies throughout the Islamic world and overlap with WM 6.

A few classes require a more extensive definition and explanation than could be given in the list above. "Military service" can be found on either side of the fence as a best or worst memory, loathed by some and welcomed by others as a kind of enforced holiday with enough to eat and no personal responsibilities. That it was not confined to males in Iran during the time of the Shiraz Survey and later must be borne in mind when reading the tables. Literate girls were drafted into auxiliary service in the Health and Literacy Corps in the cities and larger towns, though not in the villages and the countryside, and in fact our own field workers in Shiraz were for the most part uniformed female members of the army. Thus this rubric is applicable to literate urban female adult populations and to larger groups of which they form a constituent part. Neither can the various rubrics concerned with marriage and divorce, pregnancy and childbirth, connubial life and loss of children be restricted to adults. As mentioned earlier, the National Iranian Census takes counts of such life events and alterations in civil status from the age of ten. It was by no means impossible for a girl to have been engaged, borne and lost a child and been divorced all before fifteen. BM 12 and 25, WM 3 and 25 could nearly coincide in the rural areas but were kept separate for the sake of the urban. BM 13 was specifically aimed at the educated. Perhaps the distinction between BM 14 and 15 caused the most difficulty and was the most arbitrary because much of the by no means infrequent travel of the poorer classes consists of a pilgrimage to a shrine near or far and, like unpenitential pilgrimages throughout the world, does not exclude having a good time. BM 18 and 19 like WM 18 and 19 obviously apply only to the literate, just as BM-WM 25 and BM 26 have no relevance in the city. BM 26 might have been subsumed under BM 21 but, though not excessively frequent, was such a conspicuous and characteristic feature of the time that we awarded it a rubric unto itself.

In the first set of tables that follows, Nos. C II 1–8, we state first the number of individuals in a defined sub-population affirming a best or worst memory belonging to a particular class, then the percentage of members of the same sub-population making an affirmation of the same class. These, like the subsequent comparative tables, are not necessarily symmetrical in themselves nor are they all-inclusive. Only those for Shiraz approximate both specifications, the reason being that it seemed inappropriate to calculate percentage distributions of sub-populations or populations the members of which were scarcely more numerous than the classes into which they were to be distributed. This led to a lower limit of about 30, which we stretched to accommodate the 29 adult Qashqai males and consciously transgressed in the case of the illiterate Shirazi children because only there did we have substantial literate children's groups of both sexes with which to compare them. A good case could be made for setting the limit higher, but we preferred to err on the side of over-inclusion, leaving the reader to omit or disregard whatever groups he considers unjustifiably meager. In the comparison of percentages, the small denominators of certain groups are automatically taken into account.

While frequencies and percentages are stated where and as they were found, not all are statistically compared. Estimates of differential probability become misleading or meaningless when one member represents an impossibility. Zero frequency and thus probability can mean two things: either that the event did not occur or that it could not occur. In the first case we have to do with probability or improbability, in the second with intrinsic impossibility. Thus a person who has never been to school cannot experience unhappiness as a result of failure in school, a child can have no happy or unhappy recollection of his own military service (though mayhap of his fathers), etc. On the other hand we have pointed above to a number of seeming impossibilities that are not such, though their probabilities may be low. In the data tables we have used a 0 for both null frequency and impossibility, since they come numerically to the same thing. In the comparative tables, on the contrary, we have omitted zeros or other signs where the comparisons were statistically insignificant in order to avoid congesting them superfluously, but we have set a dash – where the comparison would have been intrinsically false or illegitimate even though numerically highly "significant". Similarly, in order to reduce the effect of chance, false or unclear recording, misinterpretation or misclassification we have stated no rates of significance for comparisons between frequencies that differed only by 1 on either side (including 1:0 and 0:1) even where calculation showed the difference to be "significant" by usual statistical criteria.

Table C II 1. Affirmations of Best Memories: Shiraz

	Illiterate Adults				Children				Literate Adults				Children			
	Male		Female		Male		Female		Male		Female		Male		Female	
	N	Perc.	N	Perc.	N	Perc.	N	Perc.	N	Perc.	N	Perc.	N	Perc.	N	Perc.
1.	3	2.9	5	3.1	0	0	0	0	7	3.3	3	1.9	0	0	0	2
2.	0	0	0	0	3	21.4	3	17.6	0	0	0	0	12	8.5	6	4.3
3.	0	0	2	1.3	0	0	0	0	1	0.5	3	1.9	0	0	0	0
4.	7	6.8	13	8.2	0	0	0	0	29	13.6	17	11.0	0	0	0	0
5.	15	14.6	29	18.2	1	7.1	0	0	19	8.9	23	14.9	0	0	0	0
6.	0	0	0	0	0	0	0	0	0	0	0	0	0	0	3	2.2
7.	1	1.0	5	3.1	0	0	0	0	2	1.0	2	1.3	0	0	1	0.7
8.	0	0	1	0.6	0	0	0	0	3	1.4	1	0.6	3	2.1	0	0
9.	3	2.9	0	0	0	0	0	0	1	0.5	1	0.6	1	0.7	1	0.7
10.	0	0	7	4.4	0	0	1	5.9	5	2.3	7	4.5	1	0.7	5	3.6
11.	6	5.8	21	13.2	0	0	3	17.6	7	3.3	10	6.5	6	4.3	17	12.3
12.	6	5.8	0	0	0	0	0	0	4	1.9	1	0.6	0	0	0	0
13.	0	0	0	0	0	0	0	0	10	4.7	0	0	2	1.4	0	0
14.	4	3.9	4	2.5	1	7.1	0	0	17	7.9	15	9.7	15	10.7	10	7.2
15.	13	12.6	22	13.8	0	0	1	5.9	28	13.8	8	5.2	11	7.6	6	4.3
16.	0	0	0	0	0	0	0	0	3	1.4	0	0	0	0	0	0
17.	2	1.9	0	0	0	0	0	0	4	1.9	1	0.6	0	0	0	0
18.	1	1.0	0	0	0	0	1	5.9	13	6.1	11	7.1	22	15.7	23	16.7
19.	0	0	0	0	0	0	0	0	21	9.8	13	8.4	34	24.3	38	27.5
20.	4	3.9	0	0	0	0	0	0	4	1.9	5	3.2	0	0	0	0
21.	8	7.8	5	3.1	0	0	1	5.9	9	4.2	5	3.2	10	7.1	12	8.7
22.	27	26.2	44	27.7	7	50.0	4	23.5	23	10.7	23	14.9	20	14.3	10	7.2
23.	3	2.9	0	0	2	14.3	1	5.9	2	0.9	1	0.6	2	1.4	5	3.6
24.	0	0	1	0.6	0	0	2	11.8	2	0.9	4	2.6	1	0.7	1	0.7
25.	0	0	0	0	0	0	0	0	0	0	0	0	0	0	0	0
26.	0	0	0	0	0	0	0	0	0	0	0	0	0	0	0	0
Sum	103		159		14		17		214		154		140		138	
% of pop.		11.0		16.9		1.5		1.8		22.8		16.4		14.9		14.7
% of males					39.9								54.8			
% of females					60.1								45.2			

Table C II 2. Affirmations of Worst Memories: Shiraz

	Illiterate Adults Male		Female		Children Male		Female		Literate Adults Male		Female		Children Male		Female	
	N	Perc.	N	Perc.	N	Perc.	N	Perc.	N	Perc.	N	Perc.	N	Perc.	N	Perc.
1.	3	2.9	6	3.8	0	0	0	0	4	1.9	4	2.6	0	0	2	2.9
2.	4	3.9	1	0.6	1	7.1	0	0	13	6.1	3	1.9	13	9.3	0	0
3.	3	2.9	5	3.1	0	0	0	0	14	6.5	2	1.3	7	5.0	3	2.2
4.	0	0	1	0.6	0	0	0	0	0	0	2	1.3	0	0	0	0
5.	0	0	6	3.8	0	0	2	11.8	0	0	5	3.2	0	0	7	5.1
6.	16	15.5	8	5.0	0	0	0	0	31	14.5	7	4.6	6	4.3	14	10.1
7.	5	4.8	21	13.2	1	7.1	0	0	4	1.9	6	3.9	0	0	0	0
8.	1	1.0	4	2.5	0	0	0	0	7	3.3	10	6.5	6	4.3	7	5.1
9.	10	9.7	53	33.3	1	7.1	0	0	17	7.9	42	27.3	3	2.1	5	3.6
10.	0	0	0	0	2	14.3	0	0	2	0.9	0	0	5	3.6	0	0
11.	0	0	4	2.5	0	0	1	5.9	1	0.5	6	3.9	1	0.7	5	3.6
12.	0	0	0	0	0	0	0	0	4	1.9	2	1.3	0	0	0	0
13.	11	10.7	0	0	0	0	0	0	6	2.8	0	0	0	0	0	0
14.	3	2.9	6	3.8	0	0	0	0	7	3.3	6	3.9	1	0.7	4	2.9
15.	5	4.8	0	0	0	0	0	0	6	2.8	0	0	1	0.7	0	0
16.	1	1.0	0	0	0	0	0	0	2	0.9	1	0.6	0	0	0	0
17.	0	0	1	0.6	0	0	0	0	1	0.5	1	0.6	0	0	0	0
18.	0	0	1	0.6	0	0	0	0	3	1.4	3	1.9	1	0.7	0	0
19.	0	0	0	0	0	0	0	0	22	10.3	15	9.7	19	13.6	27	19.6
20.	1	1.0	1	0.6	0	0	0	0	2	0.9	1	0.6	1	0.7	0	0
21.	3	2.9	5	3.1	0	0	1	5.9	14	6.5	7	4.7	6	4.3	12	8.7
22.	30	29.1	34	21.4	8	57.1	11	64.7	49	22.9	30	19.5	65	46.4	48	34.8
23.	5	4.8	1	0.6	1	7.1	1	5.9	4	1.9	1	0.6	3	2.1	2	1.4
24.	2	1.9	1	0.6	0	0	1	5.9	1	0.5	0	0	2	1.4	0	0
25.	0	0	0	0	0	0	0	0	0	0	0	0	0	0	0	0
Sum	103		159		14		17		214		154		140		138	
% of pop.		11.0		16.9		1.5		1.8		22.8		16.4		14.9		14.7
% of males					39.9								54.8			
% of females					60.1								45.2			

Table C II 3. Affirmations of Best Memories: Marvdasht

	Illiterate Adults Male		Female		Children Male		Female		Literate Male Adults		Children	
	N	Perc.	N	Perc.	N	Perc.	N	Perc.	N	Perc.	N	Perc.
1.	8	5.8	10	6.1	0	0	2	3.6	2	5.7	0	0
2.	0	0	0	0	0	0	2	3.6	0	0	2	3.2
3.	0	0	0	0	0	0	0	0	0	0	0	0
4.	9	6.5	14	8.5	0	0	0	0	1	2.9	0	0
5.	9	6.5	8	4.9	0	0	0	0	0	0	0	0
6.	0	0	0	0	0	0	0	0	0	0	0	0
7.	2	1.4	8	4.9	0	0	0	0	1	2.9	0	0
8.	0	0	1	0.6	1	3.1	2	3.6	0	0	0	0
9.	2	1.4	4	2.4	0	0	2	3.6	1	2.9	0	0
10.	2	1.4	5	3.0	2	6.2	3	5.4	0	0	0	0
11.	2	1.4	6	3.7	1	3.1	1	1.8	6	17.1	8	12.9
12.	2	1.4	0	0	0	0	0	0	1	2.9	1	1.6
13.	0	0	0	0	0	0	0	0	0	0	1	1.6
14.	4	2.9	0	0	2	6.2	0	0	2	5.7	2	3.2
15.	3	2.2	0	0	0	0	0	0	0	0	1	1.6
16.	2	1.4	0	0	0	0	0	0	0	0	0	0
17.	1	0.7	0	0	0	0	0	0	0	0	0	0
18.	0	0	1	0.6	1	3.1	0	0	4	11.4	17	27.4
19.	0	0	0	0	0	0	0	0	1	2.9	2	3.2
20.	0	0	2	1.2	0	0	1	1.8	0	0	0	0
21.	16	11.5	2	1.2	3	9.4	3	5.4	2	5.7	3	4.8
22.	66	47.5	100	61.0	20	62.5	35	63.6	8	22.9	22	35.5
23.	0	0	0	0	2	6.2	3	5.4	0	0	2	3.2
24.	1	0.7	0	0	0	0	0	0	0	0	0	0
25.	3	2.2	3	1.8	0	0	0	0	3	8.6	0	0
26.	7	5.0	0	0	0	0	1	1.8	3	8.6	1	1.6
Sum	139		164		32		55		35		62	
% of pop.		27.9		33.0		6.4		11.1		7.0		12.5
% of males					43.8						90.6	
% of females					56.2						9.4	

Minuscule pseudo-significances seem rather worse than useless, while field experience impresses upon one the danger of arriving at them when too much trust is placed in statistical manipulation.

Since columns of frequencies and percentages tell nothing except about the population on which the column is based, and since the comparison of many columns across a page and over pages is cumbersome, fraught with possibilities of error and inconclusive as to the significance of the comparison, we shall attend at once to the comparative tables Nos. C II 9–10 and 12–13, leaving the data sheets Nos. C II 1–8 to be referred to at need. The comparative tables carry no figures. Their one purpose is to show where differences conventionally regarded as statistically significant can be demonstrated and what the direction of the inequality as well as its degree of significance is. The degree is commonly indicated according to the Snedecore convention by asterisks, and this serves well enough when only two columns are to be compared. Not so, when the column sought for comparison may lie a couple of pages

Table C II 4. Affirmations of Worst Memories: Marvdasht

	Illiterate Adults Male		Female		Children Male		Female		Literate Male Adults		Children	
	N	Perc.	N	Perc.	N	Perc.	N	Perc.	N	Perc.	N	Perc.
1.	2	1.4	11	6.7	0	0	1	1.8	1	2.9	0	0
2.	3	2.2	1	0.6	0	0	0	0	1	2.9	0	0
3.	2	1.4	0	0	0	0	2	3.6	1	2.9	1	1.6
4.	0	0	3	1.8	0	0	0	0	0	0	0	0
5.	0	0	4	3.7	0	0	0	0	0	0	0	0
6.	14	10.1	20	12.2	2	6.2	2	3.6	6	17.1	3	4.8
7.	9	6.5	17	10.4	0	0	0	0	0	0	0	0
8.	4	2.9	3	1.8	1	3.1	0	0	1	2.9	0	0
9.	12	8.6	8	4.9	4	12.5	4	7.3	5	14.3	3	4.8
10.	0	0	3	1.8	0	0	1	1.8	0	0	0	0
11.	0	0	0	0	1	3.1	1	1.8	0	0	1	1.6
12.	4	2.9	0	0	1	3.1	0	0	0	0	0	0
13.	21	15.1	12	7.3	0	0	0	0	1	2.9	0	0
14.	1	0.7	0	0	0	0	0	0	0	0	0	0
15.	0	0	0	0	0	0	0	0	0	0	1	1.6
16.	1	0.7	0	0	0	0	0	0	0	0	0	0
17.	5	3.6	4	2.4	1	3.1	0	0	1	2.9	0	0
18.	0	0	0	0	0	0	0	0	0	0	0	0
19.	0	0	0	0	0	0	0	0	2	5.7	6	9.7
20.	4	2.9	5	3.0	0	0	1	1.8	0	0	1	1.6
21.	12	8.6	6	3.7	0	0	4	7.3	5	14.3	4	6.4
22.	43	30.9	67	40.8	20	62.5	36	65.4	9	25.7	41	66.1
23.	0	0	0	0	2	6.2	3	5.4	0	0	1	1.6
24.	0	0	0	0	0	0	0	0	0	0	0	0
25.	2	1.4	0	0	0	0	0	0	2	5.7	0	0
Sum	139		164		32		55		35		62	
% of pop.		27.9		33.0		6.4		11.1		7.0		12.5
% of males					43.8						90.6	
% of females					56.2						9.4	

ahead. Repeating the columns each time would have clogged the book. Therefore chevrons < ,> are used here in place of asterisks, the number of chevrons denoting the level of significance just as the customary asterisks do and their direction that of the gradient. Those who wish fuller, numerical information can refer at will to the basic tables. Cf. "Signs and Abbreviations" at the beginning of this book.

Just as we have refrained from tabulating all data when groups or populations became too small, we have refrained from making all the multitudinous possible comparisons of columns where the comparison seemed inapt. Within a survey population it has little meaning to compare and analyse statistically the best or worst memories of e.g. illiterate female adults with those of schoolboys, but it has unquestionable meaning to compare them with those of adult illiterate men, their mates and complements. As between survey populations, comparison of memories between Shiraz schoolboys and illiterate youths in villages and in the desert yields little information of psychological or sociological value beyond the obvious, whereas a comparison between children in Shiraz who attend and who do not attend school is

Table C II 5. Affirmations of Best Memories: Khuzestan

	Illiterate Adults Male		Female		Children Male		Female		Literate Children Male	
	N	Perc.	N	Perc.	N	Perc.	N	Perc.	N	Perc.
1.	5	3.4	11	7.3	1	2.3	2	3.1	4	6.9
2.	2	1.4	2	1.3	8	18.6	9	14.1	6	10.3
3.	0	0	0	0	0	0	0	0	0	0
4.	50	34.0	27	17.9	0	0	5	7.8	0	0
5.	7	4.8	3	2.0	0	0	0	0	0	0
6.	0	0	1	0.7	0	0	1	1.6	0	0
7.	2	1.4	4	2.7	0	0	0	0	0	0
8.	0	0	1	0.7	0	0	0	0	0	0
9.	3	2.0	0	0	1	2.3	0	0	0	0
10.	1	0.7	3	2.0	0	0	1	1.6	0	0
11.	14	9.5	24	15.9	11	25.6	16	25.0	5	8.6
12.	0	0	1	0.7	0	0	0	0	0	0
13.	0	0	1	0.7	0	0	0	0	0	0
14.	2	1.4	0	0	1	2.3	0	0	0	0
15.	11	7.5	7	4.6	4	9.3	6	9.4	5	8.6
16.	2	1.4	0	0	0	0	0	0	0	0
17.	0	0	0	0	0	0	0	0	0	0
18.	0	0	0	0	0	0	0	0	18	31.0
19.	0	0	0	0	0	0	0	0	1	1.7
20.	4	2.7	26	17.2	4	9.3	9	14.1	1	1.7
21.	8	5.4	4	2.7	3	7.0	5	7.8	5	8.6
22.	30	20.4	32	21.2	9	20.9	8	12.5	12	20.7
23.	2	1.4	4	2.7	1	2.3	2	3.1	1	1.7
24.	.0	0	0	0	0	0	0	0	0	0
25.	1	0.7	0	0	0	0	0	0	0	0
26.	3	2.0	0	0	0	0	0	0	0	0
Sum	147		151		43		64		58	
% of pop.		30.5		31.3		8.9		13.3		12.0
% of males					46.9					90.6
% of females					53.1					

apposite and may be revealing. The tables thus can be kept within manageable dimensions and meaningful bounds. Other comparisons that would have been both meaningful and desirable could not be performed because of too small sub-populations, for example between literate and illiterate women outside Shiraz. There was barely a sprinkling of the former, and schoolgirls too were rare outside the city, though less so. Gaps in the comparative tables therefore exist by necessity, though we hope not by negligence, for here again it has been our policy to over- rather than under-include.

Before entering into more detailed and systematic consideration it will be well to reflect upon what the answers to our questions, the affirmations of best and worst memories, their rates and differences may mean or imply. Certainly not altogether biographical and factual statements to be taken at their face value. One may ask whether there is any such thing as a "factual" statement of a best or worst memory at all. The answer to such a question always rests upon a subjective judgment, which may vary considerably according to time, place, circumstances and inquirer. What I recall as my happiest or unhappiest memory today may not be what I recollect as such tomorrow.

Table C II 6. Affirmations of Worst Memories: Khuzestan

	Illiterate Adults Male		Female		Children Male		Female		Literate Children Male	
	N	Perc.	N	Perc.	N	Perc.	N	Perc.	N	Perc.
1.	1	0.7	4	2.6	0	0	1	1.6	0	0
2.	6	4.1	2	1.3	4	9.3	6	9.4	3	5.2
3.	3	2.0	1	0.7	3	7.0	0	0	1	1.7
4.	0	0	2	1.3	0	0	0	0	0	0
5.	0	0	3	2.0	0	0	0	0	0	0
6.	21	14.3	26	17.2	6	13.9	4	6.2	7	12.1
7.	7	4.8	9	6.0	0	0	0	0	0	0
8.	3	2.0	0	0	0	0	0	0	1	1.7
9.	17	11.6	10	6.6	2	4.6	3	4.7	1	1.7
10.	1	0.7	1	0.7	0	0	2	3.1	1	1.7
11.	0	0	1	0.7	1	2.3	0	0	2	3.4
12.	0	0	0	0	0	0	0	0	0	0
13.	14	9.5	7	4.6	1	2.3	0	0	0	0
14.	0	0	0	0	0	0	0	0	1	1.7
15.	0	0	0	0	0	0	0	0	0	0
16.	0	0	0	0	0	0	0	0	0	0
17.	1	0.7	0	0	0	0	0	0	1	1.7
18.	0	0	0	0	0	0	0	0	0	0
19.	0	0	0	0	0	0	0	0	1	1.7
20.	4	2.7	3	2.0	0	0	0	0	1	1.7
21.	11	7.5	3	2.0	4	9.3	2	3.1	4	6.9
22.	56	38.1	71	47.0	21	48.8	44	68.8	33	56.9
23.	2	1.4	7	4.6	1	2.3	2	3.1	1	1.7
24.	0	0	1	0.7	0	0	0	0	0	0
25.	0	0	0	0	0	0	0	0	0	0
Sum	147		151		43		64		58	
% of pop.	30.5			31.3		8.9		13.3		12.0
% of males				46.9						90.6
% of females				53.1						

Furthermore, there is no objective criterion for the "correctness" of such a recollection. Wishes can be projected backwards as well as forwards. Cover memories are familiar to to every analyst. Moreover, the cover may be conscious or unconscious. Many a subject, confronted suddenly with an inquisitive intruder, may deliberately hide his deeper personal satisfactions and frustrations and comply by a superficial response. All these and other sources of error are possible and doubtless play their part. Nevertheless this form of question probably remains closer both to the subjective and objective realities of life than many others do and yields information of no mean worth about the relation in our respondents between these two kinds of reality. Even where the answer is unconsciously distorted or deliberately feigned, it tells us something about the subject's emotional set and hedonistic evaluation at the moment he articulates it and relates this information quite directly to the world in which he actually lives. The replies to questions in this and the following chapter are meaningful through their content even where the content may not reflect "the truth, the whole truth and nothing but the truth", just as an invented dream or a fanciful lie may reveal as much about the teller as

Table C II 7. Affirmations of Best Memories: Qalandari and Qashqai

	Qalandari Illiterate Adults Male		Female		Literate Children Male		Qashqai Illiterate Adults Male		Female		Literate Children Male	
	N	Perc.	N	Perc.	N	Perc.	N	Perc.	N	Perc.	N	Perc.
1.	4	13.8	3	7.3	0	0	1	2.6	1	1.5	0	0
2.	0	0	0	0	2	7.4	0	0	0	0	1	2.2
3.	0	0	0	0	0	0	0	0	0	0	0	0
4.	7	24.1	12	29.3	0	0	11	28.2	11	16.4	0	0
5.	3	10.3	10	24.4	0	0	0	0	9	13.4	0	0
6.	0	0	0	0	0	0	0	0	0	0	0	0
7.	1	3.4	0	0	0	0	0	0	2	3.0	0	0
8.	0	0	0	0	0	0	3	7.7	0	0	0	0
9.	0	0	0	0	0	0	0	0	1	1.5	0	0
10.	1	3.4	0	0	1	3.7	0	0	0	0	1	2.2
11.	0	0	3	7.3	1	3.7	2	5.1	2	3.0	0	0
12.	0	0	0	0	0	0	1	2.6	0	0	0	0
13.	0	0	0	0	0	0	0	0	0	0	0	0
14.	0	0	3	7.3	1	3.7	0	0	0	0	1	2.2
15.	1	3.4	1	2.4	0	0	0	0	0	0	0	0
16.	0	0	0	0	0	0	0	0	0	0	0	0
17.	0	0	0	0	0	0	0	0	0	0	0	0
18.	1	3.4	0	0	12	44.4	0	0	0	0	16	34.8
19.	0	0	0	0	6	22.2	0	0	0	0	3	6.5
20.	1	3.4	2	4.9	1	3.7	2	5.1	2	3.0	0	0
21.	0	0	1	2.4	2	7.4	5	12.8	10	14.9	2	4.3
22.	10	34.5	6	14.6	1	3.7	6	15.4	24	35.8	7	15.2
23.	0	0	0	0	0	0	1	2.6	4	6.0	15	32.6
24.	0	0	0	0	0	0	0	0	0	0	0	0
25.	0	0	0	0	0	0	7	18.0	1	1.5	0	0
26.	0	0	0	0	0	0	0	0	0	0	0	0
Sum	29		41		27		39		67		46	
% of pop.		20.1		28.5		18.8		20.6		35.4		24.3
% of males		41.4						36.8				
% of females		58.6						63.2				

a raw product of his unconscious. In this respect they differ sharply from the responses to the Z Test, which we shall consider at some length in the chapter after next. Each set complements the other, and through the comparison of them we hope to delve deeper than would otherwise be possible.

In interpreting tentatively the demonstrably significant group differences in best and worst memories we can sometimes fall back upon hard facts, but must rely often upon experience gained from our field work and from life in Iran and must frequently take refuge in conjecture. Many of our interpretations have the character of hypotheses that could be confirmed or rejected only by further research. Through them we hope to stimulate such research not only in Iran. After these precautionary words, let us address ourselves to the findings.

b. Intralocal Comparisons. We regard the intralocal comparisons first, beginning with Shiraz and taking the best and worst memories together.

Table C II 8. Affirmations of Worst Memories: Qalandari and Qashqai

	Qalandari Illiterate Adults Male N	Perc.	Female N	Perc.	Literate Children Male N	Perc.	Qashqai Illiterate Adults Male N	Perc.	Female N	Perc.	Literate Children Male N	Perc.
1.	0	0	0	0	0	0	0	0	2	3.0	0	0
2.	0	0	0	0	2	7.4	6	15.4	16	23.9	6	13.0
3.	0	0	0	0	0	0	1	2.6	0	0	0	0
4.	0	0	0	0	0	0	0	0	0	0	0	0
5.	0	0	0	0	0	0	0	0	1	1.5	0	0
6.	6	20.7	11	26.8	1	3.7	2	5.1	7	10.4	1	2.2
7.	1	3.4	3	7.3	1	3.7	0	0	1	1.5	0	0
8.	0	0	1	2.4	0	0	1	2.6	1	1.5	0	0
9.	0	0	4	9.8	2	7.4	1	2.6	2	3.0	3	6.5
10.	0	0	1	2.4	0	0	1	2.6	0	0	0	0
11.	0	0	0	0	0	0	0	0	0	0	1	2.2
12.	0	0	0	0	0	0	0	0	0	0	0	0
13.	3	10.3	2	4.9	0	0	7	18.0	4	6.0	0	0
14.	0	0	0	0	0	0	3	7.7	2	3.0	1	2.2
15.	1	3.4	0	0	0	0	1	2.6	0	0	0	0
16.	0	0	0	0	0	0	0	0	0	0	0	0
17.	0	0	0	0	0	0	0	0	0	0	0	0
18.	0	0	0	0	0	0	0	0	0	0	1	2.2
19.	0	0	0	0	1	3.7	0	0	0	0	0	0
20.	1	3.4	0	0	0	0	0	0	2	3.0	0	0
21.	3	10.3	4	9.8	3	11.1	2	5.1	1	1.5	4	8.7
22.	14	48.3	15	36.6	16	59.3	11	28.2	21	31.3	7	15.2
23.	0	0	0	0	1	3.7	0	0	5	7.5	21	45.6
24.	0	0	0	0	0	0	0	0	0	0	1	2.2
25.	0	0	0	0	0	0	3	7.7	2	3.0	0	0
Sum	29		41		27		39		67		46	
% of pop.		20.1		28.5		18.8		20.6		35.4		24.3
% of males		41.4						36.8				
% of females		58.6						63.2				

The city, owning a much larger share of literates of both sexes than any of the rural surveys, afforded us opportunities for comparisons that could be made validly nowhere else. The first left-hand column in Tables C II 9–10 is an instance of this. Males and females of all ages were combined together, then compared by literacy or illiteracy, there being enough literates to preclude this becoming in effect a comparison of men and boys as a whole against illiterate women and girls. We hoped thus to isolate the factor of literacy, independent of sex and age, and to see what influence it may have exercised upon our subjects' recollections besides the obvious ones registered in items 18 and 19, whether good or bad. Such an influence suggests itself already in the higher valuation of engagement and marriage (BM 4) by the literate over pregnancy and childbirth (BM 5) by the illiterate. In the former the personal relation takes precedence over the biological fact, and the latter finds its complement to a certain extent in the very significantly greater frequency with which the loss of a child is recalled as their worst memory by the illiterate (WM 7). One's own bodily accident or ill health is oftener the worst memory among the illiterate (WM 9), but that of family or friends

Table C II 9. Affirmations of Best Memories: Significance of Intralocal Comparisons

	Shiraz						Marvdasht		Khuzestan			Qalandari	Qashqai
	Adults			Literate			Illiterate		Illiterate		m	Illiterate	
	m + f	Illit.	Lit.	Child.	Male	Female	Adults	Child.	Adults	Child.	Child.	Adults	
	ill. : lit.	m : f	m : f	m : f	Ad. : Ch.	Ad. : Ch.	m : f	m : f	m : f	m : f	ill. : lit.	m : f	m : f
1.					›	›			(‹)				
2.				(›)	‹‹‹	‹‹							
3.						›							
4.	‹				›››	›››			››	‹			(›)
5.	›		‹		›››	›››			(›)			(‹)	‹‹
6.				‹		‹							
7.							‹						
8.				›									›
9.		›							›				
10.		‹	‹										
11.	››	‹	(‹)	‹‹		‹			‹		›	(‹)	
12.		››			(›)		(›)						
13.	‹‹		››	(›)	›								
14.	‹‹						›	›	(›)			(‹)	
15.	(›)		››		(›)		›						
16.	(‹)	—	(›)	—	—	—	—	—	—	—	—	—	—
17.		—		—	—	—	—	—	—	—	—	—	—
18.	—	—			‹‹	‹‹	—	—	—	—	—	—	—
19.	—	—			‹‹‹	‹‹‹	—	—	—	—	—	—	—
20.		››			›	›	(‹)		‹‹‹		››		
21.		›				‹	›››						
22.	›››			›		›	‹‹					›	‹
23.		›				‹							
24.	(‹)												
25.	—	—	—	—	—	—							››
26.	—	—	—	—	—	—	››		›				

Table C II 10. Affirmations of Worst Memories: Significance of Intralocal Comparisons

	Shiraz						Marvdasht		Khuzestan			Qalandari	Qashqai
	Adults			Literate			Illiterate		Illiterate		m	Illiterate	
	m + f	Illit.	Lit.	Child.	Male	Female	Adults	Child.	Adults	Child.	Child.	Adults	
	ill. : lit.	m : f	m : f	m : f	Ad. : Ch.	Ad. : Ch.	m : f	m : f	m : f	m : f	ill. : lit.	m : f	m : f
1.				‹	›		‹		(‹)				
2.	‹	›	›	›››		›			(›)				
3.			››				(›)			›	(›)		
4.			‹			(›)	(‹)		(‹)				
5.		‹	‹‹	‹‹			‹		‹				
6.		››	››	‹	››	‹				(›)			
7.	›››	‹			›	››							
8.	‹		(‹)						›				
9.	››	‹‹‹	‹‹‹		››	›››	(›)		(›)			‹	
10.				›	‹		(‹)						
11.		(‹)	‹‹	‹									
12.	‹				›	(›)	›						
13.	›	›››	›		›		›		›				›
14.				(‹)	(›)								
15.		››	›		(›)								
16.	—	—		—			—	—	—	—	—	—	—
17.													
18.	—	—				›	—	—	—	—	—	—	—
19.	—	—		(‹)		‹‹	—	—	—	—	—	—	—
20.													
21.	(‹)			(‹)		(‹)	›	(‹)	›	(›)			
22.		(›)		›	‹‹‹	‹‹	‹		(‹)	‹			
23.		›							‹				‹
24.	(›)			(›)									
25.	—	—	—	—	—	—	(›)						

among the literate (WM 8). Apart from the fact that the illiterate are generally poorer, more fecund (and thus have more children to lose), probably also less resourceful and certainly profit from less safeguards against illness and untimely death, this cluster of findings allows the inference that the wider horizon of the literate leads them to attribute more weight to life events that are less strictly corporeal and egocentric. They are less concerned than the illiterate with family and other feasts (BM 11), more so with job satisfaction (BM 12) and naturally also less with financial difficulties and debt (WM 13). An anticipated difference emerges very clearly and with high significance in BM 13, where the literate much more often cite as their happiest recollection some form of accomplishment beyond the necessities of labor and survival, likewise in BM 14, where they recall more joy in travel and repose for their own sake (for which, of course, they possess more opportunities as well, though observation has convinced us that this factor by itself is far from sufficient to account for the difference). The illiterate furnish counterweight and confirmation in their responses to BM 15 (pilgrimage). We were not wholly prepared to find that the literate tend more often to find satisfaction in military service (BM 16), which may be due to a number of officers' careers. A greater differentiation may be reflected in the fact that the literate more often cite other bad memories than those on the list (WM 21) and more unspecific ones (WM 24, both tendencies only). It can surprise no one that the illiterate, on the other hand, very significantly more often deny having any pleasurable memory whatever (BM 22). By all these accounts the universe of the literate appears to be wider, less egocentric and less concrete as reflected in their concerns with actually experienced events. Though the finding could be expected, its confirmation in this realistic form seems not devoid of interest.

The next column is one which repeats itself throughout all surveys and the only one that does: a comparison of male and female adult illiterates by which we hoped to cast more light on (not only or necessarily biological) sex difference. As we glance across the pages, these seem to be more regular and consistent among the bad memories than among the good ones. So in WM 2, where in Shiraz boys and men, but at the highest level of significance the literate Shirazi boys, complain, as do the men in Khuzestan, of ill treatment at other's hands. One wonders why precisely the schoolboys until one notices in the records how often being beaten by the teacher is mentioned. Getting playthings and presents pleases all alike (BM 2), but more specifically the children of both sexes among the urban literate, whereas the adults of the same class presumably treasure other sources of enjoyment more. External mishaps and catastrophes (to which they are probably more subject) affect the men in Marvdasht and the boys in Khuzestan more than the women and girls (WM 3) and in Shiraz unexpectedly impress themselves more upon the male than the female literate and less upon the illiterate males, who on the other hand suffer more than their mates under poverty and unemployment (WM 13, 15). Engagement and marriage leave happiest recollections about equally in the two sexes (BM 4), except in Khuzestan, where the men's good memories significantly predominate, and among the Qashqai, where they show a tendency to do so. The highly significant differences between adults and children are self-explanatory. Divorce (WM 4), though, leaves on the whole more lasting effects upon the women and especially the literate women in Shiraz, whereas we encounter in the city no significant difference between the illiterate male and female divorced. The lack of such sex-specific differences where one might expect them among the Qashqais and in Qalandari is probably a statistical artefact referable to the smallness of the samples. Just here, though, pregnancy and childbirth (BM 5) reveal themselves as more often impressive for rural women than for rural men. Unwanted pregnancy and childbirth (WM 5) is the woman's misery in country and city.

Going again down the columns, as we shall return to cross-comparisons later, the birth of a sibling (BM 6) is typically the city girl's happiest memory. In its counterpart bereavement (WM 6) we were not prepared to find that in Shiraz it is significantly the men's and not the women's memory. Sometimes bereavement means loss of a parent, and here the usually strong attachment between father and son in Islamic cultures may offer a partial explanation. More often, though, it implies widowhood. While on the one hand it is not easy for the Iranian woman to remarry, on the other she ordinarily finds refuge more readily in her enlarged family or kinship than does the widow in the West, which is less available to the usually elder husband. Being married very often young and concerned perhaps more with her children than with her mate, it may be questioned whether the Iranian wife in general forms as deep an attachment to him as he does to her, but we have no means of answering the question, of measuring the respective affections and must rest content with recording the findings. The mention of connubial life as best memory (BM 7) brings no clarification, for at least in Shiraz it displays no significant sexual gradient. In Marvdasht alone it occurs significantly more frequently among the women. Loss of children (WM 7) seems to affect the sexes equally except among the illiterate Shirazis, where the women mention it more often than the men. Among the same group we observe a rather sexually typical pattern in BM 9–12, which tends to be reflected in the literates and to some extent outside the city, in as much as the men more often place their own good health and achievement at the head of their lists (BM 9 and 12), the women more often reunion with their relatives and friends, also weddings, celebrations and festivals, which are mostly family affairs (BM 10–11). The gradients between adults and children in these respects, where significant, are as expected and require no comment. The worst memories in the same fields group themselves rather differently and interestingly. If the Shirazi and Khuzestani illiterate men emphasized their own good health or recovery from ill health, it is the Shirazi women, illiterate and literate alike, who at a very highly significant level recalled their own illness as their worst memory more often than the men (WM 9). The relationship shows a tendency, but only a tendency to reversal in Marvdasht and Khuzestan, but holds again in Qalandari. Where children can be compared we observe no significant sex differential in complaints of illness, but an age differential that is again obvious as the adult has more opportunity to have suffered a grave illness by sheer reason of his age. Separation from relatives (WM 10) affects literate boys more than girls and to some extent children as a whole more than adults: we recall what was said about father-son attachments. Literate and illiterate women and girls in Shiraz more often recall phobic fears (WM 11). WM 13 (poverty and debt) cannot be regarded as a true contrast to BM 13 (joy in successful work), and it requires no explanation for its preponderance among the men, though the women may be no less affected. Debt above all strikes the man more directly.

BM 14 (travel, excursion, repose, etc.) shows little sex difference except in Marvdasht, and its importance in relation to literacy has been discussed already. BM 15 (religious experience, principally pilgrimage) turns out to be not so much of a man's affair (pilgrimage) as might be expected except for the literate Shirazis, who are much more apt than the illiterate or the rural groups to undertake long pilgrimages, e.g. to Mecca or to Meshed. The non-polar WM 14 and 15 follow WM 13 where they show any significant differences at all and can be considered in the same way. BM and WM 16 (military service) also have been discussed above, while BM and WM 17 display no significant differences throughout the intralocal tables.

The differential school memories 18 and 19 are inapplicable to the illiterates and to sub-populations in which literates and illiterates are commingled (first left-hand column). The only sex difference discoverable among them is a mere tendency for the Shirazi girls to take failure in school or examination more to heart (WM 19). Unsurprisingly, success in school leaves relatively more best memories behind in children than in adults of both sexes (BM 18 and 19). Being compelled to stop school (WM 18) impresses the adult women more than their daughters, lingering often as a recollection of harsh frustration, as we have been informed directly many times. In contemporary Iran a girl is much more likely than a boy to be pulled suddenly out of school when the parents feel she is needed at home or when they suffer a financial pinch (many city children are sent to private schools) or to be denied further education after the primary level. There is a tendency for girls to be more sensitive to scholastic failure than boys (WM 19). The same mishap seems to impress the men no less than the boys (though the men were less concerned with success, cf. above), but the girls quite significantly more than their mothers. Since we are dealing with relative proportions, the circumstance that fewer grown women have attended school is irrelevant here, but the difference may be caused by the present generation taking education more seriously, whereas some years back it was mostly regarded as a superfluous luxury for women and failure or success in it were of no consequence (this does injustice to the little group of girls and young women who were seriously pursuing education already a couple of decades ago, but they were so few that they hardly influence statistical summaries such as this). Outside the city we lack adequate data.

Remembrance of good harvest has no relevance in Shiraz and shows a significant difference only among the Qashqai (BM 25) in favor of the men. As most of them are really not harvesters at all, this may be taken to refer rather to a prosperous year, the direct consequences of which in a monetary economy they felt more immediately than the women. The same sex difference applies to land reform (BM 26) and is apparent in the villages where it was effected. Ill harvest as a worst memory (WM 25) tends to affect the men of Marvdasht somewhat more than the women, elsewhere both sexes alike.

Finally we revert to the more general, now strictly paired items 20 to 24. "Always happy" (BM 20) is recalled in Shiraz more by the illiterate men, but among the illiterates of Marvdasht and Khuzestan by the women, in Khuzestan also more by the illiterate than by the literate male children and among the literate Shirazis of both sexes more by the adult than by the children. This stands as a whole in rather sharp contradiction to the usual notion of blithe schoolchildren and would appear to thwart hopes that education in general would conduce to greater happiness, though the latter conclusion is supported only by the Khuzestani boys and not by comparison of the much larger illiterate and literate groups in Shiraz, where no difference appears. Further reflection indicates, however, that according to their replies to BM 18 the children are truly eager for education, but that by WM 18 and 19 for girls at least this very zeal leads to disappointments such that an affirmation of being "always happy" becomes impossible. The marked preponderance of the "always happy" illiterate women in Khuzestan over the men and the tendency thereto in Marvdasht arrest attention and call for explanation. The only one we can offer is based on the especially disadvantageous and sorry situation of the economically poor illiterate women in Shiraz, which we shall find confirmed repeatedly in the analysis of socio-psychiatric results. The rural women, then, would be carefreer by contrast. Be it noted that no significant differences for sex and age are registered in regard to WM 20, i.e. being always unhappy.

The illiterate men of Shiraz and to an even higher degree those of Marvdasht report significantly more "other pleasurable memories" (BM 21) and by implication a greater variety of such than women do, which probably corresponds to the simple circumstance that especially on the lower socio-economic levels, which are generally more conservative also, the men are privileged by a wider range of opportunities for enjoying themselves than the women. As a good many school girls are more emancipated than their (literate) mothers, we see this tendency reversed in the literate Shirazi females. Whether conversely the men or women report a wider range of "other" worst memories (WM 21) varies a good deal. The slight differences do not amount statistically to more than a tendency except in Marvdasht and Khuzestan. In the former the men are more various in their worst as in their best memories, while the difference obtains in Khuzestan only for the worst.

A word of caution seems called for here before discussing the items No. 22 and 23 more fully. The number of true non-responders, reflected in BM and WM 23, was low. The assertion that the respondent possessed no good or bad memory (BM 22 and WM 22) need not imply a refusal of response (though it can), but rather in a larger proportion of cases an attitude toward life that may be called achronological, abiographic or ahistorical – an attitude that has impressed us over and again among the illiterate and, among other things, does not facilitate the taking of case histories. Like the outright "no response" (item 23) it is commoner in children throughout, who have less biography and are also, especially the little ones, often shy.

The numerically and percentually frequent items 22, no happy and no unhappy memories, logically should be complementary to item 20 but in fact are far from being so. BM and WM 20 occur much less often. In the table of intralocal best memories the signs of BM 20 and 22 are not reversed in any column and flatly contradict each other in the literate Shirazi females, where the women claim more often to have always good recollections (BM 20) but also no good ones (BM 22) than the girls. A tendency to contradiction is suggested in the illiterate Marvdasht adults also, the men claiming slightly less "always good", but much less "always bad" memories than the women. As the actual numbers are small and the apparent contradiction is not confirmed in the much larger Shirazi illiterate groups we shall not lay excessive weight on it. We recur to the very significantly higher rate of BM 22 in the Shiraz illiterates as compared with the literate as a whole, find no confirmation of it in WM 20 and conclude that we therefore lack justification for interpreting the affirmation of BM 22 as one of unrelieved misery. For reasons already elucidated we take BM 22 rather to be a sign of unreflectiveness, of confinement to the present, of undifferentiation (though not of indifference). The investigator may become dismayed when some 20–30 % of his subjects assert they have no happy memory whatsoever, but his dismay is mitigated when he realizes that a similar percentage disclaims any unhappy memory and that only a much smaller percentage (0–3 %) claims to recall naught but sorrow (WM 20). The interpretation accorded to BM 22 therefore seems the more justified.

The Shiraz illiterates as a whole show no sex differential for BM 22, but among the literate boys on the one hand and the adult women on the other both deny any happy memory oftener than the girls do. Where the boys are involved one may guess, but only guess at the often harsh and competitive demands of the school. In regard to the women we can refer to what was said before about the greater emancipation and diminished frustration of the younger female generation. In Marvdasht and among the Qashqais it is the women (all illiterate) who more often deny any pleasurable memory than the men, and there can be little doubt that on the whole their lot is harder and their life, as mentioned, more monotonous. The sign is reversed in Qalandari, probably reflecting in the special situation in this new village composed of tribal inhabitants from the same stock as the Qashqai nomads, but subsisting in a more liberal environment than Marvdasht, one that they themselves have created. Paradoxically too the men's more frequent assertion that they own no happy memory may mean precisely the opposite, because in all likelihood not a few of them hark back to the nomad life they have abandoned but decline to admit it. We shall meet further support for this conjecture in subsequent chapters.

When we come to WM 22 ("no bad memory", the polar opposite of BM 22 and in itself a contradiction of a "bad" memory) the tendency of the illiterate Shirazi males to assert they had none more often than the illiterate females hardly requires further comment. Comment is called for, though, when we observe in the fourth column (literate children) that the same difference and direction of sign prevail for the declared absence of bad as of good memories (cf. above). The boys disclaim both more than the girls. The most probable explanation seems to lie in the typically different training and expected social role of the sexes in Iran as in the West, where girls may admit strong emotional experiences and boys are discouraged from doing so. The same consideration might also apply to the difference already noted in the illiterate adults and help to explain why the significance there, in spite of larger numbers, is weaker. Between literate male and female adults in Shiraz it does not appear at all. One may speculate on whether in these for Iran rather special groups the traditional differences in gender roles are not tending to become equalized in some respects at least. Our findings would be compatible with this, though the speculation would need more socio-anthropological support. While the same field in the table of best memories remained blank, there is a surprisingly highly significant difference in regard to WM 22 between literate Shirazi men and boys, the latter affirming far more often that they have no bad memories. This is confirmed to an only slightly less significant degree by the literate females also. It would be easy to refer this to the age factor, since bad experiences (but sometimes also good) accumulate with the years, but we observe that the converse in BM 22 obtains for the girls only, whereas in respect to WM 22 the difference is far more marked for the boys and men. Could this simply mean that the lot of children of both sexes, as social and educational trends become more liberal and less tradition-bound, less grounded upon the absolute authority of the parent and the blind obedience of the child, is growing happier? It would be agreeable to think so, and if the supposition is true, it is only natural that this gradient should emerge among the literate.

Adult-child differentials have not been tabulated for illiterates, but when we do tabulate them in special regard to BM and WM 22 as in Table C II 11 we notice that the

Table C II 11. Shiraz, Marvdasht and Khuzestan Surveys: "No Good" and "No Bad" Memories (BM and WM 22) by Age Class, Sex and Literacy: Significance of Comparisons

	Male Adults		Male Children	Female Adults		Female Children
Shiraz literate	%		%	%		%
No good memory (BM 22)	10.7	—	14.3	14.9	›	7.2
No bad memory (WM 22)	22.9	‹‹‹	46.4	19.5	‹‹	34.8
Shiraz illiterate						
No good memory (BM 22)	26.2	‹	50.0	27.7	—	23.5
No bad memory (WM 22)	29.1	‹	57.1	21.4	‹‹‹	64.7
Marvdasht illiterate						
No good memory (BM 22)	47.5	(‹)	62.5	61.0	—	63.6
No bad memory (WM 22)	30.9	‹‹‹	62.5	40.8	‹‹	65.4
Khuzestan illiterate						
No good memory (BM 22)	20.4	—	20.9	21.2	(›)	12.5
No bad memory (WM 22)	38.1	(‹)	48.8	47.0	‹‹	68.8

illiterate boys in Shiraz deny any pleasurable memory significantly more often than the men – once more hardly a picture of happy childhood, but quite consonant both with a strict, authoritative upbringing and with the fact that many sons of the illiterate poor are put to hard work at a tender age. Less so the girls, whose employment is confined to domestic tasks and sometimes carpet weaving, and whose deficit in pleasurable memories is neither significantly greater nor significantly less than that of their equally illiterate mothers. In respect to WM 22, the denial of any bad memory, the differences for age within the same sex are essentially the same in Shiraz for illiterates as for literates, with some shiftings in the degrees of significance. Children of both sexes deny evil recollections more frequently throughout. The explanation by age suggests itself immediately and probably is valid in part, since it repeats itself over and over, but it does not harmonize at first sight with the differences in BM 22 that we have just discussed. If upbringing is on the whole stricter, severer among the illiterate, as our observations seem to confirm, this together with the other factors adduced can explain why the illiterate boys particularly are poor in happy recollections, but there remains the apparent contradiction that they are also poor – poorer than their fathers – in unhappy ones. Yet this type of child training with all its concomitants is so wide-spread, so much a matter of course still among the majority of the illiterate and so continuous throughout the span of childhood that we may surmise it is hardly remembered and recalled as an outstanding bad experience except by a few, so that it is not registered and does not emerge except in BM rather than in WM 22, though it may and probably does contribute to WM 22 also. Put more simply our hypothesis is that frustrated youth, when asked, more easily articulates its lack of pleasurable memories (BM 22) while ignoring or repressing an abundance of unhappy ones, which are a continual feature of its socio-cultural environment. It is easy to see why changes should take place in respect to BM 22 in literate, generally more liberal and more articulate surroundings. The hypothesis receives some support from the already remarked tendency of the reciprocal negations BM 22 and WM 22 to balance each other out, and considerably more from the highly significant difference between illiterates and literates as a whole in their report of B 22 (first column, discussed above) and the absence of corresponding difference in respect to WM 22.

For further clarification we can calculate the significances of differences between various classes of children, which are not stated in the main tables. There exist sufficient basic data for both sexes only in Shiraz and for the boys beside in Khuzestan. The illiterate children of both sexes in Shiraz affirm they have no pleasurable memory significantly more often than the literate ($p < 0.01$ % for boys, < 5 % for girls). The two classes of boys show no significant difference in denial of bad memories (WM 22), but the girls do ($p < 0.1$ %). Thus the illiterate girls more often have no good, but also more often less bad memories: a by no means startling finding, since the literate on the whole no doubt are exposed to a richer, more variegated environment in which more things happen, including school attendance and failure themselves. Why do the boys, then, display only a one-sided difference (more BM 22)? The question must be placed in a wider context. The same sex difference manifests itself both between the illiterate (m:f 10 % $>$ p $>$ 5 %) and the literate ($p < 5$ %). Again the illiterate boys do not differ significantly from the illiterate girls in respect to WM 22, but the literate boys do exceed the literate girls in this regard ($p < 5$ %). In Khuzestan too the illiterate boys deny a good memory more than the illiterate girls, also a bad one ($p < 5$ % in both cases). It seems to confirm the already suspected generally greater emotional reticence of the boys and youths, for we find the sex difference in at least three paired groups of children both literate and illiterate. Denial of good and bad recollections by the illiterate Shirazi girls more than by the literate could be accounted for hypothetically as above (the literate have more varied experience of both kinds). If the literate boys in Shiraz likewise report less poignant memories of both varieties than the literate girls, this can be referred to the sex difference already surmised. In Khuzestan BM and WM 22 stand in the postulated logical contradiction for the illiterate, corresponding to our hypothesis above. Finally, we must add that differences for BM and WM 20 could not be calculated for the many children's groups because both occurred too seldom, as again may be expected from the shorter life of still young people.

In Marvdasht the pattern of significant differences between the elder and younger male and female illiterates follows that in Shiraz, again with slight shifts in the degrees of significance. In Khuzestan it is rather closer to that of the Shiraz literates or somewhere between both, for the difference between women and girls in respect to BM 22 amounts only to a tendency ($D/SD_D = 1.50$) and the difference between men and boys in respect to WM 22 hardly to that ($D/SD_D = 1.26$, critical value for $p < 10$ % being 1.30). From such marginal differences we should hesitate to derive any far reaching conclusions, but we can refer to a certain "openness" of the Khuzestan DIPA at the time of our survey with a tangible readiness to accept change that was already on its way. Comparing now the sexes rather than the age groups within one or the other sex, we see that it is the women in Marvdasht, the women and girls in Khuzestan who deny any bad memories more often than their male counterparts: a behavior contrary to that of the illiterate females in the city. Maybe that the countrywoman's life in Iran is truly more monotonous and even more abiographic, more unreflecting as we have suggested already; maybe also that the particularly unhappy plight of the uneducated woman in the city, ill equipped to deal with its greater complications and difficulties and at a more obvious disadvantage against her educated sisters, makes its influence felt here. In all likelihood both work together.

There remain the non-responders in both directions, BM and WM 23. The illiterate men figure more than the illiterate women for both in Shiraz, where, in common with most places the world over, the men as a group seem less ready to talk about themselves and among the illiterates are probably less articulate, wherefore we do not encounter the same statistical difference among the literates. The literate Shirazi girls also decline response more frequently than their mothers. One recalls here the numerous extremely shy little schoolchildren of both sexes who often plunged us into doubt whether to class them as pathological or not. When asking about worst memories we got no response significantly more often from the Khuzestani and Qashqai adult women in contradistinction to the illiterate women of the city. Here either a certain lack of biography or, as we strongly suspect, some fear of uttering concrete complaints before one's neighbors (who were too often within earshot, as explained in the introduction) could account for the difference.

We have endeavored to cull from the intralocal comparisons what good and bad memories or their opposites are roughly specific for dichotomous sex, age and literacy classes and summarize the results below, omitting the comparison between the illiterates and literates that has already been drawn at the beginning of the chapter. In the summary we take account of characteristic differences that are fairly regular and consistent, though they may not be always present and may even be contradicted in certain columns. Where contradictions do appear, they rest generally upon relatively small populations and have low to medium significance. It must be recalled again that the absence of a statistically demonstrable significant difference does not necessarily mean that a true and factually significant difference does not exist, but may be an artefact of small numbers, types of distribution, etc.:

Sex Differences

Best Memories		*Worst Memories*	
Males more than females:		Males more than females:	
BM 9	Own good health or recovery	WM 2	Ill treatment at others' hands
BM 12	Activity, achievement, success in work	WM 6	Bereavement other than loss of child
BM 25	Good harvest	WM 13	Financial difficulties, poverty, debt, etc.
BM 26	Land reform	WM 15	Unemployment
		BM 22	No pleasurable memory (children only)
Females more than males:		Females more than males:	
BM 5	Pregnancy and childbirth (rural only)	WM 4	Divorce
BM 6	Birth of siblings (urban only)	WM 5	Unwanted pregnancy or child
BM 10	Reunion with relatives or friends	WM 11	Fear of animals or situations
		WM 19	Failure in school or other examinations

Age Differences

Best Memories		*Worst Memories*	
Adults more than children:		Adults more than children:	
BM 4	Engagement and marriage	WM 9	Own illness or accident
		BM 22	No pleasurable memory (females only)
Children more than adults:		Children more than adults:	
BM 2	Getting playthings or presents	WM 10	Separation from relatives or friends
BM 11	Family weddings, festivals, feasts		
BM 19	Success in school or other examinations		
WM 22	No ill memories (literates only)		

c. **Interlocal Comparisons.** In interlocal comparisons (Tables C II 12–13) our main interest is directed to such significant differences as may typically emerge between peasant, nomad and urban populations, but we must be prepared also to encounter more complicated patterns. The three villages or village clusters of Marvdasht, Khuzestan and Qalandari are not identical. Differences may also occur that cannot be referred simply to one or another of these three main types of socio-cultural environment, but may be occasioned by local customs and circumstances, of which we are far from possessing sufficient knowledge.

BM 1: childhood, youth, life with parents is approximately equally represented in Shiraz and Marvdasht, higher in Khuzestan than in Shiraz for the illiterate women and the literate boys, higher again for the literate boys in Khuzestan than in Marvdasht and higher for the illiterate men in Qalandari than in Marvdasht (tendency only), Khuzestan and among the Qashqai. A strong male attachment to the parental family stands out thus as a characteristic of the village of Qalandari and is accentuated in the schoolboys. Among females local differences are much less pronounced and their significance, where found, is low throughout, attaining the 5 % level only once (illiterate Khuzestani women over Shirazi) with a similar tendency once more for the women of Qalandari over those of the Qashqai and a sole reversal of tendency in that the women of Marvdasht claim such a memory as their best slightly more often than those of the Qashqai. Thus we have a fairly clear male gradient for this recollection from the Qashqai over Qalandari, from Qalandari over Khuzestan and Marvdasht without significant distinction between Marvdasht and Shiraz. Filial affection, at least in retrospect, thus appears strong indeed in the tribally structured nomads, not quite so strong in their settled, but still tribally organized cousins, weaker in Khuzestan, but weaker again in Shiraz and Marvdasht, which, different though they are, both are typical constituents of Fars (Qalandari, though in Fars, is not). Does attendance at school make the boys more aware of this? We can only put the question as it suggests itself but not answer it. Not clear is why the illiterate city women less often hark back to their childhood than those of Khuzestan and those of the Qashqai less than both the Khuzestani and Marvdashti, whereas it is precisely the Qashqai and Qalandari men (themselves Qashqais) who do so most often. One could suspect that the tribal

Table C II 12 a. Affirmations of Worst Memories: Significance of Interlocal Comparisons

	Shiraz: Marvdasht				Shiraz: Khuzestan			Shiraz: Qalandari		Shiraz: Qashqai	
	Adults			Children	Adults		Children	Illiterate Adults			
	Illiterate		Literate		Illiterate		Literate				
	m	f	m	m	m	f	m	m	f	m	f
1.						‹	‹‹	‹			
2.				(›)		(‹)					
3.		(›)				(›)					
4.			›		‹‹‹	‹‹		‹‹	‹‹‹	‹‹‹	‹
5.	›	›››	›		››	›››				››	
6.											
7.											
8.										‹‹	
9.		‹									
10.									(›)		›
11.	›	››	‹‹‹	‹				(›)			››
12.	›				››			(›)			
13.			(›)								
14.		›		›		›	››		(‹)		(›)
15.	›››	›››	›	›	(›)	››		(›)	›	››	››
16.		—		—		—	—		—		—
17.		—		—		—	—		—		—
18.	—	—		‹	—	—	‹‹	—	—	—	—
19.	—	—	(›)	›››	—	—	›››	—	—	—	—
20.	››	(‹)				‹‹‹			‹‹		‹
21.								(›)			‹‹‹
22.	‹‹‹	‹‹‹	‹	‹‹‹		(›)			›	(›)	
23.	›					‹					‹‹
24.											
25.	—	—	—	—	—	—	—	—	—	—	—
26.	—	—	—	—	—	—	—	—	—	—	—

Table C II 12 b. Affirmations of Best Memories: Significance of Interlocal Comparisons

	Marvdasht: Khuzestan					Marvdasht: Qalandari		Marvdasht: Qashqai		Khuzestan: Qalandari		Khuzestan: Qashqai		Qashqai: Qalandari	
	Illiterate				Literate	Illiterate Adults									
	Adults		Children		Children										
	m	f	m	f	m	m	f	m	f	m	f	m	f	m	f
1.					‹	(‹)			(›)	‹‹			›	‹	(‹)
2.	(‹)	(‹)	‹‹	‹	(‹)										
3.															
4.	‹‹‹	‹‹		‹		‹‹	‹‹‹	‹‹‹	‹		‹				(‹)
5.		(›)					‹‹‹	›	‹		‹‹‹	(›)	‹‹‹	‹	(‹)
6.															
7.							(›)								
8.				(›)				‹‹‹				‹‹‹		(›)	
9.		›		(›)											
10.			›						(›)						
11.	‹‹	‹‹‹	‹‹	‹‹‹				(‹)		›	(›)		››		
12.	(›)														
13.															
14.					(›)		‹‹‹				‹‹‹				‹
15.	‹	‹‹	‹	‹‹	‹							›	›		
16.		—	—	—	—		—		—		—		—		—
17.		—	—	—	—		—		—		—		—		—
18.	—	—	—	—		—	—	—	—	—	—	—	—	—	—
19.	—	—	—	—		—	—	—	—	—	—	—	—	—	—
20.	‹	‹‹‹	‹	‹‹			(‹)	‹‹			›		››		
21.	›					›			‹‹‹	›		‹	‹‹‹	›	›
22.	›››	›››	›››	›››	›	(›)	›››	›››	›››	‹			‹	‹	››
23.	(‹)	‹							‹‹						(›)
24.															
25.		›						‹‹‹				‹‹‹		››	
26.	(›)							(›)							

Table C II 13 a. Affirmations of Worst Memories: Significance of Interlocal Comparisons

	Shiraz: Marvdasht				Shiraz: Khuzestan			Shiraz: Qalandari		Shiraz: Qashqai	
	Adults			Children	Adults		Children	Illiterate Adults			
	Illiterate		Literate		Illiterate		Literate				
	m	f	m	m	m	f	m	m	f	m	f
1.					(›)						
2.				››						‹‹	‹‹‹
3.		›				(›)					(›)
4.											
5.											
6.	(›)	‹				‹‹‹	‹		‹‹‹	›	(‹)
7.						›				(›)	››
8.				›		›					
9.		›››				›››		›	››	(›)	›››
10.		‹									
11.		›				(›)	(‹)				
12.	‹										
13.		‹‹‹				‹‹			‹‹		‹‹
14.	(›)	››			›	››					
15.	››				››						
16.		—		—		—			—		—
17.	‹	(‹)									
18.	—	—			—	—		—	—	—	—
19.	—	—			—	—	››	—	—	—	—
20.		‹									
21.	‹		(‹)		(‹)			‹			
22.		‹‹‹		‹‹	(‹)	‹‹‹	(‹)	‹	‹		(‹)
23.	››				›	‹				(›)	‹‹
24.	›				›						
25.	—	—	—	—	—	—	—	—	—	—	—

Table C II 13 b. Affirmations of Worst Memories: Significance of Interlocal Comparisons

	Marvdasht: Khuzestan					Marvdasht: Qalandari		Marvdasht: Qashqai		Khuzestan: Qalandari		Khuzestan: Qashqai		Qashqai: Qalandari	
	Illiterate				Literate	Illiterate Adults									
	Adults		Children		Children										
	m	f	m	f	m	m	f	m	f	m	f	m	f	m	f
1.		›					›								
2.			‹	‹‹	‹			‹‹‹	‹‹‹			‹‹	‹‹‹	›	›››
3.			(‹)	(›)											
4.															
5.															
6.					(‹)	‹	‹‹				(‹)	(›)	(›)	‹	‹
7.		(›)						›	›			(›)	(›)		(‹)
8.		›													
9.						›		(›)		›		›			(‹)
10.															
11.															
12.	›														
13.	(›)											(‹)			
14.								‹‹	‹			‹‹‹	‹	(›)	
15.															
16.		—	—	—	—		—		—		—		—		—
17.	›	›							›						
18.	—	—	—	—		—	—	—	—	—	—	—	—	—	—
19.	—	—	—	—	›	—	—	—	—	—	—	—	—	—	—
20.															
21.			‹				‹				‹‹				‹
22.						‹			(›)					‹	
23.	(‹)	‹‹							‹‹‹		(›)		›		›
24.															
25.	(›)							‹	‹			‹‹‹	‹	(›)	

affiliation in both senses of this word held a stronger and more enduring emotional value for the male sex, whereas in the female it could be supplanted on the scale of values by other loyalties such as those to spouse and marital family.

The converse, WM 1, family conflict, shows it slightly more than those of Khuzestan, but significant differences among the women appear only between those of Marvdasht on the one hand and those of both Khuzestan and Qalandari on the other. Still other indications will emerge that the women of Marvdasht in 1963 on the whole had no very happy lot.

BM 2, getting playthings or presents, is typically a child's memory, as the higher significances in the children's columns show and as is apparent from the figures (otherwise here not specifically compared but obvious from the data tables). It confronts us with some surprises. Minor and inconsistent trends between city and village are hardly conclusive and may reflect, for example, a better economic status of the parents of literate boys in Shiraz who could thus buy more presents, or a more concrete, less mature attitude in the women of Khuzestan. No significant or even tendential differences come to light between the various rural-nomad pairs except a remarkably consistent and unexpected series of such between Marvdasht and Khuzestan, with adults and children of both sexes quoting such a memory as their happiest in Khuzestan regularly more often than in Marvdasht. We can only hazard a guess here that we cannot confirm. By our impression the cluster of villages in the DIPA in Khuzestan was financially better off than the villages of Marvdasht at the time we studied both. Money was beginning to flow, so to speak, from the newly erected Dez Dam into the development area, some men were finding work outside it at the dam site itself, in Dezful, in the sugar refinery of Haft Tapeh and even in Ahwaz, and such things as bicycles, watches, pocket knives, better oil lamps and the like were beginning to be noticeable in the development area as they were not in the yet economically backward villages of Marvdasht. This again could mean concretely: more presents. Such an economical differential did not exist, as far as our impression goes, between Marvdasht and the Qashqai when they were studied roughly a year apart, while the surveys of Marvdasht and Qalandari were separated by several (6–7) years and the numbers in Qalandari were probably too small to yield significant differences.

WM 2, the converse of BM 2, is in fact more comprehensive and by no means necessarily or even mainly a childish memory. Among children, as remarked above, it generally implied a beating, among schoolchildren often at the teacher's hands. Shiraz leads the rest in the number of schoolboys whose worst memory was some form of ill treatment, followed by Khuzestan and with Marvdasht last, so far as our data go. The difference between Khuzestan and Marvdasht holds for illiterate children also. When we look at the adults, it is evident at once that the Qashqai of both sexes report the memory of ill treatment as their worst far more often and with very much higher significance than any others. The obvious reason for this is to be found in our description of the Qashqai Survey, just prior to which the Qashqai and other tribal peoples of the South had endeavored to revolt against the far-reaching reforms, especially the land reform of 1963, and had been put down by military action. The "ill treatment" several times included seeing their sons, brothers or husbands shot, more often outright robbery whether by troops or brigands pretending to be such, generally with some physical mishandling thrown in. The pronounced difference requires no psychological conjectures to account for it.

Success of relatives, family or friends (BM 3) shows hardly any interlocal differences. Where it does, these are tendencies in favor of the city women and are likely to relate to a child's success in school or in getting a job. Worst memories of accident or mishap (WM 3) to others or oneself accumulate in the same categories, i.e. among the illiterate city women. We have no data on accident frequency and proneness but would risk the guess that the slightly higher frequency of this worst memory among illiterate city women, with no corresponding differentials in the countryside, might well be due to the frequency of accidents in the building trades, in which quite a number of illiterate men find occupation and in which safety precautions are minimal, in industry and even in city traffic, all which affect these women much more than the women of the villages.

BM 4, engagement and marriage, and BM 5, pregnancy and childbirth, are best considered together. Before doing so, the reader must be reminded that a great interval may elapse between betrothal and the consummation of marriage and that after betrothal the bride may live for a long time in her own family before moving to that of her parents-in-law or setting up housekeeping on her own. Practice varies, and this may explain some rather marked differences in the memorial statistics. Looking across BM 4 we observe that for illiterate adults of both sexes this memory is about equally important in Shiraz and Marvdasht and in both places decidedly less so than in Khuzestan, Qalandari and the Qashqai. This precludes any explanation in terms of urban-rural or urban-tribal differences. What Shiraz and Marvdasht have in common is that they belong to the sub-culture of Fars, while Qalandari remains to some extent an exclave in that province. This would give rise to the suspicion of some psychologically quite meaningful difference in engagement and marriage customs between the people in Fars, both urban and rural, and those of the other communities under consideration, a difference that we must confess our inability to define. These statistically highly significant differences have emerged only as our data have been worked up in detail years after the surveys were performed, and at the time of writing local sources which could well furnish the necessary information are not accessible. A question arises here that must be left to future research. The tendencies in regard to BM 5 diverge from those in BM 4. For the illiterate of both sexes pregnancy and childbirth constitute significantly more often the happiest memory in Shiraz than in Marvdasht: city and village no longer affirm the same values. Shiraz also preponderates in this respect over Khuzestan, and male Shiraz (not the women, be it noted) over the Qashqai. An explanation that comes to mind at once is that childbirth in the city on the whole is a substantially less dangerous and perhaps less painful (narcosis) affair than in the country or the desert, more and better medical facilities, including some trained midwives, being available. When we look at the mothers only we note that the Qashqai women, whether nomadic or sedentary (Qalandari) more often report pregnancy and childbirth as their happiest memory than the women of either Marvdasht or Khuzestan and that those of Marvdasht show only a tendency to do so more than those of Khuzestan. This can be attributed either to a tribal pride in childbirth or to its presumably less dangers in the two tribal communities, whose health is on the whole better (the latter has been demonstrated for the Qashqai nomads and by our own observations seems likely for Qalandari, though we have no figures to prove it except for mental health). The difference between illiterates and literates and for literates between the sexes has been commented upon already in the intralocal comparisons at the only site where they could be carried out: in the city of Shiraz.

The contrary worst memories WM 4 and 5, divorce and unwanted pregnancy or childbirth, display no interlocal differences at all. Neither are they often mentioned, certainly not as often as one would expect in a European survey, although divorce is by no means rare and by Islamic law is much easier, so that almost every married woman lives in fear of it. A moderate to good frequentation of the family planning centers in Shiraz proved that not all pregnancies are wanted, but the weight of custom is such that few women in the rather open survey situation will be prepared to admit an undesired pregnancy, much less the actual birth of a child as their worst memory.

BM 6 and 7 are closely related inasmuch as they apply to intimate familial association (birth of siblings, connubial life). Both show either no (BM 6) or hardly any (BM 7) interlocal variation. The minimal differential tendency between the women of Marvdasht and Qalandari in respect to BM 7 can be neglected in preference to over-interpretation. Many more sizeable and in part highly significant differences appear when we address ourselves to WM 6 and 7, which to be sure are not their polar opposites. Bereavement apart from loss of child (WM 6) does not by any means always imply widowhood, but frequently refers to the death of parents or siblings, for which reason it was paired against BM 6. All differences of more than 5 % significance lie here between adult female populations. This is true of the women of Khuzestan and Qalandari over those of Shiraz and the women of Qalandari over those of Marvdasht, as in other comparisons too the women of Qalandari cite bereavement as their worst memory more often than those of all other surveys, though the level of significance is lower. We know no reason for this, particularly since the nomadic Qashqai in recent years (as far as our information goes) were exposed to more violence than the settled, and the settlement presented a more favorable health picture. The same trend is substantiated, moreover, by the men of Qalandari as against those of Marvdasht and of the nomadic Qashqai. One might speculate about local epidemics or circumstances that led this Qashqai group to its decision to settle, but again we lack information and at the time of writing have no opportunity to procure it. Noticeable, though, is that the differentials are generally female, although in Shiraz both literate and illiterate men recalled bereavement as their worst memory more often than women. There is a tendency too for the illiterate Shirazi men to recall bereavement more than the men of Marvdasht, whereas in the adult females of the two communities the gradient is reversed. This seems to lend credibility to the theory advanced in the interlocal comparison: that the city men have less kinship resources to fall back on when they lose a mate.

Differences in reaction to loss of child (WM 7) are fairly numerous, but not large and only once reach significance above the 5 % level, namely between the Shirazi and Qashqai women. At this point a rather striking difference manifests itself: a reversal of sign in the city women's reaction to loss of child as against other bereavement in comparison to the rural women (except Marvdasht). If the country women complain substantially more of bereavement, the city women do so more about loss of child. They bear fewer children (mean number of pregnancies per urban family 4.6, rural 8.1 nationwide by census of 1976) and lose fewer (mortality rate for children up to 5 years: urban 62 per 100, rural 120 per 1000) [155], which suggests that the rural women become more hardened and indifferent to single loss.

Items 8 and 9 relate to health, either one's family's (BM and WM 8) or one's own (BM and WM 9), and the best and worst memories are strictly polar. All highly significant differences for BM 8 are supplied by the Quashqai, and this time by the Qashqai men. Since we have no indication that the health risk of the Qashqai families, particularly the women, is greater than that of other non-urban groups, but rather the contrary, we must attribute this in all likelihood to a psychological or socio-cultural factor. A factor intrinsic in the nomadic way of life suggests itself easily: if the nomad woman is disabled or falls ill her family and the tribe are seriously hindered when they prepare to move on, and the hindrance is more sensible than in a sedentary community. Equally, though, the better mental health of the nomads would accord well with a greater mutual concern that showed itself not only in grief, but also in joy at the improvement of a partner's condition. Here, at any rate, the Qashqai stand out conspicuously and alone. Own good health, on the other hand, seems to enforce itself upon the memory of more women in Shiraz than in Marvdasht and more in Marvdasht than in Khuzestan. The first difference can be put in parallel to the city women's greater tendency to hypochondria and hysteria which we have met in Part B, Chap. IV 3 and a clue to the second may be proposed when we add together the female prevalence rates for hypochondric and hysteric neurosis and for psychosomatic disorders and notice that the sum amounts to 21.8 per 1000 in Marvdasht, but only to 16.4 in Khuzestan. All three imply enhanced self-observation, tend to fluctuating courses and therefore may on recovery oftener leave behind them conscious memories of relief than graver physical illnesses do. The explanation remains hypothetical but accords at least with the first, demonstrable finding. The men show no interlocal differences.

The women of Shiraz and Marvdasht both bewail illness and accidents in their families (WM 8) more often than those of Khuzestan, and once more we are driven to ask whether this is not grounded in the habits of Fars, since the health level of Marvdasht approaches much more nearly that of Khuzestan than of the city. The only other difference lies between the literate male children of Shiraz and Marvdasht to the favor of the former, whose urban environment may sensitize them more to the woes of others. The Shirazi women (n. b. here as above the illiterate women) also bewail their own real or imagined ill health significantly and emphatically more often than the rural or nomad women do and are joined this time as against Qalandari and the Qashqai by the city men, though with lower rates of difference and significance. On the other hand they do not as in WM 8 go along with the women of Marvdasht, but display a very highly significant difference from them with a great deal more worst memories of bad health. Though we lack hard data, nothing in our experience seems to offer any objective basis for this. We take it to be a phenomenon of urbanization in accordance with others such as we have mentioned above and one which in the city affects the female sex especially. This becomes the more evident when we inspect the differences outside the city. They pertain almost exclusively to the men. The men of Marvdasht and Khuzestan have more to say about their own ill health than those of Qalandari and the Qashqai, between whom there is no significant difference (and between the women only a tendency for the Qashqai to register more such evil memory). More plainly perhaps than in any item hitherto we can observe clear cut differences between city residents, non-tribal villagers and tribal members, whether these be sedentary or not. Summarily: illiterate city people in Iran register ill health as their worst memory a good deal more frequently than others, the women much more than the men, as the intralocal comparison confirms, villagers more than members of tribes and village men more than village women (again confirmed by intralocal comparison), while a sex difference (women more than men) obtains only in the Qashqai village and not among the Qashqai nomads (intralocal). It is hard to interpret this otherwise than as a socio-cultural phenomenon even though we do not have precise and comparable public health data for the three groups. Moreover, this interpretation fits nearly into the psychiatric-epidemiological picture that we have drawn in some detail and for which we do possess data. Many a complaint may be and undoubtedly is voiced and remembered in the city that is passed over or at least left unrecalled in the more robust countryside and desert, and this is unquestionably done in the city a great deal more by the women than by the men. That the sex difference becomes reversed in the villages need imply nothing about real prevalence or about relative tough-mindedness and longsuffering but may find a simple explanation in the fact that the bread-winner's illness direly affects the whole family, whereas in the case of a village wife's illness there are usually relatives and neighbors to help tide over. Finally the tribal people may be actually less ill, as we have reason to believe, and more hardy, men and women alike. The differences are the more meaningful and reliable, we submit, because the factor of literacy in the city has been eliminated and only illiterate sub-populations have been compared. Interestingly, while the sex differential is reflected in the psychiatric morbidity rates for Shiraz, it is not in the villages. In Marvdasht the female psychiatric cases outnumber the male by roughly two to one, and in Khuzestan the sexes are equally represented. This may lend support to the hypothesis advanced above: that the men's predominantly physical illnesses in the villages furnish more ground for grave and troubled recollection because of their immediate and tangible socio-economic consequences. Yet it would be altogether false to conclude from this, as some public health workers and even ministries do, that the women's sufferings are "imaginary" because immaterial and therefore inconsequential.

Reunion (BM 10) and separation (WM 10) constitute true opposites. Interlocal differences are few, pertain in three out of four cases to the women and once only to the illiterate boys (more in Marvdasht than in Khuzestan) and are of rather low significance throughout. One might surmise that the more frequent expression of BM 10 in Shiraz came from the considerable number of village women who pined there under separation from their relatives. The converse holds for WM 10: separation is more often the harshest memory for the women of Marvdasht than for those of the city. At that time, be it recalled, few people from the Marvdasht villages travelled to Shiraz at all, and hardly any women, so that separation, if any family member moved to the city or elsewhere, was likely to be long. Even if a bride e.g. changed residence from one village to another, visits were infrequent. Within the rural areas there are no significant differences in WM 10.

No true opposites are BM 11 and WM 11. Weddings and similar feasts constitute BM 11. In the villages wedding celebrations may go on for a week or more and everybody takes part. They are one of the few outstanding joyful events and probably the most prominent of all. Civil and religious holidays, the latter in the majority days of commemorative mourning, played no conspicuous part in the countryside. This was otherwise in the city, where few could stop work for the daylong celebration of matrimonial alliances but the shops and bazars closed on calender holidays. The illiterate men and still more the illiterate women of Shiraz denominate such feasts more often as their happiest memory than their counterparts in Marvdasht, but between the literate men of town and city the valuation is sharply and very significantly reversed. It is plausible to surmise that the urban literates found different sources of pleasure, the more so as the literate male children follow them. It is not so easy to say why the illiterate Shirazi adults more often cited this memory than those of Marvdasht, the Shirazi men slightly more than those of Qalandari and the Shirazi women substantially more than those of the Qashqai, except upon economic grounds, the city dwellers being on the whole somewhat better off. The same consideration may hold for the highly significant differences in all four sub-populations: men and women, boys and girls between Marvdasht and Khuzestan, the suspicion being also that the Khuzestanis were economically better situated and could afford richer feasts. Certainly they were prospering more, when surveyed, than the Qashqai, whose women too far less recalled such feasts than those of Khuzestan, and the same applies to a smaller degree to both sexes in Qalandari as compared with Khuzestan. We cannot exclude socio-cultural differences either, which might help to explain why the Khuzestani apparently paid more attention to festivals of rejoicing than others did, but neither can we prove them.

WM 11, specific fears of a more or less phobic character, is neither a true opposite to BM 11 nor does it show much variation in its distribution, contrary to expectation. Mindful of the not seldom expressed fear of wild animals, dogs, snakes and robbers in the countryside and among the nomads we had anticipated significant differences in this direction but fail to find them. This may be accounted for by the difference between notions of fear and memories of fright. The single significant difference is actually reversed; the women of Shiraz recall a fright as their worst memory more than those of Marvdasht and have a tendency to do so more than those of Khuzestan. Only the literate Khuzestani boys conform, albeit weakly, to our expectation, and from them we recall vividly hearing just such fears expressed and frights, usually encounters with an animal or snake, recounted. Here again the illiterate Shirazi women seem to reflect their general plight, which we have mentioned several times.

BM 12, activity, success in work, and BM 13, joy in accomplishment outside work, stand in such a close complementary relationship that it is preferable to regard both together. As we have seen in the intralocal comparisons, both are much more a male affair, and we are not surprised to find the significant differences in the corresponding columns. Neither is it any surprise to observe that this is regularly more often an outstanding happy memory in the city with its much greater variety of occupations than in the country. Between the non-urban surveys there are no significant differences (one is only suggested between the Marvdasht and Khuzestani men). Again as anticipated only the literate men in Shiraz recall joy in free accomplishment often enough to establish at least a differential tendency over those of Marvdasht, where alone, be it noted, the comparison is possible.

WM 12, dissatisfaction with employment, is no exact opposite to BM 12, though related and, like BM 12, implies some variety and choice of employment such as under the conditions of the 1960s was hardly to be found except in the city. Yet the only significant differences apply to the men in Marvdasht, who more often mention job dissatisfaction as their worst memory than those of Shiraz or of Khuzestan. The reason is probably not far to seek, for at the time of the Marvdasht survey construction of the petrochemical plan near Qassemabad had been nearly concluded and even some trial runs had been performed, giving temporary employment to a few men who thus got a premonition of presumably better things and more than their share of frustration when the factory did not proceed immediately into operation. Other undertakings were also underway in the Marvdasht area but had yielded little fruit as yet – only a taste, enough to whet dissatisfaction. Looking ahead to WM 15, unemployment, we realize from the statistics that this is definitely a city man's affair, since the few employees of any kind from the villages were all farmer-laborers not wholly dependent upon a paid job. Material loss and bankruptcy (WM 14) were significantly more often a worst memory for both sexes in the city and, almost at the other end of the socio-economic spectrum, of the Qashqai, but probably for different reasons. In the agricultural villages there was less bankruptcy than continual grinding impoverishment and, up to 1963, debt to the landowner registered vigorously as their worst memory by all the rural women much more than the urban (WM 13). Between the rural communities in this respect there were only minor tendencies to differ. The Qashqais, by their own memory as here registered, were not more affected than others. They were very much more, however, in respect to concrete loss (WM 14), which usually meant being robbed of all or nearly all their possessions by the various types of marauders who infested the desert. Here it was the men as the titulary owners who were harder hit or, at all events, more often said so.

Reverting to pleasanter topics such as BM 14, travel, excursion, holiday, repose, and the related BM 15, pilgrimage (with no sharp boundary against BM 14) and religion, the first is characteristically quoted by the city women as compared with their rural sisters (Qalandari being an exception) and also by the literate boys in the city. The latter without much doubt had more opportunities for such an experience, the city women probably also. As the women's lives tended to be more monotonous there was reason for them to remark such events more often than their spouses, even though such a difference does not show itself in the comparison between illiterate men and women in the city. The majority of the rural women moved about so little and so rarely in those days (the situation had changed a great deal in 1976) that the urban-rural differential in respect to that memory becomes comprehensible even though it does not hold between the sexes in Shiraz. In this respect Qalandari constitutes a conspicuous exception. Its women very significantly quote BM 14 more than those of Marvdasht or Khuzestan and with lowered significance more than those of the Qashqai or Shiraz. The explanation can only lie in the special character of the new and relatively progressive village – progressive in its housing, its modest commerce and its schools, which practically all the boys and a larger share of the girls than elsewhere outside Shiraz were attending. Their mothers had been nomad women up to a few years ago. Is it any wonder that they were happy to be back on the move again? But why not the men? For one thing they enjoyed more motility anyway, traveling frequently to the city, in the summer to outlying grazing grounds and even taking jobs outside. For another we have seen indications already and shall see more that presumed longings for a return to a nomadic way of life were rather strictly repressed in the full sense of the word. Having taken the decision to settle, they stuck to it.

Although BM 14 (travel etc.) and BM 15 (pilgrimage) overlap a good deal, our results show that they are not identical. The differences are all in the same direction with two minor exceptions, but in BM 15 the Shirazi men, so to speak, join their wives. Everywhere the city joys in pilgrimage more than the country, and Khuzestan also more than Marvdasht. For the city folk there are certainly many more opportunities; they are less tied to their fields and flocks, and bus travel is cheap. Pilgrimage may also play a greater part because there is more organized, institutionalized visible religious life.

There was neither mullah nor mosque in any of the rural communities we surveyed, let alone the Qashqai camps, but in Shiraz an abundance of both. Shiraz itself is not one of the major sites of Iranian pilgrimage such as Meshed, Ray and Qom, though the shrine of Shahcheragh stands in the odor of special holiness and can attract the pious from e.g. Marvdasht, though less from more distant places. Why then the substantial difference between Marvdasht and Khuzestan? On the borders of the DIPA near Shush, roughly some 15 km from our villages in Khuzestan, is a shrine of the Prophet Daniel of more than local reputation, much visited by pilgrims from all Khuzestan and beyond. Repeatedly in our Khuzestani records we find as best memory: "A visit to the Shrine of Daniel". For the villagers there it is within practicable traveling distance even by donkey or on foot. They love to go there and combine the outing with a picnic. The citizens of Qalandari, Marvdasht and the Qashqai have no such convenient opportunity.

From religion we turn to war. Neither in its positive nor it its negative aspects does military service (BM and WM 16) or release from it (BM 17) exhibit any demonstrable interlocal preferences, so far as comparisons can be drawn at all. For the majority of pairs they cannot. The rubric is really of interest only in the intralocal comparisons of best memories in Shiraz, where the literate display a tendency to recall their service as their best memory more often than the illiterate, and among the literate the men more than the women.

WM 17, overwork and exhaustion, is no true contrast to BM 17 and was fitted in here for convenience. It yields no significant differences either in the intra- or the interlocal comparisons and might have been dispensed with altogether if it had not already been in the matrices. Such complaints are rarely uttered directly in Iran even by those who have every ground to entertain them and come to expression either as quasi-medical symptons or in the inimitable, typically roundabout, oft repeated and endearing formula of encouragement خسته نبا شير , a cumbersome English translation of which might be "Don't (let yourself) get tired." The infrequently used, more formal and rhetorical German *Werde nicht müde* comes closer but lacks the familiar heartening tone. خستہ نبا شيير is as uniquely Iranian as the lilt of Farsi, the blue of Persian tiles, the taste of local breads.

The school items 18 and 19, important though they are, offer little in the way of interlocal comparison because comparable groups outside Shiraz are mostly lacking. BM 18, attending school, impresses itself more upon the Marvdashti and still more upon the Khuzestani boys than upon the city youth without doubt for the simple reason that schools were new in both clusters of villages, newer in Khuzestan than in Marvdasht. In correspondence thereto we see that in both places failure in school was taken very much more often to heart (WM 19) than in Shiraz. A little sadly one must resign oneself to the circumstance that it was probably more the novelty than the institution itself that created the impact.

Memories of good and bad harvests (BM and WM 25) can be compared only between the villagers and the nomads. Some of these are planters also during the winter season in the south, but on the whole "good harvest" may be taken rather to mean an agriculturally prosperous year with enough water and good pasture for their flocks. As a man's best memory this far outweighs Marvdasht, Khuzestan and Qalandari. Ill harvest as worst memory is recorded by the Qashqai of both sexes significantly more than by the villagers. The reason for the striking difference to Marvdasht is not altogether clear, for we recall that both Marvdasht and the Qashqais then camping not far from Shiraz had been visited by severe drought in the three years just before the surveys of 1963/64 and retained this as a searing recollection. The surveys of Shiraz and Qalandari were carried out five to six years later. In Qalandari we heard no special mention of climatic catastrophes. Khuzestan in 1965 had already begun to receive irrigating water from the new Dez Dam. The effect was obvious, especially since we had visited Khuzestan before, at the end of the long area of aridity that began with the Arab conquest, when the Sassanide water works fell into neglect and disrepair, and lasted until the completion of the Pahlavi Dam in 1964. Though this visibly revolutionized agriculture even to the eyes of the non-expert it was little mentioned by those benefited.

Land reform (BM 26) was, as substantial percentages of best memories outside Shiraz show. As the city was not directly affected we did not include it in our interlocal comparisons. In Marvdasht the impact had been very recent, direct and immediate, and the rates of best memories therefore tend to exceed those of Khuzestan, surveyed two and a half years later. The men mention it, though the women profit by it just as they suffer together under ill harvest and bankruptcy. There is an tendency to a difference also between Marvdasht and the Qashqai men which cannot be determined by time, for both surveys fell in the same year, albeit some months apart. Reception of the land reform by the Qashqai was negative to ambiguous. Some of the nomads did hold patches of farming land, worked them in the winter and stood to profit by the reform, but for many, as explained above, it was a new instrument of oppression, designed and often harshly used to force them into a sedentary way of life that they had no intention or desire to embrace. Such a settlement as Qalandari was a conspicuous exception rather than a rule.

The unspecific items 20–24 come last, though they often claim high percentages. The city men are or claim to be much more often "always cheerful" (BM 20) than the city women, as we have seen above, but also more than the men in Marvdasht, and one cannot but wonder whether truth, pride, stoicism, a mixture of all three or still other factors lie at the back of this. After the drought just recorded it may well be that the men of Marvdasht truly had less reason to deny any evil memories. Between the city and country women the gradient is consistently reversed in favor of the country: we recall what has been said several times about the peculiar plight of the illiterate women in the city. All sub-populations in Khuzestan, the women in Qalandari and even the much afflicted Qashqai men affirm nothing but good memories more than the Marvdasht and confirm this in BM 22 by asserting very much less often that they cherish no pleasurable memories, and they are joined in this by the Qashqai women and the men of Qalandari. By this criterion Marvdasht would be the unhappiest survey site. WM 20, always miserable, confirms this only for the Marvdasht women as against those of Shiraz and does not reveal any other significant differences. Its counterpart WM 22, no bad memory, speaks in the same sense for the males of Qalandari as compared with those of Marvdasht, but also for those of Qalandari in comparison with the male Qashqai, and there is even a contradictory tendency for the Marvdashti women to deny any bad memory oftener than the Qashqai. The substantial differences between the rural and urban women, and to a lesser degree the men, in respect to this "worst memory" 22, which is actually a denial of any bad memory, threaten to become paradoxical. They are decidedly in favor of the rural women and sometimes also of the men as were the differences in BM 20 above; here the findings confirm each other. Between rural communities however the gradients that were conspicuous in BM 20 nearly disappear. Marvdasht und Khuzestan show no difference, while in respect to BM 20 they did for both sexes and both age classes. Now it is the men of Qalandari and not the women, the Qashqai women and not the men who more often indicate that they are not bedeviled by evil memories. In the intralocal comparisons we found no sex differential for either BM 20 or WM 20 in Qalandari and the Qashqai, none for WM 20, and for WM 22 more untroubled memories in the Qalandari men and the Qashqai women, the last being in agreement with the interlocal difference just mentioned. The conspicuous disagreement, or seeming lack of agreement, lies in Marvdasht, where all classes much less often say they are always in good spirits (again in comparison with other rural surveys, but in comparison with Shiraz only the men) but do not reinforce this with a corresponding assertion that they have only bad recollections, even though the recent drought had provided material enough for these. If there is an explanation it probably consists in the absence of precise equivalence between BM 20 and WM 22, BM 22 and WM 20 already discussed in relation to the intralocal comparison above. To affirm that one has no pleasurable memory need not imply that one has only bad memories, and the converse: it may mean indifference, inhibition or inadvertence. The consciousness (or lack of it) implied in saying one has no good memory (BM 22) must by no means extend to the logical conclusion that one has only bad memories (WM 20), but may take for granted or find it superfluous to mention that all memories are bad. There is a degree of stupefaction which can produce just this result. Not improbably this is what our findings actually reflect in Marvdasht. Where the differences are most strikingly significant with $p < 0.1\ \%$, namely between the illiterate women of Shiraz and Marvdasht, we find substantiation for this view: in both BM 22 (no good memory) and WM 22 (no bad memory) the women of Marvdasht far surpass their urban sisters. That the like holds for the literate male children is less surprising and apparently paradoxical, for the city boys probably experience more in both respects than the boys of the villages.

Nevertheless the Marvdashti do not lead among the non-responders either in regard to good or bad memories (BM and WM 23). The Khuzestani adults of both sexes, very markedly however the Qashqai women, surpass them, as again the often curt Qashqai women do their tribal cousins of Qalandari. The circumstance was noticeable in the field and may have conduced to missing diagnoses in the Qashqai. In the city it is the men, on the other hand, who significantly oftener report no memory both intralocally and as against the males of Marvdasht, Khuzestan (BM only) and the Qashqai (tendency in BM only). Between the Shirazi women and those of Marvdasht there is no significant difference, but the Shirazis are more communicative than the Khuzestanis and very much more than the Qashqai in regard to both happy and unhappy recollections. This might well be not so much a local peculiarity as a reaction to the field workers in Shiraz – mainly girls, with whom the women were ready and often glad to chat, the men on the whole probably more reserved and prone to take refuge in "no recollection". It would be difficult, however, to bring confirmation for this. The trends in Khuzestan, where the interrogators were all male, seem at first sight to do so when we look at the women's answers to BM 4 and 5, but we see the same trend in the comparison between Marvdasht and Qalandari. In Marvdasht there were roughly equal numbers of field workers of both sexes, in Qalandari again mostly girls who had also worked in Shiraz.

We now attempt to summarize the interlocal or environmental differences in the same way as we have the intralocal. Here "urban" is taken to mean Shiraz, "rural" the village clusters of Marvdasht and Khuzestan together with the village of Qalandari, "nomad" the still truly nomadic Qashqai sub-tribe. Many comparisons hold only for discrete sub-populations such as one or the other sex, the illiterate or literate, etc., as will be indicated appropriately:

Environmental Differences

Best Memories		*Worst Memories*	
Rural more than Urban			
BM 20	females: "Always", i.e. no ill memory	WM 6	females: Bereavement
WM 22	No bad memory	WM 13	females: Financial difficulties, poverty, debt
Rural more than Nomad			
BM 11	females: Family weddings, feasts	WM 9	males: Own illness
Urban more than Rural			
BM 5	Pregnancy and childbirth	WM 9	females: Own illness
BM 11	illiterate: Family weddings, feasts	WM 11	females: Fear of animals or situations; phobia
BM 12	male: Activity, achievement, success in work	WM 14	Material loss, bankruptcy
BM 14	female and literate male children: Travel, excursion, holiday, repose	WM 15	males: Unemployment
BM 15	Pilgrimage, religion		
Urban more than Nomad			
BM 5	females: Pregnancy and childbirth	WM 7	Loss of own child
BM 10	females: Reunion with relatives or friends	WM 9	Own illness
BM 11	females: Family weddings, feasts		
BM 15	Pilgrimage, religion		
Nomad more than Urban			
BM 8	males: Good health or recovery of near relatives or friends	WM 2	Ill treatment

Nomad more than Rural

BM 5	females: Pregnancy and childbirth	WM 2	Ill treatment
		WM 14	Material loss, bankruptcy
BM 25	males: Good harvest	WM 25	Ill harvest

The summary tabulation makes glaringly evident what was said already: that very few categories of memories indeed are characteristic for any one of the environmental groups as a whole. For the good memories there are only four (BM 5, 11, 15, WM 22) for the bad ones five (WM 2, 7, 9, 14, 25), and frequently these too must suffer a restriction. All others are applicable, when they exhibit significant differences, usually only to one sex, sometimes only to the illiterate. Sweeping pronunciations (or attempts to make them) about differences between urban, rural and nomadic populations thus must be taken with a great deal of caution, nor can any social psychiatrist or anthropologist look in this direction for an easy job. When we strive to condense the findings still more into words for a more fluent, coherent presentation we must keep the sex and other differentials constantly in mind.

In the *villages,* the bases of Iran from which we took our start, we encounter in both sexes more than elsewhere the assertion that they have no ill memory. This is reinforced by the women, who more frequently add the positive corroborative assertion that they have been "always" happy. How much this corresponds to fact is an open question. The village women enjoy more by their own statement family festivals and suffer more under bereavement and poverty, the men under their own illnesses.

The *urban* of both sexes like the nomad women cherish pregnancy and childbirth high among their happiest memories, and the illiterate urban of both sexes join the rural women in their pleasure in family festivities. Both sexes in the city likewise recall pilgrimage etc. as their happiest memory more often than in the villages or the nomad encampments. The city women emphasize reunion with their relatives and friends and take pleasure together with the literate boys in travel and the like. For the city men activity and achievement count. On the negative side the city people without distinction of sex mention as their worst memories oftener than elsewhere their own illnesses and loss of children, the men unemployment, both sexes material loss and bankruptcy more than the villagers, but the nomads still more than these.

Outstanding among the *nomads* is the recollection in both sexes of ill treatment and ill harvest, while such mention of good harvest is confined to the men. These too display a significant difference against the urban males: they more often recall the good health or recovery of a relative or friend as their best memory. Pregnancy and childbirth are apparently dearer or more memorable to the nomadic than the village women.

Particular interest has been directed to the effects of more or less voluntary settlement on hitherto nomadic, still tribally organized people, which we have had a rare opportunity to study. Therefore the differences between the nomadic Qashqai and Qalandari are to be compared by themselves and Qalandari is to be treated separately from the other villages. We note at once that for the nomads good and ill harvest both play an outstanding role and refer to what has been remarked already concerning the drought that had visited the nomads for the last three years before the survey. This as well as suffering at the hands of robbers and the military accounts for the significant excess of "other pleasurable memories" BM 21 over the village for both sexes, for when we investigate these other memories we find that they are almost uniformally recollections of good, well-to-do or even wealthy times. The nomad women are reticent about their sufferings and losses and more often give no response (WM 23) when asked for their worst memory, the nature of which can be inferred easily enough. From the same set of dire circumstances one can account for the tendency of the men to complain more of material loss, which they had indeed sustained, but also to mention oftener as their best memory the good health or recovery of relatives (BM 8), not a few of whom had been wounded in desert skirmishes and outright military attacks. The demonstrable significant differences thus seem more due to hopefully transient oppressive causes than to basic environmental factors such as we had hoped to identify, important though such causes certainly are.

The already sedentary Qashqai are much more concerned with family and domestic affairs such as memories of childhood (BM 1), engagement and marriage (BM 4, women only), pregnancy and childbirth (BM 5, both sexes), bereavement (WM 6), among the women loss of child (WM 7), own illness (WM 9) and other bad memories (WM 21). Though the difference for the last is significant at the 5 % level, it rests on the narrow margin of 4 to 1, and therefore its importance should not be exaggerated. The four "other" bad memories are "family life", "life with the tribe", "right now" and "death of my seven year old child" erroneously scored for WM 7.

Differences Between Nomadic and Settled Qashqai[1]
("Qashquai" and Village of Qalandari)

Best Memories		*Worst Memories*	
Nomadic more than Settled			
(BM 8)	males: Good health or recovery of relatives	(WM 14)	males: Material loss, bankruptcy
BM 21	Other pleasurable memories	WM 23	females: No response
BM 25	males: Good harvest	WM 25	males: Ill harvest
Settled more than Nomadic			
BM 1	Childhood, youth, life with parents	WM 6	Bereavement
(BM 4)	females: Engagement and marriage	(WM 7)	females: Loss of own child
BM 5	Pregnancy and childbirth	(WM 9)	females: Own illness
BM 14	females: Travel, excursion, holiday, repose	WM 21	females: Other bad memories
		(BM 22)	males: No pleasurable memory

d. Belief in Magic. Belief in magic shall be discussed in this chapter together with best and worst memories as a normal phenomenon of everyday life, neither a complaint nor a symptom such as constitute the matter of the next. The query "Have you ever been

[1] Parentheses show that the difference amounts statistically only to a tendency, i.e. 10 % > p > 5 %.

put under a spell?" (Q 12) implied such a belief and was reinforced in practice with other words (jadoo, jambelat, جادو ، جمبلت) that spoke expressly of such. This form of question was chosen in order to narrow positive responses down to subjects holding a fairly concrete belief, whereas a form that implied only superstition would have invited a vast number of nebulous, equivocal and hardly meaningful positive answers.

Aware from experience that the number of such would not be large and that the few positive responses from children would almost inevitably reflect the beliefs and customs of their parents, we let the age distinction fall. On the other hand we wished to investigate the influence of literacy and education, in Shiraz also that of socio-economic status. Table C II 14 is therefore drawn up somewhat differently from preceding tables.

Table C II 14. Affirmations of Belief in Magic (Q 12)

	Male			Female			
	ill.	lit.	ill. + lit.	ill.	lit.	ill. + lit.	All
	Absolute Numbers[a]						
Shiraz	10	12	22	15	6	21	43
Poor	8	6	14	10	2	12	26
Middle class	2	4	6	5	3	8	14
Well to-do	0	2	2	0	1	1	3
Marvdasht	19	5	24	36	1	37	61
Khuzestan	5	3	8	5	1	6	14
Qalandari	0	0	0	2	0	2	2
Qashqai	3	0	3	13	0	13	16
	Percent						
Shiraz	8.5	3.4	4.7	8.5	2.1	4.5	4.6
Poor	9.5	4.6	6.5	9.0	1.8	5.4	5.9
Middle class	6.7	2.5	3.2	8.2	2.4	4.3	3.7
Well-to-do	0	3.1	3.0	0	1.8	1.7	2.4
Marvdasht	11.5	5.2	9.0	15.9	10.0	15.7	12.0
Khuzestan	2.6	0	3.1	2.3	16.7	2.7	2.9
Qalandari	0	0	0	4.3	0	3.1	1.4
Qashqai	7.0	0	3.1	14.4	0	14.1	8.5

Differences in Locality

	Male	Female	Both sexes
Shiraz : Khuzestan			›››
Shiraz : Marvdasht	‹‹	‹‹‹	‹‹
Shiraz : Qalandari	›		››
Shiraz : Qashqai		‹‹	›››
Marvdasht : Khuzestan	››	›››	›››
Marvdasht : Qalandari	››	››	›››
Marvdasht : Qashqai	›		(›)
Khuzestan : Qalandari	(›)		
Khuzestan : Qashqai		‹‹‹	‹‹‹
Qashqai : Qalandari	(›)	›	››

The only significant sex differences found were in Marvdasht with m ‹ f and among the Qashqai with m ‹‹ f.

[a]Affirmations only. Data for populations from which percentages have been derived are to be found in the respective chapters of Part B and in Table D III 1.

Shiraz city does not have the lowest rate of belief in magic, as one might perhaps expect from an urban environment where more people and especially more girls go to school, but stands neatly in the middle, as do the Shirazi women, while the Shirazi men even occupy the second highest place, though considerably behind Marvdasht. This village leads as a whole and for both sexes separately – as a whole by a wide margin, in respect to the women by a narrow one over the Qashqai, in respect to the men again by a fairly wide one over Shiraz as mentioned. The Qashqai men display a substantial and highly significant difference to the Qashqai women, the latter being the second highest among their sex, the former the second lowest and exactly equal to the men of Khuzestan. In Marvdasht too the sex difference is significant, but less so; elsewhere it is not. Khuzestan and Qalandari are low throughout, Qalandari having the lowest rate as a whole and for the men. Here a demonstrable difference between the nomadic and settled tribal people emerges.

All illiterate groups have higher rates of belief in magic than the literate with two exceptions. These are the well-to-do male Shirazis and the Khuzestani women, but the exceptions are obvious artefacts of very small numbers and therefore negligible. When we take into account the socio-economic classes in the city also a quite clear and consistent pattern appears: literacy, freedom from poverty and to some extent urbanism are correlated with diminished belief in magic and probably also in superstition generally. In the city we also observe a stronger effect of literacy in reducing belief in magic among the women (2.1 % for the literate women) than among the men (3.4 % belief), while the illiterate of both sexes have the same rate of 8.5 %. The difference is most striking between the poor illiterate (9.0 %) and literate (1.8 %) urban women.

Those who wish to know more about the forms that spells, magic and folklore take in Iran can be referred to the charming book of Bess Allen Donaldson, *The Wild Rue* [62].

2. Psychiatric Questionnaire

a. Method. There are not a few psychiatric questionnaires of both open and closed type, some well developed and widely used. They have been reviewed up to 1972 by Mombour [154]. Their main advantage, inclusiveness, is at the same time their disadvantage for surveys such as ours in which the time expendable per person was sharply limited on the one hand by our desire to collect information on both normal psychology and psychopathology, on the other by available resources. In other words, any of the better questionnaires, as far as our knowledge went or still goes, would have occupied the total time that we could devote to a subject or even more, and while it might have given us a fairly good or even better indication of psychic disorder, much other information that we regarded as essential, especially for a first study within a given cultural frame such as ours, would have had to go by the board. Moreover we had already chosen instruments for the gathering of such information that were at the same time powerful indicators of mental disorder and had added some other less powerful ones as well such as lay examiners' judgments and information from third persons. The usefulness of imported questionnaires is diminished further by the inherent difficulty of translation into the precise shade of meaning intended to be conveyed and by the typical Middle Eastern subject's rebelliousness against long rows of formal (not conversational), usually alternative questions. The Middle East does not recognize the principle of the excluded middle. Nevertheless, we felt that some more direct approach to possible psychopathology, something intermediate between the test findings and the psychiactric examination that could be performed only in a minority of cases, was needed.

The result was a questionnaire created deductively rather than inductively and pragmatically, intended neither as a test nor as a quantitative instrument, though in certain respect it is capable of quantification. It may well be one of the shortest on record, for it comprises only nine psychiatric and neuropsychiatric questions, to which three other items were added for different reasons. Each of the nine questions aimed at a target symptom of a major psychiatric disorder or group of disorders, which together encompass if not all, at least a very large part of the whole field of psychiatry. The full list reads:

Question	*Target*
1. Have you ever been paralyzed?	Paralysis of every sort, especially poliomyelitis, traumata and post-ictal conditions
2. Have you ever had (epileptic) fits?	Epilepsy, but also hysterical attacks, syncope etc.
3. Have you ever had an illness during which you had pains in your head and slept a long time?	Meningitis and meningo-encephalitis, both relatively common
4. What would you say are the things you have enjoyed most in your life so far (your best memory)?	
5. What are the things you feel have given you the most trouble or difficulty in your life so far (your worst memory)?	
6. Have you ever been so depressed that you could not work?	Serious depression of every kind, primarily endogenous
7. Have you ever been so excited that you could not work?	Mania, other states of excitation or exaltation
8. Have you ever been very afraid without knowing why?	Every kind of non-reactive anxiety state
9. Have you ever felt that most people were trying to harm you?	Paranoic conditions, paranoid schizophrenia
10. Have you ever felt that the world had become strange and different?	Schizophrenic alteration, but also depersonalization etc.
11. Have you ever heard voices of people talking to you that were not really there?	Acoustic hallucinations, mainly paranoid schizophrenic
12. Have you ever been put under a spell?	

The psychiatric questions were written in English, then translated by Mr. Ordoobadi and submitted to a number of our Persian colleagues and friends until all agreed that translation had been invested with as much simplicity, including unambiguity and closeness to popular speech, including dialect variations in Fars and Khuzestan, as might well be attainable. Inclusion of the qualification "that you could not work" superficially contradicts objections raised on p. 14 against the WHO Expert Committee's proposed criteria for a "case". The answer demanded here, however, is immediate and subjective, and its very subjectivity may tell more about the experience of the disease and thus about the specifically psychiatric disease itself than an questionably objective clarification would do. It seemed the one way to distinguish in the form of a simple question between trivial depressions and exultations such as we all experience and presumably more serious troubles.

The order of the questions is not arbitrary. It begins with one of the simplest, most easily answered and least disquieting and continues with two more also rather simple neurological inquiries that the subject recognizes as medical and to which, in our experience, he almost always replies without hesitation. The next two enter the subjective sphere, but by way of normal, universal life experience. Question 6 also appeals to common experience and to the tone of melancholy that pervades so much of Iranian life, religion and art and that may assist to form a bond of sympathy between the questioner and the questioned. The succeeding questions 7 to 11 probe ever deeper into the pathological, cause more wonderment, probably also anxiety and are less commonly answered in the affirmative, often hardly comprehended except by the unfortunates to whose lot the experience has fallen. Indeed, instant comprehension with affirmation of Questions 8–11 possesses some indicative value in itself. False positives, as we had expected, were common to all the neuropsychiatric and psychiatric questions. No affirmative answer by itself, unsupported by additional questioning or other evidence, was taken as proof of anything. Affirmations were regarded simply as indications for further inquiry, which the examiner should undertake if possible himself. If he could or did not, if comprehension failed him, if the replies elicited were inconclusive or insufficient to establish an illness or its lack and also its real nature among a variety of possibilities, the case was one for individual clinical examination. Usually the false positives could be sifted out quickly, leaving a solid residue of truly pathological cases, some of which hardly could have been identified by the other means employed. As this extremely compressed questionnaire generally did not require more than a couple of minutes, we felt that its inclusion was richly justified and have retained it unchanged throughout.

The questions are listed again in abbreviated form in Tables C II 15–17, where a key word is used to denote both the question and its target. In the following we shall refer to the questions mostly by these key words or by their numbers and prefix a Q to the number.

An overview of the positive responses to each question is given in Table C II 16. For each group, male and female, adults (≥ 15 years) and children (6–14 years), the frequency and percentage of positive answers only are recorded. For any question or group there would usually be a few who for one or another reason did not reply, who by oversight were not questioned, or whose answers were either not recorded or recorded unintelligibly. As they never amounted to more than 2–3 %, their answers were treated as negative. This has especial relevance for children of lower school age, who naturally did not comprehend most of the questions from Q 6 on and in interviewing whom the examiners were accorded discretion to omit such questions as the child obviously could not understand (information relevant to Q 1–3 was sought from the family). Only a positive affirmation could have meaning in the comparisons we were trying to make, wherefore we felt justified in regarding a non-affirmation, the inability to make an affirmation or a negation as equivalent to a negative response. Questions usually were taken by the subjects in a much wider sense than intended by the psychiatrist: a circumstance that we had anticipated. This implies that the undifferentiated affirmative or negative responses are crude indicators. Small numerical differences between group percentages tell little. The measures of statistical significance are the same as in the preceding chapter and thus automatically take account of small numbers. As in that chapter we counsel against placing excessive faith even in statistically "significant" differences when such rest on few cases or on narrow margins.

The authors and their readers will remain aware throughout that positive responses themselves comprise broad ranges of meaning and intensity, and that even when they are offered to quite precise questions (e.g. "have you ever had (epileptic) fits?") they are not to be regarded literally and are not to be accepted without further interrogation and, if possible, confirmation. This is far more the case, naturally, with less precise questions such as Q 10. Is there then any justification in grouping together and summing such heterogeneous, though uniformly positive answers at all? We hold that there is when this is done and deductions are made with the requisite caution. The mere count demonstrates the great number of false positives and shows beside that such were given very much more frequently to some queries than to others. Those responded to very often in the affirmative, in numbers far exceeding the frequency of the corresponding true psychiatric cases, touch upon common woes. The affirmative responses articulate these, and their number tells us something, albeit in a very rough way, about the number of persons ready to do so. How many more may labor under the same woes but do not voice them even upon questioning we have hardly any means of ascertaining. Even with this important reservation, which must never be forgotten, the numbers and proportions of affirmative answers become interesting and to some extent informative when they are compared to each other in different groups and where the comparison exhibits substantial differences. These may lie between the rural and urban populations as a whole, between the sexes as a whole or between them in one or the other area, or the relations may be still more complicated, as we shall see. We encounter, in any case, differential reactions to questions touching upon wide fields of human experience and emotions, the extremes of which lie within the territory of psychopathology. Because of this, and because certain tentative conclusions suggest themselves after a study of these reactions, we find it justified and rewarding to consider them in more detail. We shall not attempt, on the other hand, to specify how many of the affirmative responses were "true", as this task, except perhaps for Q 1 and 2, would have required a detailed analysis of the fifteen hundred cases for which we had neither the time nor, in some instances, sufficient information.

b. Intra- and Interlocal Comparisons. The basic data for the five surveys are presented in Tables C II 15 and C II 16, both in absolute numbers (above) and percentages (below). The base for calculating percentages is the number of subjects in a column, e.g. male adults in Shiraz. Since a person could reply affirmatively to more than one question and often did, the sum of the percentages per column is usually more than 100.

Table C II 15. Affirmative Response to Items from Psychiatric Questionnaire by Sex and Age Group: Shiraz, Marvdasht and Khuzestan

	Shiraz				Marvdasht				Khuzestan			
	Adults		Children		Adults		Children		Adults		Children	
	m	f	m	f	m	f	m	f	m	f	m	f
	Absolute Numbers											
Q 1 Paralysis	32	38	6	7	18	21	5	2	11	7	2	1
Q 2 Fits	19	21	7	3	18	21	4	3	17	9	3	4
Q 3 Headache	111	127	48	43	32	46	13	8	46	59	19	18
Q 6 Depression	182	263	31	44	114	136	22	15	58	55	16	7
Q 7 Excitement	96	125	59	76	48	45	34	14	25	29	15	9
Q 8 Anxiety	133	220	32	39	70	99	20	12	25	20	18	18
Q 9 Suspicion	41	69	13	15	56	74	9	9	8	12	3	5
Q 10 Estrangement	32	45	16	15	36	52	17	8	6	5	0	0
Q 11 Voices	63	69	30	32	41	64	20	7	23	8	8	2
Subjects	317	313	154	155	170	177	96	64	160	151	101	70
all males	471				266				261			
all females	468				241				221			
both sexes	939				507				482			
	Percent											
Q 1 Paralysis	10.1	12.1	3.9	4.5	10.6	11.9	5.2	3.1	6.9	4.6	2.0	1.4
Q 2 Fits	6.0	6.7	4.5	1.9	10.6	11.9	4.2	4.7	10.6	6.0	3.0	5.7
Q 3 Headache	35.0	40.6	31.2	27.7	18.8	26.0	13.6	12.5	28.8	39.1	18.9	25.7
Q 6 Depression	57.4	84.0	20.1	28.4	67.1	76.8	22.9	23.4	36.2	36.4	15.8	10.0
Q 7 Excitement	30.3	39.9	38.3	49.0	28.2	25.4	35.4	21.8	15.6	19.2	14.9	12.9
Q 8 Anxiety	41.6	70.3	20.8	25.2	41.2	55.9	20.8	18.8	15.6	13.2	17.8	25.7
Q 9 Suspicion	12.9	22.0	8.4	9.7	32.9	41.8	9.4	14.1	5.0	8.0	3.0	7.1
Q 10 Estrangement	10.1	14.4	10.4	9.7	21.2	29.4	17.7	12.5	3.8	3.3	0	0
Q 11 Voices	19.9	22.0	19.5	20.6	24.1	36.2	20.8	10.9	14.4	5.3	7.9	2.8
of population	33.8	33.3	16.4	16.5	33.5	34.9	18.9	12.7	33.2	31.3	21.9	14.5
all males	50.1				52.5				54.1			
all females	49.9				47.5				45.9			

The percentages "of population" in the third line from the bottom, however, state what percentage of a total survey population was constituted by the members of the column in question, e.g. the percentage of adult males out of the entire survey population of Shiraz. They are to be read horizontally and do tally to approximately 100 %.

Comparisons are carried out in the same way as for the best and worst memories, but now without regard to literacy or illiteracy, as the employment of this criterion in foregoing trials yielded little information. When sub-populations are formed only by age and sex as here throughout, the tables can be drawn up uniformly, are more condensed and easier to read. First intra- then interlocal comparisons by significant differences are carried out and shown in Tables C II 15–17 as in the chapter before. In discussing them we shall proceed somewhat differently and shall not, at first, take question by question. Certain generalities emerge almost at a glance and present so few exceptions that it is more convenient to remark those first and discuss the exceptions later.

Wherever statistically significant differences can be demonstrated, adults nearly always give more positive responses than children of both sexes except in regard to Q 7

Table C II 16. Affirmative Responses to Items from Psychiatric Questionnaire by Sex and Age Group: Qalandari and Qashqai

	Qalandari Adults m	Qalandari Adults f	Qalandari Children m	Qalandari Children f	Qashqai Adults m	Qashqai Adults f	Qashqai Children m	Qashqai Children f
	Absolute Numbers							
Q 1 Paralysis	2	2	2	0	1	6	0	2
Q 2 Fits	4	2	2	1	0	10	0	1
Q 3 Headache	9	18	4	3	6	19	1	1
Q 6 Depression	23	23	3	0	17	39	4	8
Q 7 Excitement	11	14	14	8	7	24	3	7
Q 8 Anxiety	5	13	2	1	17	26	2	3
Q 9 Suspicion	11	8	1	1	12	24	1	2
Q 10 Estrangement	5	7	3	0	8	18	1	2
Q 11 Voices	6	4	2	1	3	14	1	2
Subjects	44	43	35	22	47	66	50	26
all males		79				97		
all females		65				92		
both sexes		144				189		
	Percent							
Q 1 Paralysis	4.5	4.6	5.7	0	2.1	9.1	0	7.7
Q 2 Fits	9.1	4.6	5.7	4.5	0	15.2	0	3.8
Q 3 Headache	20.4	41.9	11.4	13.6	12.8	28.8	2.0	3.8
Q 6 Depression	52.3	53.5	8.6	0	36.2	59.1	8.0	30.8
Q 7 Excitement	25.0	32.6	40.0	36.4	14.9	36.4	6.0	26.9
Q 8 Anxiety	11.4	30.2	5.7	4.5	36.2	39.4	4.0	11.5
Q 9 Suspicion	25.0	18.6	2.8	4.5	25.5	36.4	2.0	7.7
Q 10 Estrangement	11.4	16.3	8.6	0	17.0	27.3	2.0	7.7
Q 11 Voices	13.6	9.3	5.7	4.5	6.4	21.2	2.0	7.7
of population	30.6	29.8	24.3	15.3	24.9	34.9	26.5	13.7
all males		54.9				51.3		
all females		45.1				48.7		

"excitement". The children of both sexes affirm this more than the adults of the corresponding sexes in Shiraz, and in Qalandari the boys display a tendency to do so more than the men. When we look at the children's literal answers they turn out to be harmless indeed and account with no trouble for the excess. The vast majority are of the type of "bursting with joy", "so happy I didn't know what to do", "trembling with excitement" etc. on the occasion of a visit, a feast, a trip, a present, a promotion in school and the like, with no taint of the pathological. Conversely there were others that referred to fear of animals, robbers and marauders, occasionally to threats of punishment and thus likewise fell into a normal range. They overlapped of course with other questions, especially Q 8, but we took them as they came without reassigning them. The children's excess is most noticeable in the city, where it holds for both sexes, and implies in all likelihood not that the city children are more excitable, but that the adults are more restrained. On the other hand there are more and more variegated events in the city to stir excitement than in often monotonous rural life outside.

Sex differences too are quite obvious and general. The women and girls give more positive answers to the psychiatric questions than the men and boys, and where

Table C II 17. All Surveys. Significance of Differences in Frequency of Affirmative Responses to Items from Psychiatric Questionnaire by Sex and Age Groups Interlocally Compared

	Shiraz: Marvdasht				Shiraz: Khuzestan				Shiraz: Qalandari				Shiraz: Qashqai				Qashqai: Qalandari			
	Adults		Children		Adults		Children		Adults		Children		Adults		Children		Adults		Children	
	m	f	m	f	m	f	m	f	m	f	m	f	m	f	m	f	m	f	m	f
Q 1 Paralysis						››				(›)			›		(›)				‹	(›)
Q 2 Fits	‹	‹			‹			‹					›	‹‹	(›)		‹	›	‹	
Q 3 Headache	›››	››	››	››	(›)		›		›		›	(›)	››	›	›››	››		(‹)	‹	
Q 6 Depression	‹	›			›››	›››		››		›››	›	››	››	›››	›		(‹)			››
Q 7 Excitement		››		›››	››	›››	›››	›››					›		›››	›			‹‹‹	
Q 8 Anxiety		››			›››	›››			›››	›››	›	›		›››	››	(›)	››			
Q 9 Suspicion	‹‹‹	‹‹‹			››	›››	(›)		‹				‹‹	‹‹	(›)			›		
Q 10 Estrangement	‹‹	‹‹‹	(›)		››	››	››	››				(›)	(‹)	‹‹	›			(›)		(›)
Q 11 Voices		‹‹		›	(›)	›››	››	››		›	›	›	›		››	(›)		›		

	Marvdasht: Khuzestan				Marvdasht: Qalandari				Marvdasht: Qashqai				Khuzestan: Qalandari				Khuzestan: Qashqai			
	Adults		Children		Adults		Children		Adults		Children		Adults		Children		Adults		Children	
	m	f	m	f	m	f	m	f	m	f	m	f	m	f	m	f	m	f	m	f
Q 1 Paralysis		››				(›)			›		›									(‹)
Q 2 Fits		›				(›)			››		(›)						››	(‹)		
Q 3 Headache	‹	‹‹		‹		‹					›						›	(›)	››	››
Q 6 Depression	›››	›››		›	›	››	›	››	›››	››	›		‹	‹		(›)		‹‹	(›)	‹‹
Q 7 Excitement	››	(›)	››	(›)				(‹)	›	‹	›››		(‹)	‹	‹‹	‹‹		‹‹	(›)	‹
Q 8 Anxiety	›››	›››			››	››	›	(›)		›	››			‹‹	›	›	‹‹	‹‹‹	››	›
Q 9 Suspicion	›››	›››	›	(›)		››					›		‹‹‹	‹			‹‹‹	‹‹‹		
Q 10 Estrangement	›››	›››	›››	››	(›)	›	(›)	›			››		‹	‹‹	‹‹		‹‹	‹‹‹	(‹)	‹‹
Q 11 Voices	››	›››	››	›	(›)	››	›		››	›	››						(›)	‹‹	(›)	

exceptions can be noted they rise above a tendency only in two cases out of seven. One case concerns again Q 7 "excitement". The boys in Marvdasht assert this more often than the girls although, if any sobering effect of the school be postulated, they were mostly subject to it and the girls were not. We are at loss for an explanation. The other significant difference, now at the 1 % level, is for the Khuzestani men to hear voices more than the women. The boys there show a like tendency over the girls. This time the explanation is not far to seek. A number of men and of boys also spent long lonely days on the Khuzestani plain herding their flocks, and it is in just this situation of relative isolation, monotony and potential brooding that the guardian angel calls. The men of Marvdasht were less so occupied, as far as our observation goes, and more often in sight of a village or at least a neighbor. Qalandari shows a similar numerical tendency, but it does not reach statistical significance. We should expect to encounter it among the nomads but do not, probably because the women, as we have seen in the last chapter, are rather markedly superstitious in every respect and thus equally or more likely to hear "voices" than their menfolk. The same may apply to Marvdasht, where also twice as many women as men claim to hear voices, though the difference does not reach the level of a statistical "tendency". Other such tendencies will be commented upon, where comment is possible, in considering the respective questions.

Some generalities are apparent when we look at the interlocal comparisons in Table C II 17. The most obvious of these concern the city of Shiraz, which is compared in the first four upper main columns with the villages and the nomads. In this upper half of the table the quotas of affirmative responses are usually greater in the city than in the other populations. For all four subdivisions of each population (men, women, boys, girls) they are larger, wherever a significant difference or a statistical trend above the 10 % level can be demonstrated, in four of the nine questions (Q 1, 3, 7, 8) and with a singular exception (the Shirazi men) in Q 6. For Q 2 "fits" most of the chevrons, of which there are not many in these four main columns, point in the other direction, i.e. to a greater prevalence of convulsive disorders in non-urban environments. The Qashqai men and boys constitute an exception in this respect, to which we shall return below. The relationships in Q 9 "suspicion" and Q 10 "estrangement" are so similar that they can be considered together. With the rather striking exception of the Khuzestani the villagers and nomads testify to feelings of suspicion and estrangement more than the cityfolk (though the Qashqai boys do not and the Khuzestani girls show no significant difference). Well may these two sentiments go together, as evidently do those of depression and anxiety and of excitement also.

Among the villages an even more inclusive generalization is possible in regard to Marvdasht. In eight of the nine questions its inhabitants yielded higher rates of affirmation, as far as the differences are significant, than those of Khuzestan and Qalandari, and in six of the nine higher than the Qashqai. In Q 3 "headache" the converse is true except for the Qashqai boys. As already mentioned, the Marvdasht adults in addition surpass those of Shiraz in respect to Q 9 and Q 10. Glancing back to their memories in the foregoing chapter we find indications that the Marvdashti in many respects are more troubled than the other non-urban populations. These: Khuzestan, Qalandari and the Qashqai nomads require separate consideration.

Before we begin with this, it is possible to gain a brief and comprehensive overview by tabulating the mean number of affirmative responses to all nine psychiatric questions per person for each population or survey and for certain sub-populations.

Table C II 18. All Surveys. Mean Number per Person of Affirmative Responses to Items from Psychiatric Questionnaire

	Adults		Children		All
	m	f	m	f	
Shiraz	2.2	3.1	1.6	1.8	2.3
Marvdasht	2.5	3.2	1.5	1.2	2.4
Khuzestan (total)	1.4	1.4	0.8	0.9	1.2
Well and Unremarkable	1.0	1.0	0.6	0.8	0.9
Remarkable	2.0	1.2	1.0	1.0	1.4
Pathological	3.0	2.1	1.5	1.8	2.2
Qalandari	1.6	2.1	0.9	0.6	1.4
Qashqai	1.5	2.7	0.3	1.1	1.5

For the sake of facility we may call this a complaint score, though remaining aware that not every positive answer, such as an affirmation of over-excitement out of sheer joy, constituted a complaint. The vast majority did, nonetheless, and their mean sum furnishes a convenient, though crude index of just those uneasy sentiments we enumerated above. This is *not* a symptom score, as should be evident, and thus *not* an index of psychopathology, rather an indication of subjective emotional appraisal as far as the subjects were ready to disclose this. Since it is a rough index, the figures are given in Table C II 18 to one decimal only. They are presented for surveys as wholes with the exception of Khuzestan, at which site alone we carried out the differentiation between not two, but three grades of deviation from the norm with a class of the "remarkable" between the unpathological and the outright pathological. Their pattern turned out to be so coherent and illuminating that we have refrained from calculating statistical measures of dispersion and significance.

Adults register more complaints than children, as is natural, and women more than men except in Khuzestan, where the rate for adults of both sexes is the same and for the "remarkable" and pathological men higher than for the corresponding female groups. It is noteworthy that this sex difference does not obtain among the children and youth. The differences for children are now in favor of the one, now of the other sex and are slight with the exception this time of the Qashqai nomads, where the girls score 1.1 and the boys only 0.3. The greater distress of the female sex in Iran begins evidently at adolescence, or at least not before. In Khuzestan the score rises in all four sub-populations from the well via the remarkable to the pathological: a surprise to no one, but rather a confirmation of the usefulness of the complaint score, rough measure though it is. In total scores Marvdasht leads, and Shiraz takes second place by a narrow margin. After a wide gap of 0.8 units follow the Qashqai, Qalandari and lastly Khuzestan with no great differences between them. The order for the women is the same and for the men nearly so, with Qalandari and the Qashqai exchanging places. For both boys and girls Shiraz takes the top place over Marvdasht, though again by a narrow margin only. Thereafter the boys follow their fathers in ranking order (i.e. Qalandari, Qashqai, Khuzestan), while the girls deviate somewhat, their rank order from highest to lowest score being: Shiraz, Marvdasht, Qashqai, Khuzestan, Qalandari. They constitute the only sub-population for which Khuzestan is not lowest in rank. Slight shifts, usually by about 0.1, probably do not mean much. It is apparent, though, that the five surveys fall into two distinct categories with a sizeable and by no means negligible difference between them. Marvdasht and Shiraz compose a category with high complaint scores, the other three sites a category with low ones, and the differences between members of one or the other category tend to remain small. In respect to BM 4, engagement and marriage, we have seen already that Shiraz and Marvdasht go together inasmuch as both sexes at these two sites significantly less often mention this as their happiest memory than elsewhere. Whether there is any true relation between these parallel findings we have no means of saying. The easy but specious explanation that a paucity of marital joys conducts to a multitude of complaints leaves too many other possible factors uncontrolled.

Finally we compare again the still nomadic and the sedentary Qashqai populations. In the fifth upper main column of Table C II 17 it strikes the eye immediately that the valid differences for children all have opposite signs for the two sexes. The Qalandari boys give higher ratings for Q 1, 2 and 3 and a very much higher one for Q 7 than the Qashqai. The first three have in common that they are physical or psychosomatic complaints. In the adults' replies to Q 2 the men of Qalandari likewise surpass those of the Qashqai, whereas between the women of the two groups the difference is reversed just as the children's differences are (though these are not paired except for Q 1). The large difference for the boys on Q 7 has been remarked above and a tentative explanation for it has been offered which applies more to the city. The second hypothesis developed there may hold in this case too, for the folk of Qalandari live in houses that are not larger than the usual poorer city dwelling, while the nomadic Qashqai live in tents, implying that lively youngsters can vent their excitement more easily and above all with less annoyance to the rest of the family. The excess of the Qalandari boys and to some extent the men in "somatic" complaints calls for an explanation. One can be proposed here very tentatively, for which support can be adduced in the next chapter from the Z Test results. It can be safely assumed that the great majority of positive answers to Q 1, 2 and 3 reflect psychosomatic disorders and only a small but important minority true neurological illnesses. A further commonly made assumption, of which we shall have more to say later, is that psychosomatic disorders involve deep or twofold repression. The people of Qalandari have adopted consciously a new and hitherto foreign way of life, to which they steadfastly adhere. It seems not unlikely here that a certain amount of repression evolves out of this, is indeed a necessary condition and becomes an unconscious family pattern passed from fathers to their sons. Why should this not apply to the girls also? We suspect that they, or rather their mothers, are less deeply affected by this transition, as their basic tasks remain much the same, while at the same time they become less subject to suspicion and feelings of estrangement in the securer village than in the exposed camp. The predominance of anxiety among the male nomads has been mentioned above: they have good reason for it! So too do the Qashqai girls for their higher rate of depressive responses: they have lost, or seen suffer, too many members of their families. The boys have also, but the hypothesis of repression could also account for the lack of difference here.

c. Comparisons of Responses to Single Questions. We turn now to the several questions and discuss, where possible and meaningful, the exceptions already noted.

Q 1: Paralysis. The principal intention was to identify cases with paralysis or paresis that was real in the neurological sense, or that had existed at some time in the past and might contribute a clue to an illness that had left psychiatric residues and could be elicited by further interrogation. The question did fulfill this expectation as well as harvesting a crop of false positives that could be referred to a wide variety of causes such as injuries, rheumatic and arthritic pains with temporary impairment of use of the member, ulcera crurum, periarthritis humero-scapularis, abscesses and so on up to conversion symptoms and beyond to ordinary numbness and "going to sleep" of the limbs. Usually little additional questioning was needed to put the matter straight, and often the proband's own formulation proved that his affirmation was false in the sense stated above.

Sex differences do not appear directly within the intralocal comparisons except in the Qashqai, where the girls dominate significantly and the women tend to do so. Adults dominate over children, and a sex difference manifests itself indirectly inasmuch as the local differences in most pairs of sites apply to the women and girls rather than to the boys and men. The converse is true when we compare Shiraz and Marvdasht with the Qashqai among whom by themselves, as we have seen, the females lead. The explanation for these exceptions remains obscure, while the other trends fit into the observed general pattern.

Q 2: Fits. Though the Persian formulation connoted specifically epileptic fits, there was hardly any kind of episodic illness that did not occur among the positive answers. Simple dizziness and faints led the list, followed by increasingly serious circulatory disorders, gastric and diabetic crises, sunstroke, etc. Several hysterics of course affirmed. So too presumably did all our verified cases of epilepsy, though one questionnaire was lost.

Sex and age differences conform to the expected trends with the exceptions already noted that the Shirazi boys and the Khuzestani men tended, but only tended, to assert they had fits more often than the girls and women. It seems pointless to indulge in speculations about these minimal reversals. Our few cases of true epilepsy afford no basis for them. As we have observed above, the interlocal comparisons point to a greater prevalence of positive replies to Q 2 outside the city rather than within it, as in the majority of other psychiatric questions, and with the exception of the Qashqai men and boys. Marvdasht again leads over the other surveys, the adult male Khuzestani over those of the Qashqai. These might be herdsmen subject to dizziness and sunstroke under the blazing sun of the Khuzestani plain. For the reversed difference between Shiraz and Marvdasht another explanation suggests itself. Adults of both sexes in Marvdasht report "fits" about twice as often as do the adults in the city. Since "fits" carry such a wide connotation and are basically generalized phenomena affecting the whole body (special instances such as Jacksonian attacks can be disregarded), one might refer this to a tendency toward generalized neurasthenic complaints in the country as against one to more localized hypochondric symptoms in the city, which we shall meet when we come to discuss the reactive disorders in Part D.

Q 3: Headache. The keyword is too inclusive. The precise phrasing of the question ("Have you ever had an illness during which you had pains in your head and slept a long time?") was intended to make it apply to the meningo-encephalitic illnesses so common in Iran, the sequelae of which not too seldom are a pseudo-psychopathy. The qualification "slept a long time" tended to be ignored. The most trivial headache often received mention, but on the other hand the question elicited besides the expected post-encephalitic and post-typhoid conditions a number of cases of migraine and thus was highly useful despite the large number of false positives. The inevitable pursuit of questioning led to the discovery of other chronic and residual states as well.

The now familiar pattern of age, sex and local distribution is fulfilled with the notable exception that Marvdasht lagged behind the other non-urban surveys instead of leading them, and with the secondary exception of the Marvdasht boys, who complained more of "headache" than the Qashqais. All four sub-populations in Khuzestan remark this complaint more than their Qashqai counterparts, the nomad women and boys less also than in Qalandari. The same explanation for the relatively high prevalence in Khuzestan may be proposed here as for the often concomitant "fits": the extreme heat in Khuzestan, bedeviled moreover in summer by daylong scorching winds and sandstorms that sweep unhindered from the Persian Gulf over the plain until checked by the south flanks of the Zagros Mountains. All Fars is hot in summer too, but the difference must be experienced to be appreciated, as it is by the wealthy of Saudi Arabia and the Gulf States who took up their "cool" summer residences in Shiraz long before air conditioning was invented. Climatic conditions cannot be invoked to account for the difference between Shiraz and Marvdasht. Exposure to the hot sun is surely more prevalent among the farmers, who on the whole also live under poorer hygienic conditions and thus might have more reason for somatically caused headaches and infectious diseases of the nervous system, as they actually do exhibit proportionally more organic residual states. As we shall see later, though, the prevalence rates for hypochondria and conversion hysteria are much higher in the city, and in the city also we meet with tension headaches among the men that are practically absent in the villages. The presumed psychological reasons for this will be discussed in connection with the general pathological findings. We suspect that they operate to cause the difference just mentioned. This leaves us with secondary, rather small differences between the boys (significant) and women (tendency) of the Qashqai and Qalandari for which we cannot readily account.

Q 6: depression leads us into the field of psychiatry proper, though clearly not every positive answer to it denotes a depression of psychiatric proportion. Yet the abundance of positive responses to this question among adults is greater than to any other question of the nine and must give food for reflection. Everywhere the differences between adults and children are high, and their significances are seldom lower than 1 %. Truism though it be that childhood is mostly cheerful and the cares of life begin to weigh with age, it is not without interest to observe to what a ponderous degree this is confirmed by the replies to such a simple question. A more detailed analysis by smaller age classes probably would be even more revealing but cannot be carried out here.

The expected sex differential likewise appears throughout with the exception of the children in Qalandari, where the boys have a tendency to respond positively more often than the girls. Other exceptions occur in the interlocal comparisons. They follow the usual order except for the city men, who less often affirm depression than those in Marvdasht (the women more). Marvdasht once more tops all the villages, and the nomad women and girls complain of depression quite significantly more than those of Khuzestan. The Qashqai girls too have more to say about this than the girls in Qalandari, and the Qashqai women show a numerical trend in the same direction that does not reach statistical significance. In comparison with Khuzestan both the nomadic Qashqais and the adult settled ones of Qalandari register depression significantly more often. On the whole, if we risk generalizing somewhat, it does not appear that city life reduces the frequency of depressive complaints, but perhaps rather augments them, while the pattern in the villages is mixed and the people of Qashqai stock stand somewhere between the rural extremes.

Q 7: Excitement. The converse of pathological depression is manic excitation, and this was one of the targets at which the present question was directed. Pathological excitation, however, can arise from many causes and assume a variety of forms. We hoped to and did obtain information about them through this query and also about many others that must be reckoned, as the high percentages of positive responses show, to the normal scale of psychological states and reactions. The limiting clause: "Have you ever been so . . . . that you could not work?" was heeded as little by the respondents as in the case of depression or else interpreted liberally as applying to any minimal subjective impairment of performance. Despite this liberality a fairly consistent pattern of responses emerges.

Shiraz again leads wherever significant differences can be demonstrated, and the level of significance is high throughout. Females lead over males where a sex difference is found except among the children of Marvdasht. This village leads again over Khuzestan and the male Qashqai, but the Qashqai women and the girls of Qalandari (tendency only) both remark excitement more often. The excitation level of Khuzestan is low by this criterion. Between the Qashqai and Qalandari we find a difference, but a highly significant one, only in relation to the boys, whose quota in Qalandari is much higher. This could lend support to those who claim that urban life is generally, in an unfavorable sense, more "exciting" and disquieting. If the boys of Qalandari seem to stand out as a peculiarly "excitable" lot by affirming Q 7 in some 40 %, it must be observed that other sub-populations come close to this (e.g. Shiraz and Marvdasht boys and Qashqai women) or even exceed it (Shirazi girls with 49 %), but that the numbers in these or their paired sub-populations are too small to allow statistically significant differences to emerge.

Returning to the excess of the children of both sexes in the city, one is hardly surprised to observe that children are more excitable (if this is what the affirmative response really measures) than adults, but wonders why only the urban children appear to be so. If we assume tentatively that rural life on the whole may be psychologically more tranquil, why is there no statistically demonstrable difference between the adults and the children such as we encounter in the town (in Qalandari, to be sure, we observe a tendency for the boys to surpass their fathers, but no more)? One explanation has been offered: that several of the children's groups are small, but this does not hold everywhere. Another might lie in the circumstance that the transition from childhood to adulthood is sharper, more critical for many urban children, particularly for those who attend school. Most of the village children grew gradually into their adult roles and did not even assume them fully upon their early marriage, after which they commonly remained for some time under the tutelage of the enlarged family. Thus the already lower rate of overt excitability was subject to no very keen attrition such as the transition from schoolchild to candidate for employment might exercise upon the urban youth. The transition was sobering, for at that time there was unemployment in Shiraz and no assurance of a job, whereas the village youth nearly always could work along with his family and be sure of at least a meager sustenance which all shared alike. Still another explanation is hardly less probable. Nearly all the poor and most of the lower middle class in Shiraz live in close, sometimes cramped quarters, sleeping several to a room, in which any manifestation of excitement affects the others more than it does in the village. Living quarters there may be just as cramped, but motor excitement, noise, temper and the like can be vented better into the open countryside. Since parents and relatives not seldom answered the questions for the younger children, the higher rate of positive answers for the city may equally well reflect the adults' own tension, annoyance and excitability. The very friction engendered by enforced proximity in city life, especially in the densely populated poorer districts, may operate to raise the share of positive answers.

Q 8: Anxiety. It is the psychiatrist's sometimes infelicitous province to investigate almost exclusively the negative affects, and of these depression and anxiety are by far the most common, as both everyday experience and the answers to the questionnaire confirm. Half or more of the adults in Shiraz and Marvdasht admitted to an anxiety that was by definition causeless, though their replies in very many cases pointed directly to the cause, which a little interrogation soon elicited from most of the rest. Free floating anxiety, at which the question was aimed, seldom appeared, although it did so enough to lead us several times to a true anxiety neurosis.

If half the adults in Shiraz and Marvdasht confessed to a disturbing anxiety, it was less than a quarter of the children who did so, and the difference applies to other surveys as well. Where one can be confirmed statistically, the adults of both sexes show more anxiety with the one exception of the Khuzestani women. Their daughters, by our figures, are significantly more anxious (28 % as against 13 % positive replies, $p < 5\ \%$). Wherever sex differences can be shown statistically to be significant (and this is not everywhere) women confess to more anxiety than men, but no such difference can be demonstrated anywhere between boys and girls: a circumstance that should give food for reflection. We have mentioned already that there is a great discrepancy between adults and children in Shiraz and Marvdasht and must add that these two sites boast an emphatic, sorry supremacy over the others in this respect, Shiraz also over Marvdasht for the women, and that not only does the general rate for anxiety fall off in Khuzestan, Qalandari and to some extent among the Qashqai, but that the age gradient also tends to diminish. The adult Qashqai of both sexes and the women of Qalandari have more to say about anxiety than the corresponding classes in Khuzestan, which in the case of the Qashqai is easily explainable by their actual situation and in the Qalandari women perhaps by their recollection of it, and the like doubtless applies to the decided predominance of the Qashqai men over those of Qalandari. The nomad men were still directly exposed to a multitude of dangers that gave them good ground for anxiety. So were the people of Marvdasht as compared with the Khuzestani, to whom the Development Area with its many activities and improved means of access afforded some protection.

Q 9: Suspicion. With the formulation: "Have you ever felt that most people were trying to harm you?" we strove to and did obtain indications of paranoic and paranoid conditions, but of much else as well. Affirmation was afforded by a host of subjects who could not even remotely be considered paranoic in the psychiatric sense. This word having been misused and misunderstood a good deal through its irresponsible application to non-psychiatric cases and even to whole cultures, we take as our heading the ordinary term "suspicion". "Distrust" might have served as well.

The pattern of differences is similar to that of Q 8. It reflects the common experience that children are less given to suspicion and distrust than their parents. An unquestionable sex difference again manifests itself only in Shiraz and Marvdasht, but a numerical difference in the same direction is to be found between the men and women of Khuzestan and the Qashqai. It is reversed in Qalandari, but by no very great number and is remote from significance. Where they differ demonstrably, the women more often admit suspicion than the men. As in Q 8 there is nowhere a significant difference between girls and boys. Here lies food for more reflection. If the adult woman's greater share of anxiety may be rooted in a perception of her lesser physical powers, which up to adolescence may match those of the male, no such explanation can be advanced to account for her larger share of suspicion albeit indirectly. The weaker in a robust, little mechanized culture must fear the stronger, learn anxiety and from anxiety suspicion.

The interlocal comparisons present a rather different picture, however, from Q 8. The city does not lead over the country except for Khuzestan. Marvdasht surpasses all the rest by a wide margin, but the Qashqai adults and the men of Qalandari also surpass the Shirazi. The adults of Qalandari and the Qashqai both admit to feelings of suspicion much more than those of Khuzestan. Between the two groups from the Qashqai tribe there is only a minor difference in that the nomad women present more testimony of suspicion than the women of the new village. The children show few interlocal differences, and even these do not rise above tendencies except again in regard to Marvdasht boys. This fits not at all into storybook depictions of trustful countryfolk and wary urbanites. The striking absence of substantial differences either intra- or interlocal between the children of both sexes can be taken, if one is so inclined, nevertheless as a Wordsworthian hint of a certain common innocence or trustfulness of the young. They become disabused of this in different degrees according to sex and situation, as we have seen. Why more so in the village, which Wordsworth and his contemporaries also were pleased to imagine as innocent? A tentative answer is easy to offer. Life in the village is compacter as regards both relatives and neighbors. Everyone peers into everybody else's cooking pots (we are thinking here of the highly suspicious womankind), above all the omnipresent mother-in-law under whose wings or claws the village bride so often lives. The net of picayune intrigue is closer meshed. The city provides more channels of escape on the one hand and perhaps of objective rectification on the other, though the second point may be debated. We do not have enough pathological subjects with paranoid trends to illuminate the conjectures we have advanced. The high rank of Marvdasht in regard to suspicion may be referred to the special circumstances obtaining when we surveyed it. Land reform had been promulgated and was being carried out, while everybody was keen to obtain a few more sqare meters than his neighbor and to get as much out of the dispossessed and nearly always distrusted landlord as he could contrive. Suspicion was naturally rife. As these problems and sources of contention had been more or less solved for several years before we progressed to Khuzestan, it seems equally unsurprising that suspicion rated lowest there. It is superfluous to repeat what has been said about the Qashqai and Qalandari.

Q 10: Estrangement. The question "Have you ever felt that the world had become strange and different?" could encompass a great many things. At the center of our target lay, a minute bullseye, the typically schizophrenic apprehension of a generally threatening or malevolent alteration of the universe that A. E. Housman's forlorn lines suggest better than any textbook can describe:

> "I, a stranger and afraid
> In a world I never made".

We could not expect enough schizophrenics in our samples to justify the inclusion of the question on this ground alone. Concentrically around it, so to speak, lay nevertheless circles of depersonalisation and, more peripherally, not consciously accountable shifts of mood such as everyone, but the organically damaged or neurotic patient more particularly, experiences. Patients' answers have led us to such cases.

A significant sex difference was to be found only in Shiraz and Marvdasht, the women outnumbering the men as in nearly all questions involving subjective states. As the numerical and percentual differences on the whole were not large this may be a statistical artefact referable to the larger populations in these two places. A sex difference in the children is suggested only once, the Qalandari boys tending to speak of estrangement somewhat more than the girls and thus, for reasons unclear to us, reversing the trend just mentioned. The age difference that holds for most of the psychiatric questions appears in respect to this one less regularly and convincingly and possesses on the whole a lower degree of statistical significance. It attains a confidence level of 1 % only in two places: the women of Marvdasht and the Qashqai men (the women also at the 5 % level to be sure) confess to estrangement more than the girls or the boys. Interlocally Marvdasht leads as in Q 9; one reflects that suspicion and estrangement are psychologically contiguous. Just as with Q 9 also, the Qashqai lead over the Shirazi, these over the Khuzestani, and between Shiraz and Qalandari there is hardly any difference. The Khuzestani seem least subject to estrangement in every category. The Qashqai women and girls show only a tendency to surpass those of Qalandari, and for the male sex there are no demonstrable differences between them.

The general sex and the specific local differences probably can be explained as before, especially with regard to Q 9, but the relative paucity and slight degree of age differences leaves us with a question. Could it be that children, on the whole less accustomed to analyze, differentiate and articulate their feelings, take refuge more readily in a positive reply to this apparently vague and widely encompassing question when they have need to express some deviant quality of emotivity? Or is the child, to whom the world is newer, simply more full of wonder?

Q 11: Voices. We had aimed only at the auditory hallucinations relatively common in psychosis with this question and were surprised at the number of affirmations it provoked, the more so as our first field experience was gained in Marvdasht, where a third of the grown women asserted they had heard a voice of someone who was not there. The great majority of affirmative answers reduced themselves quickly upon a little interrogation to the common illusions of mistaking some chance sound for a call or signal. Beside a few genuinely schizophrenic hallucinations there remained, nevertheless, a hard and more than negligible core of those who, as described in the introductory chapter, quietly and confidently insisted that they had heard their names called by their فرشته at night. The abundance of women just mentioned was reflected in a significant sex difference in Marvdasht and a less significant one among the Qashqai, but the direction of the difference was reversed in Khuzestan, this time also in the children. We have no doubt that this was due to the influence of the shepherd boys alone upon the plain and of their fathers also as we have described it above. It is to be noted also that the Marvdasht and Qashqai women gave by far the highest rates for belief in magic. Age differences do not appear uniformly and are really significant only for the Marvdasht females: the mothers claim to hear voices thrice as often as their daughters. Marvdasht as a whole is at the top of the list except for the girls. Those of

Shiraz report double their frequency, and the difference is significant at the 5 % level. Nevertheless, the Shirazi women stay substantially behind those of Marvdasht. This becomes plausible when we reflect that roughly half of the city women were literate, but in Marvdasht practically none. The correlation between literacy and freedom from superstition is clear from Table C II 14 of the foregoing chapter. We suspect that a like influence may be responsible for the significant differences between the Qashqai women on the one hand and those of Khuzestan and Qalandari on the other. In both the latter sites, to be sure, few women were literate, but they were more exposed to the influence of the schools and of their daughters, whereas the tent school of the Qashqais was very much a male affair. The fact that there are no significant differences between Khuzestan and Qalandari for Q 11 and no other between Qalandari and the Qashqai tends to confirm this. While there are fewer interlocal differences of significant magnitude in regard to Q 11, their distribution and direction generally agrees, where they do occur, with those for estrangement Q 10.

The similar differential patterns that emerge for suspicion, estrangement and the hearing of voices are probably neither superficial nor fortuitous. Suspicion and estrangement conduce to isolation whether psychological or physical, and isolation can lead, as clinical experience and experiments on sensory deprivation show, to quasi-hallucinatory experiences that may be referred to projection and to the need for re-establishing communication that is felt to be lost. The village women are either equally or more prone to hearing voices than the men except in Khuzestan, as they have been shown by their differential responses to most of our other questions from Q 6 onward to be more prone to other forms of intense emotional experience (they may also only be more prone to speak of such). The correlation with belief in magic is evident. This probably explains, as reference to the personal records confirms, the great majority of "voices", which are readily apparent as the common, banal illusions of everyday life, in no way pathological, but the more easily perceived and credited where superstition invites them. The "voices" of the desert, by which is meant in this case almost exclusively the bitterly inclement desert of Khuzestan, constitute a category more or less to themselves. The Khuzestani rate low in belief in magic, but their belief in the guardian angel is firm (though not peculiar to this province), and the greater isolation of their shepherd men and boys together with the extraordinary harshness of the climate does the rest. Perusal of our records makes this clear. The subject might reward a further study.

The hallucination of hearing one's name called is not confined to Iran by any means and just as little is it a proof of psychosis. In days of more leisurely psychiatry before the First World War Dr. Max Löwy in Prague devoted a monograph to it [126]. Analyzing 41 cases he found only ten referable to a psychosis (5 manic-depressive, 2 schizophrenic, 3 organic), but nine hysteric and another nine called "dyshumoral", the rest with a wide range of neurotic and psychosomatic complaints. Their common premise he found to consist in a state of inner disquiet (*Unruhe*) or tension such as normally follows upon hearing one's name called unexpectedly, but in these cases for various reasons preceded it. Women outnumbered men by about two to one as in Marvdasht, but not in Shiraz. Among the men 77 % were below 40, among the women 57 %. Löwy refers the difference in the age distribution to the greater exposure of the younger man in the struggle for existence. He gives no figures for juveniles or children.

3. The Z Test

a. Previous Studies with Tests of Personality in Iran. So far as we have been able to find, the first study on personality testing in Iran was published in 1958 by Klar [113], who spent six years as a physician in the country. Klar tried and rejected such graphic methods as the Wartegg Drawing Test and the Koch Tree Test because, as he rightly observes, "only a very few Persians were able to handle a pencil", the Rorschach Test as being too circumstantial, graphology because of the different character of the Arabic script and so settled upon the Lüscher Color Test in its short form, which appealed to all. As this test [130] is little known in the English speaking countries, it seems useful to quote (in translation) Klar's own succinct description. "In the Lüscher Short Test the subject is presented with two cards, the gray card and the 8 color card. On the gray card we find the following gray shades: black, dark gray, medium gray, light gray and white. One asks which is the most sympathetic 'color' and notes the sequence of these gray tones. Then one presents the 8 color card. Here the 4 primary colors blue, green, red and yellow are mixed among the colors violet, brown, medium gray and black. Again here one goes through them from the most to the least sympathetic color . . . According to Lüscher's color theory the choice of a color in first, second, etc. place up to the last possesses a quite specific meaning. The combination of colors, the first and second place, etc. is important for the evaluation especially the contrast between the most and least sympathetic colors, . . .". The choice of a shade of gray yields information about the subject's basic mood. On the 8 color card he experiences the differences betweeen the primary colors, mixed with four achromatic colors, all the more strongly. A marked sympathy for a color shows the direction of his claims and wishes, antipathy the direction of his frustrations; and out of the combinations a great deal can be read, according to Lüscher, about his personal conflicts and inter tensions.

Klar tested by this method one thousand adult male Persians and 140 Europeans living in Persia and found as a rule complementary sequences of choice in the two groups. On the gray card the first and last choices were exchanged: the Persians chose black first and light gray last, the Europeans in Persia exactly the opposite. On the 8 color card the Persians gave their first choice to green, the second to violet, while the Europeans preferred first blue, then gray (it must be remembered, though, what Klar does not mention, that green is the sacred color of Islam). Space forbids entering into the rather complicated details, which have little meaning apart from Lüscher's theory. They lead to a very different overall personality picture: an emphasis upon defensive self-withdrawal among the Persians combined with watchfulness for small advantages and opportunities for ingratiation while remaining essentially uninfluenceable; among the Europeans in Persia also withdrawal, but combined here with sudden outbursts of energy and action and with a deep craving for affective resonance and attachment. This condensation of Klar's differentiated findings represents a gross over-simplification. We have undertaken it because the author (probably rightly) offers no generalizing summary and because it seemed proper to point out that the Lüscher Color Test does respond to ethnic differences. Astonishingly enough, in one of the very few English-language studies on the Lüscher Test Braun and Bonta [46] quite recently have asserted that this fact in their opinion invalidates the test after they found differences between their American and Canadian, male and female subjects! The Lüscher Test has been subject to sharp criticism in Europe, but on more relevant grounds. When it is used in the Middle East, one would have to inquire whether the symbolic values of and psychological responses to colors are the same there as in Europe (as they probably, and in the case of green as mentioned above certainly, are not, and as we shall see in connection with the color responses to the Z Test in Iran below).

In 1959 Klar followed his first study by a second [114] on seventy opium addicts, administering the Lüscher Test before smoking and shortly afterwards, when the drug had taken effect. Under the influence of opium he found in his subjects evidence of what he calls a (temporary and drug-induced) *névrose de banalisation* in 83 %, but of *névroses conflictuelles* in only 43 %, while he emphasizes that the majority of his subjects under ordinary circumstances were not pathological at all.

In the same year and in the same paper already quoted in regard to intelligence testing Max Valentine [195] published results of personality testing with other methods. His first population was composed of 115 candidates for admission to the Medical Faculty of Shiraz University in 1957 and of 60 candidates for the Faculty of Agriculture. To these a Ranking Rorschach Test, the multiple choice version of Harrower-Erickson and Steiner [92] was given. The only data reported are comprised in a distribution histogram of total scores. Valentine comments succinctly: "The distribution, and the median scores, seem to resemble Western norms sufficiently to enable one to pay some attention to the results. It will be noted that the median scores (194 for the agricultural, 203 for the medical candidates: remark of the present authors) are lower than Eysenck's [73] findings, which were generally about 230. This could be interpreted as a tendency on the part of the students to show more neuroticism than corresponding Western groups" (loc. cit., p. 99). The same groups took a "Study of Values Test" devised by Vernon and Allport [197], exhibiting thereon strong theoretical and social interest with a "marked uniformity" in the results.

Over one hundred medical students filled out the Maudsley Medical Questionnaire [74] and the Character Trait (Self) Rating Scales of Goldman-Eisler [84]. Their mean score of 11.0 on the MMQ was slightly higher than Eysenck's published norm for an average British population, but very high when it was taken into consideration that they were a stringently selected group of young students in presumably good health and of superior intelligence. Valentine contrasts it with Eysenck's mean of 2.81 for a "supernormal group of officers". He enters into a rather detailed discussion of the findings on the MMQ and the Goldman-Eisler Rating Scale and summarizes as follows (loc. cit, p. 107): "Personality testing shows a tendency to uniformity of response. Students are gregarious, unaggressive and protective and show a trait resembling 'oral optimism' which elsewhere has been claimed to be related to prolonged suckling, but at adolescence these beneficent traits tend to be offset by frustrations and inhibitions due to other causes. In general there is more neuroticism than might be expected but it mainly takes the form of pre-occupation with feelings of humiliation, inferiority and sensitiveness, with adjustment difficulties in the field of relationship with power figures and authority-systems . . . In the general population a different type of neuroticism, with features of anxiety and hysteria, is found to be very common." The last sentence is an observation from Valentine's general experience, not a test finding. The foregoing sentences recall the contention of the first author's counterpart and friend, Dr. M. H. Sahebo'z-Zamani, that Adler's theory of neurosis was far more suitable for Iran than Freud's as the basic question and struggle throughout Iranian history and in contemporary Iranian society was that of power.

In the decade after Valentine's work research on personality testing in Iran seems to have stagnated. Then, in the years from 1970 to 1973, follows a burst of publications from a group of Shirazi psychologists headed by Mehryar. They are based on the same or closely similar large and probably representative populations of secondary school and university students in Shiraz which we have mentioned in connection with intelligence testing (cf. Part C, Chap. I 1) and therefore will not describe again here. One of the first was concerned with "Some Normative Data on a Persian Form of the New Junior Maudsley Inventory" [145] derived from a sample of 592 secondary school students, the majority of whom were between 13 and 15 years old. The results were, briefly, that the Iranian youths and maidens were much more introverted than their British and Canadian counterparts, more homogeneous in their test scores and showed at the most trifling sex differences. Neither did their neuroticism scores differ significantly from those reported by Western workers. (In this and other papers Mehryar and his colleagues discuss in some detail their findings on Eysenck's Lie Scale, but since its effectiveness and even its very meaning in Iran are not altogether clear and since we have no comparable data to offer we refrain from further reference to this.) The three psychological dimensions (extraversion, neuroticism, lying) showed practically no correlation with each other either among the juniors or among the college students whom Mehryar studied at the same time [138] with the Eysenck Personality Inventory (EPI). Male and female Iranian students were closely similar to each other and to Eysenck's normal group as a whole in regard to extraversion, but were significantly more extraverted than British students and also, by the Inventory, more neurotic. An Iranian patient group of 50 persons from a private mental hospital was both much less extraverted and much more neurotic than the group of Iranian students. After commenting on the correlation data Mehryar remarks (loc. cit., p. 259): "It would appear that, under the cultural circumstances represented by our subjects, the two dimensions of extraversion and neuroticism approach orthogonality much closer than they do in Britain or the U.S.A. It is of some interest that even though our mentally ill subjects tend to be highly introverted and neurotic, this overall trend is not accompanied by any correlations between the two variates."

In 1972 Mehryar followed up with a study on "Personality Patterns of Iranian Boys and Girls on Cattel's 16 Personality Factor Test" [55, 141] based on the same secondary school population as before. In the following quotations from Mehryar, the abbreviations for the factors are Cattel's. The former writes (loc. cit., p. 258 ff.): "Comparing the means of Iranian boys and girls, a number of differences are of interest. Iranian girls score higher than Iranian boys on factors A, I, M, O and Q. In other words, as compared with Iranian boys, Iranian girls of this sample would appear to be more outgoing and warm (A+), more tender-minded, sensitive and over-protected (I+), more imaginative and interested in arts (M+), more apprehensive and guilt-prone (O+), as well as more frustrated, tense and overwrought (Q_4+). Boys, on their part, score higher than girls on factors C, E, H and L. Thus Iranian boys . . . would appear to be less emotional (C+), more dominant (E+), more adventurous and uninhibited (H+), and somewhat more suspecting, jealous and hard to fool (L+). All these differences are statistically significant ($p < 0.05$)." The sexes were equal on the extraversion factor, but lower on this than comparable American groups. Comparing now raw scores for Iranians and Americans, "the Iranian boys of this study would emerge as the more intelligent (B+), conscientious (G+), suspicious (L+), shrewd

(N+) and controlled of the two groups. American boys, on the other hand, score higher than Iranian boys on factors E (Dominance), F (Surgency or liveliness), Q_2 (Self-sufficiency), Q_4 (Ergic tension) and, to a smaller extent, M (Bohemianism) . . . Iranian girls emerge as the more intelligent (B+), conscientious (G+), jealous (L+), shrewd (N+), apprehensive (O+) and controlled (Q_3+) of the two groups. American girls, on their part, surpass their Iranian counterparts in terms of being easy-going (A+), surgency (F+), social boldness (H+), tender-mindedness (I+) and tenseness (Q_4+). In view of the brevity and untested nature of the 16 PF intelligence scale (factor B), however, group differences in this respect may better be ignored." The first set of findings is, as Mehryar notes, "well in accord with the sex differences reported for many different parts of the world" and with the results of the EPI in Iran. The 16 PF differentiated among groups of boys following different courses of pre-academic specialization (mathematics, natural science, arts and letters) but not among the like feminine groups.

Finally, Mehryar and co-workers published in 1973 two papers partly replicating their previous studies with the EPI, but now including Eysenck's dimension of "Psychoticism" [77, 144]. The sample was larger, over one thousand, and according to the authors less selected. It emerged as both less extraverted and less neurotic, the girls being still less extraverted (i.e. more introverted) but more neurotic than the boys. Differences to Eysenck's British means were smaller except for the new dimensions of psychoticism, on which the Iranian groups scored considerably higher. The meaning of this is not clear, but Mehryar, quoting our own findings that mental disturbances among Iranian peasants and tribesmen were not scarcer on the whole than in Western Europe and reflecting that his sample was predominantly urban, inclines to refer it to "the known association between urbanism, social upheaval, and psychotic breakdown" [100, p. 204]. Under the specific conditions of the study the authors conclude that "the findings . . . seem to leave little doubt as to the relative efficacy of psychoticism as compared with both extraversion and neuroticism and parental education in differentiating between good and poor performers on intelligence and aptitude tests" [144, p. 7]. They do not, on the other hand, altogether support the negative relationship between psychoticism and social class as reported by Eysenck [78].

Working independently of Mehryar, Baraheni conducted a psychometric study of the Eysenck Personality Inventory using a sample of 165 female and 166 male undergraduate students of the University of Tehran, a further 66 students under treatment at Tehran University Counseling Center for various neurotic disorders and 50 schizophrenic patients from mental hospitals [13]. Statistical analysis showed normal distribution of the scores on the dimensions of extraversion and neuroticism, orthogonality of these two dimensions, high coefficients of reliability, moderate validity when the normal was tested against the combined pathological groups, but failure to discriminate between these. Referring now to the presumably "normal" student group only, its total neuroticism score was significantly lower than what Mehryar had found and not significantly higher than that of Eysenck's British students, while the sex differential in Mehryar's findings was confirmed (females higher on N). The Tehran students on the whole were significantly more extraverted than the British, but not more than the Shirazis. Both mentally disturbed groups were, as Mehryar had found, significantly less extraverted than the controls. There was no demonstrable sex difference on this dimension.

Okhowat et al. had published "An Investigation on the Diagnostic Value of the MMPI Short Form in Iran" in Persian in 1973 [162] and reported on this in English, as Baraheni had done, at the memorable International Symposium on Epidemiological Studies in Psychiatry convened by the World Psychiatric Association and the Psychiatric Society of Iran in 1974 in Tehran [163]. The short form of the MMPI contained 71 items. The subjects were 30 hospitalized male addicts, 42 hospitalized male schizophrenics and a control group of 35 normal individuals. Okhowat summarizes: "Significant differences in the mean values of all the clinical scales, K and F were found [as between addicts and non-addicts: the present authors]. . . . The result partially supported discriminability of the measure, schizophrenics scoring higher as Sc, Pa, Pd, Hy and Pt."

At the same symposium Nowparast and Tarighati [159] presented what, so far as we know, is the sole paper published by Iranian authors on the Rorschach Test in Iran (although Ordoobadi had been using it with exceptional skill for years in diagnosis and counseling in Shiraz). Their subjects were 145 Iranian college students (88 male and 57 female, not treated separately) who volunteered at the National University of Iran in Tehran and thus constituted, as the authors are careful to point out, a highly selected and by no means representative, though none the less interesting sample. Using Beck's scoring system [33] Nowparast and Tarighati present means, standard deviations, ranges, medians and O's for 23 scoring categories sufficiently represented and compare these with the means and SDs of Beck's American sample. Both in quantity and quality the means and SDs for the two groups were not strikingly different except for a few categories. These were, in the intellectual sphere:

1. W, of which the Iranians gave twice as many (11.71 ± 6.49 as against the Americans' 5.50 ± 3.76).
2. Z (Beck's "Organization") with a similar difference (Iranians 57.12 ± 33.37, Americans 22.48 ± 14.91).
3. A %, somewhat smaller in the Iranian group (41.58 ± 14.88, in the American 46.45 ± 13.12).
4. P: Iranians 8.44 ± 3.56, Americans 6.79 ± 2.41.

The authors believed that "independent of Z, such an excessive W association points to the fact that the sample is certainly escaping into abstraction as the means of intellectualizing the inferior aspects of the personality . . . A mean score of 41.58 for percent of A, even though lower than that found in Beck's sample, seems high enough to indicate a slightly cautious adaptivity. The sample appears to be clinging to the most familiar stimuli in the socio-cultural environment. The finding of a mean score of 8.44 for P variable seems to be consistent with such interpretation" (loc. cit., p. 266 ff.).

Turning to the affective sphere, it is only the kinesthetic sum that forms an exception to Beck's norms, but an outstanding one. Sum M among the Iranians is 8.01 ± 4.76, among the Americans 3.50 ± 3.24. Sum C with 2.42 ± 1.72 is only slightly lower than Beck's 3.11 ± 2.74. The extraordinarily high M score "indicates a rather active and dominant fantasy life for our sample. . . . As will be pointed out, it is probable that our group as a whole is highly productive in M due to its intense use of fantasy as a defensive mechanism. It is clear, however, that the population represented by our sample is more orientated toward an 'autistic living'", conclude the Iranian authors. They carry their analysis considerably further, but we refrain from a detailed discussion of it here because of the very special nature of the sample itself and our lack of any comparable one. After presenting our results we shall return to its most striking feature, the extraordinarily introversive experience balance, and shall discuss how far the measurements of introversion-extraversion by questionnaires and by projective techniques are comparable.

b. Method, Popular Responses, Scoring. Both for the exploration of personality in its many facets and for psychiatric diagnosis the Rorschach Test in the authors' experience is an unrivaled instrument. Here is not the place to discuss the criticisms, partly justified and partly specious, that have been leveled against it: we shall allow the facts, in this case the results, to speak for themselves. Our choice of a Rorschach derivative was determined, however, not only by long clinical experience and teaching, including disappointment with other tests advocated as replacements for the Rorschach, but by other considerations as well.

The Rorschach type of test, which uses accidental forms and has no right or wrong answers, is probably as little biased culturally as any test of personality in use or even less so than the rest. Beginning with the Bleulers' investigations in Morocco [40] there is a substantial body of literature, mostly reviewed in [124], which shows that the method can be applied transculturally with meaningful results. Our own preliminary trials with the Zulliger Test confirmed these. Interpretations, while not wholly free from subjectivity, are based principally on formal and structural criteria that can be and are judged by experienced workers with roughly the same margin of subjectivity that enters unavoidably into clinical medical findings. The laboratory and the computer cannot supplant these yet, though they may supplement them. While its administration by lay assistants presents some problems, they are not insurmountable.

The full Rorschach Test with ten cards demanded more time per person than we could afford, to say nothing of the time necessitated for its scoring and evaluation. Fortunately the deceased Hans Zulliger, editor of the parallel Behn-Rorschach series [208], had developed during World War II a three card inkblot test based on the same principles, which had already proven its worth [210–212]. In its first form it was composed of slides [209] and used as a group test for the selection of officer candidates in the Swiss Army. Later the three plates were published on cards like the Rorschach cards, to be used in the same fashion [212]. The group form has continued to find employment for personnel selection and the like, while the individual form has attained wide use in Swiss and other Central European psychiatric policlinics, counseling centers and elsewhere where time presses and a good short test of personality is needed. It accommodated itself excellently to our requirements for brevity, while our own experience, confirmed by such experts as W. Morgenthaler and M. Loosli-Usteri (personal communications) convinced us that the Zulliger Test, when used with the circumspection and care demanded by any micro-method, with its three cards yielded results only slightly inferior in reliability and fullness of detail to those from the Rorschach with its ten. F. Salomon's report of his favorable experience with the Zulliger Test as applied to North African Jewish children waiting in France for emigration to Israel [173], a cross-cultural usage similar to that which we intended, confirmed our decision to try it first, and as preliminary field trials showed an evident good differentiation both of intelligence and of personality the issue was settled. We have no reason to regret it.

In another sense also we arrived at the Rorschach or Zulliger Test by elimination. So-called "objective" tests of personality tend to be objective in scoring but in little else. The subjective implications of their seemingly so simple questions even in the cultural settings for which they are designed and in the language in which they are written are multifarious and become far more so in translation and in transplantation to other cultures. They are time-consuming even in their shorter forms. With their usual demands for clear-cut alternative answers they are completely foreign to Middle Eastern mentality and are apt to call forth confusion, refusal or perhaps most often superficial but meaningless compliance, the answers falling haphazardly. Sentence and picture completion tests are strongly culturally bound, present the same difficulties in translation and do not cover as wide a range of personality variables as the inkblot tests do. Others of the TAT or Four Picture type require redrawing and restandardization besides leaning heavily on content interpretation rather than on the more objective analysis of formal factors. For all these reasons a test of the Rorschach type seemed clearly more advantageous.

The test was administered according to the usual instructions and recorded in Persian for subsequent scoring by the authors or other competent persons. The instructions included measurement of initial time (from handing over a card to the subject's first response) in seconds, since the examiners were provided with stop watches for the block design test and because we hoped in this way to obtain more objective information on shocks, but these measurements were done on the whole rather erratically except in Khuzestan, where the authors were present at and personally supervised all testing, and are of somewhat dubious value. In interpretation we have relied mainly on other shock indicators to guide us. Examiners were required to use location sheets for every response that was not whole or could not be indicated unambiguously by some short standardized designation. At the end, they should describe the subject's test behavior in a couple of words. Questioning for determinants naturally was beyond their capacities.

Evaluation took place in two phases: for screening by rapid inspection by one or both of the two authors (except in Marvdasht, q.v.) and with an eye more to the pathological or non-pathological character of the test than to a precise diagnosis, and for statistical treatment at any time, extending up to years, thereafter. For formal scoring and statistics it was necessary to establish a new list of popular responses.

By Rorschach's classical definition [170, p. 189], to which Zulliger adheres, a response is scored as popular (abbreviated P) "when one meets it in about every third record," i.e. in about 33 % of all records. Rorschach introduced this category only in a paper written shortly before his untimely death, which his friend Oberholzer edited and published posthumously (included in [170] as *Zur Auswertung des Formdeutversuchs)*. From it 7 popular answers can be gleaned. In a later publication of his own, no doubt in agreement with Rorschach, Oberholzer [160] added several new Ps and appears to have discarded some of Rorschach's. He claims, and Bohm [41, p. 53] confirms, that there are only about 9 internationally recognized popular responses, "international" referring to European and Anglo-Saxon practice. In Bohm's own compilation of Rorschach's and Oberholzer's scorings in the same work he lists 16 Ps. Rorschach's original material, on which he based his *Psychodiagnostik,* was composed of 405 records, 117 of them from normal, the rest from pathological subjects. In an unpublished count of common responses in 210 Swiss records, all pathological, we found that only four met Rorschach's 33 % criterion. They were:

Card I	Butterfly, bat	44 %
Card III	Two human beings	41 %
Card V	Butterfly, bat	61 %
Card VIII	Two animals (lateral red)	78 %

The 7 most common responses were defined by a lower frequency limit of 16 %. Quoting M. Ford, Bohm [41, p. 52] remarks "that in the USA today one reckons with every sixth rather than with every third person."

In his original German publication Zulliger [208], probably following Rorschach, lists 6 popular responses. In the English translation [212], which Salomon has edited and to which he has added a number of comments and some material of his own, there occurs a seventh: the buffalo, steer or ox to the brown of Card II. Zulliger originally based his "List of Responses and Scores" upon a material of "1000 subjects of both sexes and the most various ages" [212, p. 31], which he increased to 8000 up to the end of 1961. Apart from mentioning that they included 300 applicants for jobs with the streetcar company of a large Swiss city and 60 police recruits, Zulliger provided no further numerical information. Salomon, emending Zulliger, comments in a footnote [212, p. 49 fn.): "The original list of responses has been greatly expanded. It now contains a number of responses based upon approximately 5000 tests administered to Frenchmen in Paris as well as some 1000 tests recorded in the U.S. The scoring of all these responses was discussed with Dr. Zulliger, both by correspondence and in person. It appeared quite clear that the scores obtained in the above-mentioned countries did not differ from those obtained in Switzerland. Even the popular responses proved to be the same." Yet, although Salomon mentions "extensive statistical research", neither of the authors gives any figures for the absolute or percentual frequencies or even for the rank orders of their popular responses at all.

The demand is frequently and justly made that "populars" must be standardized afresh for new populations outside the Anglo-European groups on which most investigations have been conducted and possibly even on sub-groups for the latter, but it has not been complied with too often, as far as we can gather from the available literature. Furthermore, the problem seems hardly to have been discussed with any thoroughness at all just where the re-determination of the populars should begin – with groups of what size, heterogeneity or presumed degree of difference from the Anglo-European, within which, as Salomon suggests and our own experience tends to confirm, a rather high degree of basic homogeneity as regards the Ps can be postulated. The tendency has not been to make age and sex distinctions. Should distinctions be made for groups of different ethnic origin in countries such as e.g. the United States and Switzerland? We do not know, and the frequent omission of such banal counting gives rise to reflections when reading treatises in which the Rorschach and Z Tests are subjected to elaborate statistical treatment. Be that as it may, our initial experiences in Iran convinced us that the Zulliger Ps could not simply be taken over. In our first paper on Z Test findings in Iran [27] we examined the tests of 482 Khuzestani peasants of both sexes and all ages from six years upward, the great majority illiterate, and discovered that of the seven most common responses only two corresponded to Zulliger's. More than that, Zulliger designates one of the less frequent Khuzestani Ps (Card I: human being or demon) as an original, i.e. a response found in less than one percent of all records!

It was therefore clearly necessary to determine our own list(s) of populars, and it seemed equally clear that we could not, at least without prior empirical inquiry, take the Khuzestani P list as representative for the Shiraz city dwellers, the majority of whom were literate and enjoyed upon the whole better socio-economic conditions besides being exposed to many more stimuli and experiences than the villagers. In order to keep the labor within manageable bounds we did accept the Khuzestani as representative for the Iranian rural population within the compass of our surveys and found grounds for doing so both in the inspection of the Z Tests themselves and in the comparison of the intelligence test results [28]. Stated more explicitly, separate P lists were not drawn up for the Marvdasht and Qashqai nomad groups.

We deliberated first whether we should draw a random sample of comparable size from the Shiraz psychiatric survey population, taking for example every other member of that population as we in fact did later for other purposes. Several considerations weighed against it. The structure of such a sample within a sample would have been only superficially similar to that of the Khuzestani population in that it would have been unselected (we recall that the Khuzestan survey was a census study). Since in Khuzestan and other rural areas the vast majority of subjects were both poor and illiterate, we wished to see whether the popular responses that the literate and better-off gave would be different, while on the other hand we were by no means confident that we could simply equate the urban with the rural illiterate and poor. We also wished to see whether differences would appear between children and youths (6 to 14 years) on the one hand and adults (from 15 upwards) on the other. Therefore we purposely drew the following samples from the city:

200 adults, non-poor
150 adults, poor
75 children, non-poor
75 children, poor.

In order to maximize possible environmental differences, the poor were all drawn from the densely populated and generally poor district in the traditional center of the city, the non-poor from the residential districts that contained their own, somewhat smaller quota of poor as well, but also a relatively larger proportion of medium or well-to-do households. With only these restrictions the samples were drawn at random without regard to sex or literacy under the presumption that these factors would be distributed within the samples approximately as they were within the strata or districts from which they were taken. For each of these four intra-urban samples the popular responses were determined separately with the results shown in Table C II 19. The populars are arranged for each sub-group in their order of frequency, the frequencies being given as percentages of all records in the respective sub-group. We retained Zulliger's standard of seven popular responses, which, as can be seen, corresponds by no intention to the standard of one in six quoted above. The four lists are nearly identical as to content and differ mainly in their respective orders of frequency, though these, too, often vary only by a rank or two and by a few percent. The range of frequencies is wide, from 83 % to 17 %. Among the poor adults two responses tied for last place with 17 % each, so both are listed. This is also the only group in our Shiraz material in which Card I appears with a popular response, reaching it by the narrowest of margins. On the basis of these findings we decided that we could indeed adopt a common set of popular responses for the Shiraz population.

Table C II 19. Popular Responses to Z Test in Four Shiraz Sub-groups[a] Arranged by Frequencies

	200 adults, non-poor		*150 adults, poor*		*75 children, non-poor*		*75 children, poor*	
1.	III Butterfly (central red)	83 %	III Butterfly (central red)	61 %	III Butterfly (central red)	81 %	III Butterfly (central red)	73 %
2.	III Human being (large black)	44 %	III Worm, snake, fish (small black)	41 %	III Human being (large black)	40 %	III Human being (large black)	36 %
3.	III Worm, snake, fish (small black)	43 %	II Qadruped (brown)	34 %	III Worm, snake, fish (small black)	33 %	II Insect (brown)	36 %
4.	II Insect (brown)	28 %	III Human being (large black)	29 %	II Tree, shrub (green)	33 %	III Worm, snake, fish (small black)	35 %
5.	III Quadruped (lateral red)	21 %	III Quadruped (lateral red)	26 %	II Insect (brown)	32 %	II Tree, shrub (green)	35 %
6.	III Human being (lateral red)	20 %	II Insect (brown)	24 %	II Quadruped (brown)	32 %	II Quadruped (brown)	29 %
7.	II Quadruped (brown)	19 %	II Tree, bush (green)	17 %	III Human being (lateral red)	17 %	III Human being (lateral red)	29 %
			I Human being	17 %				

[a] Roman numerals refer to Z Test cards.

Table C II 20. Popular Responses to Z Test in Four Geographical Areas

Shiraz (Bash)			Khuzestan (Bash)			Indonesia (v. d. Meulen)		Switzerland (Zulliger)	
Card I			*Card I*			*Card I*		*Card I*	
Whole			Whole			Whole		Whole	
0. (Human being)		(14 %)	7. Human being		12 %	6. Head (human or animal)	40 %	Insect	WF+ A
0. (Crab)		(12 %)						Crab	WF+ A
Card II			*Card II*			*Card II*		*Card II*	
Brown			Brown			Brown		Brown	
4. Quadruped	DFC+ A	27 %	1. Quadruped	DFC+ A	53 %	1. Quadruped	79 %	Buffalo, bull	DFC+ A
5. Insect	DFC+ A	27 %						Insect	DFC+ A
Green			Green			Green		Green	
7. Tree, bush	DFC+ Pl	20 %	3. Tree, bush	DFC+ Pl	20 %	—		—	
Central white			Central white			Central white		Central white	
—			—			5. Flower	45 %	—	
Card III			*Card III*			*Card III*		*Card III*	
Large black			Large black			Large black		Large black	
3. Human being	WM+ H	38 %	—			4. Human being	54 %	Human being	WM+ H
Central red			Central red			Central red		Central red	
1. Butterfly	DF+ A	75 %	4. Butterfly	DF+ A	17 %	2. Butterfly	71 %	Insect, moth	DF+ A
			5. Aeroplane	DF+ ObjM	17 %				
Lateral red			Lateral red			Lateral red		Lateral red	
0. (Human being)		(18 %)				3. Human being	61 %	Human being	DM+ H
6. Quadruped	DF+ A	22 %	6. Quadruped	DF+ A	15 %				
Small black			Small black			Small black		Small black	
2. Worm, snake, fish	DF+ A	40 %	2. Worm, snake, fish	DF+ A	33 %	7. Caterpillar	24 %	—	

[a] Explanation cf. text.

This list is shown under "Shiraz" in the first column ofTable C II 20, but the Ps are now arranged for readier reference by card rather than by frequency. In the second column follows our list from Khuzestan. The only comparable data for a non-Anglo-European population that we could find are van der Meulen's [119] from 433 Indonesians, whom he describes as mostly between 18 and 35 with at least three years of schooling. In the fourth column appear Zulliger's seven Swiss populars, confirmed by Salomon in France and the U.S.A., but without the regrettably missing information about frequency and rank order. The table is so arranged that like locations and like or very similar contents appear on the same horizontal line. Percentage frequencies are given at the right of each column, ranks within columns by arabic numerals on the left, in both cases excepting Column 4. Three responses that do not qualify as popular are included in Column 1 for comparison; they are enclosed in parentheses and are given rank of zero. Here we can observe how nearly the "human being" to Card 1, which did qualify as a P among the poor adults and in Khuzestan (though with an even lower percentage), comes to qualifying in the city as a whole.

Zulliger's scores for his own Ps are reproduced, omitting the self-evident "P" after the content. We have retained them for our own Ps as far as applicable. Zulliger and Salomon offer the alternative of pure form (F) or form-color (FC) for the "animal" or "insect" to the brown spots of Card II. This is altogether justifiable and desirable where records are taken and subjects are questioned by experts, but impracticable under survey conditions with lay field workers. Since the vast majority of the Iranian domestic and desert animals (including the innumerable curs) and insects are in fact brown or a grayish-brown, we have thought it a reasonable approximation to give the score FC uniformly, just as we have assumed, following Rorschach and Zulliger, that the "human being" to the large black spots of Card III represents a kinesthetic response. Evident exceptions such as "statues" etc. were allowed for in individual scoring (F instead of M), while the P was retained.

The brief denominations of content categories in the tables naturally represent generalizations. The "human beings" to Card I or to the large black spots of Card III could be and frequently were "spirits", "demons" (div, دیو), "negroes" and the like (scored MC when appropriate), as the "quadrupeds" covered almost any four-footed animal including Zulliger's "buffalo" (to be found in Switzerland only in zoological gardens, whereas in southern Iran water-buffalo are commonplace), "steer" and "ox", and the "insect" again almost any kind of similar creature as also the "worm", "snake" and in Card III the superficially similar "fish". Two contents require special comment and warn against all too ready generalization. One is the "aeroplane" or "jet" to the central red of Card III in Khuzestan – a local "popular" determined by the proximity of a military airfield to the villages under investigation and by the circumstance that they also lay on the commercial air traffic route between Tehran and the Gulf. More important and certainly not merely local is the central white area of Card II as "flower" in Indonesia, occurring in nearly half the records. Van der Meulen quotes Zulliger to the effect that "normally no attention at all is paid to the white space" (sc. in the red of Card II) and emphasizes this great difference between the Indonesian and the Swiss findings. Fundamentally we can only confirm him; although the "flower" response does not qualify as popular in Iran. On the other hand we find abundant, though contentually divergent responses to precisely this area as well as to its subdivisions, which van der Meulen also mentions. Only the diversity of content prevents it from becoming popular in Iran, where it is more often a "lamp" or "candle", sometimes also a "statue" and is not rarely combined with the surrounding red as e.g. "a figure (or candle) in a shrine" (not to be confused with the figures familiar in Catholic regions of Central and Southern Europe). Van der Meulen points out, in our experience altogether correctly, that such a white space or even a combined white space and blot interpretation as the initial response to Card II is not uncommon (22 % in Indonesia) and is to be interpreted as a rule as a masked color shock. The Indonesian and the Iranian findings agree here. A specialty of the Iranian records, on the other hand, is the "popularity" of the "tree" or "shrub", sometimes also "grass" to the green of Card II, found neither in Indonesia nor in Switzerland. One reason for this in a predominantly arid, desert country is obvious: green is not only optically obtrusive, but marks the presence of vital, life-giving water. Another, which reconciles one with the FC+, is that straggly shrubs not unlike the green spots of Card II in form do occur frequently along the almost dry water-courses. Greenery is moreover not a decorative attribute, but an essential precondition for a city, which accounts for the communality of the response between Shiraz and Khuzestan. At the edge of Shiraz the desert begins. The city can expand as far as irrigation reaches and no farther.

The following Tables C II 21 and C II 22 facilitate comparison of the number of popular responses common between various pairs of populations or sub-populations.

Table C II 21. Number of Common Popular Z Test Responses in Pairs of Populations

	Shiraz	Khuzestan	Indonesia
Khuzestan	5		
Indonesia	4	3	
Switzerland	4	2	4

Table C II 22. Number of Common Popular Z Test Responses in Pairs of Shiraz Sub-populations

	Adult, non-poor	Adult, poor	Children, non-poor
Adult, poor	6		
Children, non-poor	6	6	
Children, poor	6	6	7

The comparisons are only rough because no account is taken of the differences in rank and percentual frequency of the popular responses, but they show at a glance the much greater homogeneity of the Shiraz sub-populations as against the populations derived from Iran, Indonesia and Europe. They show also, not surprisingly, that Shiraz and Khuzestan have more in common than either does with a non-Iranian population, and that the greatest difference is found between an Iranian rural and a European, predominantly urban population.

Here is evidently no place for an introduction to projective tests in general or to the Rorschach and Z Tests in particular. The reader who is unfamiliar with them had best skip this section. For the rest we must mention a few particulars.

The tests were scored basically according to the classical Swiss system of Rorschach [41, 170] and Binder [41, 37]. We did not follow Zulliger in giving frequently several scores to one response. This has the advantage of lending greater depth and detail but is statistically manageable only with excessive difficulty. Rather have we tended in the other direction so that the sum of scores in each main category (approach, determinants, contents, figure-ground) should be the same as the number of responses and, where percentages are involved, should total 100 %. These necessitated some modifications in traditional scoring, which the first author has employed for many years in teaching the Rorschach and Z Tests. In order to keep the number of variables within a convenient and intelligible size, we have omitted some of the less common from the tables and have combined certain others, as presently shall be explained. We list below the variables to be found in our tables, adding explanations and comments as needful, giving first the signum or abbreviation for easy reference, then the full name.

1. T: total time in minutes from handing over the first card to end of the test. Initial time, though recorded, is not stated here. Measurement to seconds would have implied a spurious exactitude in a test of this kind administered by only partially skilled workers.
2. R: number of responses. Cf. above. As a rule each integral response received one score, but in certain cases combined responses were analyzed into their components and scored separately as in ordinary Rorschach practice. The R was then increased accordingly, not retained in spite of multiple scoring as with Zulliger.
3. W: whole response.
4. W+: well-seen whole response.
5. DW: detail-whole or confabulated (secondary) whole response.
6. D: detail response.
7. Dd: small detail response.
8. Do: oligophrenic detail.
9. S: white space detail, using the white or very light gray spaces only.
10. Sc: combinatory white space detail, using the white or light gray intermediary space together with the whole or a portion of the blot. This category has received quite a number of signa in different books, often together with a W, D or Dd. As it has nothing to do with size of the response, we have separated it from these confusing and inappropriate combinations and referred it exclusively to the figure-ground relationship. In the S, this is reversed, usually indicating unequivocally oppositional tendencies. The Sc is a compromise with all that this implies.
11. F: form response.
12. F+: well-seen form response.

13. f%: form percent or percentual share of the form determinant in the total of responses. It is *not* equal to ΣF/R and is not to be confused with the frequently used F+% = ΣF+/R, which can be computed very simply from the tables and therefore is not given here as a separate variable. It is the sum of all pure form responses (F) plus the weighted sums of all other responses in which the form determinant participates significantly, as will be explained in connection with the following variables, divided by R or the total number of responses. It shows what role the form determinant plays in the whole test performance of an individual as against the non-formal determinants (color, movement, shading) and thus affords a rough measure of general affectivity, to which it is inversely proportional. It says nothing about the acuity of form perception and interpretation, as does the F+%.

14. FC+: form-color response, well-seen. It is weighted with half a point for form and half a point for color, following Rorschach.

15. FC–: form-color, not well or sharply seen. Weighted as above.

16. CF: color-form response, weighted with one point for color and none for form.

17. C: pure color response, weighted with one and one-half points for color and minus one-half point for form.

18. MC: movement-color response, weighted with one-half point for kinesthesia and one-half point for color, none for form (though form, in fact, may enter into it to some extent).

19. SUM KINA: sum of all kinesthetic values. In this as in the following sums we deviate somewhat from ordinary Rorschach practice for comparative and statistical reasons. SUM KINA comprises, of course, all kinesthetic responses, weighted with one point for kinesthesia and none for form (though here too form may enter into them), again following Rorschach. To these are added, each with a weighted value of one-half a point for kinesthesia, the sums of the following, usually not very numerous categories: Small M or small movement responses (Rorschach's Bkl; here we follow Loosli-Usteri [129]), MC as above, also MChia or movement-chiaroscuro, but not animal or object movement. It will be noted that in our tables no sum M appears. Its function in measuring, or at least estimating, the role the kinesthetic determinant plays we believe to be better, more precisely fulfilled by SUM KINA than by sum M alone. In clinical Rorschach practice as well as in such field work as here we enter SUM KINA in the left side of the experience balance where ordinarily sum M appears.

20. SUM CHRO: sum of all chromatic values on the usual scale as Rorschach has described it and as we have taken it for a model above (item 19) and below (item 22). The unit is the CF response, corresponding to one chromatic point. FC receives one-half chromatic and one-half form point. C receives one and one-half chromatic points and minus one-half form point. One-half a chromatic point each is given to the MC and the ChiaC. Note that black and white, when used as colors, are counted among the chromatic responses. SUM CHRO forms the right side of the experience balance.

21. AV: attitudinal value. This is derived from the experience balance by dividing SUM KINA by SUM CHRO and taking the arcus tangentis of the quotient. This latter, an intermediate step in computation without intrinsic psychological value, may be called the experience quotient and abbreviated EQ. It eliminates the factor of dilatation or constriction of the experience balance and reduces this from a two-dimensional to a one-dimensional expression. Where the data for SUM KINA and SUM CHRO are not available, as in the vast majority of publications they are not, a

generally sufficient approximation may be obtained for the EQ and what follows by taking the customary sum M as the dividend and sum C as divisor.

The EQ being actually a tangent, all extratensive values in which SUM KINA < SUM CHRO lie between 0 and 1, all introversive values in which SUM KINA > SUM CHRO between 1 and 00. Its graph is curvilinear and approaches maximal introversive values asymptotically. The EQ is thus altogether unsuitable for scoring and must be transformed into a simple rectilinear function, an axis along which the steps are equal.

This is accomplished by taking the arc tan EQ = arc tan (SUM KINA: SUM CHRO), which can be read off easily from trigonometric tables or from any pocket computer with trigonometric functions and their inverses. The results are best given in degrees of arc from 0 to 90 (decimals or minutes of arc are nearly always superfluous just as in the case of intelligence quotients and are stated below in certain tables only for the sake of statistical comparison of fairly large groups). Introversive values are to be found between 90 and 45, extratensive values between 45 and 0 degrees of arc. Wholly extraversive, i.e. introversionless experience balances of the type O:X have AV = 0. Wholly introversive, i.e. extraversionless experience balances of the type X:0 have AV = 90. Ambiequality lies at AV 45. Since the steps are regular and equal, AVs can be compared with each other directly and can be grouped for statistical treatment as the customary experience balances cannot.

The theoretical notation by degrees of arc as hitherto exployed, which we shall designate by AV_t, is inconvenient, however, for ordinary use. Its value run from low to high in a direction counter to that of all customary scales of "extraversion" (introversion usually receiving no mention) on which low extraversive values are to be found at the left, high at the right. This is counter also to all Rorschach and related notation, in which introversive kinesthesias stand on the left of the experience balance, the extraversive chromatic colors on the right. Moreover, the examiner ordinarily is interested in how far the subject deviates from ambiequality and in order to find out this with AV_t notation has to perform some simple, but occasionally confusing mental arithmetic. We therefore introduce and employ wherever more suitable a practical notation (AV_p) which takes the point of ambiequality at $AV_t = 45$ as the reference point for a scale extending equally far, i.e. 45 degrees, in both directions and call this reference point A. Introversive values are then given by $AV_t - 45$ and receive a letter i to show in which direction they lie. Correspondingly, extratensive values are given by $45 - AV_t$ and receive a letter e. The extreme values 0 and 90 can be designated conveniently by the majuscules E (for one-sided extraversion) and I (for one-sided introversion). E and I stand equidistant from the point of ambiequality A. A few examples may serve:

AV_t	AV_p
0	= E
1	=44e
5	=40e
19	=26e
45	= A
53	= 8i
85	=40i
90	= I

The extreme values 0 and 90 or E and I confront us with a problem that carries, happily, a greater theoretical than practical weight. They indicate that the subject lies at one end or the other or a finite scale, but the scale is theoretically infinite and extends to both sides of the terminal marks. In the not uncommon introversionless experience balance O:X, X may assume any value, but the AV score will always be 0 or E. The converse hold for X:O, where the score can only be 90 or I. Theoretically again there is no limit to the number of movement or color responses a subject can give in the absence of the other determinant or even with it, though there are well known empirical boundaries. The AV cannot show how far an individual completely lacking in either introversion or extraversion (as far the test is concerned) goes over the edge. The extreme values can be treated statistically using the limiting or asymptotic values 0 and 90, but at first glance they seem to constitute a graver practical problem than they do in fact. A second glance shows that the same problem is inherent in all scales of extraversion based on questionnaires, etc, for they too are finite and have cut-off points sanctioned by statistical practice and custom. Once a subject has answered e.g. all Eysenck's 24 extraversion questions in the sense of extraversion, there is no way for him to demonstrate on the test that he is more or less extraversive than another who has also scored the maximum in extraversion, and conversely. The most seclusive introvert can do no more than deny all the questions that are supposed to reveal extraversion unless he rejects the test. Proponents of such scales nevertheless find them acceptable and useful, as we do the method of attitudinal values, which has the advantage over the scales that in the single case one can count the Ms and Cs. If the dimension of dilatation or coarctation or the experience balance, lost in the EQ and AV, needs to be recovered, this can be performed very simply and easily by adding SUM KINA and SUM CHRO. Even better seems to us the f% or, as preferred, 100-f%, which gives a measure of all the formal, or in its second form the non-formal, determinants and takes account of the shading as well as of the kinesthesia and color.

There remains one case that cannot be represented in the AV system: the absolutely constricted record with the experience balance 0:0. This is indeterminate. In a graph it corresponds simply to the point of origin and possesses no dimension. When working with clusters of AV it is therefore necessary to eliminate all records with absolutely constricted or coarctated experience balance, though other variables in these records naturally can be utilized as desired. This correction has been performed in all the following representations and is one of the main reasons why the number of cases or subjects within certain defined groups is not consistent throughout.

22. SUM CHIA: sum of all chiaroscuro values, composed in the same manner as SUM KINA and SUM CHRO. The unit is the ChiaF response, like the CF. FChia is treated like FC, and pure Chia like pure C. For MChia see above under item 19. The F(C) or shading response (Binder's F (Fb)) is given half a point for chiaroscuro and half a point for form.

The SUM CHIA does not enter into the AV, but it does enter into the f%, or rather into its complement for

$$f\% = \frac{R - (\text{SUM KINA} + \text{SUM CHRO} + \text{SUM CHIA})}{R} \times 100$$

23. P: popular response. Cf. above and Tables C II 19–20.

24. O+: good original response by Rorschach's definition. Their recognition, of course, requires considerable practice in the respective culture, which holds for the following as well.

25. O–: poor original response, cf. above.

26. H: human whole figure.

27. Hd: human detail.

28. A: animal whole figure.

29. Ad: animal detail.

30. Pl: plant, flower, bush, tree shrub.

While all the usual content categories occurred and were duly noted in the individual records, they have not been included in this statistical tabulation because of their generally small numbers. Plant responses, much more frequent than in Western protocols and attaining in Card II to the status of a P, had to be. We shall not try to enter into content analysis except in certain special cases.

Since our weighting of all determinants is not a part of common Rorschach practice, though it is only a logical extension of Rorschach's own way of handling color responses, and since lack of acquaintance sometimes makes it appear far more complicated than it really is, we adjoin a complete tabulation in Table C II 23 of all determinant scorings with their weights as distributed among the four determinants.

c. Intra- and Interlocal Comparisons. The manner in which the Z Test groups have been formed, evaluated and collated is not altogether homogeneous and requires some description. Because the first author moved from Tehran to Bern in 1964, just after finishing the Marvdasht Survey, and had scanty time in Bern for working up his data from Iran, the Z Test data from Marvdasht never were systematically evaluated, though the test had proved itself extremely useful in the field for screening and diagnosis. A new opportunity presented itself at the end of 1965 when, with the second

Table C II 23. Weighting of Determinants for Zulliger and Rorschach Tests

Response	Form	Kinesthesia	Color	Chiaroscuro
F	1			
Small M	$^1/_2$	$^1/_2$		
M		1		
M Chia		$^1/_2$		$^1/_2$
MC		$^1/_2$	$^1/_2$	
FC	$^1/_2$		$^1/_2$	
CF			1	
C	$-^1/_2$		$1 + ^1/_2$	
C Chia			$^1/_2$	$^1/_2$
F (C)	$^1/_2$			$^1/_2$
F Chia	$^1/_2$			$^1/_2$
Chia F				1
Chia	$-^1/_2$			$1 + ^1/_2$

With this aid there should be no difficulty in filling out the formula.

$$f\,\% = \frac{\text{weighted sum F}}{\text{R}} \times 100$$ or its complementary form under item 22

author, he was called back to Khuzestan to carry out the survey already planned there a number of years before. When he was invited to present a paper at the VIIth International Congress of Rorschach and other Projective Techniques in London in 1968 comparing projective test findings in ethnic groups, the Qashqai, studied at the same time as Marvdasht in 1963/64, were an obvious choice as culturally, sociologically and ethnically distinct from the majority of the Iranian population, as nomads on the point of abandoning or being forced to abandon their traditional way of life with all that this implied. We wanted a sedentary, also rural and agricultural population for comparison and decided upon the Khuzestani instead of the Marvdasht because we placed more reliance in the comprehensiveness and thoroughness of the study in Khuzestan. On their wanderings the Qashqai did regularly traverse the Marvdasht, as we have seen them, but they were no more a part of this area than of Khuzestan, in and through which moved other tribes of the Khamseh Confederation such as the Basseri [14]. There was, therefore, no intrinsic reason to prefer one of the groups of villages to the other. (It will be recalled that Qalandari, the Qashqai village, had not yet been surveyed.) In contrast to the situation in 1964, there was now also someone who could and would give us the necessary technical assistance in the processing of the data: Mr. George Lukacs of the University of Bern, to whom we are much indebted. Because of limited time and resources we had to confine ourselves to adults only and to combine the sexes for statistical treatment. Means and standard deviations were calculated for a large number of Z Test variables, then those represented only by very small means or often totally absent were eliminated, as also were those the standard deviations of which were excessive in relation to their means so that no significant differences could be anticipated. The list of remaining variables came close to that described above and employed here, but certain differences that are still apparent must be mentioned and explained.

In the publication of 1970 [27] we had treated each of the pairs S and Sc, FC+ and FC– as a single variable. Experience impressed upon us the usefulness of separating them, as we have done since and do here. The totals for S and Sc, corresponding to the customary space responses, as well as for FC+ and FC–, corresponding to the customary sum FC, can be obtained by addition. Certain statistical computations of significance in comparison with other populations, however, cannot be carried out where the Qashqai and Khuzestan are involved. The same hold for SUM KINA, SUM CHRO and SUM CHIA in these two places, the means for which were later obtained by adding the means of their components. Listing all these would have complicated the tables and increased the computer work excessively. The reader will also notice that under the Qashqai and Khuzestani mean values are given for O+, O–, H, Hd, A, Ad and Pl, but no SDs. This is an artefact caused by a computer breakdown only a few days before the deadline for the publication, forcing us to reckon some last mean values by hand count. In re-tabulating these data we have come to the conclusion that the time and labor involved in partly recording and recomputing them (with computer facilities by no means always available) could not possibly stand in any reasonable relation to the results that might be expected. We beg our readers to exercise forbearance with these conscious faults and shall gladly place the original data at the disposal of whosoever feels impelled to process them.

With the much larger populations of Shiraz and Qalandari and with the computer facilities of the WHO at our disposal, it became reasonable and indeed incumbent to undertake more extensive analyses than we had been able to perform hitherto – to investigate the test difference, if any, between adults and children, between the sexes, between the well and ill as well as between local populations as a whole. The main basis of this was, of course, the Shiraz Mental Health Survey. Evaluating all the nearly 3000 Z Tests was out of the question. The obvious sub-group to take was the Psychiatric Survey Population, but again scoring and coding all the nearly 900 tests was beyond our powers if we were to extract anything from the remaining masses of data. We could not sacrifice the pathological cases, but just as clearly it was unreasonable, unpsychological and rather worse than meaningless to cast them all together into a potpourri of "pathological Z Tests" with no common denominator except their (clinically demonstrated) pathology. A glance at our diagnostic tables showed that the majority of the 154 "pathological" (91 or 59.1 %) were reactive and thus did have a common denominator: a reactive, essentially affective disturbance and either a neurotic (neuroses and psychosomatic cases) or usually marked neurotoid (simple reactions) personality structure, to which the Z and Rorschach Tests are exquisitely sensitive. They can be placed meaningfully and reasonably in a category which (in order to avoid over-working the word "pathological" and to eliminate the term "neurotic", which is misleading to the point of havoc in its over-inclusive Anglo-American usage) we have called that of the "Reactively Disordered", abbreviated Dr. The remaining 63 pathological cases from Shiraz are too heterogeneous for statistically useful sub-grouping in respect to their Z Test findings, though of course diagnostically highly meaningful and valuable. Even the largest of them, e.g. the oligophrenics (12 cases), the psychopathies (11 cases) and the senile-arteriosclerotic dementias (11 cases) are too small for test-statistical treatment. We contrast, therefore, the Non-Disordered (abbr. ND) or "well" against the Reactively Disordered in the sense defined and omit (with an exception to be noted) the 63 pathological whose disorder is not primarily reactive. The table headings are to be read accordingly. Qalandari offered us too few disordered for inclusion or for separate treatment, wherefore such are not to be found in the present set of tables.

After subtracting the 154 pathological cases from the 928 subjects of the Psychiatric Survey Population, we were left with 774, of whom all but a very few (mostly blind) had been given a Z Test. As again the time-devouring labor of scoring and coding the whole number seemed disproportionate to the probable results and in any case beyond our powers, we determined to use half the sample, taking all odd-numbered non-disordered subjects. They were 383. We submit that doubling the number would hardly have changed the results, perhaps adding here and there a marginal statistical significance of slight or no psychological meaning, as can happen when a basic population is multiplied out of reasonable measure. The normal group was still sizeable, even when subdivided by sex and age, as compared with all the rest.

In Tables C II 24 a–c we list the means and standard deviations for 29 Z Test characteristics or variables for the Non-Disordered and Reactively Disordered in Shiraz separately and for the Non-Disordered in Qalandari with the quarternary subdivision just mentioned. Table C II 24 d gives similar data for the Qashqai and for Khuzestan as well, but for all four populations the non-disordered and disordered of both sexes have been combined and the children omitted. Our aim therein was to offer a display of data that was directly comparable with that of our earlier publication on "Z Test Findings Among Iranian Peasants and Nomads" [27] and is in fact an extension

Table C II 24 a. Z Test Characteristics: Shiraz, Non-disordered

	Adults 131 male Mean	 SD	 127 female Mean	 SD	Children 52 male Mean	 SD	 73 female Mean	 SD
T	9.23	4.92	11.19	6.57	11.00	7.54	10.59	5.47
R	8.99	2.27	9.35	2.38	9.23	2.27	8.99	2.40
W	1.27	1.01	1.21	1.04	1.38	0.75	1.41	0.88
W +	1.06	0.90	0.93	0.82	1.25	0.74	1.23	0.81
DW	0.05	0.21	0.06	0.24	0.08	0.33	0.03	0.16
D	7.48	2.04	7.57	2.13	7.02	1.73	6.89	2.25
Dd	0.18	0.46	0.24	0.59	0.58	1.27	0.47	1.18
Do	0.15	0.42	0.26	0.58	0.17	0.47	0.19	0.49
S	0.55	0.60	0.43	0.54	0.56	0.64	0.52	0.58
Sc	0.27	0.49	0.32	0.49	0.15	0.46	0.23	0.46
F	7.10	1.95	7.17	2.09	6.81	2.32	6.43	2.66
F +	3.95	1.46	3.77	1.66	3.96	1.48	3.77	1.60
f%	77.78	13.84	77.09	14.03	73.63	14.32	69.37	16.97
FC +	0.85	0.65	0.91	0.77	1.17	0.94	1.30	0.68
FC –	0.15	0.35	0.14	0.39	0.21	0.50	0.12	0.33
CF	0.58	0.73	0.69	0.75	0.38	0.60	0.45	0.60
C	0.02	0.15	0.04	0.20	0.08	0.33	0.04	0.20
MC	0.02	0.15	0.03	0.18	0.04	0.19	0.05	0.23
SUM KINA	0.76	0.86	0.69	0.90	0.94	0.93	0.97	0.88
SUM CHRO	1.13	0.86	1.31	0.91	1.19	0.84	1.26	0.70
AV	30.63	31.24	24.27	28.24	35.00	31.83	35.51	29.63
SUM CHIA	0.14	0.37	0.20	0.52	0.21	0.40	0.30	0.51
P	2.31	1.11	2.24	1.17	2.65	1.12	2.75	1.00
O +	0.32	0.57	0.17	0.44	0.17	0.43	0.19	0.40
O –	1.12	0.98	1.16	1.06	1.00	0.95	0.92	1.04
H	0.91	1.02	1.00	1.05	0.98	1.08	1.26	1.11
Hd	0.32	0.64	0.54	1.06	0.27	0.60	0.23	0.74
A	5.40	3.52	4.98	2.03	5.08	1.69	4.52	1.89
Ad	0.18	0.48	0.17	0.42	0.35	1.03	0.30	0.83
Pl	0.88	1.00	0.98	0.94	1.08	1.13	1.37	1.31

of this, including now the city, to condense our data into fairly large categories that could be compared at a glance and would be likely to yield statistically valid differences and to see whether anything like Z Test personality pictures of the respective populations emerged as they already had in the peasant-nomad comparison.

Which data were now to be compared with which? Out of the enormous number of mathematically possible comparisons we have tried to select those that appeared psychologically most meaningful: first intralocal comparisons by sex and age, then interlocal comparisons in part by the same criteria as in Table C II 24 a–c, then by comparing all adults as in Table C II 24 d. Since we were searching now for local, possibly ethno-geographic and cultural differences it seemed legitimate and in fact necessary to include the disordered together with the non-disordered, as every local culture is likely to possess in some measure both its own etio-genetic factors (which can, but must not be, social and cultural in nature, as the example of pockets of inbreeding shows) and its margins of tolerance for their consequences. As no population anywhere in the world yet has been demonstrated conclusively to be entirely free of any and all mental disturbance (we do not except our remarkably healthy nomad group for reasons

Table C II 24 b. Z Test Characteristics: Shiraz, Reactively Disordered

	Adults 19 male		51 female		Children 13 male		8 female	
	Mean	SD	Mean	SD	Mean	SD	Mean	SD
T	8.74	5.25	10.02	4.03	13.85	5.98	10.38	4.24
R	8.58	2.39	9.04	2.97	8.23	2.68	10.63	2.07
W	2.11	1.37	1.10	0.91	1.23	0.93	1.38	0.52
W+	1.38	0.89	0.88	0.82	1.15	0.99	1.00	0.76
DW	0.0	0.0	0.08	0.27	0.0	0.0	0.0	0.0
D	6.11	1.79	7.10	2.06	6.46	2.37	8.88	2.03
Dd	0.11	0.32	0.64	1.52	0.15	0.38	0.38	0.74
Do	0.26	0.56	0.26	0.53	0.38	0.87	0.0	0.0
S	0.58	0.61	0.52	0.65	0.31	0.48	0.25	0.46
Sc	0.37	0.50	0.22	0.42	0.15	0.38	0.38	0.52
F	6.74	1.96	7.04	2.72	5.96	2.70	8.00	2.74
F+	3.71	1.32	3.33	1.70	3.65	1.51	3.88	1.62
f%	79.37	12.40	75.44	13.57	70.92	12.87	73.63	16.38
FC+	0.95	0.78	0.70	0.65	0.92	0.76	1.25	0.71
FC−	0.05	0.23	0.18	0.48	0.15	0.38	0.13	0.35
CF	0.32	0.58	0.82	0.83	0.31	0.48	0.63	0.74
C	0.0	0.0	0.04	0.20	0.08	0.28	0.13	0.35
MC	0.0	0.0	0.04	0.20	0.08	0.28	0.0	0.0
SUM KINA	0.82	0.87	0.69	0.77	1.04	0.78	0.75	1.04
SUM CHRO	0.84	0.55	1.34	0.93	1.04	0.63	1.50	0.65
AV	34.11	31.88	29.15	29.66	41.92	28.56	19.50	24.24
SUM CHIA	0.18	0.30	0.11	0.27	0.19	0.38	0.25	0.27
P	2.58	1.17	2.02	1.29	2.23	1.17	2.63	1.06
O+	0.26	0.45	0.12	0.33	0.08	0.28	0.13	0.35
O−	1.11	0.94	1.20	1.50	1.08	1.04	1.25	1.28
H	0.74	0.87	0.96	0.90	1.85	1.41	1.00	1.31
Hd	0.58	0.84	0.52	0.97	0.54	1.20	0.25	0.71
A	5.00	1.63	4.84	2.35	3.85	1.63	6.38	2.62
Ad	0.16	0.50	0.30	0.79	0.15	0.55	0.25	0.71
Pl	0.37	0.60	1.00	1.25	0.62	0.65	1.38	1.19

given in the relèvant chapter) we take the disordered and pathological to be a natural part of their respective wholes.

Comparisons of paired data were made by the t test where near equality of the SDs permitted and by the Welch-Aspen Test where such equality was lacking. We have not listed the respective values, which are available upon request or can be calculated by anyone who wishes, as they convey little information by themselves and render the tables large and cumbersome. Rather we have listed all significant differences, and these only are listed in Table C II 25 and C II 26, which follow in their construction the preceding Table C II 24 but state no numerals.

As our largest local group is from Shiraz, we begin with this and look first for differences between non-disordered adults of the two sexes. They are few. The men take quite significantly less time: 9.23 as against 11.19 minutes for the women. This may mean no more than that the majority of the women were tested in the more leisurely atmosphere of their homes and by girls with whom they were not averse to passing the time. If the men were tested at home it was usually in the evening when they and their families naturally wished to gather together. It is noticeable and probably corroborative

Table C II 24 c. Z Test Characteristics: Qalandari, Non-disordered

	Adults 41 male Mean	SD	38 female Mean	SD	Children 34 male Mean	SD	22 female Mean	SD
T	7.44	2.18	7.45	2.75	7.12	2.92	7.77	2.94
R	9.12	1.62	9.39	1.85	9.32	3.10	8.77	2.18
W	0.90	0.80	1.08	0.85	0.79	0.86	1.45	0.96
W +	0.56	0.74	0.82	0.77	0.39	0.61	0.86	0.71
DW	0.07	0.26	0.08	0.27	0.03	0.17	0.0	0.0
D	7.73	1.58	7.92	1.99	8.27	2.36	7.18	2.20
Dd	0.15	0.53	0.13	0.34	0.36	1.03	0.0	0.0
Do	0.29	0.46	0.13	0.34	0.15	0.36	0.14	0.35
S	0.44	0.55	0.37	0.49	0.58	0.61	0.41	0.50
Sc	0.34	0.48	0.24	0.43	0.30	0.53	0.05	0.21
F	6.79	1.77	6.87	2.08	6.97	2.15	6.00	2.41
F +	3.30	1.37	3.37	1.82	3.55	1.51	3.05	1.60
f%	74.73	14.64	72.39	14.23	72.79	12.41	67.64	17.59
FC +	0.76	0.66	1.05	0.77	1.15	0.83	1.32	0.72
FC -	0.17	0.38	0.21	0.58	0.15	0.44	0.23	0.43
CF	0.66	0.79	0.95	0.77	0.76	0.83	0.45	0.61
C	0.12	0.33	0.03	0.16	0.03	0.17	0.05	0.21
MC	0.0	0.0	0.0	0.0	0.0	0.0	0.0	0.0
SUM KINA	0.56	0.81	0.72	0.79	1.67	0.78	1.23	1.02
SUM CHRO	1.29	0.94	1.63	0.84	1.53	0.73	1.23	0.65
AV	21.05	29.64	24.66	26.76	19.00	22.40	40.91	24.41
SUM CHIA	0.44	0.67	0.16	0.35	0.39	0.63	0.27	0.61
P	2.15	1.26	2.66	1.36	2.58	1.28	2.50	1.06
O +	0.17	0.38	0.16	0.37	0.30	0.59	0.09	0.29
O -	1.39	0.83	1.03	0.85	1.03	1.05	1.27	1.20
H	0.71	0.87	0.89	0.86	1.12	1.02	1.23	1.31
Hd	0.63	0.94	0.50	1.37	0.45	0.71	0.27	0.46
A	4.39	1.74	5.21	2.18	4.52	2.15	4.32	2.21
Ad	0.20	0.46	0.16	0.44	0.06	0.24	0.05	0.21
Pl	1.39	1.09	1.79	1.09	1.88	1.24	1.68	1.46

that this difference in test time did not appear in Qalandari, where all testing was performed during the day and the men, generally farmers, were less bound to working hours. The Shirazi men gave more O+ and less Hd than the women – findings that can be taken together as suggestive of somewhat greater originality and less stereotypy in their habits of thought. This sex differential fails in Qalandari, where indeed the only one to be found among adults is a tendency of the men to give more chiaroscuro responses (0.44 as against only 0.16 for adult women and 0.14 for men in the city; the difference between the two adult male groups now becomes highly significant). An interpretation for this apparently isolated finding will be offered later. Nowhere among the Z Test characteristics is a significant difference between the Shirazi boys and girls manifested. The boys' fathers give less Dd and thus may have lost some of childhood's indulgence in the fascination of unessential detail, but also less FC+ and thus may have sacrificed at the same time some of the easy affective adaptation of youth that finds its expression in play. If the differences between male youth and adulthood are few and not especially marked as far as the Z Test reflects them in the city (nor in Qalandari either, where we encounter the same decrease of FC+ in the men together with an even

Table C II 24 d. Z Test Characteristics of Four Iranian Survey Populations: Adults of Both Sexes, Non-disordered and Disordered Combined

	Shiraz (half) 318 subjects		Khuzestan 296 subjects		Qalandari 87 subjects		Qashqai 112 subjects	
	Mean	SD	Mean	SD	Mean	SD	Mean	SD
T	9.94	5.64	9.09	3.80	7.48	2.53	3.63	3.24
R	8.93	2.63	9.83	3.68	9.28	2.12	8.20	9.11
W	1.24	1.05	0.60	0.71	0.92	0.83	1.90	1.18
W +	0.95	0.88	0.51	0.64	0.64	0.75	0.97	0.86
DW	0.05	0.23	0.03	0.18	0.07	0.26	0.12	0.32
D	7.18	2.35	8.14	3.08	7.99	1.93	5.88	2.57
Dd	0.25	0.67	0.88	1.19	0.15	0.45	0.21	0.63
Do	0.22	0.52	0.18	0.45	0.24	0.43	0.04	0.21
S	0.48	0.58			0.41	0.52		
S + Sc			0.94				0.44	
Sc	0.27	0.48			0.28	0.45		
F	6.87	2.35	7.34	3.42	6.90	1.99	5.27	2.33
F +	3.66	1.70	3.45		3.31	1.58	2.21	
f%	75.39	17.63	81.08	13.56	73.40	14.67	71.32	17.93
FC +	0.85	0.70			0.91	0.73		
FC			1.27	0.85			1.17	1.03
FC −	0.14	0.37			0.20	0.48		
CF	0.65	0.78	0.39	0.69	0.81	0.82	0.59	0.71
C	0.03	0.18	0.04	0.19	0.08	0.28	0.08	0.41
MC	0.02	0.16	0.01	0.08	0.0	0.0	0.14	0.35
SUM KINA	0.68	0.85	0.48		0.63	0.79	0.69	
SUM CHRO	1.21	0.92	1.09		1.48	0.92	1.37	
AV	27.47	29.92	24.23	25.75	22.76	28.05	25.21	28.84
SUM CHIA	0.17	0.43	0.20		0.34	0.61	0.22	
P	2.15	1.19	1.81	1.09	2.37	1.28	1.27	0.93
O +	0.22	0.49			0.16	0.37		
O			0.43				0.10	
O −	1.15	1.04			1.29	0.97		
H	0.92	1.41	0.58		0.77	0.86	0.79	
Hd	0.43	0.86	0.36		0.58	1.12	0.16	
A	4.92	3.28	5.80		4.86	2.07	4.29	
Ad	0.19	0.44	0.41		0.17	0.44	0.21	
Pl	0.91	0.98	1.10		1.60	1.14	0.96	1.04

more pronounced decrease in SUM KINA), they are nowhere so numerous and highly significant as between the urban women and girls. With them it is not the Dd that diminish in adulthood, but the W, and the D increase compensatorily, resulting in a numerically slight but nevertheless significant constriction of the type of approach, an increasing matter-of-factness. That this is something more than a conjecture is shown by the higher F and f% of the adult women and their correspondingly lower FC+ (but higher CF), MC, SUM KINA and Pl, i.e. in a constriction of the experience balance as well, which moreover shifts in the direction of extraversion from AV_p = 10e in girlhood to 21e in womanhood. A forced preoccupation with environmental necessities seems to take place more than in the case of the city men at the cost of internal affective resources. More Hd from the grown women fits with no difficulty into this pattern and is complementary to the loss of kinesthesia. One would expect, then, more signs of conformity in the shape of P in the adults but finds the reverse. We shall propose an explanation later for this, though one might reflect here already that constriction must not necessarily lead to more than superficial conformity. In the higher prevalence of

Table C II 25 a. Z Test Characteristics Compared for Significant Differences: Shiraz

	Shiraz, Non-Disordered				Shiraz, Reactively Disordered				Shiraz, Non-Disordered: Shiraz, Reactively Disordered			
	Adults m : f	Children m : f	Male Ad. : Ch.	Female Ad. : Ch.	Adults m : f	Children m : f	Male Ad. : Ch.	Female Ad. : Ch.	Adults Male	Female	Children Male	Female
T	«						‹					
R						‹						
W				‹	»				«			
W +					›							
DW												
D				›		‹		‹	»			‹
Dd			‹		‹						›	
Do												
S												
Sc												
F				›								
F +												
f %				»								
FC +			‹	«				‹				
FC –												
CF				›	«							
C												
MC				«								
SUM KINA				‹								
SUM CHRO												
AV				«	»							
SUM CHIA												
P				«								
O +	›											
O –												
H											‹	
Hd	‹			›								
A						‹					›	‹
Ad												
Pl				‹	«				»			

Table C II 25 b. Z Test Characteristics Compared for Significant Differences: Qalandari and Shiraz

	Qalandari, Non-Disordered				Shiraz, Non-Disordered: Qalandari, Non-Disordered			
	Adults m : f	Children m : f	Male Ad. : Ch.	Female Ad. : Ch.	Adults Male	Female	Children Male	Female
T					››	››	››	››
R								
W		‹‹			›		››	
W +		‹			››		››	
DW								
D							‹	
Dd								
Do								
S								
Sc		›		›				›
F								
F +					›			
f %								
FC +			‹					
FC –								
CF				›			‹	
C								
MC								
SUM KINA			‹‹	‹			‹‹	
SUM CHRO								
AV		‹‹		‹			›	
SUM CHIA	›				‹‹			
P								
O +								
O –								
H								
Hd								
A					›			
Ad								›
Pl					‹‹	‹‹	‹‹	

reactive disorders among the female sex in Shiraz we have some indication that the constriction we observe in the devolution of the Z Test variables is not always a smooth process and that outward conformity may not go together with inner. There are no significant differences in the space responses as measures of opposition or in the O+ and O– to help us, though the high rate of Sc for the women in Qalandari is suggestive. Otherwise, in this village we meet the same, though a less boldly structured pattern of growing up from girlhood to womanhood with loss of kinesthesias and paradoxically of extraversion also, but with increase of undifferentiated CF in the adults. A similar, though less pronounced pattern is recognizable in the transition from male youth to adulthood in the village, during which there is a significant loss of FC+ as in the city, but an even more significant diminution of SUM KINA such as found already in the opposite sex. Constriction on both sides of the experience balance seems to proceed in the male sex at a roughly even pace, since the attitudinal value is not significantly

Table C II 26. Z Test Characteristics of Four Iranian Survey Populations Compared for Significant Differences: Adults of Both Sexes, Non-disordered and Disordered Combined (Number of subjects in parentheses)

	Shiraz (318): Khuzestan (296)	Shiraz (318): Qalandari (87)	Shiraz (318): Qashqai (112)	Khuzestan (296): Qalandari (87)	Khuzestan (296): Qashqai (112)	Qashqai (112): Qalandari (87)
T	›	››	››	››	››	‹‹
R	‹‹					
W	››	››	‹‹	‹‹	‹‹	››
W +	››	››			‹‹	››
DW			‹		‹‹	
D	‹‹	‹‹	››		››	‹‹
Dd	‹‹				››	
Do			››	‹‹	››	‹‹
S						
Sc						
F	‹		››		››	‹‹
F +						
f %	‹‹		›	››	››	
FC + / FC – FC	‹‹		(‹)			
CF	››			‹‹	‹	‹
C				(‹)	‹‹	
MC			‹‹		‹‹	
SUM KINA					(‹)	
SUM CHRO		‹‹				
AV						
SUM CHIA		‹				
P	››		››	‹‹	››	‹‹
O +						
O –						
H						
Hd						
A						
Ad						
Pl		‹‹				‹‹

altered (though it is numerically in Shiraz from 10e for boys to 14e for men, while in Qalandari it remains practically unchanged with 26e for boys and 24e for men). It remains only to mention, while confining ourselves to Table C II 24 a–c, that in distinction to Shiraz the boys of Qalandari give very significantly less W and significantly less W+ than the girls, whereas we find no sex difference in this respect in the urban youth, and that the boys of the village are very much more extraverted with AV = 26e than the girls with only 4e, i.e. the girls are practically ambiaequal. Other differences between Shiraz and Qalandari appear in Table C II 24 d, but as the populations compared are different we shall not discuss them here.

More sex, but less age differences are to be found in the reactively disordered from Shiraz. The disordered Shirazi men give more W and W+ than the disordered women at the cost of their Dd. Since organic pathology is excluded by definition and in any case W+ is significantly increased, this cannot be explained by the tendency of organically deteriorated patients to produce diffuse wholes, even though in our total pathological population there are more organic illnesses and their sequelae among males than among females. In the reactively disordered the male:female ratio is 1:1.8 or roughly 1:2. This holds again almost exactly for the sub-category of the true neuroses, is 1:7 for the simple pathological developments, but reverses to 1:0.90 for the psychosomatic disorders. It would be fair to ask whether psychosomatic illness in general furthers holistic tendencies in projective tests and simple pathological development reduces them. The second question can be answered cautiously in the affirmative, as the tendency of anxiety and depression – almost the only types of simple development involved here – to Dd and D at the cost of W is familiar and will be confirmed by any Rorschach text. Not so easy is an answer to the first. Bratt-Oestergaard [45] has given some evidence for an increase of W in psychosomatically ill children, but we find it here in our adult group. The available literature, concerned almost always with delimited psychosomatic disturbances, offers no hint. Indirectly, however, we may come upon one. It has been shown in Part B, Chap. IV 2 that in the Shiraz Psychiatric Survey Population psychosomatic illnesses are significantly more prevalent in the upper socio-economic strata, and it has likewise been shown in Part C, Chap. I 6 that the mean IQ is higher in these very strata. A high IQ goes well together with a high number of both W and W+. An explanation might lie here, but it must be admitted that the chain of argument is tenuous. It is much easier to understand, though, why the disordered women give more CF than the men when we look at the diagnostic tables and observe that the female cases of hysteria and hypochondria predominate by far over the male. Probably in accord therewith the males give less Pl, which are frequently CF, especially in disturbed cases. Finally, the disordered men turn out to be significantly less extraversive (11e) than the women (16e) in a statistical sense, which fits well into the diagnostic and test findings just discussed. Between adults and children the differences are few and scattered. In the male sex there is only one: the men take less time than the boys. As between the women and the girls we find the same difference in the FC+ (diminished in adults) as among the non-disordered, but the gradient of the D is reversed, the adults giving slightly less rather than more. Why must probably remain an open question since we encounter no other significant shifts in the type of approach or in other variables to help explain it.

In the preceding paragraph we have considered the reactively disordered Shirazi by themselves and turn now to a different type of comparison: that between the non-disordered and the disordered in Shiraz as shown in the third main column of Table C II 25. Here the overall effects of reactive disturbance, if there are such, should become more apparent. Not too many do. In the disordered adult males we see a highly significant increase of W from 1.27 to 2.11, and the same interpretation suggests itself as was offered above to account for the increase of W in disordered men as compared to women. The no less significant preponderance of D in the non-disordered men is most easily understood as a simple corollary of this, with the unsurprising implication of a closer adaptation to concrete reality in the well. The one more highly significant tendency of the non-disordered Shirazi men to give more Pl (0.88) than the disordered (0.37) must be viewed in connection with the preceding main column, where it became manifest that the disordered men gave much less Pl (0.37) than the disordered women (1.00). Plant responses are typical of first and second childhood among other things, but both are excluded here. Often they are chromatic responses, but we find no diminution in SUM CHRO or its components. Is their loss, whether chromatically determined or not, a sign of contentual impoverishment in the disordered men, of a restriction in their degrees of freedom to which by culture, custom and education they may be more subject than the women and (as the table suggests) the children of both sexes? Even though our "disordered" are expressly not psychotic, the familiar differences between male and female wards in mental hospitals throughout the world, and in Iran also, come to mind: the barrenness of the former and usually at least some minimal attempt at decoration, including flowers, in the latter. That there can be quite other probable reasons for gross differences in Pl we shall see shortly in the comparison between Shiraz and Qalandari. The women's column remains empty. The boys' poses problems. Why do the non-disordered boys give more Dd than the disordered? Loosli-Usteri, than whom no one is more expert in children's Rorschach and Z Tests, remarks that "In children the Dd seem to occur more frequently than in adults. According to the overall picture one must see in them an expression either of inner insecurity or of a still very infantile autistic manner of thinking" [129, p. 34]. Either interpretation would lead one to expect an increase rather than a decrease of Dd in psychological disorder. On the other hand, Loosli-Usteri immediately thereafter restricts these rather wide interpretations and adds others depending upon the type and location of the Dd, the plates on which they occur and the age of the child, into which we cannot enter here and which, as applied to our 13 disordered Shirazi boys, would require a separate case study. In Bohm's textbook [41] we discover a useful hint from D. Merian [148, quoted from Bohm p. 354]. The author investigated 34 children between 5 ½ and 13 years remarkable for their sauciness and insolence (*Frechheit*) and found "instead of the usual displacement of the type of approach in younger children toward the Dd side relatively few Dd and in their place more but unsharp W." She used the Z Test, not the Rorschach. Unfortunately, the sex of the children is not stated in Bohm's quotation, but more boys are likely to be reported for insolence than girls. This leaves us with the apparently paradoxical problem of why the disordered boys give more H and less A than non-disordered. Their increment of H does not, however, lead to a significant increment of SUM KINA. The H remain unproductive, in a sense "lifeless" and therefore might replace the A as indicators of impoverishment and stereotypy. Again, case analysis, for which there is no place here, would be required. The girls reverse the A tendency of the boys. Loosli-Usteri (loc. cit., p. 76) refers in this regard to Griffiths [89], who "had found in her little subjects the same preference for animal forms [sc. as

Cotte: the authors]. 'The inkblots are a comfortable means for the subjects to project their subjective anxieties and desires. That explains perhaps why the subjects interpret so many animals, birds and other living creatures, for many of them are symbols of danger or of anxiety-producing ideas.'"The quotation becomes more meaningful in our context when we add to it another of Loosli's from her preceding page, where she discusses animal responses in general and their commonly accepted meaning as indicators of stereotypy in particular: "This 'stereotypy' is a measure of the capacity to employ automatized mechanisms of thought that run off without reflection. It is evident that a certain degree of automatization is indispensable for the good, and especially for the quick functioning of thought, for instance for the use of language, . . ." She cites the nearly identical quartile limits of the A% in the adults of both sexes and continues: "With children the lower limit lies around 45% for boys and 40% for girls, the upper limit around 72 or 60%. One sees from this that in girls as in women the automatization is a little weaker than in boys and grown men."This would constitute the normal case, whereas the indispensable automatization might well be weaker still in the disordered girls, and the difference in cultural and educational demands upon the youth of both sexes could be nicely reflected in the difference of the signs for direction of A excess in the two disordered groups as compared with the non-disordered.

A discussion of the fourth main column of Table C II 25 "Qalandari: Non-Disordered" having been anticipated, we pass to the fifth, a comparison of the Non-Disordered in Shiraz and Qalandari, which leads over to generalized comparisons between localities and their adult populations including the disordered.

It strikes the eye at once that every category of subjects in Shiraz, men and women, adults and children, took more time for the Z Test than the same categories in the Qashqai village. The difference is even more striking when one compares the city with the nomad Qashqai, as will appear, and it holds for the city too against the villages of Khuzestan. City life is supposed to be hectic and often is, but Shiraz has a reputation for leisureliness among the cities of Iran that at least is not contradicted by these figures. More time does not produce more answers (the R values are not significantly different), but it does seem that in the men and the boys more reflection does produce more W and also W+. A slight reversal of the D in the boys may well be a corollary of that. As a group of the same testers worked under the same supervision in Qalandari as in Shiraz we see no reason to suspect an artefact. Certain differences in the Shiraz test situation have been cited above, but they refer to the adults of the two sexes and thus are not applicable to the generality of the T differences observed here. May what is popularly regarded as a local characteristic, but is generally banned by science into the realm of imagination, find its confirmation here? We have no data from other Iranian cities for comparison. It may be added that popular opinion often rates the Shirazis as leisurely, with an inclination to the arts, but never as stupid (a certain city on the Caspian coast has a well-known reputation for that and is the butt of countless jokes!) and thus does not controvert the W and W+.

At the bottom of the column we meet another nearly common characteristic of the well Shirazi as against the farmers of Qalandari: with the exception of the girls they give substantially fewer plant responses. The most likely explanation seems to be that this is simply a reflection of the countrymen's natural interests, and we shall find confirmation of this when we come to compare Qalandari with the nomadic Qashqai.

Certain differences between paired sub-categories of the non-disordered in Shiraz and Qalandari remain for consideration. The men of Shiraz give more F+, which probably accords with their increased W+ and may not reach significance in the boys, who also have a higher W+ rate, because of their smaller numbers. They also give more A, perhaps reflecting more "automatization" in Loosli-Usteri's sense in the urban environment, though this explanation is far from certain. It is striking that SUM CHIA is very significantly lower for the men, and for the men alone, in the town, and that this difference is even reflected, though to a lesser degree of significance, when the whole adult population of Shiraz (as represented in the survey sample) is compared in Table C II 26 with that of Qalandari. The mean value for the men of Qalandari (0.44) is more than thrice that of the same category in Shiraz (0.14) and the highest of any group, disordered or not, that we have had occasion to observe. Since we cannot refer it to overt pathology, the group being non-disordered by definition, we are forced back upon speculation. One offers itself. The village of Qalandari, it will be recalled, was formed of nomads who had settled there only eight years before the survey. Thus practically all the men had been bred to and had practiced a nomadic life. Might the loss of this, voluntary or involuntary, more sensible probably to the men than to the women, have precipitated some trait of covert melancholy, at least of unarticulated and vocally denied wistfulness and longing in the sedentary former nomads? A multiplicity of chiaroscuro responses in a group of displaced, homesick persons would surprise nobody. The argument is again tenuous. We can only offer it for what it may be worth and regret that we have no comparable group against which to test it (the resettled residents of Wadi Halfa would be a case in point, but Dr. Baasher's plan to re-examine them after his first survey of Wadi Halfa [11], so far as we know, has never been executed, and if so almost certainly without the aid of Z or Rorschach Tests). Samples of the numberless refugee populations that are a pitiable and disgraceful feature of contemporary history have been studied by projective methods, but we cannot regard them as a valid basis for comparison, as too many other factors, especially violence of no slight degree, are involved. A finding of Salomon's, though derived from children, may lend some support [173]. With the Slide Z Test he examined Algerian children waiting for months in France for resettlement in Israel. Obviously pathological cases were excluded from the study. His group A had been at most two weeks in France, group B at least six months. Both consisted of one hundred subjects. The new arrivals were mostly wild and undisciplined, unschooled and came from the lowest socio-economic strata. Half a year under affectionate and paedagogically skilled care transformed them, according to Salomon's description, so that they could be compared with any other normally educated juvenile population in regard to behavior and social adaptation. Salomon remarks briefly: "As a result of their education we must take . . . the percentual differences in their FChia, A = 2 %, B = 4 %. They confirm the enhanced voluntary effort toward an intellectual and affective adjustment to reality." ChiaF rose somewhat from 0.4 % in A to 1.0 % in B. (Salomon administered the test twice in a single sitting: we quote his figures for both times together and eliminate the double data from the quotation for the sake of simplicity without significantly altering the result.)

The adult females do not present any features for discussion except those already mentioned in a general way: the T and Pl. In the boys of Qalandari we find CF doubled over Shiraz (0.76 to 0.38) and SUM KINA increased from 0.94 to 1.67, the result of which, besides an enrichment of the experience balance as a whole, is a shift from an attitudinal value of 10e in Shiraz to 26e in Qalandari, i.e. towards rather marked extraversion in the village boys. To be noted is that this does not hold for the girls, where none of the three variables is significantly affected. The non-disordered Qalandari girls, whose mean AV is only 4e, "catch up" with their mothers' 24e later. More struggle is involved in the village, if we may so interpret the increment of Sc there over the city. A similar increment of animal detail (Ad) may point to acquiescence in facile solutions, as refuge to Ad often does.

Table C II 25 has given us intralocal, Table C II 26 gives us interlocal comparisons. Shiraz and Qalandari are here again, but now Khuzestan and the Qashqai also. The four populations are matched in the six possible ways. Their intrinsic composition is different from that in Table C II 25, comprising for each population all the adults (or a representative sample of them), non-disordered and disordered, of both sexes, but excluding the children. The tabulations are confessedly risky attempts to catch "local color", to sketch briefly local character. Many objections have been and are raised, sometimes vehemently, against this. To abandon it implies, however, abandoning comparative ethnology, anthropology, sociology and psychiatry, for which we are not ready. Proceeding cautiously, let us rather see what emerges from the data themselves.

Several differences between Shiraz and Qalandari have been discussed already, have been partly localized in sub-categories of the non-disordered and re-emerge here with sufficient penetration to color the whole picture. Such are the higher T and lower Pl in Shiraz. More attributable to the male sex in Shiraz but significantly affecting the composite sum here we find again in the city more W and W+, but in the present table correspondingly less D. The men's high SUM CHIA in the village is confirmed, though with a smaller degree of significance, since the women are now included in the reference population. Their inclusion and the omission of the children may well account for the larger SUM CHRO in Qalandari, since the women there give significantly more CF than their daughters and at least numerically more than their husbands. Besides this, the enhanced SUM CHRO might be a rather simple corollary of the greater number of Pl and this again a natural corollary of subsistence upon agriculture.

We turn our attention now from the second to the fifth column of Table C II 26, the comparison between the Khuzestan villagers and the nomad Qashqai. It was not only the first socio-ethnic comparison of this kind, based on a projective test of personality, that we have undertaken and published [27], but has remained one of the most interesting, rewarding and one of the richest in significant differences, as a glance at the table proves. Moreover, the nomadic Qashqai are in many ways a key, the only strictly nomadic population we have been able to study, in their whole way of life and social structure a sharp contrast to the sedentary townsmen and urbanites. The differences and similarities between the settled Qashqais of Qalandari and the still nomadic Qashqais can be displayed and analyzed better if we compare the nomads with permanently settled villagers first.

The peasants gave 9.8 responses on the average, the nomads slightly less with 8.2, but the discrepancy does not reach statistical significance. That for the total time does: 9.1 minutes for the sedentary group, but only 3.6 for the itinerant, less than half as long. Something may be due here to an artefact of the situation, since we knew the nomads would move on after three days, were pressed to examine as many as possible and did not tend to linger long over hesitant subjects. We believe, however, that this factor cannot explain the entire difference, since other test findings, as we shall see, accord well with the notion of quick reaction. One of the first of these is the strongly differing number of whole responses: 0.60 in the peasants, but three times this, 1.9 in the nomads. On the other hand, only 1.0 of these 1.9 nomadic global responses could be scored as well perceived, that is roughly half, whereas five sixths of the peasants' (0.51) were judged positive. The two findings together might be interpreted as an inclination to rapid, but not overly critical general appraisal on the part of the nomads, to something like a snap judgment of new situations as a whole. Running through the other apperceptive modes, we find that the peasants average 8.1 details, the nomads 5.9. This highly significant difference stands out more markedly, and in the expected direction, when we look to the small and oligophrenic details, both of which, like the D also, are significantly more numerous in the village. Taken together Dd + Do amount to 1.06 among the peasants and only to 0.25 in the nomads: cf. Table C II 28, where the apperceptive types are listed for comparison. The sedentary person appears more concerned with the minutiae of things, at least of unfamiliar things, possibly more cautious, less bold – an unsurprising difference when one considers the two ways of life. It now becomes interesting to inquire after the F+% (not given in Table C II 24 d). Even after a rather lenient judgment of what forms may be regarded as well perceived the figures for both populations are low: 47 F+% for the farmers, 42 % for the nomads. Though the difference appears slight, it is statistically highly significant. It corroborates the tendency to less exacting appraisal among the nomads that we have suspected on other grounds before. How are the well-seen forms achieved? As we might surmise in records of this type, to a considerable extent through popular responses, which make up 17 % – 18 % of the total. Originals are few, 1.7 %; more among the peasants with 4.4 % (ns), though not often of good quality.

From the more formal and intellectual aspects of the tests let us turn to those which reflect emotions and manners of experience: the determinants other than form. We are not surprised to find that their total share in the nomads' responses is higher than in the peasants', f% being 71 in the former and 81 in the latter, the difference statistically highly assured. The mean number of FC responses is almost identical in both populations, around 1.2. In the desert the color type shifts somewhat to the right, the CF increasing significantly to 0.6 over 0.4 in the villages, and we also come upon a modest but highly significant number of pure color answers such as the peasants hardly give at all. The like holds for the scarce, but very meaningful MC. Chiaroscuro responses are rare, amounting to about 0.27 in both groups alike.

It is the kinesthesias, of course, that now claim our attention, and it seems a little disappointing that no statistically significant differences emerge in SUM KINA and AV. Yet the question is worth pursuing further. While movement responses are not frequent in our two populations, neither are they lacking, though they do not appear where the Western trained specialist expects to meet them. Zulliger's popular M's for Card III are a rarity in Iran, as pointed out before, but conversely Card I was seen by 12 % of our people as a human or at least anthropomorphic creature, so often with a suggestion of at least attitudinal kinesthesia that we have scored it routinely as M in default of an indication to the contrary (such as "picture", "statue" and the like). Zulliger mentions it as an original! Be that as it may, our nomads brought forth on the average 0.69 movement responses, including the weighted MC. The farmers gave no MC, and their kinesthetic average was restricted to 0.50. The difference in the movement score rests such a small step below the 5 % confidence level that we cannot disregard it. Are the nomads, then, more introversive? Their experience balance is less coarctated on both sides than that of their sedentary brethren. In round figures the balance is for the nomads 0.7 : 1.4, for the farmers 0.5 : 1.1. It is tempting to conceive both the broader range of experiential possibilities and the much stronger tendency to global apperception as functions of the open desert and its wide-ranging denizens. Is man's regard directed more inward beneath the stars? By a single statistically insignificant AV point only, if at all (21e for Khuzestan, 20e for the Qashqai). Probably of more psychological importance is the wider compass of the experience balance in the nomads, corresponding to the lower f% that we have already noticed. More affectivity, it would seem, dwells in the black tents than in the dun houses.

If interest in external things predominates, to what is it directed? More than two thirds of the contents are animate, human or animal, and are complemented by another 11–12 % of plants. These together occasion the bulk of the color responses also, the brown animals or green trees to Card II, while the bold red blotch of the same card is not much used as color, calling to mind all that Rorschach and later authors have said about the avoidance of red. The number of animal responses differs percentually between tent (55 %) and farmhouse (63 %), but the difference does not sustain any test of significance. The large share of A + Ad may reflect conceptual stereotypy, which no one acquainted with rural Iran would be likely to doubt, but also simply occupational preoccupation. Other content categories are scattered and allow no conclusions. One is conspicuous by its absence. With a mere handful of exceptions we have encountered no sexual responses at all in either of these Iranian rural populations. Are they, then, inhibited in respect to the foreigner, or even without his or her presence? Our experience elsewhere in Iran does not lead us to believe so. There was no dearth of sexual responses in trial tests performed at dispensaries on the outskirts of Tehran and Isfahan, nor later in Shiraz, whether the subjects were male or female.

The bold differences in P speaks for more conformity, more stereotypy and conceptual automatization in Loosli's sense in the village, a wholly unsurprising result when one reflects that the nomad is constantly exposed to and must improvise against the whims of an inclement nature (whether he is less bound by convention is a matter for ethnologists to decide, and we prefer not to indulge in the risks of romanticism, having experienced whither they lead in the usual cityman's view of the "idyllic" countryside that he has at most visited on a picnic). The city dwellers have more P than the villagers of Khuzestan just mentioned and therefore more than the nomads with whom we have contrasted these, and again it is not difficult to conceive that more conceptual automatization may be required to cope with the greater, but also more systematized complexity of urban life. Qalandari is a problem unto itself. One might expect its P average to stand between that of the persistent nomads and the long settled villagers and townsmen, but it actually tops all the rest with 2.37 P. When analyzing responses to the psychiatric questionnaire we found reason to believe that tendencies to repression might be stronger in Qalandari than elsewhere, and data on shocks in the Z Test to be presented at the end of this chapter will provide confirmation for this. Repression, though, can lead easily into stereotypy. The excess of Do in Qalandari over both Khuzestan and the Qashqai would harmonize with this conclusion as would the deficit of W in comparison with the nomadic Qashqai, while some remnant of nomad habits might explain why the people of Qalandari nevertheless give more W than those of Khuzestan. Finally, the numerical difference in the mean P values between Qalandari (2.37) and Shiraz (2.15) is neither large nor statistically significant. At the time of our surveys (1970) there was a lively traffic between Qalandari and the city, facilitating the acquisition of urban stereotypy by the new villagers.

A phalanx of double chevrons, all pointing to the right except in one case, sweeps across the page on line T, and another phalanx, but with mixed signs, is visible on line W. Indeed, the mean test times vary within no inconsiderable bounds, as we observe when we list them in order from large to small in the first column of Table C II 27. Comparison with the means of the P's (third column) turns out to be intriguing. Their sequence is the same except again for Qalandari. Be it noted that the number of responses R (second column of Table C II 27 and first column of Table C II 26) differs significantly only between Shiraz and Khuzestan, though it is low, but not significantly so, in the Qashqai as one would expect from the very much shorter total time. If P means stereotypy and stereotypy in the favorable case (there are quite different ones) means economy and facilitation of thought, but P and T run parallel, we are confronted by a seeming paradox. Could it be that the Shirazis are not only in fact leisurely, as they are popularly reported to be, but also a little complacent, even dull and therefore make more use of convenient stereotypes in their perceptual judgments? Yet whenever and wherever local differences in intelligence quotients have been demonstrated (cf. Part C, Chap. I 6) they have been in the favor of the Shirazis as against the villagers and nomads, and their increment of W and W+, both commonly correlated with intelligence, has been observed. Their F+% is the highest of all. When we compare the reaction times as in the fourth column of Table C II 27, dividing T by R, we encounter the same sequence as before. The Shirazis take not only more time on the whole, but more time per answer. A solution presents itself when we calculate the P% (fifth column). The sequence becomes almost reversed, at least sharply dichotomized, Shiraz and Khuzestan having in common a relatively low, Qalandari and the Qashqai – fellow tribesmen – a relatively high and approximately equal P%. This can only imply that the apparently complacent slow reactors are not simply reposing, as it were, upon their stereotypes and automatisms. If not, they must be producing other, presumably more differentiated responses, and the surplus of W and W+ in Shiraz suggests which. Our rather coarse classification of variables does not permit a more precise answer, but the problem would deserve further study.

The converse holds for the sum of the white space responses S + Sc, whether by number or by percent. Comparing them with P% it appears that Shiraz and Khuzestan are (relatively) high in oppositional tendencies, but low in compliance (P), Qalandari

Table C II 27. Comparison of Certain Z Test Variables and Ratios: All Surveys Except Marvdasht

	T	R	P	T/R	P%	F+%	S + Sc N	%
Shiraz	9.94	8.93	2.15	1.13	24	41	0.75	8.4
Khuzestan	9.09	9.83	1.81	0.92	20	35	0.94	9.6
Qalandari	7.48	9.28	2.37	0.81	32	36	0.68	7.3
Qashqai	3.63	8.20	1.27	0.44	35	27	0.44	5.4

and the Qashqai the contrary. The complementary relationship between the two variables appears altogether logical, though it does not always obtain in practice. Their pairing suggests a common ethnic trait, whether its origin lie in heredity, culture or outward circumstance (the Qashqai were, on the whole, a minority under pressure).

It may be and should be mentioned here, with a glance back to p. 274, that not only are W, W+ and F+% as well as the other so-called "intelligence factors" of the Rorschach and Z Tests "commonly correlated with intelligence" in the sense of textbooks on projective techniques, including Rorschach's own *Psychodiagnostik* [170], but are directly and statistically so. S. Heydarian, using our material, has studied the correlations of a large number of Z Test variables with IQ in our adult Shiraz sample of 386 both non-disordered and disordered subjects. The following emerge as significant:

Variable	*r*	*Significance of r*
T	–0.22	0.001
W	0.12	0.010
W+	0.15	0.002
F+	0.11	0.021
C	–0.09	0.034
P	0.09	0.039
0–	–0.21	0.001

The kinesthesias and the good originals are missing, probably because of the heterogeneous implications of the first and the numerical scarcity of both. The M imply both intelligence and introversion, but ours was a predominantly extraverted population.

In Table C II 27 Qalandari stands out in other respects as the exception which it is, with a P% close to that of the nomads to which the citizens of Qalandari belong by origin and no very remote experience, but with a mean number of P close to and even above that of the not distant city, to which many new ties bind them. Their reaction time has slowed down remarkably when compared to that of the mobile nomads, and their oppositional tendencies as reflected in the space answers have risen. It is hard not to surmise that one witnesses here the mixed and somewhat discordant effects of a profound alteration in way of life, with reliance on stereotypy to help bridge the gap, with latent opposition or at least reluctance and with some deceleration of the quick wits of the wanderers who, more than the settled, are constrained to rely often upon a well-nigh instant judgment. We recall too that it was the men of Qalandari and these alone who produced a significantly increased SUM CHIA, a phenomenon appropriate to the conclusions we have tentatively drawn.

From the viewpoint thus far gained it becomes convenient to reflect upon the oversprung sixth column of Table C II 26 and to analyze in more detail the differences between the Qashqai and Qalandari. Other things, particularly the ethnic factor, being equal, we may hope to read off here fairly directly the consequences of voluntary settlement on a nomad population. The factors T, W, W+, D and F have been discussed already. Together with the drop of W after settlement may go the rise of Do that we find not only in this column, but also in the third and fifth. There is no ground to believe that these Do are actually oligophrenic, and it has become well known that this original meaning which Rorschach himself assigned them applies only to a fraction of cases.

Likewise it would exceed reasonable bounds to conjure up spectres of anxiety, melancholy and fear such as the Do may express in frankly pathological cases, but they may well adumbrate such qualities in the form of reserve, caution and constriction just as the increase of the D at the cost of the W and the excess of F in the same columns also does. If the dwellers in Qalandari as "new villagers" (Qalandari in fact was more often called simply *deh-e-nou* or literally "the new village" than by its proper name) are apperceptually more constricted than the Qashqai nomads, it is slight wonder that the Khuzestani (fifth column) and the Shirazi (third) are likewise or more so, and that the Khuzestani as "old" villagers are more so than those of Qalandari (f%, in the fourth column, here reaches its maximum as does the percentage of S + Sc). This constriction, now less apperceptual than affective, is reflected in the sixth column presently under consideration as it is in the third, fourth (W!) and fifth. In the sixth the signs of the apperceptive variables on the whole become reversed as against column two. We take this to be related to traits of the Shirazi character (if one may speak of such) that we have endeavored to elaborate above. The CF rise in Qalandari as against the nomads, just as the Pl do – in all probability correlative, environmentally determined phenomena. Following this lead, we note them rising substantially also in Shiraz as against Khuzestan, but without accompanying increase of Pl, for which the urban environment (even though Shiraz has been entitled the "city of flowers and nightingales" for centuries) proffers dwindling occasion. We observe here not so much rural adaptation, but rather urbanite expansion of mental horizons, confirmed by the apperceptive factors in the first column. Yet some residual boldness of the nomads seems reflected in the higher rate for CF, partly also for C and MC, in the Qashqais as compared with Khuzestan and Shiraz and in the comparison between Khuzestan and Qalandari. In this last pair we find again the old villagers more constricted than the new in T and in f%, whereas the new seem to retain some of their nomad heritage in W, CF and perhaps also in C.

For the sake of a quick overview from a slightly different point of vantage Table C II 28 recapitulates the apperceptive types in round percentages according to the scheme of Tables C II 24 a–d. In place of misleading zeros we have left rubrics open when the representation in them was substantially less than one percent. Objections may be raised justly against this reductive form of presentation because, as is well known, the absolute W values for instance are more informative and decisive than the percentages. Nevertheless, such an overview has advantages, even virtues of its own, and the absolute figures are given for all who wish to consult them in the foregoing tables. For like reasons we give no standard deviations here. The table is intended for easy comparison at a glance. Therefore we include in it also the practical notations of the attitudinal values. These can be derived from the theoretical notations employed in Tables C II 29 a–b for statistical reasons by a trigonometrical transformation, unless special tables such as Bohm gives [41, p. 462, reprinted there by consent from the first author} are at hand. As certain features stand out more clearly and conspicuously than in the preceding tables, we shall risk repetition and comment upon them briefly.

The apperceptive patterns, with few exceptions such as 2b, 3c, 4b and 4c, do not vary greatly. Nonetheless, in the Shiraz non-disordered a consistent and characteristic shift is noticeable between the young and the adults of both sexes, the former having slightly more wholes in relation to the total, the latter distinctly more details, while the

Table C II 28. Apperceptive Types as Percentage of Total Responses: Attitudinal Values in Practical Notation

	N	W	DW	D	Dd	Do	AV_p
1. Shiraz, Non-Disordered							
a. Men	131	14		82	2	2	14e
b. Women	127	13		81	3	3	21e
c. Boys	52	15	1	76	6	2	10e
d. Girls	73	16		77	5	2	11e
2. Shiraz, Reactively Disordered							
a. Men	19	25		71	1	3	11e
b. Women	51	12	1	78	7	2	16e
c. Boys	13	15		78	2	5	3e
d. Girls	8	13		84	3		25e
3. Qalandari, Non-Disordered							
a. Men	41	10		85	2	3	24e
b. Women	38	12	1	85	1	1	20e
c. Boys	34	7		88	3	2	26e
d. Girls	22	17		81		2	4e
4. Adult Populations, Non-Disordered and Disordered							
a. Shiraz (half)	318	14		81	3	2	18e
b. Khuzestan	296	6		83	9	1	21e
c. Qalandari	87	10		85	2	3	22e
d. Qashqai	112	23	1	73	3		20e

sum of Dd + Do decreases with adulthood. The children, especially the girls, are less extraverted. A sizable sex difference appears only between the men with 14e and the women with 21e, but even then is statistically not significant. Disregarding for the present the question of statistical significances of differences between pairs of data and looking more to the configurations, we can remark that those just mentioned accord well with the known tendency of children to give global, undifferentiated, often diffuse and rather reiterative wholes beside their Dd's in the Rorschach and Z Tests, which increasingly evolve into fewer but better W+ and into D. It seems to correspond to a natural process of maturation and adaption to reality, as we have remarked before. There is some confirmation for this in that such a shift is reversed for the D's in the disordered group and for the W's in the disordered males. Their W's rise from 15 % to 25 %, and their D's sink from 78 % to 71 %, accompanied by a paradoxical increase in extraversion from near ambiequality at 3e to 11e (paradoxical, that is, if we hypothesize that both detailed apperception and extratensive attitude be related in some way to a "reality principle"). Among the disordered Shirazi girls the reverse displacement is confined to the D's (from 84 % to 78 %), while the attitudinal value surprises us by being much more on the extratensive side in the girls (25e) than in the women (16e). We have seen in Table C II 24 a–b that this takes place at the cost of the adaptive FC+ in the disordered women, as we have observed and analyzed the price paid by the non-disordered women for their adaptation.

We should now expect to find a confirmation in the non-disordered of Qalandari but do so only in the female sex, where the W's drop from 17 % in girlhood to 12 % in womanhood, the D's rise from 81 % to 85 % and extraversion from practical

Table C II 29. Distribution of Attitudinal Values in Shiraz

AV_t[a]	Males Ad.	Males Ch.	Males Ad. + Ch.	Males Ad. Dr	Females Ad.	Females Ch.	Females Ad. + Ch.	Females Ad. Dr	Males and Females Ad.	Males and Females Ch.	Males and Females Ad. + Ch.	Males and Females Ad. Dr
	Absolute Numbers											
0 : 0	13	3	16	2	9	4	13	4	22	7	29	6
0	49	18	67	7	58	23	81	21	107	41	148	28
1 – 9	0	0	0	0	0	0	0	0	0	0	0	0
10 – 19	5	1	6	0	2	1	3	0	7	2	9	0
20 – 29	8	3	11	0	11	6	17	2	19	9	28	2
30 – 39	14	4	18	2	14	5	19	6	28	9	37	8
40 – 49	7	6	13	2	11	9	20	5	18	15	33	7
50 – 59	3	3	6	0	5	4	9	2	8	7	15	2
60 – 69	14	7	21	3	5	12	17	8	19	19	38	11
70 – 79	10	2	12	3	7	7	14	1	17	9	26	4
80 – 89	2	1	3	0	0	0	0	0	2	1	3	0
90	6	4	10	0	5	2	7	2	11	6	17	2
Sum A[a]	118	49	167	17	118	69	187	47	236	118	354	64
Sum B[a]	131	52	183	19	127	73	200	51	258	125	383	70
	Percent											
0	41.5	36.7	40.1	41.9	49.1	33.3	43.3	44.7	45.3	34.7	41.8	43.7
1 – 9	0	0	0	0	0	0	0	0	0	0	0	0
10 – 19	4.2	2.0	3.6	0	1.7	1.4	1.6	0	3.0	1.7	2.5	0
20 – 29	6.8	6.1	6.6	0	9.3	8.7	9.1	4.3	8.0	7.6	7.9	3.1
30 – 39	11.9	8.2	10.8	12.0	11.9	7.2	10.2	12.8	11.9	7.6	10.4	12.5
40 – 49	5.9	12.2	7.8	12.0	9.3	13.0	10.7	10.6	7.6	12.7	9.3	10.9
50 – 59	2.5	6.1	3.6	0	4.2	5.8	4.8	4.3	3.4	5.9	4.2	3.1
60 – 69	11.9	14.3	12.6	18.0	4.2	17.4	9.1	17.0	8.0	16.1	10.7	17.2
70 – 79	8.5	4.1	7.2	18.0	5.9	10.1	7.5	2.1	7.2	7.6	7.3	6.2
80 – 89	1.7	2.0	1.8	0	0	0	0	0	0.8	0.8	0.8	0
90	5.1	8.2	6.0	0	4.2	2.9	3.7	4.3	4.7	5.1	4.8	3.1
Mean	30.6	35.0	31.9	34.1	24.3	35.5	28.4	29.1	27.1	35.3	30.1	30.5
SD	31.2	31.8	31.4	31.9	28.2	29.6	29.2	29.7	30.1	30.4	30.2	30.1
AV_p[a]	14e	10e	13e	11e	21e	10e	17e	16e	18e	10e	15e	15e

[a] For explanation see text.

ambiequality at 4e (like the disordered Shirazi boys!) to 20e. In the males the share of W's, already small, increases slightly from 7 % to 10 % and that of the D's drops equally slightly from 88 % to 85 %, i.e. the apperceptive type remains essentially unchanged from childhood to adulthood, and the same holds for the attitudinal value with a shift of only two points from 26e to 24e. Deliberately overstating the question we could ask: do the non-disordered grown men of Qalandari remain in a sense big boys, while their wives mature into women? Some light might be thrown upon this problem by data from juvenile Z Tests in Khuzestan, the Qashqai and Marvdasht and by adult data from Marvdasht by comparison, all of which have yet to be processed. The disordered of Qalandari are too few to permit even an estimate of what share of each sex in their disparate course of development falls by the wayside. Probably only an anthropological study could come near to answering the basic questions. We do know, though, that the non-disordered Shirazi girls undergo quite considerably more psychological processes of constriction and restriction as reflected in the Z Test while growing up than the boys of the city do, more also than the girls of Qalandari (Table C II 24 c) and that in Shiraz the proportion of reactively disordered females to males is nearly two to one. Further we know that the over-all mental health of Qalandari at the time of the surveys was substantially and significantly better than that of Shiraz. Has the persistence of the "big boys" (*sit venia verbo!*) contributed to make it so? This raises fundamental problems of social and mental health, including education, which it would be worth while, even at considerable expense, to investigate more closely.

The adult bisexual populations show quite uniform extraversive attitudinal values from 20–22e. The Qashqai stand out by their holistic apperceptive type (approximated, remarkably enough, by the disordered Shirazi men) as we have seen already and find a contrast in the Khuzestani, who in addition display a percentage of Dd higher than all the rest. It would be easy to point out that the Khuzestani have their roughly 15 % of psychiatric morbidity, while the Qashqai had none, but the Shirazi also have a prevalence rate of 17 % and contrast in the distribution of their apperceptive modes less sharply with the Qashqai. Qalandari as usual stands in almost every respect in between except in regard to its D%, which is not markedly different from the 83 % of Khuzestan or the 81 % of Shiraz, and its morbidity rate lies in between also. As remarked already, a rather striking parallel exists between the apperceptive types of Khuzestani adults in general and non-disordered Qalandari boys in particular, which might at least engender an hypothesis if there was a one-sided distribution of psychiatric morbidity in Khuzestan, but there is no such predilection either in total prevalence or in reactive disorder. Rather, the figures for both sexes are exactly the same. This leaves the question open, as far as we see, except for the rather tentative hypothesis advanced in connection with Table C II 28.

We now attempt to summarize age, sex and environmental differences in the major Z Test variables as we have done in the two preceding chapters for items from the questionnaire. It must be remembered that our hitherto evaluated Z Test material is less comprehensive: Marvdasht is lacking, as are the children's groups from Khuzestan and the Qashqai.

Sex Differences

Very few of these attain statistical significance. Among the "normal", i.e. the non-disordered, the men take less time for the test than the women. In Qalandari, but not in Shiraz, they give more human details. Boys and girls present no significant differences.

Among the reactively disordered in Shiraz there are more differences. The men give more W and W+, less Dd, less plant responses (Pl). With a mean AV_p = 11e they are on the whole less extratensive than the women with a mean of 16e. The women also give more color-form responses (CF).

Comparing the non-disordered with the reactively disordered by sex and age categories we find that the disordered give:

Men	*Women*
more W	no significant differences
less Pl	
Boys	*Girls*
less Dd	more A
more H	
less A	

Age Differences

These are tabulated for the "normal" or non-disordered only. No numerical values are stated. The adult group is always taken as the first, the children's as the second member of the comparison. The chevrons indicate here only the direction of the gradient: a chevron pointing to the right implies that the adults have higher values for the variable in question, a chevron pointing to the left means that the children do. The degrees of significance of the differences as well as the numerical values of the means can be found in the basic Tables C II 24 a–d, C II 25 and C II 26.

	Shiraz		*Qalandari*	
	m	f	m	f
W		<		
D		>		
Dd	<			
SC				>
F, f%		>		
FC+	<	<	<	
CF		>		>
MC		<		
SUM KINA		<	<	<
AV_t		<		<
P		<		
Hd		>		

When the sexes are combined, it is found that the adults in Shiraz give significantly less W, but more D, Dd and Do than the children, whereas this difference is reversed in Qalandari. Thus we observe in the city at least an adult tendency to apperceptive constriction. This applies in part to the affective factors as well. The children (except the Shirazi boys) lose some of their kinesthesias and (except now for the Qalandari girls) some of their adaptive color responses (FC+). The adult women in both Shiraz and Qalandari seem to compensate this by an increase of less differentiated and thus less adaptive color responses (CF) and, corresponding thereto, by a shift toward extraversion (AV). The men show fewer significant changes.

Environmental Differences

Comparisons are drawn here between adult non-disordered groups only, corresponding to Table C II 26. The sexes are combined, as are several related Z Test variables for brevity and convenience. As in the preceding table, the chevrons indicate only the direction of the significant gradient.

The first pair of columns serves to compare the city of Shiraz with the two villages of Khuzestan and Qalandari, the second pair to compare these villages with the nomadic Qashqai, the fourth colum being at the same time a comparison between the already settled and the still nomadic tribesmen.

	Shiraz: Khuzestan	Shiraz: Qalandari	Khuzestan: Qashqai	Qalandari: Qashqai
T	>	>	>	>
W,W+	>	>	<	<
D(Dd, Do)	<	<	>	>
F, f%	<		>	>
FC	<			
CF	>		<	>
C			<	
MC			<	
SUM CHRO		<		
SUM KINA			<	
SUM CHIA	<			
P	>		>	>
Pl		<		

Comparison of both villages with the city shows excellent agreement with regard to total time and to apperceptive type: the urbanites take more time and produce more wholes, including more good wholes; the country folk are quicker and give more details. One might conclude that the city people on the whole were somewhat more deliberate and thoughtful, and this would fit well with their higher mean IQ. After this, there are no more pairs of significant inequalities in the first two columns, but the train of thought can be pursued further. The Shirazi give less FC, but more CF than the Khuzestani and logically therefore have a smaller f% (since the CF weigh more than the FC as non-formal determinants). This can be interpreted as a certain deficiency in affective differentiation and adaptation complementary to their intellectual appreciation (and perhaps a price for it, though one would like to believe that it must not always be purchased at such cost?). In the larger SUMS CHRO and CHIA we see evidence again that the village people in Qalandari rely more on emotional, less on intellectual appraisal, though we do not find corresponding differences in FC and CF (the FC tend numerically in the same direction as between Shiraz and Khuzestan, the CF in the opposite). The simplest formulation, to be used cautiously and with the reservation that data for Marvdasht are still lacking, would be that, as far as our information goes in this time and place, urban life seems to favor intellectual at the cost of affective adaptation.

The second two columns contrast the two villages with the nomads and exhibit again a rather striking agreement in respect to the first four variables: time, apperceptive type and use of formal determinants. Though the villagers take more time than the nomads, they, unlike the city dwellers, give more detail and less wholes, and they make more use of form than the nomads do. They also see more popular responses. In psychological terms this could lead us to expect from the nomads quicker, more global, less formal, perhaps more intuitive appraisals and reactions with less stereotypy, more swift and independent judgment – no surprise when one considers the different environments in which the two groups live. Something of this independence seems to be sacrificed in the villages. Looking now for differences between the Qashqai villagers in Qalandari and the nomadic Qashqai we meet with only one variable in which the difference is significant: the CF. This is probably best understood here as an indication of less impulsive emotionality among the nomads, though they would seem to have more of it than the long-settled Khuzestani. They also, however, have both more MC and SUM KINA than these, indicating a better affective balance and capacity for synthesis.

d. Attitudinal Values. The attitudinal value has been treated hitherto globally as a single characteristic of populations and sub-populations and has shown us some interesting, though not startling differences between them. Its use instead of the classical experience balance, from which it is derived, renders a more detailed and penetrating analysis possible. As it consists of a single, one or two digit figure designating equal intervals along a linear scale, its distribution as well as its mean values and their measures of dispersion can be studied in the several groups and compared between them. For this, however, it is desirable to have rather large populations as a basis for comparison. We therefore take Shiraz as our point of reference and proceed cautiously to some smaller groups. The data are presented in Tables C II 29 and C II 30, their main components again as histograms in Diagrams C II 1 and C II 2. The tables themselves require some explanation before we enter upon the results.

As described on p. 264 ff. a totally constricted experience balance 0:0 cannot be represented by an attitudinal value, and such cases must be eliminated from group calculations. Their number is shown in the first line of the table against 0:0. It is then subtracted from the total number of valid records in the relevant category (sum B), leaving the number of records with AV_t from 0 to 90 (sum A) of which the distribution is shown in the upper half by absolute frequencies, in the lower half by percentages. For calculating these sum A has been used as the divisor. The number of records shown in the foregoing Table C II 28 for each category corresponds to sum B, but the AV's in that table have been corrected to sum A as in the Tables C II 29 and C II 30. Sum A includes the extreme values with the intrinsic limitations already discussed. Because of these limitations the extreme values can be represented graphically only as one-

Table C II 30. Distributions of Attitudinal Values Outside Shiraz: Non-disordered Subjects Only

AV_t[a]	Khuzestan Males Ad.	Ch.	Females Ad.	Ch.	Qalandari Adults m	f	Qashqai Adults m	f
	Absolute Numbers							
0 : 0	9	3	11	5	1	0	5	8
0	76	46	58	34	23	19	11	28
1–9	0	0	0	0	0	0	0	0
10–19	0	1	0	0	1	2	0	1
20–29	8	1	4	4	3	7	6	6
30–39	7	2	4	5	1	1	5	6
40–49	12	5	10	5	3	6	7	6
50–59	3	2	2	0	3	1	0	1
60–69	15	11	16	7	4	4	4	5
70–79	2	4	7	2	1	0	2	1
80–89	1	3	1	0	0	1	1	0
90	2	6	1	2	2	1	4	3
Sum A[a]	126	81	103	59	41	42	40	57
Sum B[a]	135	84	114	64	42	42	45	65
	Percent							
0	60.3	56.9	56.3	57.5	56.2	45.1	27.5	49.1
1–9	0	0	0	0	0	0	0	0
10–19	0	1.2	0	0	2.4	4.8	0	1.8
20–29	6.3	1.2	3.9	6.8	7.3	16.7	15.0	10.5
30–39	5.6	2.4	3.9	8.5	2.4	2.4	12.5	10.5
40–49	9.5	6.2	9.7	8.5	7.3	14.3	17.5	10.5
50–59	2.4	2.4	1.9	0	7.3	2.4	0	1.8
60–69	11.9	13.7	15.5	11.9	9.8	9.5	10.0	8.8
70–79	1.6	4.9	6.8	3.4	2.4	0	5.0	1.8
80–89	0.8	3.7	1.0	0	0	2.4	2.5	0
90	1.6	7.4	1.0	3.4	4.9	2.4	10.0	5.3
Mean	20.2	27.8	24.7	21.8	22.9	23.8	37.4	24.0
SD	27.4	34.6	30.2	28.7	29.8	26.9	30.4	28.2
AV_p[a]	25e	17e	20e	23e	22e	21e	7e	21e

[a] For explanation see text.

dimensional, the dimension being their absolute or relative frequency. Therefore they are shown in Diagrams C II 1–2 not by histogram columns, but by thin cross-hatched bars. Because of their sometimes excessive length the E bars at the right are drawn to half scale. The width of the true columns is set naturally and conveniently at ten degrees of arc, since the range comprises ninety degrees. Again for the sake of convenience we shall take usually the mid-value of each column as a short designation for the range of values spanned by the column and speak of values around 0, 5, 15, . . . 45, . . . 75, 85, 90 degrees when the values 0, 1–9, 10–19 etc. are meant, and correspondingly in practical notation. In this, the letter E corresponds to 0, A to 45 and I to 90. Be it recalled again that the theoretical notation runs from right to left along the abscissa, i.e. contrary to the usual extraversive values on other scales, and that the practical notation runs from the ambiequal point A to both sides.

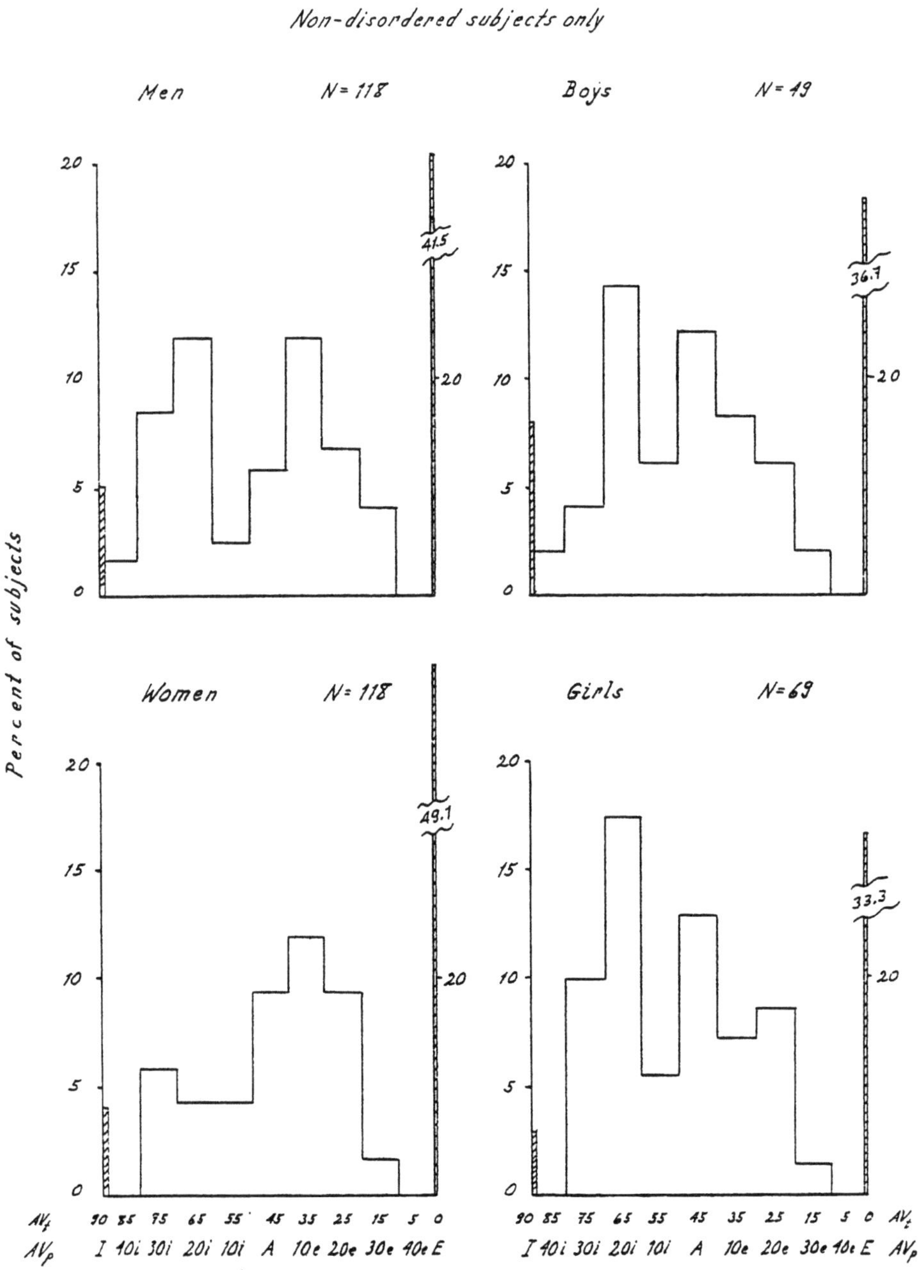

Diagram C II 1. Distributions of Attitudinal Values in Shiraz

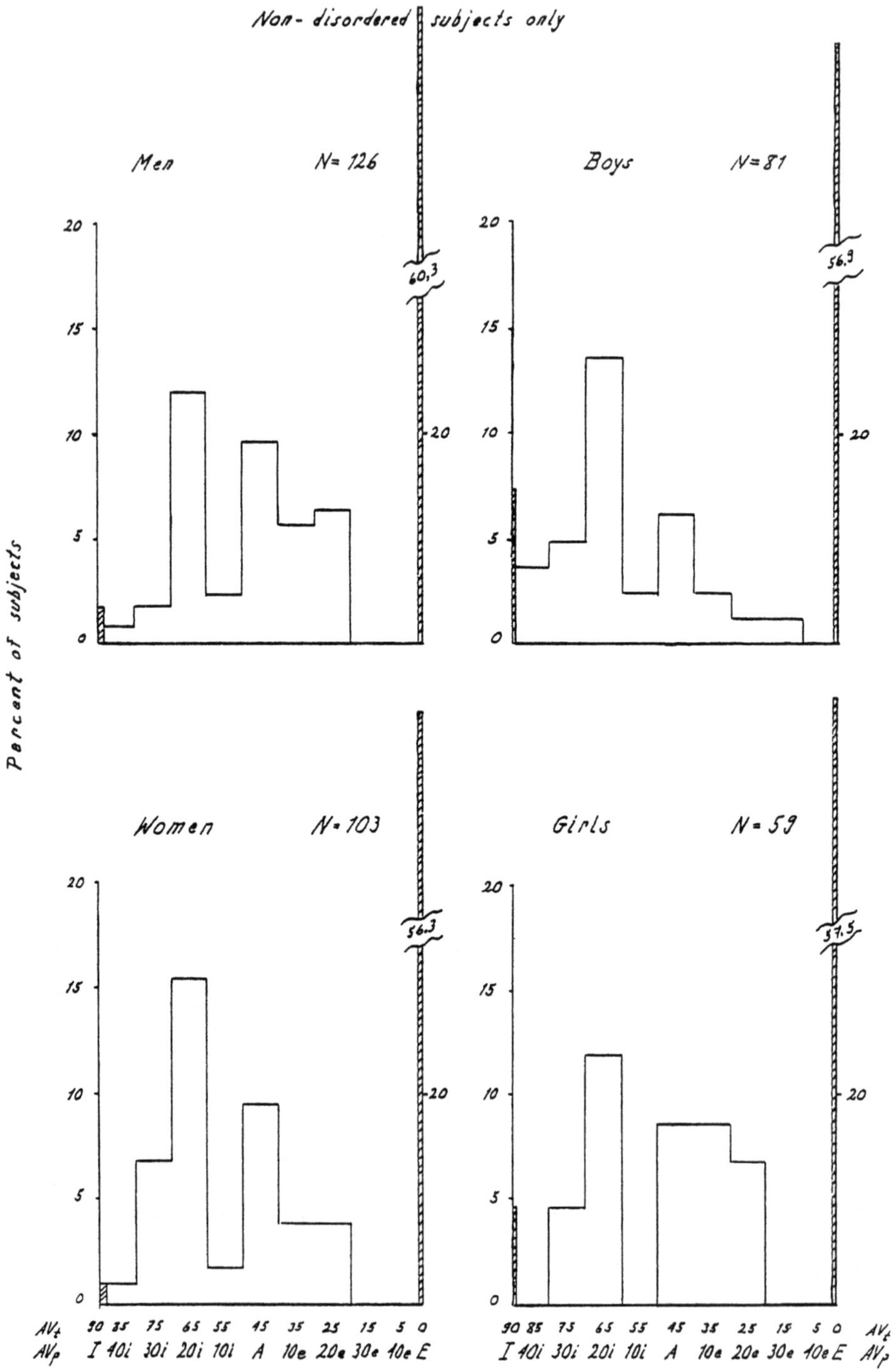

Diagramm C II 2. Distributions of Attitudinal Values in Khuzestan

In Table C II 29 we have retained the same quadruple division of the basic population as hitherto into male and female adults and children or into men, women, boys and girls. For the non-disordered cases it rests upon one randomized half of the Shiraz Psychiatric Survey Population (all cases with odd numbers), but for the reactively disordered upon all the cases of this category. In this way we have sought to obtain a sufficiently comprehensive initial population so that its principal sub-groups could be compared with each other while circumventing the formidable and probably unrewarding task of scoring and tabulating all the over nine hundred records. Even so, the children's groups have become rather slight. The non-reactively disordered of all ages have been excluded as too heterogeneous for our purpose, the two groups of reactively disordered children as too small. For the sexes separately non-disordered adults and children have been combined, and in a third main category the sexes also. As in Tables C II 24 a–c we were looking for differences related to age and sex and have found several. Fusion of the sub-populations then becomes questionable, but we have carried it out in the table to enable comparison with data from the literature, which are by no means regularly broken down by sex and age. Diagrams C II 1–2 show only the four main categories, the fusion of which tends to obliterate differences of, we are inclined to think, no inconsiderable psychological significance.

Glancing across the top rows of absolute numbers in Table C II 29 we observe that the absolutely coarcted cases (0:0) make up roughly 10 % of the total (sum B). The introversionless (AV = 0) are seen in the top row of the percentage table to constitute 40–50 % of the adult cases and around 35 % of the children's. They account in substantial measure for the uniform and rather marked tendency to extraversion that is evident throughout the last line (AV_p). The circumstance is worthy of note for two reasons. The share of such cases in the Central European populations to be mentioned below was usually, like that of the 0:0 cases above, around 10 %, while that of the 0:0 cases in Europe was much lower on the whole. Secondly, Nowparast [159] has reported mean experience balances from Tehran students that were strongly introversive, as we have seen in Section a of this chapter. We encounter only zeros in the range of AV_t = 1–9 and many zeros in the range 80–89. In both these ranges the percent values are usually low and sometimes nil, but their radical disappearance here especially in the range 1–9 we take to be an artefact of the Z Test with its rather coarse scale determined by the intrinsically smaller number of responses, since they do not as a rule vanish when similar histograms are drawn for the Rorschach Test. On the other hand, the generally high extraversion values are not an artefact of the Z Test, as it is known that the Z yields proportionally both more kinesthetic and more color responses than the Rorschach [cf. Bohm, 12]. If there are many introversionless subjects, there are also not a few without extraversion, as the two rows with AV = 90 prove.

Looking down the columns and keeping also Diagram C II 1–2 in mind, we remark that with one important exception the attitudinal value distributes bi- or multimodally in Shiraz, as we have already observed in Qalandari. This is no Iranian peculiarity, since the first author has shown in several studies [15, 16, 25] that it does so no less in Central Europe. Flückiger's [80] data confirm this independently. She gave the Slide Z Test to 140 male students of a Swiss teacher's college and states the sum M and sum C for each. There was only a single absolutely coarctated experience type. When the rest are re-calculated to attitudinal values we get the same bimodal histogram with peaks at 20i and 10e as for the men in Shiraz, though with a shallower trough between them and with only 5.1 % E and 2.1 % I. The mean AV_p turns out to be 2i, the proportion of introversive to extraversive subjects (i:e ratio, see below) 53:47. This contradicts the almost universally assumed and asserted, but by no means universally demonstrated "normal" distribution of introversion-extraversion in non-projective tests. Both Anastasi [6] and Eysenck [74] have published distribution curves on the dimension of extraversion that they claim to be "normal", but that in fact suggest bimodality. Anastasi has even noticed this but has dismissed the uncomfortable finding with the remark (loc. cit., p. 86 fn.): "The slight bimodality near the center of the scale might result from larger 'gaps' between the items designed to sample intermediate degrees of this behavior" without offering any evidence for this, and Eysenck has preferred to disregard the fact entirely. Other studies of intro- and extraversion, usually mentioning only the latter, by questionnaire techniques do come close to a normal distribution. One such is the Freiburg Personality Inventory, basically similar in its questionnaire and factor-analytic method to Eysenck's several scales and to the MMPI, but developed and standardized independently in Germany by Fahrenberg and Selg [79]. Its most valid scale is said to be that for extraversion. Flückiger, after grouping her subjective by experience types into introverts, extraverts, ambiequals, dilated and coarctated (few), has correlated their Z Test status with their scores on the Freiburg Inventory and has found such low correlations (r –0.093 for extratension and –0.124 for introversion) that she concludes (loc. cit., p. 181): "Extraversion in the Freiburg Personality Inventory and extratension as attitudinal type evidently encompass different dimensions of personality and therefore are not comparable with each other." This should be borne in mind when reading the summary of investigations carried out by means of extraversion scales in Iran at the beginning of the chapter. On the other hand, bimodality accords with Jung's theory of attitudinal types [109]. Anastasi has argued against this that, if there are two distinct types, their values must pile up at both ends of the distribution, and this seems to be met in part here, where many values do pile up at E, sometimes also at I (especially in the boys' histogram). The argument, though, is in itself far from valid, for the scores equally well can pile up and do pile up around two eccentric modes within the extremes. Considering the large numbers at the extremes, especially the extraversive extremes, one might speak with more justification of tri- or even quadrimodality. Whatever terminology one may prefer, the fact remains that no concentration of attitudinal values around a central mode occurs. The trough between the two types lies at AV_t 55 or AV_p 10i for all Shirazi groups and for many, but not all Central European. The peaks also shift, e.g. from AV_t 45 in the boys to 35 in the men, showing that we have not to do with a constant artefact caused by the relative coarseness of the measure. We must add that it has been demonstrated, using the Rorschach Test, the Lüscher Color Test and the Freiburg Personality Inventory on identical subjects that the Rorschach AV's distribute bimodally, the other measures normally [25]. The histograms usually suggest and sometimes exhibit quite clearly a bell-shaped or Gaussian distribution about each of the two eccentric modes. This fact of bi- or multimodality renders measures of central tendency and dispersion rather questionable. A mean attitudinal value may nevertheless indicate a predilection of the population in question as a whole, but the validity of its comparison with other means by the usual procedure involving standard deviations from "means" that are no true measures of central tendency seem doubtful. The SD's are nevertheless stated for those who wish to use them.

The category of adult males may be taken first as a satisfactorily good-sized group representative of the active population. Besides its 41.5 % of subjects at E, it has two quite distinct modes of equal prominence at 20i and 10e. The extraversionless at I with 5.1 % are not many, yet more than the 1.7 % around 40i and the 2.5 % around 10i. Especially the distribution around the mode at 10e has a "normal" or Gaussian configuration. The mean AV_p is 14e, but when the two extreme categories E and I are omitted the area under the histogram on the introversive side as against that on the extraversive, which we can denominate as i:e is as 52:48 %, i.e. nearly ambiequal with a slight tendency to introversion.

The boys' histogram is superficially similar and (without extremes) obviously bimodal, but on closer examination presents some interesting differences. The introversive mode is again represented by 20i, but the percentage is higher with 14.3 % rather than the men's 11.9 %. The trough likewise follows immediately at 10i, but the second and hardly less pronounced mode (12.2 %) tends more to the introversive side, though actually found at A. Thereafter steps fall off regularly toward E, which with 36.7 % is somewhat lower than the men's 41.5 %. The mean AV_p = 10e is correspondingly less extratensive than the 14e of the adults. Comparison of the areas gives a ratio of 59:41 % for intro- to extraversion. The percentage of I is fairly high with 8.2. By all measures it is therefore manifest that in growing up from boyhood to male adulthood in Shiraz bimodality of attitudinal types is preserved, but with an unequivocal shift to the extratensive side.

The girls' distribution is quite similar to the boys'. Modes and troughs lie at the same places. The drop from the second mode at A towards E is less regular, with a slight rise at 20e. Both I and E are represented by somewhat smaller percentages. The overall mean value is identical and the ratio of the areas is similar, being 62:38 %. No sex differences worthy of note emerge.

They do, however, emphatically between the adult women and the men. The women's histogram is practically unimodal around 10e, the slight second elevation around 30i being of doubtful relevance. I has its lowest percentage value with 2.9, E its highest with 49.1. The introversive mode that was so noticeable a feature of the men's histogram has vanished. Corresponding thereto the overall mean is 21e and the area ratio is 41:59 %. Growing up in Shiraz means for girls a very much more pronounced apparent shift to extraversion than for the boys, for all but few an abandonment of it or perhaps a transformation. This has shown itself already in Table C II 24 a in a general way and corresponds doubtlessly to the diminution there of SUM KINA, FC+ and MC in the adult females, the significant increase of f% and CF in the same category as against their daughters, but can be analyzed in more detail with the help of the AV. Here a sharp difference in the maturation of the two sexes exposes itself very clearly: the males drift as a group towards extraversion, probably under the pressure of environmental exigencies, but retain their bimodality, whereas the girls, starting from the same basis as the boys, are impelled into a unimodal, unilateral extratension of formidable degree – if it be a true extratension. Binder's "introversive color responses" come to mind. According to Rorschach and Binder the introvert in general is more or less inhibited in his capacity to respond to peripheral affective stimuli such as the chromatic blots represent. Binder writes [37, p. 88]: ". . . since introversive inhibition tends to reduce peripheral emotional responsiveness, the number of color responses in general is depressed. Rorschach and subsequent investigators in full agreement with him have emphasized that this is really the case in decidedly introverted subjects. Such subjects when contemplating the colored cards succeed mainly in the intellectual abstraction of certain forms, but preserve a constant and rather poorly regulated inhibition with regard to the colors. Not seldom then a phenomenon occurs that is analogous to the already mentioned brusque and clumsy, jerky movements of the introverts: when for once a more strongly exciting color (especially red or yellow) forces a more intensive emotional reaction upon them in spite of their tendency to rejection and therefore, in contrast to normal experience of color, carries with it a keen note of displeasure, then this 'penetrating' feeling disturbs and disrupts rational interpretations of form, since these are no longer subject to the tendency to plastic formulation inherent in normal regulation, which restrains too strong emotions through flexible modulation and restricts their consequences. This explains a finding that we have not seldom encountered in the records of markedly introverted subjects: small number of color responses in general and total absence of FC answers as a consequence of introversive inhibition, together with these however occasional C or CF answers (which do not belong to the already mentioned intellectual color responses) as a result of 'disruptive' emotions and insufficient normal regulation. Enke [68] has observed exactly the same thing in his studies, and we agree with him entirely when he emphasizes that one cannot regard such occasional C responses in the presence of general color inhibition as signs of extratensive experience. Enke is looking for a psychological explanation of these responses in the same direction as ourselves when he says that such interpretations occur when the color 'forces itself upon the subject against his will'." A few lines further follows a sentence of particular importance for our present inference: "In the daily life of introverts we meet with corresponding occurrences: together with general rejection of emotional contact with the environment they are helpless against singular strongly emotionally toned impressions, which the introvert either dissociates so that they become crystallisation points for neurotic complexes, or in reference to which he abandons his initial rejection so that he can even enter into an exclusive, exaggerated relation to the respective singular phenomena of his environment."

It seems to us very likely that both occur in the maturation of the Shirazi girls and are reflected in the women's diagnoses. As mentioned, these show as against the men a preponderance of reactive disorders in general and of simple pathological reactions and developments in particular (14 simple cases to 2, 59 cases of reactive disorder to 32). The girls do not as against the boys. This would imply that the involuntary, disproportionate affective responses to environmental stimuli in naturally introversive girls and young women are indeed potential "crystallisation points for neurotic complexes", but that the crystallisation does not always take place. When it does not, the simple pathological development often results; when it does, the neurosis follows. Yet the majority of the women happily are not reactively disordered, at least in a manifest clinical sense. For these, we believe, Binder's second pattern of reaction holds: the typically introversive initial rejection is abandoned, and the subject enters into an exaggerated contrary relation to the phenomena of her environment – a pseudo-extraversion.

The hypothesis may seem bold, but there is more than one piece of evidence to support it. First there is the simple fact that the obtrusively evident introversive mode such as we see in the AV histograms of the men, the boys and the girls is not present in the women's, that their mean AV is the most extraversive of the four groups and their share of introversionless records with 41.9 % the highest, whereas that of the girls with only 33.3 % is the lowest. This alone would serve only to render the hypothesis interesting, but not to prove it. Secondly, however, we have the disproportionate share of reactive disorders in the adult females such as we do not find in the adult males: a circumstance that fits neatly into Binder's theory. Thirdly, we encounter among the women in significantly increased measure exactly the secondary phenomena, consequences and corollaries of their "introversive inhibition" that Binder describes: a small to vanishing number of color responses, few FC, augmentation nevertheless of CF and C. A fourth line of evidence will present itself when we discuss the shocks below. Here we must add a word of caution about the term "intellectual introversion". Binder explains his choice of it as being due to an "intellectual abstraction of certain forms" from the chromatic blots by means of which the subject circumvents a color reaction, but it carries connotations that can be misleading. The "extraction" of form or abstraction from color (the original reads "*intellektuelle Heraushebung bestimmter Formen*") is "intellectual" only in the very limited sense of not being directly emotive. Indirectly, though, it is highly, and the consequences are still more so, consisting in mild to vehement inadequately modulated and differentiated emotional reactions. The implication is certainly not that the girls, when they grow up, become more "intellectual". Such an expression as pseudo-extraversion would seem to us to fit the case better. We conclude that a majority of the introversive Shirazi girls mature into pseudo-extraverts and, in case of maladjustment, reflect this in heightened frequencies and typical forms of reactive disorder, while the extratensive go their own way. This type of development obtains by every indication much less in the male sex in Shiraz. This sex exhibits to be sure a moderate extratensive shift, but on the whole without sacrificing normal introversion to pseudo-extraversion. We shall return to this below.

The concept of pseudo-extraversion helps us to understand why the women, who by crude test criteria are more "extraverted", give significantly less popular response than the girls, as we have seen on p. 287 and in Table C II 25. Genuine extraversion should facilitate adjustment to the environment and its common modes of apperception. Pseudo-extraversion, constrained, resentful and sometimes rebellious, need do nothing of the sort and seems not unlikely to have the opposite effect.

Is this pattern of female maturation peculiar to Shiraz, to Iranian cities or to Iranian culture generally, to say nothing of other countries? The only available set of Z Test data large enough for a fair comparison are from rural Khuzestan. They are given in Table C II 30 and Diagram C II 2 in the same manner as the data from Shiraz except that, for the reasons stated, we have not recombined sub-categories such as adults and children, male and female and have not calculated AV distribution for the reactively disordered because their number, when divided again by sex, becomes too small. A first glance reveals that the proportion of the introversionless is higher throughout than in Shiraz. If it ranged around 40 % in the city, it is nowhere lower than 55 % in the countryside and climbs to 60.3 % in the case of the men. We think again of a more demanding life in the rural villages, one that is not necessarily harder than the life of the city poor, but certainly one that entails more immediate perils of all degrees, more sudden minor and perhaps also major emergencies that must be met at the moment and against which initial introversive rejection or withdrawal is unavailing. The four AV distributions on the whole are bimodal, but the extratensive mode of the boys in Khuzestan, actually around A and therefore "extratensive" only by comparison, is substantially smaller than that of the boys in Shiraz. The mean AV_p is nevertheless more rather than less extratensive with 17e as against 10e in the city. The explanation must be sought in the higher rate of E (57 % to 37 %). The i:e ratio for the Khuzestani boys is 78:22 %, for the Shirazi boys 59:41 %. We see in the male Khuzestani youth a dichotomy rather than a true bimodality of attitude, which appears to become compensated in adulthood. Cohen and Schmidt [57] have presented rather interesting evidence for such dichotomization, using the Intraversion-Extraversion scale of the Eysenck Personality Questionnaire [75] with one hundred college students almost equally divided between the sexes. They hypothesized that on the IE scale "the midrange might include at least three types of individuals: a) those who fall into the midrange because of an indifference towards the types of activities described on the scale, here called indifferent types (IT); b) those who fall in the midrange because of strong, conflicting attitudes towards the various activities described, being very extraverted in some ways and introverted in others, called here the mixed type (MT); and c) those who fall in the midrange because of a genuine commitment to a midrange response . . . called here the ambiverted type." The "midrange" was defined as extending one standard deviation from the mean on the IE scale in either direction. Sixty-nine of the hundred participants fell into it. They were further evaluated on the neuroticism and "psychoticism" scales of the EPQ and by an activity preference scale. The latter "was constructed by converting each of the 21 items from EPQ IE scale from a question format into a statement format," to which the subject had to reply in two ways, indicating on a five point scale how frequently the statement was felt to be true for himself and how much disturbed he would feel if forced to change the frequency of the activity described by the statement. The first score was used to differentiate between ambivalent and moderate responsiveness, i.e. between the MT and the other groups, the second to differentiate between degrees of upsettingness, i.e. between the IT and the remaining groups. The 25 subjects assigned to the mixed type group scored significantly higher on the neuroticism scale than the combined two others, supporting the existence of this group as distinct from the ambiverted or indifferent. The authors do not refer to the possibility of true bimodality nor mention the literature dealing with it. The men's histogram is bimodal as in Shiraz, but the "extratensive" mode remains at A instead of piling up at 10e as it does in the city, and the extraversive shift from 17e in boyhood to 25e in manhood is greater than the displacement from 10e to 14e in Shiraz. E claims 60 %, little more than in boyhood, but the i:e ratio becomes 56:44 %, proving that the general increase in extraversion does not lie principally in its extreme or introversionless form. A certain counterbalance is not only maintained, but augmented. This may be reflected in a lower rate of reactive disorders in the adult men (6.3 %) than in the women (11.9 %; $0.20 > p > 0.10$) when the numbers in each sex and age group are taken as divisors rather than the total population. We shall return to this and propose an explanation when we have discussed the females.

Their distributions are bimodal in both age categories, but in the grown women the scales of introversion-extraversion have tipped as compared with Shiraz. If the Shirazi women had lost a large share of their introversion since girlhood, the Khuzestanis have rather gained or regained it. This is hardly reflected in the mean AV_p, which only shifts from 23e to 20e, but very decidedly in the change of the i:e ratio from 50:50 % to 70:30 %. In contrast to Shiraz, the Khuzestani women do not recruit pseudo-extraverts from the oncoming generation. The already high percentage of E remains practically unchanged at 56–57 %, while in the city it mounts from 33 % to 49 %. The difference is striking, demonstrates that generalization from Shiraz to the rest of Iran is inadmissible and calls for explanation. One socio-cultural difference is obvious and seems apt to provide it. The great majority of the Shirazi girls are literate (87 %), but an even greater majority of the village girls are not (in 1965 only 6 girls out of 70 = 8.5 % were literate). Moreover, the women of Shiraz at the same time were 50 % literate, while in our Khuzestani sample not one of the 308 grown women could read and write. All schools of Western type (and the Iranian public schools are basically of Western type, whatever differences may exist) conduce to extraversion and usually further or enforce it deliberately, often under the title of "adjustment". Rarely indeed are the gentle arts of introversion tolerated and almost never taught. This implies that at least half and with years more of the Shirazi females have been subject to a powerful extraverting influence that their sisters in the village, according to one's preference in the choice of terms, have missed or escaped. Therefore we find in them the traits of pseudo-extraversion described above. Are the Khuzestani women free of these? With their high E% such would be altogether unlikely. In regard to simple reactive disorder which we have taken as one sign we find practically no difference to the Shirazi. (In the following percentage comparisons we take, as explained above, the number of persons in the respective category as the divisor, not the total population, for which reason the rates do not agree with those in the general prevalence tables.) The Khuzestani women, however, display less neurotic plus psychosomatic disorder (7.9 %) than the Shirazi (12.0 %). When they do become neurotically or psychosomatically disturbed, on the other hand, they tend to become more severely so, the proportion of P_1 to P_2 cases in Khuzestan being 5:9 and in Shiraz 28:17 (there are no reactive cases of degree P_3 in these samples). The numbers are too small throughout to suffice for statistical significance (in the comparison of P_1 with P_2 X^2 is 2.05 and $0.20 > p > 0.10$), but the pattern is interesting, possibly meaningful and accords well with the equivocal influence of introversion. Preservation and cultivation of natural introversion is a necessary condition for mental health in persons of introversive disposition, and the consequences of its thwarting we have observed. On the other hand natural introversion facilitates repression and dissociation once these begin and thus is likely to lead to severer disturbance than when the same defense mechanisms become pathological in the extravert.

What, now, of the men in Khuzestan? In 1965 only 8 % of them were literate, in contrast to 57 % of the boys and youths by modest standards and to 89 % of the men in Shiraz. Neither for the men nor for the boys can any influence of the school in the direction of pseudo-extraversion be affirmed, for most of the men have never gone to school, and the girls, who seldom went, show the same rate for E as the boys, of whom over half attended. The high level of E must be attributed to some other factor acting on the whole Khuzestani population, a factor that may well be environmental as we have suggested above but could also be genetic. It is noticeable too that in spite of high E values CF is significantly less in the Khuzestani adults than in Shiraz. The boys in Khuzestan show on the whole more reactive disorders than the men (10.9 % as against 6.3 %), the women however (as in the city) more than the girls (11.9 % for the former, 4.3 % for the latter). Though the differences do not attain statistical significance, they give food for thought. In Khuzestan both female generations were still going through much the same process of maturation as far as formal education was concerned and in

Shiraz likewise, though not quite to the same extent. Not so the males. The men were almost wholly analphabetic, the boys divided. Besides this, the whole Dez Irrigation Pilot Area was on the threshold of a new phase of questionably assimilated development. It would not be difficult to see in such divergent educational influences, with all that they imply far beyond the schoolroom, at least one factor that could help to account for patterns of attitudinal development in Khuzestan that deviate from those we have met in the capital of Fars. Certainly the city too was undergoing change, but as the figures for literacy demonstrate the change, at least in this respect, had affected the generations and the sexes more equably. Despite this we observe that on the whole the Khuzestani youths shift in the same way as do the youths of Shiraz to enhanced extraversion in manhood and retain, apart from the introversionless, their essential bimodality. Their literate and illiterate components would require separate study if one were to venture any further conclusions, but they are too small for valid statistical comparison.

Our hypotheses concerning the effect of formal education on Iranian youth receive support from the work of previous investigators quoted in Section a of this chapter. Mehryar and his colleagues, it will be remembered, found that both youths and maidens from 13–15 years showed more introversion than their British counterparts on the Junior Maudsley Inventory, but as college students were both more extraverted and more neurotic than the British. Baraheni confirmed their greater extraversion, using the Eysenck Personality Inventory, did not find them more neurotic than the British, but like Mehryar did discover a sex difference inasmuch as the females had higher neuroticism scores. As we were working with primary and secondary school pupils, our Persian colleagues with secondary pupils and college students, the effect does not appear bound to any specific educational level.

Not without reservation we append kindred findings from the nomadic Qashqai and from Qalandari adults in Table C II 30. (Be it recalled that the inhabitants of Qalandari were themselves Qashqais who had settled there eight years before the survey and that our data represent a nearly complete census study of the little village, whereas our sample from the nomads comprised only about one-fifth of the sub-tribe and for extraneous reasons could not be drawn as systematically as we should have liked.) The numbers are themselves small for a distribution, and those for the children are omitted as being smaller yet. Both populations claim special interest because the morbidity rate in Qalandari was significantly lower than anywhere else in our investigations hitherto and because in the nomad sample we encountered no pathological case at all. It would be intriguing to discover a common denominator, but we have not found one in this table (a common denominator of tribal origin and structure nevertheless exists). It is remarkable that in Qalandari there is only one totally coarctated adult subject, but this paucity does not apply to the nomads. The AV distributions are bimodal throughout with a tendency to extraversion as strong as elsewhere except in the Qashqai men, who also yield the lowest E percent among our various collectives. This does not hold for the women, but we cannot be sure that this is not an artefact of sampling. Only one of the four groups has been subject directly to much schooling: the men of Qalandari. Thirty-nine percent of them had become literate, largely as a result of an intensive adult education program in the village. Only two of the 43 boys and youths in Qalandari were not attending school. Thus among the men in Qalandari we find a distribution not unlike that in Khuzestan: a high E%, but an i:e ratio of 64:36 %, suggesting that one part has succumbed to pseudo-extraversion while another has preserved its introversive resources. Both, according to our epidemiological findings, have remained largely free from manifest mental disorder. Most of the girls (16 out of 22) were attending school in Qalandari, but only 5 % of the grown women were literate. In the nomad sample none were. Since the two adult female groups are predominantly extratensive both in their mean AV and in their i:e ratio (Qashqai 38:62, Qalandari 41:59) it would be easy to construe out of this a contradiction to our hypothesis about the influence of non-education on girls in Khuzestan. It must be recalled, however, that the conditions of the nomad and the village woman's life are vastly different. Few of the Qashqai girls attended the tent school, but 46 of the 50 boys did.

When boys and men are combined in Shiraz the pattern of AV distribution changes little, fundamentally hardly at all. Fusion of the girls and women leads to apparent bimodality because of the numerical overweight of the latter but confuses or disguises the highly important difference. The like holds for the combination of adult men and women, whereas boys and girls together display the same bimodality that they do separately. Lastly, when we take the whole urban non-disordered sample we find bimodality as in three of its four principal components with a common AV_p = 15e. Over-inclusive pictures such as this, however, must be regarded with caution and treated with discrimination.

As the question naturally had presented itself whether reactive mental disorder would influence either the representative attitudinal values, as schizophrenia has been shown to do [182], or their distribution in comparison with the undisordered members of the same urban population, we have treated these values apart from the rest, omitting the few childhood cases. Both for male and female adults we find the same bimodality as in the non-disordered, modes and troughs at the same places, but mean attitudinal values that in both sexes are several points less extratensive than those of the corresponding non-disordered adult groups (male ND 14e, Dr 11e; female ND 21e, Dr 16e). As in both sexes we have observed a shift towards extraversion in adulthood, this can be understood in general as a manifestation of regression.

A word of caution must be added regarding the shift toward extraversion just mentioned. While studies by the AV method are lacking, a number of competent authors have commented on the experience balance in children. We summarize their findings and opinions from Bohm's *Vademecum* [42], where the sources are stated. Rorschach himself found a tendency to coarctation in children of school age and to ambiequality in puberty, followed by variability in adulthood and inclination to introversion around 30 and 50–55 years. Loosli-Usteri finds children's experience balances to be on the whole extratensive-coarctative. According to her the introversionless balance (O:X or E) is much more common in children than in adults, which does not hold for our Shiraz findings, and an introversive balance is said to be rare. Weber remarks merely that the balance is more labile in children than in adults. Dworetzki finds from about 8 years on a gradual decrease of color and increase of movement responses – a tendency rather the opposite to what we have observed in Shiraz. Van Krevelen confirms Loosli-Usteri in the age classes from 7 to 14 years, after which he finds an introversive-coarctative experience balance with a mean of 1.1 : 0.6 (= 16i). Generalizations from the Shirazi data therefore are inadmissible, and explanations for them must be sought in the specific socio-cultural circumstances under which they were obtained.

In Table C II 31 we offer comparative mean attitudinal values from various Iranian and foreign populations for what they are worth. Where the sexes are treated separately, the attitudinal values have been corrected by elimination of the totally coarctated, as explained. This accounts for some rather odd Ns such as 1a, 1b and 2a, where the number of subjects tested were 100, 100 and 50 respectively. Both of Loosli-Usteri's groups are noteworthy because this author took unusual care to exclude abnormal subjects, whereas many statistics pertaining to "normals" are derived more or less from whosoever volunteered and was not obviously disturbed. The correction was possible because the respective authors and institutions kindly placed their original data at the disposal of the first writer, for which he renders due thanks. Wittenberg's data he received by personal communication. They were obtained by having each subject lay three color pyramids according to Pfister-Heiss [167] composed of fifteen squares of colored paper apiece, then counting the "introversive" (blue and green) and the "extraversive" colors (red and yellow).

Table C II 31. Mean Attitudinal Values for Comparison: Theoretical and Practical Notation

	N	AV_t	SD	AV_p	Test[a]
1. Male					
a. Institute of Applied Psychology, Zürich. Police aspirants.	93	47.8	29.0	3i	Ro
b. Loosli-Usteri. Normal Swiss adults.	99	43.1	26.6	2e	Ro
c. R. Kuhn. Swiss army recruits.	1205	41.1	28.2	4e	Ro
d. J. J. Wittenberg. Dutch KLM employees.	471	32.5		12e	Pf
e. Bash. Non-disordered adults from Shiraz.	118	30.6	31.2	14e	Z
f. Bash. Non-disordered adults from Qalandari.	41	21.0	29.6	22e	Z
2. Female					
a. Institute of Applied Psychology, Zürich. Applicants for vocational guidance.	49	48.1	24.7	3i	Ro
b. Loosli-Usteri. Normal Swiss adults.	57	44.6	25.4	A	Ro
c. J. J. Wittenberg. Dutch KLM employees.	190	41.4		4e	Pf
d. Bash. Non-disordered adults from Shiraz.	118	24.3	28.2	21e	Z
e. Bash. Non-disordered adults from Qalandari.	42	24.4	26.7	21e	Z
3. Both sexes, non-disordered and disordered					
a. Bash. Shiraz adults.	318	27.5	29.9	17e	Z
b. Bash. Qalandari adults.	87	22.8	28.0	22e	Z
c. Bash. Qashqai adults.	112	25.2	28.8	20e	Z
d. Bash. Khuzestan adults.	296	24.2	25.8	21e	Z
e. Nowparast. Tehran students.	145	73.2		281	Ro
f. Beck. American norms.		48.4		3i	Ro

[a] Ro = Rorschach; Z = Zulliger or Z Test; Pf = Pfister-Heiss Color Pyramid Test.

Our own data for the sexes combined in Part 3 of Table C II 31 are corrected, while those of Nowparast and Beck are not. Nowparast mentions that 88 of his volunteer student group were male and 57 female but does not give separate values for the two sexes. From his summarily stated "composite experience balance" of 8.01:2.42 we have derived the AV of 23i in our table. It is remarkable for its high rate of introversion such as is not even approximated anywhere else so far as we know, though not so remarkable when one has become acquainted with a considerable number of Iranian students. One would like very much to know how many of his volunteers were extraversionless, not only introversionless, and what sex differences, if any, appeared. For comparison we have sought out the Z Tests of the seven students in our Shiraz sample. Four were women, three men, and one of each sex had a totally constricted experience balance. The male student who did was also a pathological case, a neurotic of degree P_1. The mean for the remaining two male students was AV_p = 3i, for the three female students 5e, for the five together 1e or practically ambiequal.

The succession could not be satisfactorily determined in such a large majority of the records with their relatively few responses that we have abandoned any attempt to relate its several types statistically to our groups and categories.

e. Shock. This brings us to the subject of shock. Rorschach knew and described shock as it occurred in his test and realized that it could exhibit varying degrees. His friend and collaborator Oberholzer introduced the expression "*larvierter Schock*", which can be translated as masked or disguised shock, in a publication a few years after Rorschach's death [160]. The distinction between manifest and disguised shock is generally accepted in European practice, though it is not always well defined and has engendered some controversy, to enter into which would be beyond the scope of this book. Binder has preferred to speak of "masked complexes" and has argued that the so-called masked or disguised shock is really no shock at all, but an evasion of color or shading (*Farbenflucht*). It seems agreed on the whole that manifest shock, whether pertaining to color, shading, kinesthesia or white space, is one of the best indications of neurosis, with the reservation that not every neurosis must exhibit shock. Disguised shock too may point to neurosis, though of lighter degree, but mainly to neurotic tendency or to what Schultz-Hencke [177] has aptly called neurotoid structure – the matrix of neuroses. The distinction again is not altogether sharp, but in practice useful nonetheless. We have retained it here, taking as signs of manifest shock open verbal or obvious non-verbal expressions of aversion to one of the determinants just mentioned, to white space, to a new card or a new content in general, a startle reaction, a rejection or, on the contrary and as so-called compensated manifest shock, equally open and obvious expressions of liking followed by inability to come to terms with the card. For disguised shock there are a large number of signs which can be found singly or more often in combination such as prolonged reaction time, facial expressions or gestures of dislike, use of the white space instead of the blot for the first answer to a card, sudden drop in number and quality of responses in comparison to those preceding and succeeding, manifestations of embarrassment, singular sexual responses as first answer to a card and many more, for which the reader must be referred to the standard literature.

Since shock accurs usually on the presentation of a card (though there is also a "delayed shock" as second answer) and the Z Test comprises only three cards it offers

Table C II 32. Frequency of Shocks in Z Test Records from Shiraz and Qalandari

	Shiraz Non-Disordered			Shiraz React. Disordered			Qalandari Non-Disordered			Sign. Diff.	
	N	n	%	N	n	%	N	n	%	SH ND: SH Dr	SH ND: QL ND
	One Shock, Disguised										
Men	131	33	25	19	10	53	41	18	44	‹‹	‹
Women	127	34	27	51	21	41	38	12	32	‹	
Boys	52	12	23	13	4	31	33	13	39		‹
Girls	73	20	27	8	4	50	22	5	23	(‹)	
All	383	99	26	91	39	43	134	48	36	‹‹‹	‹
	All Shocks, Manifest and Disguised										
Men	131	56	42	19	15	79	41	27	66	‹‹	‹‹
Women	127	54	43	51	29	57	38	14	37	‹	
Boys	52	19	37	13	8	62	33	17	52	‹	(‹)
Girls	73	30	41	8	7	87	22	9	41	‹‹	
All	383	159	42	91	59	65	134	67	50	‹‹‹	‹

Key: SH = Shiraz; QL = Qalandari; ND = Non-Disordered; Dr = Reactively Disordered; N = number of subjects whose tests were evaluated; n = number of subjects exhibiting specified shock phenomena (explanation see text); % = (n x 100) : N.

less opportunity for detailed analysis of shocks by number, place, kind and degree and of their interference with each other than does the Rorschach Test, in which such analysis plays a role of the highest importance. After trying a number of categorical schemes for statistical treatment of shock phenomena in the Z Test we reduced them to three: 1. records with no indications of shock, 2. records with indications of one disguised or masked shock, 3. records with more than one disguised shock, with manifest shock(s) or with both. Actually this implies only two categories, for the first category is given by subtraction of the other two from the total. Furthermore, the second category can be subtracted from the third to give the number of more seriously disturbed records. For simplicity's sake therefore we show in Table C II 32 only the second and third categories. Be it noted that no regard is taken to the presumptive origin of the shock in a reaction to color, shading, kinesthesia, white space or specific content. Important though this is in invidual diagnostic practice, it proved impracticable in records taken by lay workers. For brevity and convenience we shall speak below of subjects with "one shock" (upper half of the table) and imply thereby a single disguised shock, and of subjects with "all shocks" (lower half) with the implication that the single disguised shock of the upper half is included in the lower.

Several working assumptions must be made explicit. One of these is that the disguised shock especially in its lighter forms often corresponds to the mere evasion of color (or shading etc.) that Binder, not without good grounds, declines to call a "shock" at all and that he, again with good grounds, considers to be a sign of repression, but not of dissociation. Only when the firm barrier of dissociation is broken through, he argues, is such an abrupt and vehement disturbance manifested in the record that one is justified in speaking of a "shock". This carries theoretical and practical implications, for it will be remembered that according to Binder's definition, which we follow on the whole, the two defenses of repression and dissociation constitute the necessary and sufficient conditions for a neurosis. Both are necessary, but neither by itself is sufficient. Repression alone, often expressed as color evasion, conduces to simple pathological development but does not suffice for neurosis, for which the further condition of dissociation must be fulfilled. Neurosis must not lead to shock in the Rorschach or Z Test, but a manifest shock, according to Binder, is always a sign of neurosis.

For several practical reasons we deviate somewhat from this strict interpretation. We find more manifest shocks than manifest neuroses (about double the number) and more disguised shocks than relevant simple pathological developments. This does not invalidate Binder's theoretical position but probably reflects only our inevitably more superficial examination of subjects and some reticence, such as seems called for in epidemiology, in adjudgment of open psychopathology. Binder's views were derived from intensive study of clinical cases. We do not controvert, but rather modify them to apply to a probably large number of sub-clinical cases which, under the given conditions and limitations, we did not and could not identify. Another reason for modification is the now well established fact that shock phenomena of all kinds are so widely spread and so frequent in undoubted normals that they are neither pathological in themselves nor, in all probability, pathognomonic. Thus Loosli-Usteri [127, 128] found shocks of all degrees, including very slight and disguised ones, in some 50 % of her normal men and even in 70 % of her normal women.

The absence of shock seems on the whole to tell us rather more than does its presence, though in our own experience Binder seems to be in the right when he holds that a neurosis must not manifest itself in a shock. An investigation into these questions on the basis of our own material will have to be reserved for the future. Our working hypothesis may be stated as follows: A disguised shock proves neither a simple pathological reaction or development nor a neurosis, but is suggestive of proneness to both, especially the former. It is an indication of the neurotoid structure referred to already, which like complexes, every person has, but in different degrees. The degree is presumably higher in the case of manifest shock, higher still in the presence of more than one, and may be estimated in the individual case by the intensity of the disguised shock and its approximation to a manifest one. For statistical treatment the inclusion of such nuances is unsuitable. The term "latent neurosis" carries far-reaching and dangerous implications, and we therefore eschew it. Rather do we look upon disguised shocks as tentative indicators of a more strongly neurotoid structure, of a reduction in natural immunity, of a certain liability first to simple pathological reactions and developments, which may have taken place already, then on the basis of these to true neurosis. Conversely manifest shock or an accumulation of disguised shocks raise the suspicion of at least sub-clinical neurosis but do not demonstrate it. What is "sub-clinical" depends, of course, on the "clinic". The threshold will be lower in the true clinic than in the field.

Turning at last to our own table we find in both halves an unmistakable corroboration of our main thesis that shock of all kinds, disguised or manifest, is a valid indicator of reactive emotional disturbance. This is evident from the last line of both halves, where the frequency of shock in the reactively disordered of Shiraz proves to be very significantly higher than in the non-disordered as a whole. It is higher too for "all shocks" in all sub-populations defined by age and sex, as it is for the adult in regard to "one shock", whereas there is no significant difference in regard to "one shock" for the boys and only a tendency for the girls. The numbers in both children's groups, however, are small. On the other hand the non-disordered, as mentioned above, are by no means free of shock either manifest or disguised, though the total percentages are somewhat lower than Loosli's, especially for the women. In Shiraz the frequency of "one shock" is nearly the same for all four sex and age categories and lies around one quarter. In Qalandari it is higher, especially for the men, with an overall frequency of 36 % as against 26 % for Shiraz, and this difference is significant at the 5 % level. For "all shocks" the rates in the non-disordered of Shiraz are again fairly uniform and range slightly over 40 % (the difference between the boys' rate of 37 % and the girls' of 41 % is not significant). In Qalandari they are distinctly higher for the men, with a tendency for the boys, and this is enough to constitute a significant difference at the 5 % level for the two non-disordered populations compared with each other. The fact that this difference obtains only between the men is interesting, and we shall revert to it below. Returning to Shiraz, it is noteworthy that in both half-tables the shocks among the disordered women are not more numerous than among the men (the two percent difference for "one shock" is insignificant). Since there are proportionally nearly twice as many neurotic females as males in Shiraz, one could argue from this that the women's pseudo-extraversion is not an essentially neurotic phenomenon, the more so as the percentage of reactively disordered men with more than one or a disguised shock reaches 79, but that of the women only 57, and the difference is significant at the 5 % level of confidence. The difference between boys and girls runs in the opposite direction and approaches a so-called "tendency" with $p < 0.11$. In the reactively disordered with more than one shock the Shirazi girls not only have a strikingly higher percentage (87) of records with such shocks than the women (57 %), but the difference, although based on only 8 children's cases, turns out to be significant with $p < 0.05$. It would be inconsistent and illogical to deny any connection between the facts and the hypothesized tendency of at least a major part of the female sex in Shiraz to develop from introversion into pseudo-extraversion, but this confronts us immediately with a seeming contradiction: the just mentioned substantial preponderance, in Shiraz, of female over male neurotics. The contradiction resolves itself when we analyze the distribution of all reactive disorders, not only of neuroticism, in the city. The sexes share about equally in the psychosomatic disturbances. Females have nearly twice as much neurosis as males, but seven times as many simple reactive developments (2 male cases to 14 female). Furthermore, all the simple developments were diagnosed in adults, whereas instances of childhood neurosis were by no means lacking in either sex. This harmonizes very well both with the significant drop in frequency of "all shocks" in the disordered between girlhood and womanhood (the numerical rise from boyhood to manhood in the disordered and the minor age shifts among the non-disordered are not statistically significant or even close to that) and with the statistically demonstrable tendency to a difference in "all shocks" between disordered boys and girls (the girls leading). Re-stated theoretically: the tendency to neuroticism as indicated by shocks of all kinds and degrees in the Z Test is greater in the Shirazi girls than in the boys, but during maturation a considerable part of the girls make or undergo an attitudinal transition from introversion into pseudo-extraversion. Therefore if they fall into reactive disorder, this constitutes much more often than among the men a simple development and not a neurosis. We may quote again Binder's remark that "they (sc.

the introverts) are helpless against singular strongly emotionally toned impressions, which the introvert either dissociates so that they become crystallization points for neurotic complexes, or in reference to which he abandons his inital rejection so that he can even enter into an exclusive, exaggerated relation to the respective singular phenomena of his environment" (cf. p 296). The latter is exactly what occurs in the simple reactive development. Needless to say, not all the pseudo-extraversive women take the one or the other of these unhappy courses, though it would require a more detailed study, e.g. a comparison with their answers to the psychiatric questionnaire, to determine whether in general they attained a level of mental health and freedom from complaint equal to the rest.

The "well" or non-disordered of Qalandari now present us with some problems and surprises of their own. (There are not enough disordered to permit comparison either intra- or interlocally.) Whereas the non-disordered men and women of Shiraz have approximately the same number of disguised shocks, the men and boys of Qalandari have significantly more than those of Shiraz (44 % as against 25 %). Their difference to the women of the same village falls short of statistical significance but reaches it comfortably when all shocks are considered. Nearly the converse holds among the village children, where the boys display at least a statistical tendency toward more "one shock" than the girls, but the difference between boys and girls for "all shocks" together is insignificant. A similar constellation obtains for "all shocks" as compared between village and city, but is more accentuated: the men's difference becomes more highly significant, the boys' less, and the overall interlocal difference remains significant at the 5 % level as before. As psychiatric prevalence rates are significantly lower for Qalandari than for Shiraz, it would be natural to expect a lower rather than higher shock frequency also, but the expectation is not fulfilled. The explanation, according to Tables C II 24 d and C II 25, must be sought among the men. It will be recalled that both in respect to other Z Test variables such as T, W, W+, FC (all diminished) and Do, Pl, SUM CHRO (all increased) and to responses on the psychiatric questionnaire we encountered a number of indications of latent tensions, of mostly sublimated and compensated conflicts in Qalandari such as frequently show themselves already in a disguised or single shock. The on the whole voluntary profound alteration of the Qalandari villagers' way of life from nomadic to sedentary within (then) recent time seems to have been accomplished successfully, even highly successfully as far as overt mental disturbance goes, but it would be a matter for wonder if it left no traces. The Z Test, we contend, reveals these. It is natural that they should appear more in the adults, to whom this change in life is a conscious vivid memory, than in the children, to the younger of whom it is at most a dim one, and more in the men, who are more affected, than in the women. In regard to such socio-cultural changes Louise Spindler [184; quoted from Bourguignon 43, p. 318] "found that significant differences exist between the adaptations of men and women. . . . Women experience less conflict and turmoil in the acculturation process than men do, as shown in life history interviews and test data. Combining the data for men and women distorts the picture [185]. Because women continue to play traditional roles to a much greater extent than men, their roles and values are much less directly challenged by the acculturation process. In contrast, the men must, to a significantly greater extent, acquire new skills and new value orientations. Moreover, among the Menomini, even under traditional conditions, the roles of women were much more flexible than those of men.

As a result, in the new situation they experienced much greater continuity in the expectations placed on them than was true for the men. This situation in turn often has resulted in a difference in degree of acculturation among spouses, which has heightened the conflicts experienced by the men." What the Spindlers found applied to a Northern American Indian tribe applies no less, in our experience, to the Qashqai tribe of Iranian nomads, including the greater flexibility of the women's roles. Barth [14], writing on the related Basseri, is quite explicit about this, and we can confirm it from our own observation. This greater flexibility, be it noted well, does not hold for the women's roles in the Iranian villages, and in the cities at most for an extremely small well-educated upper class. Returning to the men, we recall that in this group and in this one alone we observed in Tables C II 24 c and C II 25 a highly significant increase in SUM CHIA, just as we now observe significantly more shocks. Binder's remark [37, p. 141] is relevant here: "In the case of mild occasional 'complex moods' the number of shading responses is not substantially heightened and their contents are usually emotionally indifferent. The more the number of shading responses rises, the more do affectively toned contents increase and the more noticeable becomes a slight tendency to perseveration of such responses leading over into the picture of a one-sidedly dysphoric emotional lability which, when the affectively laden shading responses multiply still further, passes without sharp boundary into the picture of an incessant neurotic moodiness. In clinical observation it corresponds to these experimental findings that the complexes react more and more frequently, intensively and perpetually and influence the mood correspondingly until a veritable displacement of it occurs." Salomon, in express agreement with Binder's phenomenological description, proposes an explanation and draws inferences from it that seem pertinent here. He seeks the genesis of the shading responses in the infant's very early diffuse sensory experience, in which the mother's face, not yet distinguished as such, is probably the first lighter visual object before a shadowy background. Anxiety arises when that relative luminosity associated with warmth and nourishment recedes and shadow occupies the field. Thus all shading answers are laden to differing degrees, from mildly dysphoric to threatening, with unconscious remniscences that imperil security and self-confidence. Salomon concludes therefore [174, p. 51] that shading responses, "wherever they occur ultimately are evidence of inner doubts of the responder's own self-esteem. They mirror in summary the history of his more or less frustrated object relations." Frustrated object relations are a common denominator of all the grown men of Qalandari. Even though the frustration was voluntarily undertaken, consciously accepted on the whole (we cannot say with how many tacit exceptions and under what pressures), has procured visible rewards and has kept manifest mental disorder on a level below that of other Iranian villages, it would be bold indeed to suppose that there were no lingering doubts, no latent questions of self-esteem when the nomad, proud of his independence and large, though not unlimited freedom, determines to become an husbandman. Should they not be reflected in the shading responses and the shocks that go with them?

Part D Comparisons and Conclusions

I. Differential Psychology

In nearly all the chapters of Part C questions of differential psychology have been treated and summarized for the respective methods of investigation. The Z Test, in itself more complex than the other methods and productive of more complex results, has remained in part an exception. These treatments have furnished us with a kind of warp, to which comparisons across methods, such as we shall attempt below, form the woof. As the threads have been strung and to some extent patterned already, we shall be brief, presenting little numerical data anew, but rather referring to partial conclusions hitherto evinced by or derived from them and endeavoring to weave them together.

The principal differential psychological questions we take to be those of sex, age, education, socio-economic status and environment. "Environment" comprises not only localities, but also and much more than this social structures, cultural frameworks and ethnic affiliations with all their manifold implications. Needless to say, we cannot enter into all of these. Our emphasis will be as heretofore principally on the differences, as far as such are ascertainable, between rural, urban and nomadic groups.

1. Sex

Immediately there comes to mind the wide and clear cut difference between the performance of male and female subjects on Western type tests of intelligence in Iran – a difference that subsists whether the test be of verbal or performance type, the latter including the simple and familiar Draw-A-Man (and Woman) and whether the subject be illiterate or literate. This latter point we take to be of particular importance, for it could be argued easily that, given equal educational opportunities including co-education, the sex difference in intelligence test performance would vanish. In Iran it does not, nor is it substantially diminished. When male norms are applied to test results of females the difference of about five IQ points remains whether we compare the illiterates or the literates of the same sex. The rather evident socio-cultural reasons for this have been discussed in Part C, Chap. 2 and need not be repeated here. It is more important to note that the ingrained cultural depreciation of female intelligence in Iran proves itself hitherto to be stronger than the emancipating effect of education even where this is provided and, as in Shiraz, fairly widely utilized. It holds also at higher educational and socio-cultural levels, though here exceptions do make their appearance. This is nearly the one finding on which all psychological investigators in Iran, native and foreign, are unanimous, the other being that Iranian subjects on the whole tend to perform very much less well on Western type tests of intelligence than

Western subjects do. The obvious consequence is a fresh standardization on any and all intelligence tests (of Western type, but are there others?) and separate standardizations for the two sexes in Iran, unjust though this is to a minority of genuinely emancipated intellectually capable women. The injustice can be compensated by applying to them the male norms.

Sex differences in best and worst memories have been summarized in Part C, Chap. II 1 b. They offer little that is surprising, corresponding mostly to stereotyped sex roles familiar throughout the patriarchal world. The men are concerned with work and sustenance in the widest sense: achievement, harvest, land reform on the pleasurable side, poverty, debt and unemployment on the other, but also with their own good health or recovery from illness and with ill treatment at others' hands. This last covers a wide range from a beating by parent or teacher over being ground down by creditor or landowner to and through robbery and thievery, sometimes by those appointed to safeguard against it. It is noticeable that bereavement other than loss of an own child stands high among the men's worst memories, but not among the women's. For these, immediate bio-social and familial relationships are more important: pregnancy and childbirth (but for the rural women only), birth of siblings (for the urban only), reunion with relatives or friends; on the sorrowful side unwanted pregnancy or child, divorce, to which come outright fears. The surprise enters when we note that fear of failure in school or examinations is one of the consistently worst memories for the (younger) women, be it that they are cowed by the oft expressed depreciation of female intelligence mentioned above, be it that the more circumspect are well aware that success in school is almost the only way out of the enthrallment that to their mothers has been a matter of course for centuries. Fewer girls than boys have an opportunity to go to school, and probably more are withdrawn before completing the rural six grades, so that failure endangers them.

On the complaint score (affirmative responses to items from the psychiatric questionnaire, Table C II 18) the adult women register markedly higher than the men everywhere except in Khuzestan (we shall return to the children in the next chapter). Regardless of age, female respondents give more positive answers to the psychiatric questions than do male except for Q 7 "excitement". It seems impossible to say whether we meet here with a fact (i.e. that the males are actually more exciteable, which we personally doubt) or with a cultural stereotype, which allows the male to confess to excitement (much more than in Anglo-European cultures), but not to fear, the more so as this reversal of the common cultural gradient is found in one place only (Marvdasht). In Qassemabad it still held in 1976 for the children, but not for the adults. The tendency to hear "voices" is stronger among the men in Khuzestan, among women in Marvdasht and among the Qashqai, but the difference is a local rather than sexual one. The city displays no sex difference in this regard. Another local difference to be commented upon below is the tendency (statistically no more than this) for the boys of Qalandari to complain more of depression and of estrangement than the girls. There is no appreciable difference between their elders.

It is interesting to observe that the women, contrary to popular belief, are not on the whole more superstitious than the men, but only in certain places (Marvdasht, Qalandari, Qashqai) and circumstances (the middle class, but neither the poor nor the well-to-do in Shiraz). To this we shall return from time to time.

The Z Test presents hardly any sex differences that are valid for all or nearly all the surveys. The non-disordered men in Shiraz took less time than the women, but this may well be an artefact of the testing situation. The Shirazi men gave more O+, the women more chiaroscuro, the men being probably less conformist, the women more subject to anxiety and fear, as indeed they tell us directly in their responses to the questionnaire. More sex differences appear among the reactively disordered. Such men in the city give more W and W+; they also have more psychosomatic disorders, the women more simple pathological developments, and in Part C, Chap. II 3 c we have endeavored to trace the connection between them. It seemed probable that the disordered women's deficit in W and W+ was really an excess of Dd and Do disguised only by the lesser numbers of the latter, and that these in turn corresponded to the women's openly expressed anxiety. In Shiraz the women were numerically more extraverted than the men, but the difference is statistically significant only among the disordered. In Qalandari the relationship is reversed by a small, insignificant margin. There are not a few indications in good agreement with each other that this apparent sex difference in Shiraz derives actually from a different pattern of maturation for boys and girls inasmuch as a substantial number of the latter assume an attitude of pseudo-extraversion. Once more the difference is environmental rather than sex-specific and shall be considered under that aspect.

2. Age

As our intelligence test was standardized as an age-grade scale, no comment is called for beyond that given in appropriate Part C, Chap. I.

So far as good and bad memories are concerned, the harvest of age differences valid across all surveys is no greater than that of sex differences and on the whole confirms the obvious. Thus it is obvious that adults significantly more than children should recall their engagement or marriage as their happiest memory, children more than adults getting playthings or presents, family celebrations, success in school, and at first glance it seems equally obvious that they should more often say that they possess no ill memories. There is food for reflection, though, in the circumstance that only the literate children affirm this significantly more than their parents as there is in the further circumstance that only the women affirm that they have no pleasurable memory more often than their daughters, but not the fathers more often than their sons. Do the literate children have less to complain of, since they come on the average from better situated homes, or do they become schooled in reticence – an hypothesis that seems by no means untenable, since practically any schooling consists of more than a simple accumulation of knowledge? The question is more complicated than its formulation here suggests, as we have shown in the relevant chapter, to which the reader must be referred. Probably both factors operate, and more besides. The sad lot of a great many adult females probably affords explanation enough for their denial of any happy memory even in childhood, for such happy childhood memories as do exist can become either heightened by contrast or obliterated. More than adults, children report as their worst memory separation – an unsurprising consequence of the breaking of tender emotional ties. Among children we naturally encounter more non-responders to our biographical question as they are endowed both with less biography and with less reflection upon it. Equivalent thereto, at least in part, is the more frequent denial among children of both happy and unhappy memories with the restrictions mentioned above.

The complaint score of children is in every instance lower than that of adults of the same sex. The difference tends to become small for the females of Khuzestan, less so for the males. In respect to the single questions of the psychiatric questionnaire this rule is broken for Q 7 "excitement", as it was broken for this same question in regard to sex. The simple reason for that lies, as we suspect and have detailed in the apposite place, in the harmless exuberance which childhood both enjoys and is more ready to confess. Other reasons may lie in children's fears and terrors such as the formulation e.g. of Q 8 tends to exclude.

Differences in Z Test variables and their patterns between youth and adulthood in both Shiraz and Qalandari are few in the male sex, but abundant in the female, as we have mentioned in passing above. The men give less Dd and less FC+: the common denominator could be some loss both of emotional adaptability and of youth's fascination with details that possess for it physiognomic attributes. The women lose not their Dd, but their W and rise compensatorily in their number of D, reflecting a matter-of-factness that is enjoined by necessity upon all but the well-to-do. This is confirmed by more F and a higher F+%, less FC+, MC, SUM KINA and Pl, i.e. a general constriction both of the type of approach and of the type of experience, which at the same times shifts from 10e in girlhood to 21e in womanhood. It has been noted above that the grown women give numerically more Hd; one need hardly be surprised if a touch of melancholy accompanies the constriction. The male sex suffers some constriction also in its progress from childhood to adulthood, but less, and with small shift of its mean attitudinal value (from only 10e to 14e), i.e. substantially less pseudo-extraversion. Among the reactively disordered of Shiraz it is noteworthy that the alteration in D is opposite to that of the non-disordered, diminishing in womanhood, while among the unpathological it increases. Girl children, but not boys, interpret significantly more popular responses than their parents.

When we calculate not the absolute values of the modes of approach, but their shares within the whole type of approach, the young of both sexes have more wholes in relation to the total, the adults more details, whereas the sum of Dd + Do decreases in adulthood. The D being prime representatives of reality, these changes together could imply if not a constriction, at any event a concentration upon that which is immediately, practically given.

Shock phenomena in the Z Test exhibit significant age differences only among the disordered of Shiraz and in Qalandari. In the former the men have more shocks, both "one" and "all", than the boys, but in the female sex the differential is reversed. We have related this to the different patterns of development and maturation for the two sexes, leading into more simple developments in the women, but more neurosis and psychosomatic illness in the men. In Qalandari the non-disordered men have more shocks than the boys, but the females show no age differential; the explanation is to be sought in the recent history of the "new village".

3. Literacy and Socio-Economic Status

These two not unrelated variables may be considered together, the more so as we have few data on the differential psychology of literacy vs. illiteracy per se.

As the intelligence tests were standardized separately for illiterates and literates, no numerical comparisons can be drawn. The scatter histograms of the intelligence quotients for males show a hump left of the mean around IQ 85–90 for the illiterates, for the literates somewhat more higher than medium scores tailing off fairly regularly to the right. For the illiterate females the peak of the skewed normal distribution is at 85–90 where the males' "hump" was and is more pronounced than the inconspicuous peak of the literate females at 95–100. Indeed their vertex is practically flat from 95–105, and again as in the literate males we see somewhat more higher scores tailing off to the right than lower scores dropping rather abruptly at 85 to the left. The "hump" just mentioned may be a deficiency of the test. For the rest it seems evident that even with separate standardization the literate exhibit a somewhat greater number and range of superior test performances.

Because of unavoidable limitations in our time and resources we have refrained from separate tabulations of the psychiatric questionnaires and the Z Test in regard to literacy as well as to SES, the more so as study of the best and worst memories in respect to literacy proved even more informative than we had hoped. The results are given in detail at the beginning of Chap. II 1 b, Part C. Briefly, when we pool sexes and ages and differentiate by literacy only we observe that as expected going to or succeeding in school was often the best, being withdrawn from or failing in school often the worst memory for the literates, though naturally not for the rest. The finding itself and the often impressive formulation of the answers demonstrate the subjective value placed upon education by those to whom it is not a matter of course. Beyond that the literate of both sexes more frequently recalled engagement and marriage than pregnancy and childbirth as their happiest memory, more often job satisfaction and also military service (officers!). Their worst memories were less often of own ill health or bodily accident, but more of such of family or friends, less often of financial difficulties or debt (here the rough correlation with SES comes into play). We remark here a tendency for the literate to attribute higher value to aspects and events of life that are less strictly corporeal and egocentric. This receives a not unexpected, but in its degree striking corroboration from the very pronounced tendency of the literate to cite as their happiest recollection some form of accomplishment beyond the direly necessary and to remember travel and repose in the same fashion. It is easy to answer that they possessed more of such amenities, as they unquestionably did, but the question is also worth asking whether on the whole their ability to look beyond the narrowest horizon did not also further their acquisition of literacy and through this of a generally better SES as well. Altogether unsurprising is that the illiterate far more often deny having any happy memory at all, further, that they much more often confess to belief in magic. Fewer literate women believe in magic than literate men.

The differential psychology of the poor could be investigated only in Shiraz, where there were enough non-poor for contrast, and was investigated only by the intelligence test for reasons given. Added to these, it seems unlikely that much could have been gained by including the memories and the psychiatric questionnaire: the answers are too obvious. More might come out of the Z Test, but for practical reasons such study will have to be postponed. The poor of every group, whether male or female, literate or illiterate, achieve significantly lower mean IQs than the non-poor. Literacy does not cancel or overweigh the effects of poverty, and poverty only by exception sharpens the wits. Poverty cannot be interpreted here as a consequence of illiteracy since we meet with the same drop in mean IQ in the poor whether they be literate or not. A seeming paradox occurs when we compare the illiterate poor with the literate poor: the former have a significantly better mean IQ by 2.6 points. The suspicion seems entirely justified that among those who remain poor despite the advantage of literacy there are disproportionately more who have barely achieved formal literacy and are in fact practically illiterate or else unable to turn their literacy to any advantage. A certain number will be prevented from doing so by ill fate, as others remain illiterate through no choice of their own, but a margin of untalented school children remains, or rather falls behind in Iran as elsewhere. The same comparison between the non-poor leaves the illiterate with a numerical advantage of 1.3 IQ points which is not even statistically significant but may suggest that the illiterate who rise above poverty are a trifle cleverer on the whole than those who do not.

4. Environment

As explained in Part C, Chap. I 6, broad comparisons of intellectual performance can be made only on the basis of Arithmetic Test A, for only this test was used alike in all surveys. When we do so for the men we come upon few significant environmental differences. Such are demonstrable for the Shirazi age class 20–39 against the Qashqai and the age class of 40–59 against the Marvdashti. We shall meet below with plentiful support for the hypothesis that city life stimulates the exercise of intelligence, but it is far from clear why the differences emerge in just these places and in just these age classes. For the nomads one could indeed surmise that they are most remote from urban influence, and for Marvdasht one could invoke the special situation of those villages at the time they were surveyed, which also will become more apparent below, but the question of the age classes remains. Very tentative answers have been proposed in the chapter just quoted.

All the illiterate rural women, from wherever they come or to whatever age class they belong, fall far behind their urban sisters in intelligence test performance. This was based for Test A, as will be recalled, on mental arithmetic, in which the city women without much doubt acquired more practice. The not always statistically significant but generally observable tendency of the rural men also to lag behind the urban confirms the above mentioned hypothesis that not merely concrete practice e.g. in buying and selling, but on the whole the more varied, stimulating and demanding urban environment forced the inhabitants of the city to exercise their intelligence and thus to improve their use of it. Marginally, to be sure, the question can be raised whether inbreeding in some rural groups with a high percentage of cousin marriages (15 % in Marvdasht, 25 % among the Qashqai) does not reduce the intellectual level.

Significant differences between rural-nomad groups were few, slight and irregular, so that a discussion of them here appears out of place. The details, together with some hypotheses, the reader will find at the close of the Chap. C I 6 already cited.

Best memories in the city that ranged consistently high for both sexes and age classes as compared to the villagers and nomads were pregnancy and childbirth, pilgrimage and religion. The single worst memory of similar generality was that of one's own illness. Thereafter restricition become necessary. Family celebrations belonged to the happiest memories in the city too, but only for the illiterate in comparison with the villages and only for the females in comparison to the nomads. The urban males more often took or recalled joy in activity, achievement, success in work than those of the villages, but this difference does not show itself to be significant when they are contrasted with those of the desert. The Shirazi women significantly more often mentioned travel, holidays or rest than the women of the countryside, more often reunion with friends or relatives than those of the tents. On the other hand there were more worst memories of material loss or bankruptcy in the city than in the country, more of the loss of an own child than among the nomads. The urban women more frequently related a worst memory of some kind of fear or phobia than the village women did, but not more than the nomad women.

The relatively sophisticated city as a whole, somewhat to our surprise, does not have the lowest quota of belief in magic. The highest for both sexes together and separately is encountered in Marvdasht, followed by the Qashqai with the exception of the men. The second position among the men is taken up by the poor of Shiraz. For both sexes the rate in the city decreases regularly as SES rises. Khuzestan stands low in superstition (the astonishing figure of 16.7 % for literate females rests on one case out of six and is therefore meaningless), Qalandari lowest of all. Since the ethnically related nomad Qashqais were high, the striking difference can be referred directly to the influence of settlement and education.

On the complaint score too the city occupies no unique or even exceptional position. Its rates for all groups run very close to those of Marvdasht, but not to those of the other villages. Shiraz and Marvdasht, both in Fars, register substantially more complaints of all kinds in both sexes and age classes than all the rest. Their citizens agree in complaining more about paralysis, depression (except the Shirazi men), excitement (except the Qashqai women), anxiety, and record more often the hearing of "voices" (except the Marvdashti women). Depression and anxiety are close neighbors; excitement may or may not be related to them. "Paralysis" rarely meant what it said, but was rather a sign of hypochondria. So were most of the "fits", which according to questionnaire were more numerous in Marvdasht than in the city and indeed than anywhere else. Similarly were suspicion and estrangement commoner in Marvdasht than elsewhere, including Shiraz. Shiraz surpassed Khuzestan in these respects and was itself surpassed by the Qashqai. The remarkable similarity between the complaint rates, both general and particular, for Shiraz and Marvdasht, with the latter sometimes leading, refutes any hypothesis that urban life at that time in Iran was necessarily less satisfying, more troubled and distressed than life in the villages or among the (Qashqai) tribe(s) on the whole, i.e. the attribution of such qualities to urban life in itself under the existing circumstances. On the contrary, the complaint score for the other villages and for the Qashqai was distinctly less, discouraging generalization.

Even more complex and less suited to generalizing do the relations become when we address ourselves to the Z Test. One generalization holds nevertheless: all subgroups of the Shirazi population took more time for it than the subjects anywhere else. No other seems possible without considerable restriction. Since the Marvdasht Z Tests are not yet available and the numbers in Qalandari and among the Qashqai are much less, we shall concentrate on a comparison between Shiraz and Khuzestan even though, as we have already seen, broad conclusions thence regarding rural-urban differences are not admissible. The Shirazi not only take more time, but also more time per response than the Khuzestani; they give more W and W+ with higher F+%, less D and Dd, less F and f%, less FC, more CF and more P. On the one hand the intelligence factors rise in Shiraz, with a greater tendency toward a more comprehensive overview and synthesis such as is sometimes termed "theoretical" intelligence, corresponding very well to the consistently higher IQs found in the city. On the other we observe some deficit in emotional adaptation and differentiation in the relation of FC to CF. This suggests sharpening of the wits, but some obtuseness of feelings in the city, something that one may be forced to call urbanization without urbanity however loaṭh one is to do that, for it flouts the great tradition of Shiraz as one of the most urbane cultural centers of the world. Yet one at least of the characteristics of urbanity is leisure, which the Shirazi in responding to the Z Test take. They produce a significantly greater number of popular responses than the Khuzestani, perhaps reflecting some urban sterotypes, but the percentage of P in both sets of records is hardly different and is below that of both the settled and nomadic Qashqai.

Another comparison between Shiraz and Khuzestan has proved unexpectedly fruitful and has been depicted in some detail in Part C, Chap. II 3 d. It concerns patterns of maturation in the two sexes as revealed by the attitudinal values and shall be recapitulated here with the help of Table D I 1. From it we see that the distribution of the AV is bimodal in both boys and men in Shiraz. Manhood brings several displacements in the direction of extraversion: in the second mode from A to 10e (while

Table D I 1. Attitudinal Values: Means and Characteristics of Distributions (Non-disordered Subjects Only): All Surveys Except Marvdasht

	Modes		E %	Ratio i : e	Mean AV
Shiraz					
Boys	20i	A	42	59:41	10e
Men	20i	10e	37	52:48	14e
Girls	20i	A	33	62:38	10e
Women	(30i)	10e	49	41:59	21e
Khuzestan					
Boys	20i	(A)	57	78:22	17e
Men	20i	A	60	56:44	25e
Girls	20i	A–10e	58	50:50	23e
Women	20i	A	57	70:30	20e
Qalandari					
Men	20i	20e	56	62:38	22e
Women	20i	A	45	41:59	21e
Qashqai					
Men	20i	10e	28	42:58	7e
Women	20i	10e	49	38:62	21e

( ) low peak, ____ broad peak.

the first remains at 20i), in the mean AV from 10e to 14e, and in the i:e ratio from 59:41 to 52:48, while on the other hand the percentage of the introversionless decreases somewhat from 42 % to 37 %, implying the acquisition of some introversive traits as well. Quite differently in the female sex, which takes its start in girlhood from the same bimodal distribution, with modes at the same points as the boys have, and from the same mean AV of 10e. The women's distribution becomes practically unimodal at 10e also. If there be a second mode it lies around 30i, though it is very low; that is, the distribution becomes more dichotomous than in girlhood. Then there were less introversionless (33 %), in womanhood there are more (49 %) than in the male sex: the gap widens, as can be seen from a comparison of the i:e ratios also, and the mean AV is displaced correspondingly toward extraversion. In Khuzestan bimodality among the boys is rather weaker than in Shiraz with a less pronounced second mode at A and with some introversive tendency evident in the i:e ratio of 78:22 despite a high proportion of introversionless subjects (57 %) and a more extratensive mean AV than in the city. The men show a distinct bimodality with a general shift towards extraversion that is apparent in all three measures: E%, i:e ratio and mean AV. Again the other sex presents another picture, but not the same one as in Shiraz: girls and women are clearly bimodal and have practically identical AV means and E%, but the i:e ratios change from 50:50 in girlhood to 70:30 in womanhood. The women, or some of the women, acquire a reserve of introversion somewhat such as the Khuzestani boys have, and even the change in the mean AV, though slight, is in this direction. As we have elaborated in Part C, Chap. II 3 d, the one unquestionable objective factor we can call upon to explain the difference is the fact that the great majority of the Shirazi boys and girls as well as the Khuzestani boys were attending school, whereas the Khuzestani girls with few exceptions were not. Moreover, the majority of the Shirazi men and about half the women had been to school, but hardly any of the Khuzestani men and none of the women. Thus in city and village the male sex seems to accomplish its transition from childhood to adulthood with a certain shift towards extraversion that is more pronounced in Khuzestan than in Shiraz while maintaining on the whole the proportions of its distribution of attitudinal values. The hypothesis seems reasonable that the shift is more pronounced in Khuzestan because in Shiraz the boys' fathers had already been through the extraverting process of education, while in Khuzestan they had not. The Shirazi girls, on the other hand, arrive at a nearly unimodal distribution from a bimodal one, losing much of their initial introversion. We interpret this as a somewhat forced assimilation into or adaptation to their extraverted environment in contradistinction to their mothers. In Khuzestan both the girls' and women's distributions are bimodal, but introversion increases among the women instead of decreasing as it does in the city. The Khuzestani women, be it noted, though not introverted are less extraverted than the men, the Shirazi women more. We tend to see here not simply a rural-urban difference, but one determined by the availability and utilization of education, i.e. formal schooling because of the easily interpretable differences described above both between the sexes and the generations. It must be emphasized further that we are attempting here to describe and analyze normal, not pathological and by no means necessarily pathogenic processes, since the populations in question were all normal by definition and the reactively disordered had been excluded from them. In the evolution of the females in Shiraz we can trace directly the rise of the intellectual or pseudo-extraversion such as we have depicted and we can contrast it with a different pattern of development in the countryside. Here, we remember, the complaint score was higher for all and higher for the women than for the men. Between the well adults of Khuzestan there was no sex difference, and in the pathological subjects of those villages the men lead! Yet, as we shall see further on, there are no statistically significant differences in the psychiatric prevalence rates between Shiraz and Khuzestan. Questions of pathogenesis arise here that would require and deserve a detailed treatment such as we, regretfully, cannot bestow upon them at the present.

Between Shiraz and Qalandari the differences on the whole are very much like those between Shiraz and Khuzestan. The F+% that was 41 in the city and 35 in Khuzestan is 36 in Qalandari. The cityfolk have more W, W+ and less D. Differences between FC and CF do not appear here, but the total SUM CHRO is significantly higher in Qalandari, as is also the SUM CHIA. The diffference in SUM CHRO can be accounted for the same way as in Khuzestan, and the agreement between the two villages now encourages one to think that some cautious generalizations about differences between town and city may be permissible after all. That the cityfolk give fewer plant responses is understandable without difficulty. Seeking an explanation for the lower SUM CHIA in the city we note that it is mainly referable to the men and that these, but not the women, exhibit significantly less shocks than in Qalandari. That and why some melancholic longing for their old nomadic way of life among the men of Qalandari constitutes the probable reason for this we have set forth in detail in Part C, Chap. II 3 e.

The comparison of the nomadic Qashqai with Shiraz turns out quite differently. The type of approach is wider, even bolder in the nomads with the W (but not the W+) leading. F+% is merely 27, the lowest of all populations. D and Do fall far behind, as do also the F and f%; the latter is likewise the lowest we have recorded. SUM CHIA tends to rise. MC increases startlingly over the city. There are many fewer populars. The pattern of these differences indicates a broad, quick, synthetic, emotionally toned rather than analytically reasoned apprehension of the world for which the word "intuitive" seems a fitting designation. This we do not find in the villages. It leads us now to consider the differences between the nomads and the village people, particularly those of their own Qashqai stock.

The nomads have been compared at some length with the citizens of the Khuzestan villages. The differences are essentially similar, though somewhat less accentuated, to those between the nomads and urbanites: more intellectual, rational apprehension in the latter, more intuitive and emotional in the former. City and village agree with each other better than either with the nomads. We come here upon a probably genuine difference between the sedentary and the mobile. Details are given in the text. In certain other respects, however, the Qashqai, whether sedentary or not, possess characteristics in common that distinguish them from the Shirazi and the Khuzestani. They take distinctly less total time and have a shorter reaction time per response, and they have a higher P% (cf. Table C II 27). We have seen reason to surmise that they make more use of stereotypes, which again can facilitate quick reaction.

What happens to the nomadic Qashqai when they settle down? There are significant changes in the form of a general constriction of the type of approach, which converges with that of the long settled villagers, displaying less W and W+, but now an F+% of 36 instead of 27, more D, Do, F and P. Reactions are slower on the average. Caution seems to mount together with more readiness for criticism and opposition: S + Sc rises from 0.44 to 0.68. On the other hand CF, and with it Pl, rises, while FC remains about the same. Some of the nomads' boldness may reside in these CF and assert itself in their increase despite other influences to the contrary. Another reason for the rise of the extraversive CF reveals itself when, with the circumspection demanded by small numbers, we compare the AV means and distributions (Table C II 30). In the Qashqai and in Qalandari these are, as elsewhere, bimodal for the adults of both sexes, though bimodality is less evident in the men of Qalandari (there are not enough children in either group to justify comparing distributions). Corresponding to the higher rate of CF in the villagers there is almost no total coarctation to be found there, while among the nomads it is encountered in both sexes in the usual proportions. The Qashqai men have a mean AV of only 7e, those of Qalandari 22e, with which the women's means of 21e in both populations are practically identical. Moreover, out of the Qashqai men only 27.5 % are wholly introversionless, but out of the three comparable populations about one half. More than half of the men of Qalandari are so, and their high rate of 56 % without introversion would seem to imply that the male population there was strongly extraverted, but the implication is contradicted to some extent by the i:e ratio of 62:38. The contradiction can be resolved when we reflect that 39 % of the men in Qalandari had acquired literacy and that the literate, following the pattern traced in Shiraz and Khuzestan, had been in all likelihood impelled into pseudo-extraversion, the illiterate not. Both were substantially represented. The Qashqai and Qalandari women alike were almost totally illiterate; their distributions and all their characteristics were very similar, and their mean AV, as we have seen, identical, i.e. strongly extratensive. There was no educational influence that could be held responsible for that fact such as was evident in both Shiraz and Khuzestan. In its absence it seems justifiable to infer that the unequivocal extraversion of the Qashqai women, whether nomadic or settled, represents a constitutional trait, be this genetic or early acquired, as does also the much slighter extratension, not far from ambiequality, of the nomadic Qashqai men and of the Shiraz boys. Both, in the process of schooling, become impelled into some degree of true or pseudo-extraversion with a corresponding rise of mean AV toward E, but the men of Qalandari retain more introversive reserves with an i:e ratio of 62:38 than those of Shiraz with 52:48.

In conclusion we may attempt, drawing upon concrete findings but not again quoting them and relying less upon statistical significances than upon coherent patternings, to sketch broadly and tentatively psychological pictures of our principal environmental groups, endeavoring at the same time to trace their evolution from the simpler to the more complex, from the nomadic over the rural to the urban. Such pictures cannot be anything but composite, constituting sweeping generalization to which there are numberless exceptions, so that their worth altogether may be cast into doubt. Nevertheless we feel that enough convergent, mutually supportive evidence has accumulated to justify such an experiment which may, after all, come somewhat closer to real life than mere heaps of figures, however elaborately processed, can attain. The reader is at liberty to disregard or to condemn them.

The nomads as a whole react swiftly, globally, intuitively and emotionally, show little inclination to reflection and critical analysis, but rather make some use of conceptual sterotypes to come to terms with an environment that is itself less complicated than that of the rural and urban goups. The men mature into a position on the extratensive side of ambiequality and retain some introversive reserves as they do so; the women grow into rather unequivocal extraversion. They are very superstitious, the men less so (extraversion furthers projection). The emotivity of both sexes is probably higher than that of any other population studied, but is vented freely and results in little conflict or opposition. Memories of the past are immediate and personal: for the women pregnancy and childbirth or else loss of a child, for the men ill harvest or ill treatment. The complaint rate is the lowest from our surveys, the mental health status probably the best.

When the nomads voluntarily settle, constriction and caution begin, but the possibility of fairly bold emotional outlet remains. The settlers become somewhat more critical and enter more readily into opposition. The attitudinal maturation of the women proceeds very much as among the nomads, but that of the men leads into a pronounced pseudo-extraversion for some, while others retain a portion of introversion. Latent psychic tensions become demonstrable in the whole population, but much more among the men, who develop a more pronounced neurotoid structure with a tendency to dysphoria and probably nostalgia. Nevertheless the complaint score remains low for both sexes. Superstition seems almost to be cast off; we find here the lowest percentages of all, lower still among the men than among the women. Mental health is good, though some cases manifest themselves that we did not discover among the nomads. The mode of readjustment seems to be effective.

In Khuzestan the type of approach is practical and concrete, already more constricted than in Qalandari and approaching in some respects that of the city, though diverging from it in other important ones such as the concreteness just mentioned. Its empirical realism is demonstrated by its minimal employment of stereotypes among all the four populations as well as by an acuity of perception only slightly below that of Shiraz. Realism may be reflected more in opposition to what is perceived as incorrect or false (S + Sc attains its maximum). The boys, who begin with a certain reservoir of introversion, grow into markedly extraverted men, while the women – alone among our samples – though on the whole extraverted, are slightly less so than their daughters and displace their second, extratensive mode back toward the introversive side; their i:e ratio also becomes distinctly introversive. A consequence of this seems to be that the women's sum of reactive disorders in Khuzestan lies below that in Shiraz, where quite a different pattern of maturation obtains for the female sex. Emotivity tends to be less copious, but more differentiated. The complaint rate is low, and more than elsewhere we hear both men and women answering that they have always been happy, have no ill memories. Those that they do possess and most occupy them are their own illness in case of the men, bereavement and poverty in case of the women. Superstition is rather low, corresponding to the realistic traits mentioned above, and it is even lower among the women than men. Khuzestan is the only place in which we have found it to be so, just as it is the only place in which the women retain or recover their normal introversion, recalling what has been said already about the relation between extraversion, projection and superstition.

That we cannot generalize from Khuzestan to all rural communities is shown by the fact that in Marvdasht both the complaint score and the belief in magic are very high, though in the resurvey of Qassemabad in 1976 they had dropped sharply.

Deliberation, broader comprehension, synthesis rather than global appraisal characterize the approach of the Shirazis. It is rational, but relatively unstereotyped.

This conforms to the pattern of test intelligence, and in Shiraz the mean intelligence test scores are regularly higher than in the country or desert. Cognitive appraisal is sharper, but at the cost of finely differentiated affectivity. Thought seems to replace intuition, consideration to replace spontaneity. The men, who move by moderate steps from low extraversion in boyhood to slightly higher in adulthood, seem to accomplish this with less tension and friction than the women. These show divergent patterns of attitudinal maturation, the larger part probably being forced into an intellectualized or pseudo-extraversion, a smaller part retaining its introversive resources. Repression, leading into a substantial number of simple reactive developments, is the consequence. The rate of such, as we have seen, exceeds that of Khuzestan. Complaint scores too are high, and higher for the women than the men, for the girls than for the boys. Belief in magic takes a middle place, is less than among the nomads, but distinctly higher than in both villages (and only a trifle less than in Marvdasht). Memories of pregnancy and childbirth are dear to the women as they are in the desert, but are joined by those of pilgrimage and religion, for which the easily accessible Shrine of Shahcheragh in Shiraz may account. Dear too are reunions with relatives and friends (often visiting from the countryside). Recollection of their own illness weighs upon the city people, upon the men that not simply of financial difficulty and poverty, but of unemployment and debt, while on the other hand they more often take joy in their own success or achievement.

Emotional intuitiveness in the nomads, practical common sense in the peasants, a degree of intellectualism, repression and conflict in the urbanites – these are truisms, one could reflect, and need no survey. A wise author, whose name we cannot find to honor, has written that many a life has to be spent in discovering that truisms are true. Yet another "truism": the belief in the simple, healthy countrymen, has proved demonstrably false. Such a weighing of truisms seems part of the province of psychology.

A question hangs over the end of this chapter that is not strictly speaking psychological. Different sex and socio-cultural groups pass through the process of additudinal maturation in different ways and with different consequences. How are these differences to be explained? Why, for instance, do the Khuzestani girls grow into mild uncomplaining introverts, the Shirazis mostly into pseudo-extraverts with a quantity of complaints, but with no significant difference in psychiatric morbidity between them? We are confident that formal education, i.e. the school of modern type (not the old Qoranic school, which girls rarely attended anyway) together with the reception of formal education by the environment, particularly by the pupil's educated or uneducated parents of both sexes, plays a part, and we have referred to the part that we suspect it to play in the appropriate places. Yet we are equally confident that it would be vain to invoke this single factor to account for all the complex differences, and that it would be unfair to place all praise or blame upon the school. The question is properly one for an ethnologist or cultural anthropologist. We could not get one, and the time when one might have been able to find answers to our questions is likely already to be past.

II. Indicators of Psychopathology

A variety of short indicators of pathology having been applied, it becomes imperative to inquire into the validity of each, into the contribution of each to the sum of pathology discovered and into the validity and general usefulness of the indicator system as a whole. We assume as the basis of validation our clinical identifications and diagnoses, well aware that they are not infallible but conscious also that we have no better. Too often it seems to be forgotten that the ultimate validation of all psychological tests, questionnaires, rating scales etc. is in practice, which for the psychiatrist means policlinical or clinical practice. The possibilities of both sampling and diagnostic errors are evident and have been discussed in the introductory chapters. They shall not be argued further in this section.

As major indicators of general, sometimes also of special psychopathology we have the Zulliger or Z Test, the psychiatric questionnaire and the examiners' judgments. They were applied and shall be considered in that order. The intelligence tests, important as they are, are not indicators of general psychopathology except in rather rare cases, but point to a large sector of special pathology in cases of oligophrenia. They will receive mention from time to time in connection with the three more widely applicable indices as well as having been treated by themselves in Chap. C I.

A more than conjectural estimate of the indicators' value and validity is only possible where their application and evaluation were performed wholly or largely independently of the clinical investigations. Strictly, the independence of one from the other should have been complete. Actually, this condition could be fulfilled only by certain indicators and in certain conditions. In three of the five surveys the needful conditions could not be met even approximately because the psychiatrists were constantly in the field together with the examiners, observing most or all the persons tested, attending to their replies to the questionnaire, plying them when appropriate with further questions and thus directly or indirectly influencing the examiners' judgments. This applies to Khuzestan, the Qashqai village of Qalandari and in part to the Qashqai nomads. The gain in information and clinical precision more than outweighed any loss in methodological stringency.

Some of this stringency could be recovered in Marvdasht and in Shiraz, where the authors, though much in the field, could not systematically and directly observe the testing of all subjects. We shall therefore confine ourselves in this chapter mainly to these two surveys which – fortunately for our present purpose – were at the same time the largest.

In Marvdasht special circumstances abetted a more detailed and exact appraisal. Before beginning field work we had inquired of teachers, headmen, demonstration agents and anyone else who seemed in a position to know, including town gossips, about persons suspect of psycho- or neuropathology in the respective villages and had taken such persons as targets among others for clinical examination. In the city, clearly, such a procedure was not possible; its role in Khuzestan has been depicted in Chap. B II. Furthermore a unique opportunity presented itself in Marvdasht inasmuch as one of the very few Persian psychologists at that time competent in projective techniques, Mr. Hushang Ordoobadi, Lecturer and Student Counselor at the Pahlavi University in Shiraz, consented to inspect all our more than five hundred Z Tests blindly, without having seen the subjects or knowing more about them than their age and sex, and to point out to us those he deemed distinctly suspect of psychopathology. The adverb is intended to imply that his criterion by agreement was somewhat stricter than that which we subsequently applied in Shiraz, where we had less opportunity for direct observation and therefore were willing to risk more false positives for the sake of missing fewer false negatives, i.e. of overlooking true cases in the psychiatric survey population. He designated 26 such, of whom on individual psychiatric examination we found 22 to be pathological to a critical degree, four not, confirming his judgment in 84 % of the probands in question. When writing up the field work the first author tried to estimate in all the 50 pathological cases which single indicator had contributed most (though not necessarily exclusively) to their identification and could ascribe this in all the 22 clinically confirmed cases to the Z Test. The share of the test in the identification of the pathological collective under the conditions described therefore could be estimated at 44 %. This is low, but must be understood in the light of the test's high validity (cf. above) and deliberately conservative evaluation as also in the light of the circumstances that here only one indicator was ascribed to each case. How the several shares of the indicators, except the questionnaire, were distributed is shown in Table D II 1 reproduced from our earliest publications [17, 20]. As shall be described below we have applied somewhat different methods and standards since, but the table remains instructive in several respects. By it the share of the Z Test (44 %) and of the examiners' judgments (46 %) in identification of cases were practically equal. In only 10 % of the cases, however, was the principal identification made by local informants, and half the time, when such informants pointed to supposed pathology, clinical examination did not confirm this. Their identifications generally referred to obviously and gravely ill individuals on the one hand or on the other to such as the psychiatrists did not judge to be pathological, but who seemed rather to be deviant or "remarkable" personalities as described in Khuzestan, to "stick out" in an inessential manner. Of the three children designated by the teachers a supposedly oligophrenic boy turned out to

Table D II 1. Marvdasht Survey: Methods of Psychiatric Case Identification and Their Effectiveness, Identification Being Ascribed in Each Case to a Single Indicator (1964)

	T	Inf.	X	Z	Sum
Designated as suspect by	3	7	30	26	66
Clinically positive	1	4	23	22	50
Clinically negative	2	3	7	4	16
Validity of the method as percent clinically positive cases	33	57	76	84	
Percent of all clinically positive cases identified by the method	2.0	8.0	46	44	

Key: T = teachers; Inf. = lay informants; X = examiners; Z = Z Test, blindly evaluated.

be myopic and hardly able to see the blackboard. A girl who was inattentive and who, the teacher thought, might be mentally retarded, was by every indication including tests especially bright and therefore bored by the not too exacting lessons, as she shyly admitted to us in the teacher's absence. These results seem worth mentioning because some surveys have relied rather heavily upon informants, further because a number of sociologists and antipsychiatrists strive to define the psychiatric patient or case exclusively as a social deviant and to impugn society as the sole cause of psychiatric disorder.

Returning to the same material a decade later we found it necessary to complement the data above. Several patently oligophrenic Z Tests had not found a place in Mr. Ordoobadi's list, they being, as it were, clear to the naked eye or having been pointed out already by teachers or other informants. This led us to review all the Z Tests of the pathological group of fifty. Applying now the somewhat more generous criterion we had been accustomed to use in Shiraz and including the cases that had been omitted previously from the list by reason of their very obviousness, beside two total rejectors, we found 37 of the 50 cases to be suspect by our own evaluation of the Z Test, i.e. 74 %. This re-evaluation was undertaken by the second author, who had not participated in the Marvdasht Survey and did not know any of the patients concerned, though she did know that the entire collective was considered to be composed of individuals with a significant degree of psychopathology. Her evaluation was thus only half blind. What of the clinically negative cases?

The validity of an indicator may be estimated in two different ways. One, as described, is the ratio of clinical confirmations to the number of cases designated by the indicator as positive or suspect. For Marvdasht we have stated these percentages for each of the indicators expect Q at the foot of Table D II 1. This, however, presents a one-sided picture suitable only for clinical work, whereas epidemiology is double-faceted. A false positive weighs as much as a false negative. We have accordingly added the false positives and false negatives together wherever practicable and have expressed their sum as a percentage of the total sample. This could be done throughout for X, and the results are compiled in Table D II 4 below, to which we shall return. Z and Q presented special problems.

In order to obtain such a total discordance rate for any given indicator, it would have been necessary to muster the entire survey population in respect to it, and by strict methodological criteria this mustering, as far as judgments and not merely counting of findings were involved, should have been conducted blindly, preferably by an independent judge. Both criteria were fulfilled in principle by Mr. Ordoobadi's estimation of the Z Test in Marvdasht. We recall that in this way 22 cases out of 50 were identified as pathological by the Z Test (Z+) and clinically confirmed (Cl+). Four were designated as Z+ but not confirmed on clinical examination (Cl–). Twenty-eight of the 50 clinically positive cases (Cl+) were not identified by the Z Test (Z–) employed in the manner described. Of the 500 persons scrutinized by the Marvdasht Survey, eight could not be given the Z Test because of blindness or severe somatic illness, leaving 492. The discordance rate for the Z Test in Marvdasht by the then criterion is thus $(28+4):492 = 6.50 \pm 1.11$ %, a very low rate indeed, which is due to the extremely small number of false positives (Cl–, Z+), in spite of a relatively large proportion of false negatives (Cl+, Z–). We could not test our later re-evaluation in the same way without reviewing all the 450 clinically negative subjects – a task which, in addition to that just to be described, we felt to be insufficiently rewarding and in any case beyond our powers.

A different situation prevailed in Shiraz. There both authors working closely together examined cursorily all Z Test records as they came in, much as Mr. Ordoobadi had done in Marvdasht, but consciously used a laxer criterion in order to miss as few clinically positive cases as possible. They had also seen some, though by no means all of the freshly tested subjects while supervising the field work and ultimately did see all who were judged on clinical grounds to be pathological. A closer scrutiny of all the more than nine hundred Z Tests was impossible under the circumstances, though we naturally paid more attention to borderline records and were generous in our ascription of suspicion, which implied going back for personal examination. During the four years after the survey while we were working up our pathological cases we reviewed all their Z Test protocols and made a definite decision on their pathological or non-pathological character, permitting ourselves no borderline or marginal classification, just as we did in regard to the clinical findings. In his year of fellowship at the Netherlands Institute for Advanced Studies the first author undertook to do the same for (clinically) non-pathological subjects, shuffling them with the pathological. The evaluation was again half or rather more than half blind, for a great many of the subjects the writer had never seen at all, though at the sight of other records recollection was instantly at hand. There was no one even remotely available to perform a truly blind evaluation. Out of the 154 cases ultimately denominated as pathological, two could not be given the Z Test. From the remaining 152 records, we held 111 to be pathological or strongly suspect, i.e. 73 %. This is almost exactly the same figure that the second author's re-evaluation of the like group in Marvdasht had yielded. Out of the 774 clinically "normal" persons five could not be given the Z Test, and 27 Z records were judged to be pathological. The discordance rate thus becomes $(41+27){:}921 = 7.38 \pm 0.86$ % for the Z Test in Shiraz, only a little higher than in Marvdasht. The difference is not significant.

The questionnaire as a whole was not amenable to psychiatric quantification, though some of its single components were, as has been shown in some detail in Part C, Chap. II 2 a. Only one question of the nine, Q 2 epileptic fits, could have yielded even theoretically a pathognomonic response and actually harvested a crop of false positives. In using the questionnaire in the field as an indicator for further examination the authors let themselves be guided not only by the number of positive answers (one could suffice), but also by their configuration, their formulation (often invalidating the positive response) and their context. We did not score the questionnaire, but judged it clinically. Where it seemed to offer a hint worth following, we usually penciled a Q on the form, but sometimes this came to be omitted when the follow-up could take place almost upon or on the spot. This was much more the case in Marvdasht that in Shiraz. Retrospectively we found that our Q markings were not consistent enough to justify a formal count and evaluation of them, though they did appear in a considerable share of the records belonging to pathological cases. We then reviewed all such records from the Marvdasht and Shiraz surveys, noted the suspicious Q where present and judged the questionnaire as a whole anew where it was absent. It seemed impracticable and indeed unjustifiable to attempt this with the records of unpathological persons whose classification as such we already knew and would have involved far more guess work than the retrospective evaluation of the Z Tests did. For these there are fairly good criteria familiar to everyone conversant with projective techniques, whereas the overall

Table D II 2. Contribution of Indicators to Identification of Cases

No. of pos. indicators	0	1				2				3	
Indicator		Z	Q	X	Sum	ZX	ZQ	QX	Sum	ZQX	
Degree of severity											Total
	Shiraz Survey										
P_1	3	11	13	2	26	2	28	8	38	13	80
P_2	3	5	5	1	11	5	12	7	24	25	63
P_3	0	0	0	1	1	0	1	0	1	9	11
Total P	6	16	18	4	38	7	41	15	63	47	154
Z pathological 111 = 73 % of 152[a] cases											
Q pathological 121 = 80 % of 152[a] cases											
X pathological 73 = 47 % of 154 cases											
	Marvdasht Survey										
P_1	1	1	0	1	2	1	6	1	8	3	14
P_2	1	2	0	2	4	2	11	6	19	6	30
P_3	0	0	0	1	1	0	1	0	1	4	6
Total P	2	3	0	4	7	3	18	7	28	13	50
Z pathological 37 = 74 % of 50 cases											
Q pathological 38 = 76 % of 50 cases											
X pathological 27 = 54 % of 50 cases											

[a] n. b. 152 = 154 cases minus two persons not testable by reason of sensory defect.

Table D II 3. Number of Indicators and Degrees of Severity

	Percentage by Row					Percentage by Column			
No. of pos. indicators	0	1	2	3	Sum	0	1	2	3
Degree of severity									
	Shiraz Survey Comparisons by per cent of 154 Cases								
P_1	4	33	47	16	100	50	68	60	28
P_2	5	17	38	40	100	50	29	38	53
P_3	0	9	9	82	100	0	3	2	19
Total P	4	25	41	30	100	100	100	100	100
	Marvdasht Survey Comparisons by per cent of 50 Cases								
P_1	7	14	57	22	100	50	29	29	23
P_2	3	13	64	20	100	50	57	68	46
P_3	0	17	17	66	100	0	14	3	31
Total P	4	14	56	26	100	100	100	100	100

appraisal of the questionnaire was a much more personal affair and lacked precedents. The results of our re-workings of the questionnaire in the pathological cases of Shiraz and Marvdasht are contained in Tables D II 2 and D II 3, which we shall discuss below. The indication afforded by the questionnaire was esteemed to be positive in 38 out of 50 cases in Marvdasht or 76 % and in 121 out of 152 cases in Shiraz or 80 %, thus

Table D II 4. Discordancy Rates of Examiner's Judgments, in Percent

Survey	Male Rate	SD	Female Rate	SD	Both Sexes Rate	SD
Shiraz	12.93	1.56	15.65	1.69	14.29	1.15
Marvdasht	8.24	1.72	10.92	2.06	9.50	1.33
Khuzestan	12.40	2.12	13.72	1.63	13.00	1.59
Qalandari	1.33	1.32	7.81	3.35	4.32	1.72
Qashqai	6.74	2.66	14.61	3.74	10.67	2.31
All Surveys	10.49	0.91	13.67	1.06	12.02	0.70

running slightly ahead of the Z Test. On the other hand, the implications were seldom specific. In only 12 cases out of the 38 with a suspicious clustering of positive answers in Marvdasht did the cluster (or single response) seem to point unequivocally to the ultimate diagnosis. No such evaluation for diagnostic specificity was undertaken for the Shiraz questionnaires and none for the Z Test at all. Under field conditions we could not spare time for more than a quick guess. A subsequent re-evaluation would have been influenced inevitably and far too strongly by our foreknowledge, gleaned from many sources, about the members of the pathological group and would have had little worth unless conducted blindly by some third person. Mr. Ordoobadi could not undertake the onerous task then, and there was no other such person.

The examiners' judgments or X had been passed already; we had only to count them. In a few cases the judgment was lacking or ambiguous; these have been subtracted from the total of subjects. The results for all five surveys are to be found in Table D II 4, for the sexes separately and together. We were interested in seeing whether men and women were judged equally by the examiners according to our clinical criteria. It is apparent immediately that they were not. The discordancy rate is higher in every survey for females than for males, and for the surveys combined the difference is significant at almost the 1 % level. This holds whether the examiners were predominantly females as in Shiraz or exclusively male as in Khuzestan and therefore cannot be referred to the sex of the examiners. Did this have any influence at all? The coding of our Shiraz data gave us an opportunity to investigate this question from another angle. When males were judged by the predominantly female cohort of examiners in Shiraz there were 12.9 % of false judgements in both directions, but when females were judged mostly by their own sex 15.7 %. The difference, however, did not approach statistical significance. Another explanation must be sought for the uniformly higher discordance rates for female subjects. We suspect it to lie in a cultural artefact. The examiners were Iranian and judged according to their own culture and customs. The psychiatrists, though not unfamilar with Iran, consciously adhered to European standards in appraising a case. Many reactions in female subjects which they considered to be pathological at least in degree and sometimes also in kind obviously were not regarded as such by our Iranian co-workers, but were simply attributed to the girls' and women's normal nature and lot. For this we have numerous examples. Yet an attempt on our part to cut our judgments according to local standards would have been fraught with uncertainty and contravened the principles set forth in the introduction. Having worked to these already, we could not arbitrarily alter them in mid-course, and doing so would have introduced new sources of error.

The discordancy rates run around 10–14 % but vary a good deal from one survey to another and drop sharply in Qalandari. The explanations on the whole are not difficult to find. The highest rates, as might be expected, occur in Shiraz, where our examiners were the youngest, least experienced and in part least motivated. They possessed no professional and too little life experience at all. The best rates (except for Qalandari) come from Marvdasht, where the examiners were all medical or paramedical people with some life experience and with generally excellent motivation. The same group worked among the Qashqai, and the discordance rate is only a little higher. The high rate in Khuzestan occasioned some surprise at first glance, for our three young men there had worked very well indeed and had no dearth of life experience, beside which two came directly from the health services. The surprise dissolved when we looked again at the discordant cases, mainly the false negatives. The tendency was quite plain for these excellent, robust workers to discount smaller deviations in the countryside and to regard as pathological only that which was quite manifestly so, the rest being attributable as in the case of the city women mentioned above simply to a hard lot or in some cases to a physical illness, as in several instances of dementia together with anemia, cardiac disease or general decrepitude. The low rate for Qalandari seems too good to be true, and is. The judgments were made not only by the pick of our Shirazi examiners, but also in the constant company of and undoubtedly, albeit unintentionally, influenced by ourselves. It would be better to disregard this figure, but we have included it for the sake of completeness and because it nevertheless possesses an instructive aspect.

Table D II 4 displays the efficiency of the examiners as a group, but there were marked individual differences. Table D II 5 is an attempt to quantify these. Twenty-nine persons contributed at least one of the 1072 sets of tests performed on the psychiatric survey population in Shiraz and Qalandari. Four of these persons – two psychologists, a nurse and a visiting social worker – carried out only a test or two apiece, altogether five sets of tests, and, as they were not required or expected to do more, are not included in the table . Out of the remaining 25, four were male students from the Red Lion and Sun School for Nursing Aides, one was an experienced social worker who voluntarily joined the survey for several weeks and took an active part in testing with a view to applying it later in her own domain, and one was a psychology student temporarily assigned from Tehran. The other 19 were all young female members of the Health Corps, the majority of whom remained with the survey throughout. We have assigned each of them an identifying number and, when they worked in a special or temporary capacity, an indication. Since every set of tests with questionnaire and examiner's judgment as to need for further psychiatric clarification was required to be signed, the number of sets of tests that each examiner contributed to the total and the agreement or disagreement of the examiner's judgment with the clinical finding could be determined. The percent of the total contributed by each examiner is set out in the first column of the table (where two examiners tested one subject, each is credited with half a test). Examiners are ranged in the order of their contributions. The first six of the 25 contributed 49.2 %, the first seven 54.2 % of the whole. The contribution of No. 1 was outstanding, and we should add that the same person cheerfully undertook a great deal of other work such as initial registration and collection of demographic data, following up reluctant subjects and, later, supervision. All this was accomplished with the zeal, reliability and skill of a professional. While we do not wish to enter into

Table D II 5. Shiraz Survey: Performance of Individual Examiners

Examiner No.	Contribution to total of 1072 tests	Concordance rate[3]
1	17.2%	83.7%
2	7.2	78.1
3[a]	6.5	87.1
4	6.3	95.6
5	6.2	93.3
6	5.8	88.8
7[a]	5.0	91.6
8	5.0	88.8
9[a]	4.7	79.2
10	4.5	82.3
11	4.2	87.9
12	4.0	79.9
13	3.6	85.9
14[a]	3.2	89.7
15[a]	3.1	88.0
16[1]	3.0	87.5
17[a]	1.8	92.5
18	1.5	87.8
19[a,1]	1.5	90.9
20[a,2]	1.1	82.6
21[a,1]	1.1	66.7
22[a,2]	1.0	90.5
23[a,1]	0.9	63.1
24[a]	0.4	100
25[a]	0.3	100

Key: [a] not full time with survey; [1] male student nurse aide; [2] psychologist and social worker; [3] explanation cf. text.

personal detail here, it would be unfair not to include a note of gratitude and appreciation for Miss Mariam Jahanmiri. No. 3 was not less eager and efficient and might well have risen to second rather than third place if she had not joined the survey about a month after the others. The contribution of Examiners Nos. 7–12 is 27.4 %, which, added to the 49.2 % executed by Nos. 1–6, accounts for 76.6 % of the whole. In other terms, roughly half the work was done by six to seven examiners out of 25 and three-quarters of it by twelve out of 25. Below No. 12 all the individual shares are less than 4.0 % and, because of the play of chance, qualitative evaluation of the examiners' work becomes more difficult and problematical, as we shall see.

The second column of the table, headed "concordance", is an attempt to evaluate the quality of the examiners' performance. It was calculated by adding together the cases in which the examiner's and the clinician's judgment, whether both positive or both negative, agreed and dividing this sum by the number of cases for which the examiner in question was responsible (cf. Table D I 5). As there was a good deal of individual variation, and as "quality", if it can be estimated in this way, did not by any means go regularly either with quantity or with the authors' judgment of the examiner's work, resort was had to the calculation of mean concordance. For the first six examiners it was 87.8 %, for the second six it was 84.9 %, for Nos. 7 to 20 it was 86.8 %, and the differences were not statistically significant. No relation between quantity and quality could be demonstrated in this manner. Another attempt was made through dividing the number of positively concordant cases by the total per examiner. This resulted not only in very widely fluctuating ratios, but also in certain conclusions that were grossly unjust in both directions and reflected an excessive influence of chance. Such chance might lead an examiner into a household with several ill members, whose illness she either did realize, earning a higher mark than another who encountered fewer pathological clusters, or did not, earning a disproportionately low one. Other examiners who saw only a handful of negative subjects might be rated zero. A nurse (not included in the table) happened to test a clinically pathological subject, recognized him as such and would have received a rating of 100 % success since she tested nobody else. This second method therefore was abandoned.

Returning to the concordance ratings, the same influence of chance becomes noticeable after the first dozen examiners with four or more percent of the total to their credit, as the number of clinically pathological subjects falling to the lot of each of the rest could only be small and a "right" or "wrong" judgment could sway the concordance rate unduly. For this reason we have not tallied Nos. 21 to 25 in our calculation of means. Among them are the experienced and able social workers mentioned above and also two of the four male nursing aid students. The contribution of these and their two companions, who are also low in the list (Nos. 16 and 19) is not fairly represented by these percentages. These young men performed not a few crucial evening home visits and thus contributed very substantially to the satisfactory coverage rate of the survey. These and many other circumstances are either not reflected in the figures or are even distorted by them, wherefore, though we should be happy to express our gratitude, we refrain from mentioning names. One thing, however, does appear clearly enough from this tabulation: that much fewer, somewhat more mature persons, none of them inadequately motivated, not only would have sufficed for the task, but in all probability would have executed it with less loss of time and cost of supervisory effort. The Khuzestan survey provides confirmation.

After looking at the indicators Z, Q and X singly, we now wish to collate them, to examine their contributions and efficiencies when used together as they were in practice. As explained above, this can be done fairly satisfactorily and without danger of gross distortion by single cases only for the Shiraz and Marvdasht Surveys. The results are set out in Tables D II 2 and D II 3. There we find in the top row of Table D II 3 the number of indicators that were positive in a given case, the cases being grouped vertically by degree of severity, with the sub-totals for each number of positive indicators at the bottom and those for the degree of severity at the right. There being three indicators, a case could have none, one, two or all three positive. To the few who actually did have none and therefore appear at first glance almost "illegitimate" we shall return. If only one indicator was positive, it could be any one of the three. A positive indication by the Z Test (here according to our own re-evaluation more than ten years later) is shown by a Z, a positive though not necessarily specific indication of psychopathology from the questionnaire by a Q, and a suspicion of pathology by the lay examiner such that professional clarification was regarded as needful by an X. Thereafter the number of cases having only one indicator positive is summed for each degree of severity separately and for the pathological collective. The arrangement in the group with two positive indicators is similar, but here of course pairs of indicators in their three possible combinations appear. For the cases in which all three indicators are positive there is naturally only one entry against each degree of severity.

In Shiraz there were six and in Marvdasht two cases in which none of the three major indicators was positive, and the reader will rightly wonder how they came to be included at all, the more so as they are not confined to the P_1 level of mild pathology. In both places, in fact, they are evenly distributed between P_1 and P_2, but do not fall into P_3. Two of the six Shirazi cases, both school children, would have drawn and did draw attention to themselves by their low intelligence test performance. In the case of the nine year old boy with a single point on the arithmetic test and zero block design score, his mother too was unintelligent but suffered mainly from a hypochondric neurosis (P_1). A 14 year old girl obtained 5 raw score points on Arithmetic Test B and one point on the Block Design Test B. Her father was an irritable psychopath (P_1) who had driven his wife into such a labile emotional development that she was rated P_2; both had pathological Z Tests. The girl herself was regarded as an anxious, irritable psychopath with a pseudo-debility probably referable to the extremely unfavorable home situation, but the Z Test even on repeated inspection was so bland that we could draw no indication from it and were influenced by this very blandness to classify the case as one of psychopathy rather than of simple or neurotic development, as the circumstances would have made it easy to do, and to rate her as P_2.

The remaining four cases were discovered by visits to their families, in all of which there were one or several pathological relatives with positive indicators. An eight year old boy hysterically copied his mother's (P_1) gastrointestinal and migrainoid psychosomatic complaints. Curiously, the second P_1 case, that of a forty year old husband, was of the same kind, but had progressed to the stage of (psycho)somatization, the wife (P_2) providing the model. A case of medium severity (P_2) was discovered upon the visit to the home of a boy suffering from the consequences of a commotio cerebri and identified as peculiar and irritable by the examiner (P_2). His mother, 37 years old, had been forced into an irritable development and near-desperation by a sequence of eleven childbirths, poverty and the care of two more children from her husband's first marriage. She had been briefly hospitalized because of her "nervousness" and was under medical treatment still. Her pathology was not apparent in the Z Test, had escaped the examiner and was not elicited by the questionnaire, but became quite clear in a short interview. The last P_2 case was that of a post-encephalitic 14 year old boy, one of whose brothers had a similar condition that showed itself in the Z Test also as P_2. Their father had undergone a simple depressive development of grade P_1.

The four cases just described would have dropped through the meshes of the survey had they not possessed pathological relatives whom the net caught. They represent a margin of 2.6 % of the psychiatric cases whose discovery was fortuitous. If they are subtracted from the 154, the morbidity rate is altered only insignificantly from 16.6 % to 16.2 %. Except by comparison with our census studies there is no way of estimating how many such cases were missed, but the comparison suggests that the number was not large. Their discovery was facilitated by the familial clustering of pathological cases, one at least of whom was likely to exhibit a positive indicator or indicators. In examining any indicated case we made it a rule to inquire carefully about all members of the household. Even the brief sketches just given illustrate on the one hand the psychic induction and transmission of psychopathology, while on the other such observations do not exclude genetic and constitutional factors by any manner of means.

One of the Marvdasht cases without indicator concerns a seven year old boy who was not only attending the first grade, but also asserted he liked school and understood "everything". His teacher, who pointed him out to us, was of a different opinion and held him for a backward pupil. On the arithmetic test he earned one raw score point (knowledge of coins) and on the block design test none. At interview he gave every indication of a dull youngster and was rated as a case of mild oligophrenia (P_1, ICD 317). He was the youngest of five siblings and the only male among them; his four sisters were not at school. The second case relates to a nine year old girl who was actually in school but not progressing, as both first the family (which ranges among the "village informants" in Table D II 1), then the teacher and finally the pupil herself confirmed. She liked school and lessons, she said, but she simply could not learn as her comrades did and was afraid of being reported to her parents as unsatisfactory. Tests (arithmetic raw score 2, block design 0) and clinical examination gave no hint of any other cause. She helped her mother at home, got along well, was not in her own view unjustly punished or beaten. We diagnosed a mild imbecility (P_2, ICD 318.0). Thus both cases possessed in fact their indicators outside the three listed, partly in informants, partly in the results of the intelligence tests. The very low scores on these naturally would have been much less striking had not both children been attending school. As pointed out in the introductory chapters, the questionnaire is not highly indicative in younger children except for neurological or symptomatic residual disorders and then usually depends on replies from relatives or other informants.

As might be expected, the proportion of cases in which only a single indicator was positive is largest for P_1 in the Shiraz survey (Table D II 3 Percentage by Column, 1) with 68 % and decreases through 29 % for P_2 to only 19 % for P_3. In this table the raw data from Table D II 2 are combined according to number of indicators and degree of pathology, expressed in percent and compared both horizontally and vertically for the Shiraz and Marvdasht surveys. Their pattern is less regular in the latter partly because of the smaller numbers with greater influence of chance fluctuations on percentage calculations, partly because of the probably too few P_1 cases as explained in the relevant chapter. Therefore we shall refer mainly to the Shiraz data. It is noticeable that a similar progression from P_1 to P_3 does not appear in Marvdasht. Neither is it regular in Shiraz when comparison is made by row (upper left). There, as in Marvdasht, half of the P_1 cases have two indicators: a circumstance that speaks for the indicators themselves. Corresponding to this, the percentage of cases in Shiraz having two positive indicators was highest (60 %) in P_1 category, though taken by row almost equal for P_2 and P_3, but lower for P_1. Where only one indicator is involved, the contributions of Z and Q in Shiraz are roughly equal, but X lags far behind. The case is different in Marvdasht, with Z and X nearly equal and no Q, but the total of 7 is too small for any conclusions to be drawn.

Anticipating somewhat, we encounter the problem of the two P_3 cases (one each in Shiraz and Marvdasht) with only a single positive indicator, whereas one would naturally expect more positive indications in the severest cases. The first concerned a twenty year old youth from Shiraz, whom the examiner recognized and the psychiatrist confirmed to be an untestable idiot, a victim of infantile jaundice. The dissimulating replies that his relatives supplied to the questionnaire seemed innocuous, so that Q had to be rated negative and Z omitted. The psychiatric examination produced the necessary confirmation. The other such case was that of a thirty year old woman from Marvdasht with a traumatic epilepsy, whom the examiner correctly judged, but whose tests and questionnaire no longer could be found, although the case notes are in our files. In default of them she had to be rubricated under X alone. Neither case was in danger of being missed.

Since Z and X do appear by themselves as single valid indicators, it may cause some surprise that the combination ZX plays a very small part in the groups of 63 and 28 cases respectively with two indicators apiece, accounting for only 7 and 3 cases respectively. The combination QX furnishes twice as much, but the lion's share is found under ZQ. This accords well with the percentages of correct identification by single indicators shown at the left below the half-tables in Table D II 2, whereby Z and Q are both correct in about three quarters, X only in about half the verified cases. This might mislead one into regarding X as no better than chance, with 50 % likelihood for right or wrong, and discarding it altogether. We recall, however, that X contributed 4 out of 7 identifications by a single sign in Marvdasht and 4 out of 38 in Shiraz, and that in each place one P_3 case was identified by X alone. Quantitatively, the loss of four cases would have diminished the overall Shirazi prevalence rate from 16.59 to 16.16 per thousand and the Marvdasht rate from 9.90 to 9.11 – the first to be sure by a trifling, the second by a not inconsiderable degree. In any instance, no one would wish to miss cases when their identification can be accomplished with so little expenditure of time and effort.

Cases with two positive indicators constitute percentually the largest group of the four with none, one, two or three indicators in both surveys. It would have been a pleasant corroboration if it had been the group with three instead, but again too good to be true. On the other hand, it would have been disquieting if the group with only one indicator had led. Analyzing the cases with three, we remark again that their share is much higher for P_3 in both surveys (comparison by row) than for P_1 and P_2, as one would expect, but that it does not increase from P_1 to P_3 when comparison is made by column. Its maximum lies in both cases at P_2. The fallibility of all indicators plays us a trick here, and we must inquire how serious this is. The discrepancy for Shiraz and for Marvdasht amounts to two cases each against a total of 11 P_3 for Shiraz and 6 P_3 for Marvdasht. At both sites one case each has two indications and one case each only one. The latter two have been described, and it has become apparent that they were very unlikely indeed to have been missed, while in the former two there exists at least a reassuring confirmation of one indicator by another. By another method of comparison we observe that in the two surveys combined there are $47+13 = 60$ cases in which all three indicators are positive or 29 % of the 204 cases altogether, but only $11+6 = 17$ P_3 cases, i.e. 8 %.

If the question be posed, finally, which of the three principal indicators should be retained and which abandoned, our answer to the latter would be: none. All are fallible. How fallible they are depends to no small extent upon working conditions, i.e. time and personnel. Under favorable circumstances the fallibility of certain indicators can be reduced substantially: cf. the examiners in Shiraz and Marvdasht. If we were forced by whatever exigency to choose one indicator only it would be the Z Test, as its discordancy rate is much the smallest, but this only under the condition of possessing adequate opportunity for reviewing the records at leisure after the field work was done.

A quick estimation of them in field likewise yields a very satisfactory discordance rate, as Mr. Ordoobadi's results prove, but misses too many true cases. For catching them, as it were, on the wing, the questionnaire, when applied flexibly, abutted by clinical judgment and supplemented wherever needful by interrogation, does as well. We should state again, however, with all emphasis that it is not an instrument to be used mechanically, as the vast majority of other psychiatric and psychological personality questionnaires are.

Our indicators, especially Z and Q, may embrace nearly equivalent areas, as the figures demonstrate, but the boundaries of these areas are *not congruent*. What one indicator points out, another may miss, and vice versa. This emerges with great clarity from the identifications by single indicators, and therein lies the incontestable advantage of using several brief indicators of widely different kinds. Multiplying basically similar indicators such as several questionnaires, as has been done in some infelicitous examples, is more likely to multiply mistakes than anything else. These remarks only repeat familiar facts of clinical practice, but we should like to re-emphasize them for purposes of epidemiological research.

Looking back upon the amount of paper consumed we found ourselves confronted with the question how much we could have learned from paper alone? In at least one oft-quoted survey the two psychiatrists never saw a patient, although they had professionally prepared detailed extracts from a 65 page questionnaire administered by experts on which to work [186]. In order to obtain an estimate we examined an additional 1535 individual records of both sexes and all ages outside our psychiatric survey population, which together covered most of the rest of the city and were drawn from all its districts but one (the survey districts naturally excepted). The rest might have been covered too, but more urgent and more profitable tasks called, so 437 records were not scrutinized for this particular purpose. We strove to draw simply from what stood in black and white on paper – personal data, test findings, responses to the psychiatric questionnaire, examiners' judgements, their and sometimes our own notes – a conclusion as to whether the individual probably was psychiatrically well or ill in the sense in which we have understood these terms throughout and to differentiate further between only a suspicion and a high probability of illness. We did not try to make diagnoses or estimates of severity. As we set to working through these records it became clear to us that an objective judgment on the basis of the papers alone was impossible and that our estimate of their efficacy could be at best a very crude one, for even three to four years after the date vivid memories of persons and whole households intruded themselves and determined the judgment after a mere glance at the file. True, these instances were in the minority, and the magnitude of the rough estimate interested us still. Working from the routinely gathered and demanded information alone, we gleaned from the 1535 files 173 that seemed to offer considered grounds for suspicion of more than trifling psychopathology and 3 more in which we could regard the suspicion as close to a certainty, i.e. 176 or 11.5 % of the non-survey group altogether. The closer, more exacting personal scrutiny given the psychiatric survey population with its 16.6 % of pathological cases thus had been quantitatively rewarding besides furnishing us qualitatively with diagnoses and information about degree and distributions of severity. In addition to the routinely, systematically gathered data we then tried to take into account the accidental, unsystematic information that had accrued to us in various ways: often on random supervisory visits during the first or testing phase throughout the city, less often by notes of other supervisors, of examiners or colleagues, in conversations about families seen and visits performed etc., occasionally through all manner of other informants. Where we had either seen a case ourselves and been able to make a prima facie diagnosis or had been given an unambiguous, convincing description, as was possible mainly in severe mental deficiencies and organic cases, epilepsies and a few schizophrenias, we classified it as "assured outside the psychiatric survey population". There were 49 such. Where our own direct or others' recorded observations outside the routinely collected information gave ground only for suspicion we classified the individual as "suspect by other (than routine) indications". Of such there were 52. The observed cases rated as assured or suspect outside the psychiatric survey population thus comprised 101 persons or 6.6 % of the 1535. Adding them to those whom we had estimated by their routine records alone as being strongly or less strongly suspect (excluding as far as was possible the influence of memory) we count altogether 277 probably pathological cases or 18.1 % of 1535 persons and exceed with this figure the 16.6 % of cases verified in the psychiatric survey population.

These percentages are no more than empirical notes without claim to scientific value and are offered for what they are worth. They may hold some interest for workers in the field or even have some use for the crude assessment of expectations. Beyond this they do not purport to go. The scientific epidemiologist will rightly wonder why we did not submit a sample of records to "blind" inspection by a third party or parties. We should have been glad to do so, had we been able to find one with the requisite time, interest and qualifications, which last include reading Persian.

III. General Psychiatric Epidemiology

General epidemiology, whether psychiatric or other, can content itself with an enumeration of cases – in itself a valuable and practically useful piece of knowledge. This basic knowledge, however, becomes more meaningful when related to such universal biological factors as sex and age and to such socio-cultural factors as socio-economic status and environment in the broad sense in which we have taken this word. Properly it should also be brought into relation with the full picture of public health and medicine, including diverse epidemiologies, but this can be done systematically only where very extensive, detailed and reliable statistical material is available. Where it is or has been in Iran, we have tried to take advantage of it, and indeed our first psychiatric survey was part of a public health survey, as the subsequent ones ideally should have been. Most of the essential demographic data we have collected ourselves. A great deal more sociological and ethnological information would have been welcome and may in part exist somewhere, but we have forced ourselves to resist the temptation of searching for it for years in the relevant special libraries without much hope of coming upon what we really needed and delaying the already much delayed publication accordingly. Let us rather try to make the best of what we have.

Table D III 1 presents an inventory of what we do have, summarizing the basic characteristics of our five main surveys according to time, place, census population, the sample intended to be taken therefrom and the sample actually scrutinized. The corresponding characteristics for Qassemabad in 1963 and 1976 are given in the local Chap. I 4 of Part B because Qassemabad 1963 is included in the Marvdasht Survey of that year. They are not essentially different from those of the two other villages, Kenareh and Zangiabad, that were surveyed at the same time except for a certain excess of female cases. The last line of the table indicates the thoroughness and to some extent the success of the survey, though it does not tell the whole story. Khuzestan and Shiraz stand out with a coverage of some 99 %, and Qalandari is not far behind. The Khuzestan survey is the one in whose results we rest the most confidence, the one in which we had the best staff and the only one in which we were not pressed for time. In Shiraz we were under great pressure after long initial delay and could only achieve coverage by reducing our goal. The results, we believe, justified doing so, and indeed we had no other choice. In Qalandari too we were pressed for time, but even a generous extension of it probably would not have enabled much better coverage, since a fraction of the population was widely scattered over the region and even over the entire country during the summer. Among the Qashqai the pressure was strongest and both coverage and randomization poorest, so that we have tended to doubt our own results until Qalandari furnished a partial corroboration for them. We still question the psychiatric morbidity rate of zero in a sample of 189 persons, but we have better grounds than in 1963–4 to believe that the true rate must be low. The most dubious results were those of

Table D III 1. Census Populations and Samples from All Surveys

	Marvdasht	Khuzestan		Shiraz	Qalandari	Qashqai Nomads
Year	1963	1965		1970	1970	1963
Census population: all ages	3984	614		346 231[a]	193	499
			Survey Population (SP)	Psychiatric Survey Population (PP)		
Intended sample of census population	820	614	3386	1153	193	499
Percent of intended sample out of census population	20.6	100	0.98	0.33	100	100
Intended sample ≥ 6 years	598	485	2941	940	153	380[b]
Percent of intended sample ≥ 6 years	72.9	79.0	86.9	81.6	79.2	76.1[b]
Actual sample ≥ 6 years	500	482	2914	928	144	189
Percent of actual out of intended sample ≥ 6 years	83.6	99.4	99.1	98.7	94.1	49.7

[a] Estimate obtained by multiplying official number of households 62723 x 5.5, this factor representing the mean household size in our Survey Population.
[b] Estimate obtained by prorating data from [166], wherein only ten-year age groups are stated.

our first survey in Marvdasht, not only because it was the first, from which we had to learn and did learn much, but also because of the special circumstances described in Part B, Chap. I.

The numerical results and the total psychiatric prevalence rates for all surveys except the Qashqai are summarized in Table D III 2 according to site, sex and degree of pathology. Here and hereinafter the Qashqai are omitted because their rates are zero throughout. In the first sub-table are listed the absolute numbers together with the size of the psychiatric survey population (PP) from which they were derived. Note that the PP here comprises both the unpathological and the pathological. In the second sub-table we have calculated the percents by row for each site separately, showing for each sex, together and severally, what percentage of cases was to be found under which degree of pathology. The last sub-table states percentages referred, for each site, to the psychiatric survey population scrutinized at that site. These are true prevalence figures, and the final column for P of males and females together contains the overall prevalence rates per hundred for the four sites (elsewhere we have stated them as a rule per thousand as more convenient, avoiding decimals). The good agreement between Shiraz and Khuzestan is immediately apparent in the third sub-table, likewise the much lower rates in Qalandari and the deviations of Marvdasht (though some items agree closely) from both. We shall now attempt to analyze these findings in more detail and apply statistical criteria to them.

Before setting out to do so, we must consider which comparisons between surveys are legitimate, meaningful and unlikely to lead us far astray. Shiraz and Khuzestan can be compared directly and fully in every respect except SES. Qalandari can be compared with both as far as its lesser numbers allow; for most subgroups such as degrees of pathology they are too small. The Qashqai, as explained, have been omitted throughout, as their inclusion would only encumber the tables. Though somewhat reassured about Marvdasht after having resurveyed Qassemabad, we have excluded the dubious P_1 category there from statistical treatment. There seemed good reason to suppose that in 1963 we had in Qassemabad and in the whole Marvdasht an over-representation of females and in both sexes, but particularly among the males, an under-representation of P_1. The resurvey of Qassemabad in 1976 under somewhat more favorable circumstances and with a better coverage (90 % instead of 82 %) brought out again a significant female surplus of cases together with a numerical, though statistically insignificant, drop in total prevalence. A strong rise of P_1 as against P_2 could be regarded as realistic, confirmed by relevant psychological measures and related to advantageous socio-economic development. Our dubiety concerning the P_1 rates from Marvdasht did not and does not extend to the sum of $P_2 + P_3$. There is a female surplus, but for it we have obtained secondary partial confirmation. The sum of 7.2 % agrees precisely with that from Khuzestan, which we have no reason to doubt, and is marginally lower than the 8.0 % of Shiraz. Observation and experience at all three sites make it wholly plausible to us that the total P rate of Marvdasht would be of the same order as in Shiraz and Khuzestan, perhaps even (judging by the complaint scores) rather more than less. Moreover, after perusing a number of epidemiological surveys such as are collated in Annex III it seems also somewhat more than likely to us that not a few investigators have classified as pathological only such cases as would be P_2 or P_3 by our standards. Their rates range around the 7–9 % that we have discovered in three of the four surveys under question (Qalandari has only 2.8 %). Comparison of the summed P_2 and P_3 frequencies therefore seems not only permissible, but even requisite, particularly in regard to other surveys. Determination of this group of "hard" cases is also without doubt attended with less uncertainty and subjectivity than that of P_1. In the following Table D III 3, where the significances of the rates set down in Table D III 2 are compared in the usual way, we have therefore included a rubric $P_2 + P_3$ which encompasses Marvdasht, while the other rubrics (P_1 and P) do not.

The prevalence rates were compared by X^2 and were not calculated when the population of the cells was 0 or 1 (nc). Besides the prevalency rates, we also compared the differential rates for the sexes in each of the specified populations and sites (right hand columns), using now both X^2 and the critical ratio, which generally, but not always, agreed. The designation to the left is to be read first, that above second, the chevrons accordingly. Thus in the first line there are significantly more P_1 cases of both sexes together in Shiraz than in Qalandari, and the level of confidence is better than 5 %. The difference is not significant for either sex alone. By critical ratio, but not by X^2, there is a tendency for more women than men in Shiraz to be psychiatrically disturbed at the P_1 level.

Far more impressive to us than the few significant differences was the near uniformity of most results, though they covered a wide range of geographical and socio-economic differences. For all P_1 there is only the single significant difference just mentioned, with a tendency (resulting from small numbers, but by our experience a fact) for Khuzestan to exceed Qalandari. Neither in P_1 nor in P_2 and P_3 combined is there any significant local difference to be found for one sex by itself. When they are combined for $P_2 + P_3$ the same pattern emerges as for P_1, together with a tendency for Qalandari to have less pathology than Marvdasht (by observation again a fact). By critical ratio more $P_2 + P_3$ females than males are to be found in Khuzestan and in Marvdasht: sex differentials will be discussed below. They vanish here for total P, while on the contrary, thanks to increased numbers, significant but generally agreeing differences for the two sexes apart do appear. They are unanimous: Shiraz and Khuzestan, as we suspected from Table D III 2, do not differ significantly anywhere, but both do highly significantly from Qalandari. As mentioned in Part B, Chap. 2 c, this difference has been confirmed by Fisher's exact probability test. The Qashqai must not be forgotten: they stand closer to Qalandari than to Khuzestan or the city. It is evident that this cannot be an urban-rural difference. The common denominator is the (then still) intact tribal structure of both the itinerant and the settled Qashqai. They enjoy on the whole substantially, demonstrably better mental health, whatever else their tribulations may be. The prevalence rates for Shiraz and Khuzestan on the other hand, diverse as these two sites are, agree very well with published rates, gained according to similar standards though with greatly differing methodology, from sites as remote from Iran and from each other as London and an Austrian city dubbed "Kleinburg".

The discussions and tables that now follow have been executed according to a unified plan. Except for a few instances, which have been treated partly in the relevant chapters and partly shall be taken up in the next, the number of cases for single psychiatric diagnoses, redivided by sex, degree of severity, site, etc. was usually too low for valid statistical comparison. We have therefore adopted the expedient of grouping them into the major categories employed in the diagnostic tables, i.e. the symptomatic, reactive and constitutional, omitting the functional psychoses again because of their

Table D III 2. All Surveys Except Qashqai: Total Prevalence Rates by Sex and Degree of Pathology

	Male				Female				Male and Female				
	P_1	P_2	P_3	P	P_1	P_2	P_3	P	P_1	P_2	P_3	P	PP
	Absolute Numbers												
Shiraz	34	28	10	72	46	35	1	82	80	63	11	154	928
Khuzestan	22	14	0	36	15	16	5	36	37	30	5	72	482
Qalandari	0	3	0	3	3	1	0	4	3	4	0	7	144
Marvdasht	4	11	3	18	10	19	3	32	14	30	6	50	500
	Percent by Row												
Shiraz	47.2	38.9	13.9	100	56.1	42.7	1.2	100	51.9	40.9	7.1	100	
Khuzestan	61.1	38.9	0	100	41.7	44.4	13.9	100	51.4	41.7	6.9	100	
Qalandari	0	100	0	100	75.0	25.0	0	100	42.9	57.1	0	100	
Marvdasht	22.2	61.1	16.7	100	31.3	59.4	9.4	100	28.0	60.0	12.0	100	
	Percent by Psychiatric Survey Population (PP)												
Shiraz	3.7	3.0	1.1	7.8	5.0	3.8	0.1	8.8	8.6	6.8	1.2	16.6	928
Khuzestan	4.6	2.9	0	7.5	3.1	3.3	1.0	7.5	7.7	6.2	1.0	14.9	482
Qalandari	0	2.1	0	2.1	2.1	0.7	0	2.8	2.1	2.8	0	4.9	144
Marvdasht	0.8	2.2	0.6	3.6	2.0	3.8	0.6	6.4	2.8	6.0	1.2	10.0	500

disproportionally small numbers. Great though their importance is, they are of a different order of magnitude. Their inclusion would only have encumbered the tables and changed no basic differences or their significances, as we have determined by calculating such tables for ourselves. When we compared e.g. the three larger surveys (Shiraz, Khuzestan, Marvdasht) in regard to the relative frequencies of the disease categories either for all P or for any grade of it, the tables contained 3 x 3 cells with 4 df. If we chose to compare any pair of surveys or any other pair of variables in regard to the same distribution there were 3 x 2 cells and thus 2 df. The same principle could be applied to the three sub-categories of one main category: that of the numerous reactive disorders with their subdivisions into simple, neurotic and psychosomatic. Therefore the Tables D III 4 and 5 are double, with the three main disease categories in the upper, the three sub-categories of reactive disorders in the lower half. Our interest lay in inquiring whether there existed significantly different patterns of frequencies for both triplets according to sex, age, SES, degree of severity and environment.

Few such comparisons including Marvdasht were possible for the reasons set forth above. Their X^2 values were all remote from significance, so they are not represented here. Qalandari was excluded because of its much smaller numbers, as of course were the Qashqai.

The remaining tables have 3 x 2 cells and 2 df. Wherever their X^2 values implied a level of confidence poorer than 10 % no further calculations were performed, as indicated by dashes – in the respective columns. If the level of confidence was 10 % or better, the paired values for each category or sub-category were compared by critical ratio in two ways, taking once as a basis of reference the sum of the column in question, once the number of subjects in the respective psychiatric survey population. The critical ratio was applicable in the not infrequent cases where the population of a cell was zero or very low and X^2 could not be employed. Chevrons were used as heretofore, and ns to show that no significance was attained. Be it noted that in these tables ns and a dash do not have the same meaning.

In Table D III 4 one sees comparisons by sex that are more detailed and textured than the global comparisons of Table D III 3. Only Shiraz and Khuzestan afforded suitable bases. Both are subdivided again into P_1, P_2 and P. The reference base for each left hand column C was the number of cases of the respective sex (C_x) and degree of pathology, for each right hand column PP_x the number of subjects (not cases) of the respective sex in the total psychiatric survey population. Trial computations based on the number of cases of both sexes and on the total PP gave nearly the same results in regard to the presence or absence of significant differences, but the degrees of significance were altered here and there. Comparison by sex based on numbers of own sex seemed more appropriate where we were inquiring not about overall sex differentials, but about difference in the distribution over categories.

Beginning with Table D III 4 we observe that in Shiraz there is no significant sex difference in the distribution over the major categories for P_1, but there is for P_2 and for all cases taken together (P). In both P_2 and P the females have very significantly more reactive disorders, and the difference is made up by a surplus of symptomatic disorders among the men, to a lesser extent also by a male surplus of constitutional disorders that reaches a not quite certain significance only in P. Briefly, the Shirazi women and girls have more reactive disorders and more severe ones than the men and boys. Turning to Khuzestan there is an indication of the same difference, but it is significant only for P_2,

Table D III 3. All Surveys Except Qashqai: Significance of Differences Between Total Prevalence Rates by Sex and Degree of Pathology

		P_1 m SH	KZ	QL	f SH	KZ	QL	m + f SH	KZ	QL	m : f χ^2	D/SD_D
Shiraz	SH		ns	ns		ns	ns		ns	›	ns	(‹)
Khuzestan	KZ			ns			nc			(›)	ns	ns
Qalandari	QL										ns	ns

		$P_2 + P_3$ m SH	KZ	QL	MD	f SH	KZ	QL	MD	m + f SH	KZ	QL	MD	m : f χ^2	D/SD_D
Shiraz	SH		ns	ns	ns		ns	nc	ns		ns	›	ns	ns	ns
Khuzestan	KZ			ns	ns			nc	ns			(›)	ns	ns	‹
Qalandari	QL				ns				nc				(‹)	ns	ns
Marvdasht	MD													ns	‹

		P m SH	KZ	QL	f SH	KZ	QL	m + f SH	KZ	QL	m : f χ^2	D/SD_D
Shiraz	SH		ns	››		ns	›		ns	›››	ns	ns
Khuzestan	KZ			›			(›)			›››	ns	ns
Qalandari	QL										ns	ns

Table D III 4. Shiraz and Khuzestan Surveys: Comparisons by Sex

	Shiraz						Khuzestan					
	P_1		P_2		P		P_1		P_2		P	
χ^2 df = 2	ns		$p < 0.05$		$p < 0.01$		ns		$p < 0.10$		ns	
D/SD_D	C_X	PP_X	C_X	PP_X	C_X	PP_X	C_X	PP_X	C_X	PP_X	C_X	PP_X
Symptomatic	–	–	›	(›)	››	›	–	–	ns	ns	–	–
Reactive	–	–	‹‹	‹	‹‹‹	‹‹	–	–	‹	‹	–	–
Constitutional	–	–	ns	ns	›	(›)	–	–	(›)	ns	–	–
χ^2 df = 2	$p > 0.05$		$p < 0.10$		$p < 0.05$		ns		ns		ns	
D/SD_D	C_X	PP_X	C_X	PP_X	C_X	PP_X	C_X	PP_X	C_X	PP_X	C_X	PP_X
Simple reac.	(‹)	‹	‹	‹	‹	‹‹	–	–	–	–	–	–
Neurotic	ns	‹‹	›	ns	ns	‹	–	–	–	–	–	–
Psychosomatic	››	(›)	ns	‹	›	ns	–	–	–	–	–	–

C_X : based on cases with respective sex.
PP_X: based on subjects of respective sex from total psychiatric survey population.

the degree of significance is lower, and we cannot conclude from the table whether the men make it up in the symptomatic or constitutional categories or in both. When we attempt further to analyze the sex differences in kind of reactive disorder we now find for Shiraz a significant difference in P_1, but one that is not altogether clear from the table because C_x and PP_x do not fully agree. They tend to in respect to the simple reactions and the psychosomatic disorders, the women having more of the first, the men more of the second. For the neurotic disorders PP_x is fully, but C_x not at all significant, but PP_x has a broader numerical basis and therefore allows more confidence. Almost the same picture holds for P, which is likewise significant at the 5 % level. P_2 manifests only a trend, but a different one. The women still lead in the simple reactions, but not in the psychosomatic disorders, and there is an indication, this time according to C_x, that the men have more severer neuroses. Khuzestan turns in a blank, in all likelihood because of the lower number of cases. Further details must be sought in the diagnostic tables.

The question how age influences mental health must be put differently. The constitutional disorders are by definition ageless, if we disregard differences in age of manifestation and in life expectancy. Symptomatic disorders obviously mount with increase of exposure and with approach to old age. Such tables as D III 4 seemed superfluous, the more so as our data only enabled a comparison between youth and adulthood. We have therefore taken recourse to a form of comparison employed in our first publication on Khuzestan [26], taking separately for the unpathological and pathological their percentages in each age group with their respective sums as bases, not the entire PP. If the percentages correspond roughly one to the other across age, there can be no influence of age per se; if they differ significantly at certain age levels there must be. As the data are already given in the relevant chapters and tables (Table B I 3 for Marvdasht, B II 2 for Khuzestan and B IV 1 for Shiraz) they shall not be tabulated again here. The interested reader easily can make his own regroupings and percentage calculations, and even these are present in Table B IV 1. As this table uses an age class of 6 to 14, whereas we shall have occasion below to use a subdivision into 6–9 and 10–14, we may state that among the former there were in Shiraz 14 pathological and 107 unpathological members, among the latter 24 pathological and 161 unpathological. We can now calculate a comparison of the pathological and unpathological for all the usual six age classes in a table with 6 x 2 cells and 5 df. For Shiraz X^2 is 16.69 and thus $p < 0.01$, for Khuzestan $X^2 = 13.28$ and $p < 0.02$, whereas for Marvdasht X^2 is only 6.51 and the difference far from significance ($p < 0.30$). Neither does a significant difference for Marvdasht appear when we calculate the sexes separately.

Where do the differences lie? In early school age and beyond middle age. In Shiraz the age class 6–9 encompasses 8.4 % of the pathological, but 13.0 % of the unpathological; in Khuzestan the percentages are 8.3 % (identical with Shiraz) and 19.4 %. For the following five year interval of 10–14 years the proportions are somewhat different: in Shiraz the unpathological still lead by a small margin (19.9 % to 16.2 %), but in Khuzestan they fall behind (16.2 % to 19.5 %). In the crucial adolescent lustrum 15–19 the percentages of the unpathological in both places are again less than those of the pathological, and in Khuzestan the pathological even fall back to the level of the 6–9 year olds: 8.3 %. In the early middle age range from 20 to 39 the percentages are nearly equal for both groups in both places. In later middle age from 40 to 59 they diverge in the opposite direction. Shiraz has 16.9 % unpathological, but 19.5 % pathological; Khuzestan 18.5 % and 29.1 %. The like discrepancy is visible over 60. The lines cross. Youth furthers mental health, middle age sustains it, more advanced age (though still remote from senility) impairs it. Noteworthy is that adolescence on the whole does not.

As between Shiraz and Khuzestan, the differences are significant at the 5 % level for the age classes 6–9 and 40–59. In age Khuzestan has a larger proportion of pathological cases, in youth of well persons. The rates for senile and arteriosclerotic dementia do not differ substantially. Whatever other interpretations may be offered, it cannot be concluded from these data that village life tends to conserve mental health past middle age.

The lack of any demonstrable age effect in Marvdasht came at first as a surprise. Upon reflection it is not difficult to explain and confirms our doubts about the validity of certain aspects of the survey. It is easy to conceive that youth was over-represented, because in the few days in the field we could catch nearly all the children in the villages, whereas then and upon our sporadic returns a number of the mature men were missed (absent in the fields, in other villages or on journeys and thus beyond our reach, even though we sent messages in advance requesting them to be at home when we arrived). This appears to have sufficed to cancel out the otherwise very pronounced and significant age effect. We have no reason to suppose that it was absent in Marvdasht any more than in Shiraz and Khuzestan.

Only in Shiraz were there appreciable group differences in socio-economic status that lent themselves to statistical analysis, though in the villages one or another person might be identified as better-off. The relation of poverty or freedom from it to mental health has been treated under a number of aspects in Part B, Chap. IV 2 on Social Psychiatry in Shiraz, to which the reader is referred. It may be recalled that there was a pronounced and significant difference in total psychiatric morbidity rates to the disadvantage of the poor, which applied also to morbidity of medium degree (P_2). The poor women were more affected than the poor men: 63.4 % of the ill women were poor, but only 45.8 % of the ill men ($p < 0.05$). Nevertheless, when we compare the poor and non-poor in the same way as the sexes across major disease categories and sub-categories of reactive disorders we encounter no X^2 value that even approaches significance. Our evidence does not suggest any configuration of disease categories or of reactive sub-categories that is peculiar to the poor. It could be argued that constitutional disorders would appear more frequently as a cause of poverty or simple developments as a reaction to it, but nothing in our data supports this. This remains true when the sexes are treated separately: no difference in pattern appears.

One would like to know whether different degrees of severity are related to or imply different categories of mental illness or reactive disorder or, in other words, whether certain types of illness tend as a whole to be lighter, others severer. They do, as can be seen from Table D III 5. Comparisons were drawn here only between P_1 and P_2, as the severest cases of degree P_3 were fortunately few. The bases of comparison by critical ratio were the number of cases of respective grade (C_p) and the total psychiatric survey population (PP). Again the Shiraz and Khuzestan surveys furnished the material, but this time we have also drawn together the results of all surveys combined from Tables D IV 1–2 in the next chapter. All three sets are highly to very highly significant for the disease categories, as are Khuzestan and the pooled surveys for the reactive sub-categories, but significance for these is wanting in Shiraz. The reactive disorders are very significantly more often P_1 and P_2 in all three comparisons. The symptomatic disorders incline with very high significance to P_2 in Khuzestan and in all surveys together, in Shiraz only by C_p and at a mere 5 % level of confidence. For the pooled surveys the constitutional disorders again tend to be graver by both criteria, while for Shiraz and Khuzestan C_p indicates no more than a tendency and PP is silent. Evidently the surplus of lighter cases among the reactive disorders is compensated mainly by a surplus of severer cases among the symptomatic, while the constitutional disorders range across various degrees with perhaps some inclination toward severity. This unsurprising result must not blind one to the fact, however, that in practice there are a great many exceptions and that, above all, the diagnosis of a reactive disorder by no means implies one that is not severe or even grave – one that does not require to be taken seriously. Psychiatrists acquainted with paralyzing obsessive-compulsive neuroses or malignant hysterias need no admonitions. Neither should it be forgotten

Table D III 5. Comparisons by Degrees of Pathology ($P_1 : P_2$): Shiraz and Khuzestan Surveys Separately and All Surveys Together

		Shiraz		Khuzestan		All Surveys	
χ^2	df = 2	$p < 0.02$		$p < 0.001$		$p < 0.001$	
D/SD$_D$		C_p	PP	C_p	PP	C_p	PP
Symptomatic		‹	ns	‹‹	‹‹	‹‹‹	‹‹
Reactive		››	››	›››	››	›››	››
Constitutional		(‹)	ns	(‹)	ns	‹	‹
χ_2	df = 2	ns		$p < 0.001$		$p < 0.02$	
D/SD$_D$		C_p	PP	C_p	PP	C_p	PP
Simple reac.		–	–	››	›››	››	›››
Neurotic		–	–	ns	›	ns	›
Psychosomatic		–	–	‹‹‹	(‹)	‹	ns

C_p: based on cases with respective degree(s) of pathology.
PP: based on total psychiatric survey population.

that there are symptomatic residual states and constitutional disorders of light, even slight degree.

Lastly we return to the question of environmental differences and ask whether there are such in patterns beside the relatively few in total prevalence rates. The scarcity of the latter does not lead one to anticipate many of the former, but it is far from proving that they do not exist. It will be remembered that all four 3 x 3 comparisons (Shiraz-Khuzestan-Marvdasht compared for P_2 and P across the three major disease categories) turned out to be statistically insignificant. By rule one might have stopped there. Impelled by certain impressions and by curiosity we nevertheless went on to compute the six possible 3 x 2 sub-tables, i.e. comparisons of paired sites over three categories. Only one emerged as significant: Marvdasht-Khuzestan for P_2, with $X^2 = 7.02$ for 2 df and $p < 0.05$. By both criteria Marvdasht had more reactive, Khuzestan more symptomatic disorders, while the rates of the constitutional disorders were not significantly different. This agrees with and confirms what was said about the surplus of P_2 symptomatic disorders in Khuzestan above. For P_1 a comparison was proper only between Shiraz and Khuzestan. It showed no valid differences.

Finally, we could make the same kind of comparisons for the sub-categories of reactive disorders. For P_1 between Shiraz and Khuzestan X^2 was 8.90, and for 2 df $p < 0.02$. Khuzestan led in the simple disorders, Shiraz in the psychosomatic, and for the neuroses there was no difference at this level of severity. Marvdasht could be included in the P_2 and P. For P_2 with now 3 x 3 cells and 4 df, X^2 was 7.64 and this very nearly attained the 10 % level of confidence (7.78). The subordinate comparisons between Shiraz-Marvdasht and Marvdasht-Khuzestan yielded no significant differences, but for Shiraz-Khuzestan X^2 with 2 df was 5.67 and p therefore near to the 5 % level (5.99). The picture was nearly the converse of P_1, as indeed was to be expected, Shiraz leading now in the simple, but more severe developments and Khuzestan in the severer psychosomatic illnesses. The frequency of severer neurosis tended statistically to be slightly higher in the city. For all P together, i.e. all degrees of severity, we found $X^2 = 6.16$ and thus $0.20 > p > 0.10$ for 4 df. Only the comparison between Shiraz and Marvdasht brought forth a subordinated X^2 value near to significance: 4.97, $0.10 > p > 0.05$ with 2 df. The city led in the neuroses, but displayed a tendency to fall behind in the simple developments, while the psychosomatic rates were roughly balanced. In sum, Marvdasht led over Khuzestan in total reactive disorders of medium degree, but was exceeded by Shiraz in neuroses of all degrees together: a finding for which we were prepared by a number of other indications. Among reactive disorders of lighter degree only there was no difference in the neuroses between Shiraz and Khuzestan (Marvdasht falling out of the comparison), but Khuzestan had more simple, Shiraz more psychosomatic illnesses.

IV. Special Psychiatric Epidemiology

1. Combined Surveys

Combining the results of all surveys enables calculations that could not be performed legitimately with lesser numbers, but is this measure justified? It can be so only if the demographic characteristics of the combined populations under scrutiny do not deviate grossly from those of the national population. We possess various indications that they do not.

Our very techniques of random sampling on the one hand, of census study on the other insured representative samples. Some doubts about this in Shiraz, where we did not succeed in sampling the whole city, could be mostly resolved. On the other hand the choice of villages and tribes was not random, but dictated in part by expediency and necessity. Linguistic minorities were not represented except by a few Turkish speaking members of the Qashqai tribe. There was some geographic diversification, but not as much as we should have liked. Tehran was excluded. None the less, comparison of our pooled data with nation-wide census findings seems encouraging.

The national male: female ratio in the census of 1966 according to Nahapatian and Khezaneh [155] was 52:48 % or 108:100. Ours for the combined surveys turned out to be precisely equal. The age structures have been compared several times and shown to be similar. After the extensive Shiraz Survey we had feared an over-representation of the city, but the national ratio of city to country dwellers could be calculated from the data of the same authors for 1966 as 42:58 %, while ours showed itself to be 41:59 % when the greater part of our field work was completed in 1970 (Qassemabad 1976 is not included because it partly overlapped with Marvdasht in 1963). There is also internal evidence. The comparisons by environment in Chap. III of this Part have shown certain differences in the distributions to be sure, but not in the total rates with the exception of the two small Qashqai populations. The agreements far overweigh the divergencies, so that we feel justified in pooling our data and making such cautious use of them in this form as we can. The results are presented in the same way as for the single sites, by degrees of severity and by all degrees together, in Tables D IV 1–4. Comment is supplied in the ensuing sections.

The same results, subdivided by sex and by sites but not by degrees, are presented for comparison in Table D IV 5 according to the ICD.

Table D IV 1. Psychiatric Diagnoses of Mild Cases (P_1)

Diagnoses	Number of cases					p. 100 of 283 cases					p. 1000 of 2243 subjects				
	m	f	m + f			m	f	m + f			m	f	m + f		
I. Funct. psychoses		2	2				0.7	0.7				0.9	0.9		
1. Schizophrenia															
2. Affect. psychoses		2		2			0.7		0.7			0.9		0.9	
II. Acute symptomatic psychoses			0					0					0		
III. Subchronic & chron. sympt. psychoses & residual states	8	6	14			2.8	2.1	4.9			3.6	2.7	6.2		
1. Epilepsy				4					1.4					1.8	
a. cryptogen.	2	2			4	0.7	0.7			1.4	0.9	0.9			1.8
b. symptomatic															
2. Sen. & arterioscl.	3	2		5		1.1	0.7		1.8		1.3	0.9		2.2	
3. post-infectious		1		1			0.3		0.3			0.4		0.4	
4. post-traumatic	1			1		0.3			0.3		0.4			0.4	
5. endocrine		1		1			0.3		0.3			0.4		0.4	
6. addiction	1			1		0.3			0.3		0.4			0.4	
7. other	1			1		0.3			0.3		0.4			0.4	
IV. Reactive disorders	43	62	105			15.2	21.9	37.1			19.2	27.6	46.8		
1. Simple path. dev.	9	21		30		3.2	7.4		10.6		4.0	9.4		13.4	
a. anxious	2	3			5	0.7	1.1			1.8	0.9	1.3			2.2
b. depressive	6	15			21	2.1	5.3			7.4	2.7	6.7			9.4
c. irritable		1			1		0.3			0.3		0.4			0.4
d. neurasthenic		1			1		0.3			0.3		0.4			0.4
e. other	1	1			2	0.3	0.3			0.7	0.4	0.4			0.9
2. Neuroses	23	31		54		8.1	10.9		19.1		10.3	13.8		24.1	
a. anxious	5	5			10	1.8	1.8			3.5	2.2	2.2			4.5
b. phobic	1	1			2	0.3	0.3			0.7	0.4	0.4			0.9
c. depressive	4	5			9	1.4	1.8			3.2	1.8	2.2			4.0
d. hysterical	4	4			8	1.4	1.4			2.8	1.8	1.8			3.6
e. hypochondriac	1	5			6	0.3	1.8			2.1	0.4	2.2			2.7
f. neurasthenic	1	1			2	0.3	0.3			0.7	0.4	0.4			0.9
g. self-insuff.		2			2		0.7			0.7		0.9			0.9
h. negativistic	1				1	0.3				0.3	0.4				0.4
i. other & polym.	6	8			14	2.1	2.8			4.9	2.7	3.6			6.2
3. Psychosomatic	11	10		21		3.9	3.5		7.4		4.9	4.5		9.4	
a. headache					14					4.9					6.2
١. migrainoid	3	6				1.1	2.1				1.3	2.7			
ب. other	4	1				1.4	0.3				1.8	0.4			
b. gastro-intest.	3	2			5	1.1	0.7			1.8	1.3	0.9			2.2
c. asthmatic															
d. other & polym.	1	1			2	0.3	0.3			0.7	0.4	0.4			0.9
V. Constitutional disord.	9	4	13			3.2	1.4	4.6			4.0	1.8	5.8		
1. Clin. oligophrenia	6	3		9		2.1	1.1		3.2		2.7	1.3		4.0	
a. cryptogenetic	6	3			9	2.1	1.1			3.2	2.7	1.3			4.0
b. genetic															
2. Psychopathy	3	1		4		1.1	0.3		1.4		1.3	0.4		1.8	
a. irritable	1				1	0.3				0.3	0.4				0.4
b. anti-social															
c. schizoid	2				2	0.7				0.7	0.9				0.9
d. other		1			1		0.3			0.3		0.4			0.4
Total	60	74	134	134		21.2	26.1	47.3	47.3		26.7	33.0	59.7	59.7	

Table D IV 2. Psychiatric Diagnoses of Medium Cases (P_2)

Diagnoses	Number of cases					p. 100 of 283 cases					p. 1000 of 2243 subjects				
	m	f	m + f			m	f	m + f			m	f	m + f		
I. Funct. psychoses		2	2				0.7	0.7				0.9	0.9		
1. Schizophrenia		1		1			0.3		0.3			0.4		0.4	
2. Affect. psychoses		1		1			0.3		0.3			0.4		0.4	
II. Acute symptomatic psychoses			0					0					0		
III. Subchronic & chron. sympt. psychoses & residual states	21	14	35			7.4	4.9	12.4			9.4	6.2	15.6		
1. Epilepsy				4					1.4					1.8	
a. cryptogen.	1				1	0.3				0.3	0.4				0.4
b. symptomatic	2	1			3	0.7	0.3			1.1	0.9	0.4			1.3
2. Sen. & arterioscl.	2	7		9		0.7	2.5		3.2		0.9	3.1		4.0	
3. post-infectious	7	2		9		2.5	0.7		3.2		3.1	0.9		4.0	
4. post-traumatic	4	1		5		1.4	0.3		1.8		1.8	0.4		2.2	
5. endocrine	1			1		0.3			0.3		0.4			0.4	
6. addiction	2			2		0.7			0.7		0.9			0.9	
7. other	2	3		5		0.7	1.1		1.8		0.9	1.3		2.2	
IV. Reactive disorders	21	46	67			7.4	16.2	23.7			9.4	20.5	29.9		
1. Simple path. dev.	1	7		8		0.3	2.5		2.8		0.4	3.1		3.6	
a. anxious		1			1		0.3			0.3		0.4			0.4
b. depressive	1	4			5	0.3	1.4			1.8	0.4	1.8			2.2
c. irritable		1			1		0.3			0.3		0.4			0.4
d. neurasthenic		1			1		0.3			0.3		0.4			0.4
e. other															
2. Neuroses	14	22		36		4.9	7.8		12.7		6.2	9.8		16.0	
a. anxious	3	2			5	1.1	0.7			1.8	1.3	0.9			2.2
b. phobic		1			1		0.3			0.3		0.4			0.4
c. depressive	2	5			7	0.7	1.8			2.5	0.9	2.2			3.1
d. hysterical	1	7			8	0.3	2.5			2.8	0.4	3.1			3.8
e. hypochondriac		3			3		1.1			1.1		1.3			1.3
f. neurasthenic															
g. self-insuff.	2	1			3	0.7	0.3			1.1	0.9	0.4			1.3
h. negativistic	1				1	0.3				0.3	0.4				0.4
i. other & polym.	5	3			8	1.8	1.1			2.8	2.2	1.3			3.6
3. Psychosomatic	6	17		23		2.1	6.0		8.1		2.7	7.6		10.3	
a. headache					13					4.6					5.8
١. migrainoid	1	11				0.3	3.9				0.4	4.9			
ب. other	1					0.3					0.4				
b. gastro-intest.	1	3			4	0.3	1.1			1.4	0.4	1.3			1.8
c. asthmatic		2			2		0.7			0.7		0.9			0.9
d. other & polym.	3	1			4	1.1	0.3			1.4	1.3	0.4			1.8
V. Constitutional disord.	14	9	23			4.9	3.2	8.1			6.2	4.0	10.3		
1. Clin. oligophrenia	7	5		12		2.5	1.8		4.2		3.1	2.2		5.3	
a. cryptogenetic	7	3			10	2.5	1.1			3.5	3.1	1.3			4.4
b. genetic		2			2		0.7			0.7		0.9			0.9
2. Psychopathy	7	4		11		2.5	1.4		3.9		3.1	1.8		4.9	
a. irritable	4	2			6	1.4	0.7			2.1	1.8	0.9			2.7
b. anti-social	2				2	0.7				0.7	0.9				0.9
c. schizoid															
d. other	1	2			3	0.3	0.7			1.1	0.4	0.9			1.3
Total	56	71	127	127		19.8	25.1	44.9	44.9		25.0	31.7	56.6	56.6	

Table D IV 3. Psychiatric Diagnoses of Severe Cases (P_3)

Diagnoses	Number of cases					p. 100 of 283 cases					p. 1000 of 2243 subjects				
	m	f	m + f			m	f	m + f			m	f	m + f		
I. Funct. psychoses	2		2			0.7		0.7			0.9		0.9		
1. Schizophrenia	2			2		0.7			0.7		0.9			0.9	
2. Affect. psychoses															
II. Acute symptomatic psychoses			0					0					0		
III. Subchronic & chron. sympt. psychoses & residual states	6	5	11			2.1	1.8	3.9			2.7	2.2	4.9		
1. Epilepsy				2					0.7					0.9	
a. cryptogen.															
b. symptomatic	1	1			2	0.3	0.3			0.7	0.4	0.4			0.9
2. Sen. & arterioscl.		2		2			0.7		0.7			0.9		0.9	
3. post-infectious															
4. post-traumatic	1	1		2		0.3	0.3		0.7		0.4	0.4		0.9	
5. endocrine															
6. addiction	4			4		1.4			1.4		1.8			1.8	
7. other		1		1			0.3		0.3			0.4		0.4	
IV. Reactive disorders	1		1			0.3		0.3			0.4		0.4		
1. Simple path. dev.	1			1		0.3			0.3		0.4			0.4	
a. anxious															
b. depressive	1				1	0.3				0.3	0.4				0.4
c. irritable															
d. neurasthenic															
e. other															
2. Neuroses															
a. anxious															
b. phobic															
c. depressive															
d. hysterical															
e. hypochondriac															
f. neurasthenic															
g. self-insuff.															
h. negativistic															
i. other & polym.															
3. Psychosomatic															
a. headache															
α. migrainoid															
β. other															
b. gastro-intest.															
c. asthmatic															
d. other & polym.															
V. Constitutional disord.	4	4	8			1.4	1.4	2.8			1.8	1.8	3.6		
1. Clin. oligophrenia	4	4		8		1.4	1.4		2.8		1.8	1.8		3.6	
a. cryptogenetic	3	3			6	1.1	1.1			2.1	1.3	1.3			2.7
b. genetic	1	1			2	0.3	0.3			0.7	0.4	0.4			0.9
2. Psychopathy				0					0					0	
a. irritable															
b. anti-social															
c. schizoid															
d. other															
Total	13	9	22	22		4.6	3.2	7.8	7.8		5.8	4.0	9.8	9.8	

Table D IV 4. Psychiatric Diagnoses of All Cases

Diagnoses	Number of cases					p. 100 of 283 cases					p. 1000 of 2243 subjects				
	m	f	m + f			m	f	m + f			m	f	m + f		
I. Funct. psychoses	2	4	6			0.7	1.4	2.1			0.9	1.8	2.7		
1. Schizophrenia	2	1		3		0.7	0.3		1.1		0.9	0.4		1.3	
2. Affect. psychoses		3		3			1.1		1.1			1.3		1.3	
II. Acute symptomatic psychoses			0					0					0		
III. Subchronic & chron. sympt. psychoses & residual states	35	25	60			12.4	8.8	21.2			15.6	11.1	26.7		
1. Epilepsy				10					3.5					4.5	
a. cryptogen.	3	2			5	1.1	0.7			1.8	1.3	0.9			2.2
b. symptomatic	3	2			5	1.1	0.7			1.8	1.3	0.9			2.2
2. Sen. & arterioscl.	5	11		16		1.8	3.9		5.6		2.2	4.9		7.1	
3. post-infectious	7	3		10		2.5	1.1		3.5		3.1	1.3		4.5	
4. post-traumatic	6	2		8		2.1	0.7		2.8		2.7	0.9		3.6	
5. endocrine	1	1		2		0.3	0.3		0.7		0.4	0.4		0.9	
6. addiction	7			7		2.5			2.5		3.1			3.1	
7. other	3	4		7		1.1	1.4		2.5		1.3	1.8		3.1	
IV. Reactive disorders	65	108	173			23.0	38.2	61.1			29.0	48.1	77.1		
1. Simple path. dev.	11	28		39		3.9	9.9		13.8		4.9	12.5		17.4	
a. anxious	2	4			6	0.7	1.4			2.1	0.9	1.8			2.7
b. depressive	8	19			27	2.8	6.7			9.5	3.5	8.5			12.0
c. irritable		2			2		0.7			0.7		0.9			0.9
d. neurasthenic		2			2		0.7			0.7		0.9			0.9
e. other	1	1			2	0.3	0.3			0.7	0.4	0.4			0.9
2. Neuroses	37	53		90		13.1	18.7		31.8		16.5	23.6		40.1	
a. anxious	8	7			15	2.8	2.5			5.3	3.5	3.1			6.7
b. phobic	1	2			3	0.3	0.7			1.1	0.4	0.9			1.3
c. depressive	6	10			16	2.1	3.5			5.6	2.7	4.4			7.1
d. hysterical	5	11			16	1.8	3.9			5.6	2.2	4.9			7.1
e. hypochondriac	1	8			9	0.3	2.8			3.2	0.4	3.6			4.0
f. neurasthenic	1	1			2	0.3	0.3			0.7	0.4	0.4			0.9
g. self-insuff.	2	3			5	0.7	1.1			1.8	0.9	1.3			2.2
h. negativistic	2	0			2	0.7				0.7	0.9				0.9
i. other & polym.	11	11			22	3.9	3.9			7.8	4.9	4.9			9.8
3. Psychosomatic	17	27		44		6.0	9.5		15.5		7.6	12.0		19.6	
a. headache					27					9.5					12.0
migrainoid	4	17				1.4	6.0				1.8	7.6			
other	5	1				1.8	0.3				2.2	0.4			
b. gastro-intest.	4	5			9	1.4	1.8			3.2	1.8	2.2			4.0
c. asthmatic		2			2		0.7			0.7		0.9			0.9
d. other & polym.	4	2			6	1.4	0.7			2.1	1.8	0.9			2.7
V. Constitutional disord.	27	17	44			9.5	6.0	15.5			12.0	7.6	19.6		
1. Clin. oligophrenia	17	12		29		6.0	4.2		10.2		7.6	5.3		12.9	
a. cryptogenetic	16	9			25	5.6	3.2			8.8	7.1	4.0			11.1
b. genetic	1	3			4	0.3	1.1			1.4	0.4	1.3			1.8
2. Psychopathy	10	5		15		3.5	1.8		5.3		4.4	2.2		6.7	
a. irritable	5	2			7	1.8	0.7			2.5	2.2	0.9			3.1
b. anti-social	2				2	0.7				0.7	0.9				0.9
c. schizoid	2				2	0.7				0.7	0.9				0.9
d. other	1	3			4	0.3	1.1			1.4	0.4	1.3			1.8
Total	129	154	283	283		45.6	54.4	100.0	100.0		57.5	68.7	126.2	126.2	

Table D IV 5. Distribution of Cases by ICD (9th Revision)

ICD No.	Marvdasht Survey m	f	m + f	Khuzestan Survey m	f	m + f	Shiraz Survey m	f	m + f	Cross Sum
290.0	0	0	0	0	0	0	2	4	6	6
.1	0	0	0	0	0	0	1	0	1	1
.4	0	0	0	0	0	0	1	2	3	3
.9	0	0	0	0	2	2	0	0	0	2
293.1	0	0	0	0	0	0	1	0	1	1
294.1	0	0	0	0	0	0	1	2	3	3
.8	0	0	0	1	0	1	1	0	1	2
295.3	0	0	0	0	0	0	0	1	1	1
.6	1	0	1	0	0	0	1	0	1	2
296.1	0	0	0	0	0	0	0	2	2	2
.2	0	0	0	0	1	1	0	0	0	1
300.0	3	0	3	4	1	5	0	3	3	11
.1	0	1	1	2	0	2	3	10	13	16
.2	0	0	0	1	1	2	0	1	1	3
.4	1	4	5	2	1	3	3	5	8	16
.5	1	1	2	0	1	1	0	0	0	3
.7	0	1	1	0	1	1	1	6	7	9
.8	0	0	0	3	2	5	3	2	5	10
.9	0	0	0	0	1	1	9	7	16	17
301.2	0	0	0	1	0	1	1	0	1	2
.3	0	0	0	1	1	2	4	2	6	8
.5	0	0	0	0	0	0	0	1	1	1
.6	0	0	0	0	0	0	0	1	1	1
.7	0	0	0	0	0	0	2	0	2	2
.8	0	0	0	1	0	1	0	0	0	1
303	0	0	0	0	0	0	1	0	1	1
304.0	0	0	0	0	0	0	6	0	6	6
306.9	1	1	2	0	0	0	0	0	0	2
307.6	0	0	0	0	0	0	0	1	1	1
.8	0	0	0	2	0	2	3	1	4	6
309.1	3	4	7	3	5	8	2	11	13	28
.2	0	1	1	0	1	1	0	2	2	4
.3	0	0	0	0	0	0	0	1	1	1
.9	0	2	2	0	0	0	0	0	0	2
310.1	0	0	0	1	4	5	0	0	0	5
.2	0	1	1	3	0	3	1	1	2	6
.8	0	0	0	1	1	2	5	1	6	8
312.3	0	0	0	1	0	1	0	0	0	1
313.0	0	1	1	2	1	3	0	0	0	4
.1	0	0	0	1	0	1	0	0	0	1
.2	0	1	1	0	0	0	0	0	0	1
314	1	0	1	0	0	0	0	0	0	1
315	1	0	1	0	0	0	0	0	0	1
316	1	6	7	0	2	2	4	3	7	16
317	1	0	1	1	0	1	1	1	2	4
318.0	1	2	3	3	2	5	2	3	5	13
.1	1	1	2	1	3	4	4	0	4	10
.2	0	0	0	0	0	0	2	0	2	2
345	1	1	2	1	0	1	4	2	6	9
346	1	4	5	0	5	5	4	6	10	20
	18	32	50	36	36	72	72	82	154	276

Qalandari m: 306.2, 310.8, 318.2	7
Qalandari f : 300.0, 345, 346, 346	0
Qashqai	283

2. Functional Psychoses[1]

No psychiatric epidemiological survey extending beyond a few hundred probands can escape the question of prevalence of the major functional psychoses, though when attempting to provide even a tentative answer to it the authors must be haunted by the feeling that they need not one or several, but tens of thousands of subjects. Caught between Scylla and Charybdis, the epidemiologist is ineluctably aware that very large numbers can be examined at best superficially and that borderline cases therefore are likely to be missed, while (mis)chance may prevent even a patent case from falling into the small, thoroughly investigated sample at all. In our five studies from 1963 to 1970, 2243 persons aged six or more were subjected to psychiatric scrutiny, and out of these 1468 were fifteen or more years old, fifteen being the lowest limit of the age of risk commonly assumed for the functional psychoses.

As schizophrenia constitutes the core of classical clinical psychiatry, we begin with a consideration of our schizophrenic cases. Three persons were diagnosed definitely as such. Besides these one male subject (Table D IV 6, Case No. 6) had almost certainly suffered schizophrenic attacks, but the disease was not active or even demonstrable at the time of examination, and he was classified as a schizoid psychopath. By most, especially elder authors he would have been included among the schizophrenics. Another schizoid psychopath (Case No. 4) presented much evidence of a paranoid-hallucinatory disorder that our Shirazi colleague did not consider schizophrenic, but that easily might have been diagnosed as such by a psychiatrist less intimately familiar

Table D IV 6. Schizophrenias

No.	Sex	Age	P	SES	ICD	Clinical Characteristics	Survey
						Definite	
1	f	31	2	w	295.3	paranoid Q 6, 8, *9*, 11	Shiraz
2	m	33	3	p	295.6	chronic paranoid Q 0	Marvdasht
3	m	48	3	p	295.1	hebephrenic Q 1, 7, *9*	Shiraz
						Suspect	
4	m	30	1	p	301.2	schizoid psychopath (paranoid-hallucinatory schizophrenia?) Q 3, 6, *9*, *10*, *11*	Shiraz
5	f	30	3	p	345.8	limbic or temporal lobe syndrome (hebephrenia?). Questionnaire missing.	Marvdasht
6	m	44	1	p	301.2	schizoid psychopath (very probably remitted paranoid-hallucinatory schizophrenia) Q 6, 7, *9*, *11*	Khuzestan

Q = Items from the psychiatric questionnaire to which the patient replied in the affirmative. Positive responses suggestive of the diagnosis are in *italics*.

[1] Crude prevalence rates for the functional psychoses and various other psychiatric categories to be discussed below from countries in the Middle and Far East and in North Africa are stated for comparison in Annex III.

with the cultural background and the nuances of the patient's own language. Not so much his vivid hallucinations (possibly pareidolia or dreams) as his composed insistence that he himself had seen poison put deliberately into his food and survived, coupled with an inappropriate flatness of affect, even then left us with lingering doubts. More anomalous was the case (No. 5) diagnosed in Marvdasht as a psychomotor epilepsy without major seizures or as a "temporal lobe" or limbic syndrome if that designation be preferred. In our own minds there was hardly any doubt even without benefit of EEG concerning the diagnosis, but there was equally little doubt that in older epidemiological compilations and probably also in some of newer date the patient would have been reckoned among the schizophrenias. We therefore include her among the three suspect cases for purposes of statistical comparison. The three definite cases all met both the ICD's [207] and M. Bleuler's criteria for the diagnosis of schizophrenia, as did the suspect case 4. Case 5 fulfilled them in respect of psychopathology, whereas a somatic cause could not be excluded and was regarded as likely. Only Case 6 fell short of them, but by his anamnesis almost certainly had been schizophrenic.

Case 2 instantly and decisively negated every item of the questionnaire in a manner that was itself a demonstration of schizophrenic negativism, hence the paradoxical result.

Using a dividend of 3 and a divisor of 1468 we obtain a crude prevalence rate for the adult population of 2.04 ± 1.18 per 1000. This approximates Shepherd's [178] rate of 2.4 per 1000 computed on the same basis for his tenfold larger London sample of 14667 subjects at risk (i.e. in his terminology from 15 years upward, with no upper limitation of age). A dividend of 6 yields a crude prevalence rate of 4.09 ± 1.66 per 1000.

Considering the various age structures of populations the age of risk must be defined and a correction must be made, for which Weinberg's "short formula" is by far the most generally used [203]. According to it, individuals below the age of risk are not counted or are substracted from the total survey population if it includes such. A divisor is formed of half the subjects at the age of risk together with all the subjects that have passed its upper boundary, the presumption being that subjects are distributed by age nearly equally over the period of risk and that at any given age within this span about half will have passed their individual critical point of risk or have been eliminated by death etc. The question then arises: what is the age of risk for schizophrenia? There is no doubt that a peak of incidence occurs in late adolescence, so the lower limit has been set generally at 15, 16 or 17 years. Under the erroneous impression created by the term "dementia praecox" the upper limit has been taken in most elder studies at 39–40, sometimes at 45, rarely at 50 or above. For the sake of comparison with a number of classical investigations we have calculated the age-corrected incidence or expectancy (the expressions are used synonymously) for schizophrenia by Weinberg's short formula, first assuming 15–39 to represent the age of risk. With 3 (definite cases) as dividend this yields an expectancy of 3.05 ± 1.76 per 1000, with 6 (definite and suspect cases) 6.11 ± 2.49 per 1000.

Lin [121] has greatly facilitated comparison by re-calculating the data of a number of authors to conform to the assumption that the age of risk for schizophrenia lies between 16 and 40 years. The reader may refer to his tables 9 and 10 (Shepherd also gives "Psychosis prevalence rates reported in a number of epidemiological surveys" in his Table 17, but they include all psychoses and do not appear to have been re-calculated to the same base, so they are not strictly comparable). The comparable rates of expectancy range between Bremer's [47] 10.0 per 1000 for Norway to Brugger's [50] 3.8 for Thuringia, the latter being the lowest rate that Lin quotes, though still a shade higher than ours if we consider only definite cases. At the time when Brugger was writing, however, there is hardly any doubt that our three suspect cases would have been regarded as unquestionably schizophrenic. As Brugger's figure was gained by a census study of no less than 37561 persons it deserves serious consideration. The same author has reported only slightly higher rates from two other census studies in Germany (3.6 per 1000 in Rosenheim [49] and 4.8 in the Allgäu, Bavaria [48]), but in Basel, using the proband method, has arrived at the astonishingly high rate of 15.3 per 1000 – one of the highest hitherto reported. The results of other studies range in between. From the older ones by the proband method Luxemburger's figure of 8.5 per 1000 from Munich has long been taken as the standard [131]. Among the newer Lin's own from Taiwan, a census study of 19931 individuals, holds an outstanding place. His overall rate comes to 5.9 per 1000. As Lin published in 1953 he could not include in his compilation Essen-Möller's findings from Sweden published in 1956 [70]. Essen-Möller states as a crude rate for his adult population of 1958 (census) 9 per 1000 for cases with an established diagnosis of schizophrenia or 11 per 1000 if four suspected cases are added. We have re-calculated his data as Lin has done for his predecessors. Counting only established cases and assuming the age of risk to lie between 15–39, the expectancy for the Swedish population turns out to be 11.2 per 1000. If age of risk is taken to be 15-59, the Swedish expectancy is 14.2 per 1000. That there is good reason for setting the upper limit higher, around sixty, has been shown in M. Bleuler's incomparably thorough book *Die schizophrenen Geistesstörungen* (The Schizophrenic Mental Disorders) [39], the culmination of a life's work. Bleuler demonstrates the by no means infrequent incidence of what are called "late schizophrenias", i.e. of cases, predominantly paranoid, between the fortieth and sixtieth year, after which they become practically indistinguishable from paranoid disorders associated with and commonly attributed to pre-senile and senile alteration (the *Altersparanoid* of German-speaking psychiatry). Assuming now, as we believe justified, the age of risk to lie between 15 and 59 years, we derive by Weinberg's formula from our data an expectancy for schizophrenia of 3.72 + 2.14 per thousand for definitely diagnosed active cases and of 7.43 + 3.02 per thousand when suspected and remitted cases are included. In older surveys remitted cases regularly have been, and it is only recently and by no means uniformly that cases of limbic or temporal lobe syndrome without manifest seizures or neurological abnormalities other than EEG findings have begun to be recognized and to be differentiated from schizophrenia. The second, larger figure is therefore more suitable for comparison with all but a few newer studies.

Among such those of Dube [63] and Shepherd [178] occupy a prominent place. Beside a crude rate of only 1.49 for active cases, Dube calculates an age-corrected expectancy, using Weinberg's method and an age range of presumably 15–40, of 6.0 per thousand for schizophrenia in India. Since our crude rate for "established" cases comes close to Shepherd's, it becomes desirable to compare the corrected expectancies. Because his published data on patients at risk place them in age classes that extend from mid-decade to mid-decade, we take, for the sake of comparison, his age classes of 15–24 and 25–44 as constituting the population at risk for schizophrenia. It comprises 7056 persons. The population of 45 and over comprises 7026 persons (615 persons of unknown age are omitted from all our calculations). Dividing his 35 cases of schizophrenia by (7056 : 2) + 7026 = 10554 one obtains an age-corrected expectancy rate of 3.32 per thousand. This is very near to ours, for which the age of risk was assumed to be 15–39. (Our Shirazi data have been machine counted to single years, five-year and ten-year groups, but doing this for the hand recorded and counted village data would have entailed excessive labor and altered the result little. Since there is a margin of error in Shepherd's data also from the group of unknown age, an exact comparison still would not have been possible. We take the figures to be approximately comparable.)

Strotzka reasonably does not calculate expectancies for his small, but carefully investigated "normal group" of 500 with its 74 psychiatric cases. In his "psychiatric cases in the norrower sense", a separate group of 100 psychiatric cases derived from general practice, he finds eight schizophrenias. By contrast we count at most six schizophrenias among 283 psychiatric cases altogether, i.e. only 2.3 percent. Baasher [10] has found 7.0 per 1000 between 16 and 50 years of age in a census study of 1860 subjects in the rural Sudan, Jayasundara and co-workers 5.0 per 1000 among 2500 Ceylonese [107]. It would be pertinent to mention large scale North American studies, but the newer ones of predominantly sociological orientation have disregarded diagnosis, whereas the varying criteria of the older ones do not allow comparison. By any standards or assumptions it appears that the prevalence and age-corrected incidence (expectancy) of schizophrenia that we have found in Iran are low.

The expectancy for the affective or manic-depressive psychoses presents fewer problems. The majority of authors find it to be about half that for schizophrenia. Lin again has recalculated the data from various epidemiological studies on the basis of a common age of risk between 20 and 50 and states as his own corrected incidence figure 2.3 per 1000. A number of others (Brugger, Bremer; Uchimura, Tsugawa, these latter quoted after Lin) record similar expectancies, all considerably below their own reported rates for schizophrenia. Scandinavian authors such as Fremming, Helgason, Strömgren and Sjoegren (tabulated in Angst [7] p. 75) report on the other hand expectancies that are both higher in themselves and roughly equal to those they report for schizophrenia. Essen-Möller counts 9 cases as either endogenous-depressive or belonging to his group of "manic, dysphoric or confusional" patients of heterogenous, but in these cases probably also manic-depressive causation. With the age of risk at 20–49 this gives an expectancy of 7.4 per 1000, at 20–59 of 8.2 per 1000, both being only a little below his rates for schizophrenia and in approximate agreement with those of his fellow Scandinavian authors except Bremer and Helgason, whose rates of 18 per 1000 for men and 24.6 for women are the highest of all. Calculated for his total adult population from 15 years upward his rate would be 4.5 per 1000. Here it must be observed that investigators are nearly unanimous in fixing the lower limit of the age of risk at 19 or 20. Many take the upper limit to be 49–50, others 59–60, the former being preferred by elder authors with an inclination to distinguish between endogenous depression and involutional melancholia. Since Angst [7] has convincingly shown by clinical, statistical and genetic evidence that there is no ground for separation between the two, we have no hesitation in taking 59 as the upper limit.

Our three cases, tabulated in Table D IV 7, hardly present any diagnostic difficulties. It is noticeable that all three cases are unipolar, female and poor. Nearly all authors report a preponderance of female patients: here it is absolute. No patient with a mania or a history of mania fell into our samples, though such certainly exist in Iran. We have a lively recollection of a manic psychopath in a Khuzestani village close to our

Table D IV 7. Endogenous Depressions

No.	Sex	Age	P	SES	ICD	Clinical Characteristics	Survey
1	f	30	1	p	296.1	monopolar (depressive) affective psychosis Q 1, *6, 10*	Khuzestan
2	f	50	2	p	296.1	involutional depression Q 1, 3, *6*, 7	Shiraz
3	f	55	1	p	296.1	involutional depression Q 1, 3, *6*, 8	Shiraz

cluster. The expectancy for affective psychosis in our pooled Iranian samples, assuming the age of risk to be 20–59, comes to 4.56 ± 2.63 per 1000. This agrees very closely with the figure that M. Bleuler [38, p. 80] gives as a result of a study performed by the proband method on 599 parents of hospitalized tuberculous patients: 4 ± 2.8 per 1000. Shepherd finds almost exactly as many affective (36) as schizophrenic (35) psychoses in his population at risk (i.e. from 15 upwards) and therefore arrives at the same rate of 2.4 per 1000 as for schizophrenics. Re-calculation of his data does not appear practicable as two (for this question important) age class boundaries cannot be brought into agreement with ours.

One of the most recent and most extensive studies in this field and one of the few that encompasses a satisfactorily large population is that of Dube and Kumar in India [64], a census study of 29468 inhabitants in the Agra region of Uttar Pradesh. All ages from five upward were included. The crude rate for the 37 cases of manic-depressive psychosis was 1.26 per thousand, corresponding closely to our own crude rate calculated from 3 : 2243 = 1.34 per thousand. The Indian authors group by decades from five years on, so a precise age-corrected comparison with our findings cannot be drawn. A rough one can, however, between their 15–54 year old group of 14627 subjects, among whom 32 cases were identified, yielding an uncorrected prevalence rate of 2.17 ± 0.38 per thousand and our own 15–59 year old group with three cases and a similar prevalence rate of 2.27 ± 1.31 per thousand. One of our cases, as will be recalled from the table, was 55 years old and thus just tipped the scale, agreeing with Dube's and Kumar's finding that the prevalence (in their survey of males only) tended to increase with age. From the data in Dube's own next publication [63] based on the same population one can calculate an age-corrected expectancy of 3.9 ± 0.64 per thousand when the age of risk is again taken to be 15–54, only a little below ours of 4.6 for the range of 20–59. If we adjust our boundaries to 15–59, the rate becomes 3.7, practically the same as in India.

For an extensive discussion of prevalence and incidence of depressive disorders both psychotic and reactive the reader may be referred to C. Silverman's *Epidemiology of Depression* [180]. In compiling large amounts of data from many and heterogeneous sources the author has conveyed regrettably little information as to how the respective investigators obtained them originally, so that comparison between the dismayingly various rates is hardly furthered.

This chapter cannot be concluded without a reference to the work of John Ionescu-Tongyonk, a Rumanian-born psychiatrist who emigrated to Thailand and has devoted his life to a study of depression in all its forms in cross-cultural perspective, since he practices in Bangkok among both oriental and occidental patients. Though his papers cover almost every aspect of depression, epidemiological data from field studies in the sense of this book are lacking. With regard to endogenous or psychotic depressions he has contributed an observation of considerable interest. In a publication of 1971 [101] he identified only 2 % of 193 oriental patients treated for depression as psychotic, but 14 % of 70 occidentals. Six years later [102] the respective percentages were 9 and 12. The percentages of somatization of depressive complaints showed a similar convergence between the two ethnic categories. In a valuable summing up of his work, which includes a review of the literature on Thai culture and personality and a great many points of social psychiatric interest, Ionescu-Tongyonk concludes [102, p. 159]: "This study established that the symptomatology of depression in Thai patients is becoming progressively similar in structure and severity to that of occidentals, apparently because of the impact of rapid westernization. The rate of suicidal ideas and attempts was the same in both groups, which seems to indicate that depressive suicidal tendencies are a direct manifestation of the depressive somatosis and are not modified by cultural factors. Although the rate of depressive psychosis remains somewhat lower in orientals, its incidence is on the increase . . ." In agreement with Kraepelin (1904), Ionescu-Tongyonk came to the conclusion that the framework of the psychopathology of depression tends to remain the same throughout the world, independent of various socio-cultural patterns.

Since the author has taken up the topic of suicide in the passage just quoted, it seems appropriate to add here the very little information that we possess. We could not find any general statistics on suicide in Iran. The Austrian ethnologist Erika Löffler, who had lived twice for periods of many months among the Boir Ahmad in Southern Iran, somewhat westward from the Qashqai territory, and has published studies of their culture, told us personally in 1974 that up to a short time before suicide had been unknown in that tribe, at least among the women, but that in the past year or two several attempts had occurred. Much grimmer is a note that B. Good appends to a paper that will be discussed in Chap. IV 4 [85, p. 55, Note 11]: "The matter of suicide in Iran deserves extended research. In the internal medicine hospital at Maragheh, which usually handled emergency suicide attempt cases, 18 % of all patients admitted (117 out of 654 cases) in the year 1352 (1973–74) were attempted suicide cases."

3. Epilepsies

Although the epilepsies are subsumed in our diagnostic tables under "III. Subchronic and Chronic Symptomatic Psychoses and Residual States", as far as they present psychiatric complications, not all do, while their variety and importance requires treatment in a separate chapter.

Since epilepsy can and does strike at any age, the calculation of "age-corrected" expectancy rates has, at least in our view, little meaning, although a number of complicated formulae have been proposed for doing so. This does not preclude awareness that certain types of epilepsy have quite definite age predilections, and that age-corrected rates for such types are indeed meaningful. Their several numerical representations in our material, however, are far too small to justify any computations of this kind. We list our 13 cases by age in Table D IV 8 as we have done for the functional psychoses and include among them one case characterized by a "temporal lobe" or, more properly, limbic syndrome without known seizures as a form of psychomotor epilepsy (identical with Case No. 5 in Table D IV 6, where the question of schizophrenia was discussed). Though certain readers and authors will take exception thereto, we hold the inclusion to be justified by the work of Slater and Beard [183], Wagner [199], and by our own experience [22]. With the exception of this single debatable case we have held to a definition of epilepsy corresponding to Hauser's and Kurland's [94, p. 14]: ". . . *seizure* was defined as the clinical manifestation of paroxysmal hyperactivity of a set of neurons in the brain . . . We defined *epilepsy* as a condition in which seizures, as defined, tend to recur chronically because of a persistent and possibly progressive structural or physiologic abnormality of brain tissue." Implications are that single seizures do not constitute proof of epilepsy, and that the febrile convulsions of childhood likewise are not to be reckoned as epileptic, though they may be precursors of true epilepsy. Few of our subjects had ever had an electroencephalogram. We relied for our diagnoses on case history and description, mindful also of the words of the authors just quoted that "normality of electroencephalographic patterns . . . does not exclude the diagnosis of epilepsy". Neither did we attempt to distinguish between active and inactive or remitted cases, contrary to the principle to which we have generally held. This would have necessitated much more full and exact anamneses than were obtainable in most instances. Our prevalence rates are thus for life-time prevalence from six years of age upward.

Referring our 13 cases to the 2243 individuals under scrutiny we obtain a crude prevalence rate of 5.80 ± 1.60 per thousand. As a total life-time prevalence rate for all forms of epilepsy this is unquestionably too low, since the numerous childhood epilepsies, the incidence of which is high in the first six years of life, are not comprised in it. Furthermore, pure petit mal epilepsies, more frequent in childhood than later, can be missed easily in such a survey as ours, either going unnoticed by the family or being attributed to mannerisms, inattention, misbehavior, etc., while the patient does not always oblige by displaying an absence in the brief time available for examination. Nevertheless Lin [121], whose investigations covered every age from the cradle to the grave, reports a crude rate of only 1.3 per thousand for Taiwan. In his already quoted compendium of other epidemiological studies up to 1953 (partly reproduced in Annex III) the crude rates are all distinctly smaller than ours, the highest being those of Akimoto (2.5 per thousand) and Tsugawa (2.6 per thousand). Among older European studies Brugger found 2.2 per 1000 epileptics in Basel, but only 0.7 per 1000 in Thuringia. In the adjacent Basel countryside (Kanton Basel-Land) M. Bleuler, working at about the same time as Brugger in the 1930s, found however 5.7 per 1000 epileptics among his probands, who were relatives of patients in a general hospital. This rather high rate, similar nonetheless to our own, is approximated by Klemperer's in Germany with 4.8, by Giel's in Ethiopia of 5.2 and exceeded, so far as we know, only by Nandi's of 10.4 in West Bengal. Janz and Scheffner, to be sure, quote an official American estimate [106] of approximately 10 per thousand.

Newer polyvalent psychiatric surveys except Lin's seem to have paid scant attention to epilepsy. Essen-Möller, Baasher, Jayasundara, Shepherd and Strotzka do not mention it. Helgason [97] calculates a life-time prevalency on Iceland of 4.3 per 1000 for males and 3.0 for females. His Icelandic colleague Gudmundsson [90], surveying epilepsy only, arrives at the overall prevalence rate of 3.6, and the annual incidence is said to be almost twice as high for males as for females [quoted from 94]. Turning to surveys of epilepsy alone, one of the most thorough is doubtless that of Hauser and Kurland [94] in Rochester, Minnesota, where they found a life-time prevalence of 6.9 per thousand in 1960 and 6.5 in 1965, to be compared with 3.8 from an earlier, less comprehensive study in the same city by Kurland [118]. These authors review the literature of special surveys and mention the following rates from investigations which they consider reasonably thorough and representative: Brewis et al. from Carlisle, England, 5.5 [48]; Matthai from the Mariana Islands 3.4 [135]; Wajsbort et al. from Northern Israel 2.3 [200].

Be it observed finally that 12 of the 13 subjects affirmed Q 2 of the questionnaire (seizures). One questionnaire (Case 12) is missing.

A glance at Table D IV 8 discloses such a sharp dichotomy between exclusively male cases from 6 to 29 of age and exclusively female from 30 to 32 that it appears artificial and is probably merely fortuitous. Why no cases older than 32 appear is less easily explained. Conjecturally one can invoke such factors as low life expectancy, high accident proneness and the nearly certain fatality of a status epilepticus in a hot climate in which emergency treatment until recently was hardly available. Certain groups of age-bound epilepsies do indeed exhibit a marked preference for one or the other sex, but this could not account for such a dichotomy as remarked above. Helgason too has found a higher prevalence for males in the ratio of about 3:2, while ours is over 2:1. Six of our 13 cases (possibly more) are symptomatic. Four, all symptomatic, are psychomotor. The distribution by degree of severity follows roughly that of our total psychiatric population with 6 P_1, 5 P_2 and 2 P_3. Ten of the thirteen cases are classified as neuropsychiatric, only three as purely neurological, i.e. without alteration of either personality or intellectual and mnestic powers of more than trifling degree, whereas at least one presented a clinical picture that easily could have been taken for schizophrenic. All but two were poor. None came from the well-to-do class. Regrettably, it was too often impossible to ascertain the diurnal type either from the patients themselves or from their relatives, though a few of the nocturnal type did emerge (according to Janz the most frequent of the three types, accounting for 44 % of clinical cases). While the total absolute number of cases is not large and does not permit a study of epilepsy by itself in Iran, the prevalence rate found, even though children below school age are not included, is among the highest reported in general epidemiological surveys and can warrant the conclusion that the epilepsies constitute a special problem within the general and mental health spectrum of Iran. This carries some consolation in the fact that the great majority of epilepsies are amenable to treatment and that the substantial proportion of symptomatic cases surely is capable of reduction through better hygiene and accident prevention.

Table D IV 8. Epilepsies

No.	Sex	Age	P	SES	Or.	DT	Clinical characteristics	NP	Survey
1	m	6	1	p	c	?	Occasional generalized major attacks	n	Khuzestan
2	m	7	2	p	c	d	Occasional generalized major attacks	n	Khuzestan
3	m	7	1	p	c	?	Petit mal	p	Shiraz
4	m	8	1	m	c	?	Occasional generalized major attacks	p	Shiraz
5	m	16	2	p	s	d	Post-infectious, psychomotor	p	Khuzestan
6	m	21	2	p	s	?	After undiagnosed disease of childhood, psychomotor with pseudopsychopathy	p	Shiraz
7	m	22	3	p	s	d	Traumatic, psychomotor	p	Marvdasht
8	m	26	2	p	c	n	Rare generalized major attacks, personality alteration	p	Shiraz
9	m	29	1	p	s	n	Traumatic, rare generalized major attacks, marked neuro-vegetative disturbance	n	Khuzestan
10	f	30	1	p	c	?	Beginning in pregnancy. Rare generalized major attacks, personality alteration	p	Shiraz
11	f	30	2	p	s	?	After typhus. Generalized attacks, personality alteration	p	Qalandari
12	f	30	3	p	s	d	Traumatic. Vegetative crises, probably psychomotor attacks. Clinical behavior remniscent of hebephrenia	p	Marvdasht
13	f	32	1	m	c	n	Beginning in pregnancy. Generalized major attacks	p	Shiraz

Key: P = Pathology by degree (1 = mild, 2 = medium, 3 = severe); SES = Socio-economic status (p = poor, m = medium); Or. = Origin (c = cryptogenetic, s = symptomatic); DT = Diurnal type (n = nocturnal, a = awakening, d = diffuse, ? = unknown); NP = predominantly neurological (n) or psychiatric (p) case.

4. Symptomatic Psychoses and Residual States

We classify the presenile, senile and cerebro-arteriosclerotic diseases together. Relatively brief epidemiological investigation in the field renders difficult such a distinction between them as even under more favorable conditions more often falls to the pathologist than the psychiatrist. By fairly common consent the age of risk for such disorders is taken to be from 60 upward. Our crude rate is 7.1 ± 1.8 per 1000, our age-corrected expectancy 110 per 1000.

Comparisons are hard to find in the older literature. There, the senile-arteriosclerotic psychoses are overlaid by rampant general paralysis and deleted by low life expectancy. If elder authors state any such figures at all, they are usually for "dementia", "deterioration", "organic psychoses" and the like – names which can cover a variety of conditions. Though we cannot affirm that all our senile-arteriosclerotic cases are pure, we have endeavored to separate them from those in which a different organic pathology seemed at least highly probable.

Assuming the age of risk to be from 60 upward as stated, Lin has arrived at an expectancy of 10.7 per 1000 for his Taiwan population. It is noticeable that his expectancies vary greatly, from 27 per 1000 in Baksa, "a small village producing fish and rice", to zero in the market center of Simpo. Brugger's older data, as Lin has recalculated them, come in Thuringia (9.3 per 1000) and Bavaria (10.9) remarkably close to his, as do Tsugawa's for Tokio (14.7). Other Japanese rates from rural areas are lower. So is Strömgren's from Bornholm (only 2.8), while Bremer by Lin's calculation finds an expectancy of 25.2 for Norway. Essen-Möller combines both light and severe cases in his Swedish population. When we recalculate them to the basis of his populations from 60 upward, we find an expectancy for men of 206 per 1000 and for women of 113 per 1000 – figures that are nearer our own. Both high and low rates are encountered in rural areas. These can as little be considered, in themselves, as conducive to serene longevity as to idyllic contentment. In two populations of about five hundred persons each we met with five cases in Khuzestan, but in Marvdasht none, none also in Qalandari and the migrating nomads. In Shiraz there were 11 cases out of 71 subjects aged 60 or more, i.e. 155 per 1000. The prevalence among the entire Shiraz Psychiatric Survey Population of 928 persons was 12 per 1000.

Shepherd refrains from stating directly any figures on senile-arteriosclerotic diseases, arguing that few people consulted a physician primarily because of such ailments (it will be recalled that his data are all drawn from those of physicians in general practice), but he does offer relevant information indirectly in his Table 45: "Medical and Social Factors Associated with Psychiatric Illness, by Psychiatric Category". There, 8.3 % of the psychotic cases are referred to senile and presenile degenerative disorders, 0.5 % of the neurotic, 0.2 % of the psychosomatic and 0.5 % of the others. Since more than one diagnosis or factor was admitted per patient, the numbers cannot be summed, but they do furnish some notion of the magnitude of the problem.

Recently Lauter [120] has reviewed the problem under somewhat different aspects. He summarizes (his Table 5, p. 281) seven studies on "psychiatric diseases of old age" and finds that for the "psychoses" the "figures, with a single exception, lie between 6 and 8 %", the lower age limit being taken by two authors at 60 and by five authors at 65. "Psychosis" is not defined, but the text speaks of "severe organic and endogenous psychoses", i.e. not only of the senile-arteriosclerotic category. If we apply the ICD definition of psychosis to our cases in this category only, we find a prevalence of 5.5 % in the population of 60 and over (8 cases). This definition, however, as the Glossary points out [207, p. 219], is considerably wider than the concept, demanding productive symptoms, in common clinical use in Central Europe. By this only two cases would qualify.

The picture of the senile-arteriosclerotic or degenerative disorders of old age thus remains somewhat contradictory and confusing. It is complicated by other chronic disorders such as depressions and schizophrenias, and it is by no means simple to draw a line between normal aging and pathological senility. Besides this, real differences due to factors such as heredity, hygiene, nutrition, environmental stress and the like seem not improbable and require careful investigation. While geriatric cases do not yet choke the Iranian mental hospitals as they do those of the West, the problem is lurking only around the corner as life expectancy rises. It urgently demands both research and preparatory action.

Having mentioned general paralysis above, we should add that throughout our survey work in Iran we came upon no case of it. All Iranian colleagues and hospitals agree that it is rare, as the first author can substantiate. Where it does occur, it is confined almost exclusively to the vicinity of the Gulf ports. Routine VDRL or similar tests for syphilis were not available except in Khuzestan, where Gremliza had introduced them. There the few positive readings all referred to bejel, a syphilis-like trepanomatosis that does not affect the central nervous or the cardiovascular system [86].

The remaining symptomatic cases of their residua give little occasion for comment. As we have seen, the majority of the post-infectious cases follow upon meningo-encephalitis of generally unknown, probably often viral etiology, both sexes being affected equally. The consequences lie in the well-known alterations of character and personality, making the victims a tribulation to their neighbors and sometimes to themselves: a pseudo-psychopathy, not a dementia. According to world-wide experience improvement in general sanitation may be expected to diminish their number. The six male posttraumatic cases to the single female reflect the greater exposure of the male population. The hazards are more rural, agricultural and elementary than in Western countries, where traffic accidents take an immensely greater toll. Even in Shiraz in 1970 the streets were seldom crowded, and traffic moved, on the whole, at a leisurely pace. As its volume increases year by year, one may hope that measures will be taken to keep its risks within bounds. The remaining smaller groups or their representatives have been described in the appropriate local chapters. It may not be out of place to emphasize once again that we have not addressed ourselves to the problem of addiction and that no general conclusions can or should be drawn from the sparing figure of only seven male urban cases.

5. Reactive Disorders

The reactive disorders constitute the bulk (61 %) of all diagnoses, with an overall prevalence rate of 77 per thousand or roughly 8 %. One might add "as expected" if one did not recall what a minute proportion they formed in earlier epidemiological surveys and if we did not still have ringing in our ears the polite mockery of those who gave us to understand that the search for reactive disorders especially among the country people was nothing more than a wild goose chase. One of the great changes that has come over psychiatry in the past half-century or more has been the recognition that the reactive disorders, which have always been there, did exist and were a part of psychiatry itself. Their rising share in epidemiological studies over the decades tells us probably less about the disorders themselves than about those whose eyes gradually opened to recognize them. Conversely, a newer fashion insists upon regarding all psychiatric illness as reactive and thus asserts a position as extreme, as hemianopic as that of the psychiatric generation to which all "insanity" was hereditary and degenerative. Not the smallest purpose or use of such an inclusive survey as we have attempted lies to our belief in obtaining a better estimate of the relative shares of different kinds of aberrations from mental health with their widely differing, not infrequently multiple etiologies and pathogeneses, their interrelations with each other, the environment and the social order. Our grounds and criteria for classification and diagnoses having been presented already in the introductory section (cf. Part A, Chap. III), we turn now to the findings as a whole.

If we accept the definitions given there and the theory of double repression as applying to the psychosomatic disorders, we have a logical progression from the simple development, in which there may be dissociation but there is little or no repression, to the neuroses, characterized per definitionem by the presence of both, and thence to the psychosomatic illnesses, in which the ever resurgent complexes have been re-repressed, as it were, so thoroughly that they force (in contrast to conversion hysteria) a concrete, patho-physiologically meaningful and persistent somatic outlet. Very roughly their proportions are about 1:2:1. Among the simple developments it is the anxious and depressive that make up the great host, and it is the women who fall prey to them more than the men and tell us so: a finding for which we were prepared by the responses to Question 6 in Chap. C II 2. Their share is more than double the men's. In the neurotic developments or, more simply, the neuroses the sex difference for this group almost vanishes. Males are trained and expected to repress. The sum of anxious, phobic and depressive neuroses together is 15 for the male subjects and 19 for the female, for the depressive neuroses alone 6 and 10 respectively. It may be remarked that all the male anxiety neuroses that we diagnosed (8 cases) came from outside Shiraz. Female preponderance manifests itself again in the hysterical neuroses (11 female to 5 male) and in the hypochondric forms, where there is a single male to compare with 8 females.

While anxieties and depressions could be both simple and neurotic, the conversion hysterias by definition can only be the latter. Out of our 16 cases, all were of urban origin save three. These were a 20 year old woman (P_2) from Marvdasht and two men, both rated P_1, from Khuzestan, one 44 and one 54 years old. In the city the three male cases were 22, 30 and 46 years old, two of degree P_1 and one of P_2, one poor and two (including the case of medium severity) somewhat surprisingly well-to-do. The ten females ranged between the ages of 8 and 60 with a mean of 29, and it was noticeable that the ages of half of them lay between 30 and 39. Only the 60 year old patient just mentioned exceeded this upper limit. In some contrast to the two comfortably situated hysterical males, 8 of the women were poor and 2 of middling socio-economic status. That conversion hysteria is no trifling disease to be shrugged off or passed over as clownery may be seen from the circumstance that we were compelled to grade more than half the females (7 cases) as P_2, whereas only 4 passed as P_1. So far as the small numbers permit any conclusion, it would seem that conversion hysteria affects the female sex more seriously but spares the poorer men who are under stress to provide for their dependents. The stress factor may also help to explain why hysteria is seldom found in Iran outside the city. Even within it 9 out of 13 cases belong to the low socio-economic level, the expectation being about 6, the same level on which the villagers and nomads with maybe a handful of expections found themselves. The middle and upper levels nevertheless were represented. Between poverty in the country and poverty in the city furthermore there is a difference, which is probably of kind more than of degree. The exigencies of life assert themselves in both places, but in the country and on the trail they may be more immediate and elementary. Adequate physical reaction may be more urgently necessary. Conversion hysteria prevents this and mayhap for this reason finds less place in the psychological economy of the directly stressed.

The numbers speak a language that is eloquent without statistical treatment. When we apply the X^2 test to the entire neurotic collective of 90 cases, distinguishing between the sexes on the one hand and the hysteric and non-hysteric neuroses on the other, the differences miss statistical significance as they do within the neurotic collective of the city by itself, but the recurring trend hardly can be ignored or dismissed. Less easy is a statistical comparison between city and village or camp. As explained in the introductory part, the conditions of the Marvdasht and the Qashqai nomad surveys differed somewhat from the rest. In Marvdasht the number of P_1 cases is certainly too low, and in the nomad camp it is not unlikely that some pathological cases of unknown degree were missed. The surveys in Khuzestan and in Qalandari do permit comparison, however, and may be combined for this purpose, totaling 482 +144 = 626 subjects among whom 72 +7 = 79 are pathological. The hysterias are only 2 from 21 neurotic cases in Khuzestan and 0 from a single neurosis in Qalandari, but they are 13 from 54 neuroses in Shiraz.

The picture of the hypochondric neuroses is even more one-sidedly feminine and urban. The unique masculine case and six of the eight feminine ones are from the city. The numerical relationships thus parallel the psychological. Conversion hysteria and hypochondria are both concerned with the body, its ailments and malfunctions. Conversion hysteria creates these, as it were, while hypochondria exaggerates traces already present and within or not far outside everyday bounds. It is therefore not surprising that their bearers are of the same sex and that they tend to congregate in the city, where not only are the consequences of physical debility less dire, but there are also physicians to be consulted. A hint, though not more than a hint that the accessibility of physicians and of traces of popular medical knowledge such as become disseminated even among the poor and ignorant in the city may play a part is offered by the circumstance that, so far as our investigations go, the kindred neurasthenias, whether simple or neurotic, do not tend to accumulate in the city. Rather is the contrary true, as all our four cases are rural. Hypochondric complaints usually are localized, neurasthenic not, and where only the vaguest notions of anatomy exist localization, at least in internal organs, becomes less probable.

The kinds of neuroses hitherto discussed are familiar, easily recognized and covered by ICD titles. They tend to cluster, the anxious, phobic and depressive having in common a tendency to withdrawal, avoidance or depreciation, the hysterical, hypochondric and neurasthenic a pre-occupation with one's own body. Notwithstanding the superfluity of psychiatric terms already in existence, we have felt constrained to introduce one more: the "neuroses of self-insufficiency" in order to avoid minute sub-classifications and to bring together a small group of cases with a common characteristic indicated by the name that might otherwise have been engulfed in the "other and polymorphous" further down the list. They are of two sorts, one consisting of neurotic pseudo-debility, the other of a neurotically exaggerated reaction to some real physical handicap such as a minor paresis after poliomyelitis. Examples have been given for these as for the negativistic neuroses typical of childhood.

The "other and polymorphous" remain. The "other" are only three: one 39 year old man with paranoic suspiciousness but no trace of psychosis, an irritable 21 year old women whose trait could be traced to repressed frustration and dissatisfaction over being compelled to abandon school, and a seven year old enuretic girl, all three being from Shiraz. In this category lurks no single case of obsessive-compulsive neurosis nor of neurotic depersonalization. Though we not infrequently came upon anankastic symptoms and noted them accordingly, in no instance that we encountered were they the leading feature of the illness, justifying a diagnosis. As the suspicion has been uttered a good many times that Islamic ritual might be conducive to compulsive traits, the absence of even one clear case in our material is a point to be mentioned. Equally, however, one must bear in mind that Islam possesses no monopoly in this respect. Jewish ritual law, Catholic prescriptions for the attainment of absolution and Protestant searchings of conscience may be not less conducive. Less remarkable to us seems the lack of any case of more than accessory neurotic depersonalisation, since even in European practice we very rarely find occasion to use this as a primary diagnosis.

The "other and polymorphous" neuroses are about equally distributed between the sexes, but in our material they are almost wholly a product of the city (three exceptions). With the exceptions mentioned under "other" and with the further exception of a pubertal crisis classified under ICN No. 300.8 they to our minds defy the demand of this international system that mixed neuroses should not be placed under this rubric but under the symptom that stands out in the foreground. In all these 15 cases we could discover no such symptom, or else the choice of one before the other would have been wholly arbitrary. Despite injunctions to use the classification 300.9 (not otherwise defineable neuroses) as sparingly as possible we have employed it for our truly polymorphous cases.

The 44 psychosomatic patients constitute 19.6 % of our total psychiatric material or roughly one quarter of the reactive cases – that quarter in which, if the theory be correct, repression is deepest. Again females preponderate, and they do so by virtue of one sub-category, that of migrainoid headache. Seventeen such cases are women; only six of them come from the city. From the four male cases three are urban. Applying the X^2 test to the psychosomatic collective divided into male and female sufferers and non-sufferers from migraine the preponderance of the women is significant with $0.05 > p > 0.02$. It is still more striking, nearly overwhelming, when we look at the villages alone. The observation was impressed upon us from the very beginning of our field work, when over again, to an extent for which European medical experience had in no way prepared us, we came upon girls and women prostrated for days on end, several times a month (in other words: by no means necessarily or even usually in connection with menstruation) by violent headaches with all the symptoms of migraine except one-sidedness. True hemicrania was hardly encountered at all. The effect on the families naturally was marked. Corresponding thereto, 6 of the female cases were graded P_1 and 11 of them P_2. Fifteen were illiterate, 14 poor. These bare numbers support the impression we gained repeatedly when conversing with the victims and inquiring into their life histories: that the majority of the rather frequent psychosomatic migrainoid headache cases represent the dumb but eloquent protest of the poor, illiterate, generally peasant woman to a harsh, traditionbound and altogether constrained life in which she is subject not only to the unrelenting demands of the elements and of village society, but also to the male sex in general and her husband in particular. As we have seen in connection with the simple developments, she may bewail her anxiety and sorrow more freely than her spouse. She will rarely raise her voice against him; she may struggle on in inbred obedience, but when the trial becomes too heavy and the harsher rural environment discourages the conversion-hysteric reaction pattern, she represses more sternly, is manifestly, incontestably ill and through her incapacitating illness gains a subtle, unconscious, effective revenge upon her taskmaster. Only one woman among our 283 patients suffered more than incidentally from another type of headache, raising the question why the migrainoid kind should take such an excessive precedence over all others. We suspect that the explanation can be found in the visibility of its manifestations. A migraine victim usually looks drawn and sick even to the most ignorant observer, acts sick and often confirms the sickness by the vomiting that generally terminates the attack. For other headaches there is little evidence but the sufferer's word. The manifestness of both hysteria and migraine may help to account for their much greater frequency in the female sex in Iran, where tradition and custom hitherto have inhibited on the woman's part any other expression of dissatisfaction except depression. If it be objected that depression, hysteria and migraine have been found more frequently among women than men in other parts of the world also, one may ask the objector to consider the position that women have held up to recently in those other parts and in some places still do.

Among the men we encountered quite a different picture. Only four in all the surveys together had migraine. Three of these were from Shiraz, all of degree P_1, all with secondary education, one poor and two from the middle class. The fourth case was that of an illiterate 36 year old farmer from Marvdasht, of degree P_2. In sharp contrast to the women, five men (but only one woman) suffered to a critical degree from other types of (mostly tension) headaches of probable psychosomatic origin. Three were from the city, all of degree P_1, all literate, and were evenly distributed over the three socio-economic classes. The other three from the villages were all poor and illiterate, one of them a mild case, the others P_2. The numbers are too small to yield statistically significant differences, but rather remarkably similar patterns emerge when we classify all the 27 cases of psychosomatic headache by sex, literacy and migrainoid or non-migrainoid type of the headache, as in Table D IV 9.

The diagnosis of psychosomatic gastro-intestinal disease must be made with caution and taken with reservation in a country where, especially in the rural areas, simply somatic gastro-intestinal disease is rife. Some cases received confirmation through radiological diagnoses of ulcer. There were only two asthma cases. Even if we add to these one of psychosomatic cardiovascular distress described under Qalandari, we cannot gainsay the impression that the participation of the pulmonary and cardiovascular systems in the whole psychosomatic group seems to be low in Iran and

Table D IV 9. Characteristics of Psychosomatic Headache Patients

	m	f	m + f		m	f	m + f
Non-migrainoid	5	1	6	Literate	6	3	9
Migrainoid	4	17	21	Illiterate	3	15	18
Total	9	18	27	Total	9	18	27

stands in some contrast to the frequent complaints about dyspnea, palpitations, thoracic oppression and the like that are so common in European practice.

It stands in contrast also to the detailed description of such complaints that B. Good [85] has given in his article "The Heart of What's the Matter". As it is based on protracted and careful observation in the city of Maragheh in East Azerbaijan (northeastern Iran) and is one of the very few field studies on such matters that have come out of Iran, it requires particular mention here. With praiseworthy perspicacity and knowledge of the local idiom (Aseri, a Turkish dialect with Farsi admixture) Good narrates and traces down the underlying meanings and implications of the innumerable allusions to "distress of the heart", نرا حتى قلب, that occur in everyday speech and, in fact, not seldom lead the sufferer to seek paramedical or medical relief. In a nearly literal extract from Good's own presentation, he found, in a survey of a stratified population of 750 persons, in nearly 40 % of the (how many?) households at least one person (but how many more, and how many altogether?) who had suffered heart distress in the preceding eight months. The majority were female, particularly women of childbearing age. Almost exactly half had been taken to a physician. From his exceedingly sparing and unhomogeneous data it is not possible even roughly, e.g. on the basis of mean family size, to estimate the incidence or prevalence of such complaints. The semantic analysis that follows is of real interest, but ends in apparent blithe indifference to the fact that "distress of the heart" may mean, among a great many other things, simply and precisely that: the pathological anatomic or pathophysiological illness of an organ of the body. The confused reader is left with the impression that a great part of the inhabitants of Maragheh were suffering or had suffered from "distress of the heart" and with some of his own over the waste of precious material. The reason for the discrepancy lies probably in the vast, though basically not unbridgeable difference between Good's linguistic-ethnological and our own medical epidemiological approach. To take literally in a medical sense every one of the countless references to "distress of the heart" in daily Aseri or Farsi dilutes even a broad psychosomatic concept far beyond usefulness or even meaningfulness. This is not to assert that it is pointless to analyze the deeper meanings of such references as Good has done and to inquire into what "semantic fields" (as the author calls them) they lead. Neither does the circumstance that half the persons using such references consulted a physician demonstrate that they must be regarded as ill. We recall what was said in Part A concerning the criteria of a "case": it is not simply anyone who walks into a doctor's office!. For further clarification one may remind oneself that such expressions as "heartsore" or "sick at heart", although now hardly current, belong to no very ancient English and as a rule did not carry any medical connotations.

For comparison one may look to Shepherd's survey [178, p. 112, Table 28] and the answers that patients consulting general practitioners gave to three relevant items of the Cornell Medical Index Health Questionnaire touching on somatic symptoms of anxiety as manifested through the heart: 1. "Do you have pains in the heart or chest?", 2. "Are you often bothered by thumping of the heart?", 3. "Does your heart often race like mad?". When the answers to all three are summed, they were affirmative in 31 % of male and 40 % of female non-psychiatric patients, and in practically 100 % of psychiatric out-patients of both sexes. For patients "who were considered by their doctors to have been suffering from a psychiatric condition at any time in the year of observation" [loc. cit., p. 109] the rates of affirmation were 61 % for males and 64 %

for females. Similarly, Strotzka [188, p. 74] mentions that among his 100 psychiatric cases in the narrower sense 41 presented cardiovascular and pulmonary complaints as primary, 44 % as secondary symptoms. This confirms the great frequency of such complaints, as Good implies, but does not establish them as cases of psychosomatic cardiovascular or pulmonary illness.

The six "other and polymorphous" comprised the cardiovascular case mentioned above, one case of probably psychically determined eczema, one of cholecystopathy , one of gross obesity in a boy without endocrinological findings (checked in Nemazee Hospital), and finally two with multiple, truly polymorphous complaints.

For comparison we have looked to Cremerius' monograph on "functional syndromes" (sc. in internal medicine; [60]). From 21500 patients who attended the medical out-patient department of the University of Munich during the years 1949–51 some 3000 were diagnosed as having functional or psychosomatic complaints without ascertainable organic foundation. For his follow-up study twenty years later the author selected six principal diagnostic groups and omitted several smaller ones. These latter included 98 cases of migraine, and the author mentions besides that a number of patients who complained of headache were classified either as purely neurotic rather than psychosomatic or else were combined because of other symptoms with the group of heterogeneous psychosomatic syndromes. When we recombine certain of his main groups and other related smaller ones for which he states total figures we can draw a rough comparison as in Table D IV 10 below.

For many reasons the comparisons cannot be made strictly, especially as Cremerius' much larger proband group was composed of patients who themselves had come seeking treatment. Even so, the relative scarcity of pulmonary and cardiovascular disorders and the abundance of headache, especially migraine and migrainoid forms, in Iran remains remarkable. Cremerius found a small, but statistically significant predominance of females among his psychosomatic cases (53 %), which is more prominent in our material (17 male to 27 female or 39 : 61 %).

6. Constitutional Disorders

Clinical oligophrenia is not identical with low psychological test performance though closely related to it and should be diagnosed only very sparingly without confirmation by the latter. On the other hand, low intelligence test performance is far from sufficing

Table D IV 10. Comparative Frequencies of Types of Psychosomatic Disorders

	Iran Number	Iran Per 100	Munich Number	Munich Per 100
Gastro-intestinal	9	20.5	1028	37.2
Pulmonary and cardiovascular	2	4.6	823	29.7
Headache (including migraine)	27	61.3	334	12.1
Polymorphous and heterogenous	6	13.6	582	21.0
	44	100	2767	100

for the diagnosis. "Life performance" rather than mere test performance might be denominated the critical criterium, though it must be employed with caution as well. It includes the subject's history beside his present state. Constant subnormal performance markedly below the expectations of the society or culture of which the subject is a true, not merely transitory, fortuitous or compulsory member can constitute an important sign of clinical oligophrenia when other factors such as mental deterioration from whatever cause, neurotic pseudo-debility, organic impairment of drive (*Antrieb*) etc., are excluded. Other criteria such as sheer undifferentiated simple-mindedness (very different from the nuanced simplicity of wise and serene spirits), persistent lagging behind the intellectual claims and accomplishments of the vast majority of one's peers both for short and long ranges, lack of acuity down to sheer obtuseness, sometimes also accessory physical signs can play their various parts. We shall discuss here the clinical diagnoses made in the course of field work with the help of raw data from (then) still unstandardized tests and refer to the test criteria in Part C, Chap. I on intelligence testing.

In all, 29 clinical cases of oligophrenia were diagnosed, which constitute 12.9 per thousand of the total population under psychiatric scrutiny in all surveys. The rates (here and hereafter to be understood per thousand) were 14.6 for the male and 11.1 for the female sex: the difference lacks any statistical significance. It must be remarked again that, as we admitted only a single diagnosis per case, these were practically "pure" oligophrenias and that the figures, as our case notes confirm, would have been higher if we had included multiple diagnoses in our statistical treatment. Modern textbooks such as M. Bleuler's or Schulte's and Tölle's [176] usually state the prevalence of oligophrenia to lie between 10 and 30 per thousand. Because of the difficult problem of the broad transitional zone between mental normalcy and deficiency, which becomes even more thorny and controversial in transcultural comparisons, the prudent tendency of the WHO is to restrict the diagnosis of oligophrenia to obvious and severe cases and thus probably to limit the acceptable frequency to around ten per thousand.

The psychiatric literature confronts us with an enormous range of figures, of which we quote only a few by way of example. The lowest we have encountered is Uchimura's of 0.6 from Hachijo Island, but his Japanese colleagues Tsugawa [191] and Akimoto [4] far surpass him with 9.6 and 10.0 respectively. In the mid-range lie Lin's figures from Taiwan of 3.4 for his survey of 1946/48 [121] and 4.9 for the survey of 1961/63 [123], the difference being significant at the 5 % level. Rates within a similar order of magnitude are reported from such diverse sources as Brugger in Basel (3.3) and in Thuringia (5.4), Strömgren in Denmark (4.2), Sjoegren in Sweden (5.7) and Baasher in the Sudan (3.8), but in Scandinavia Bremer arrives at a tenfold higher rate of 45.3 for a small isolated fishing village in Norway. Neither nationality nor geography seems to enhance approximate uniformity, and the question naturally presents itself whether any such can or should be expected. Pockets of cretinism were a well-known phenomenon in Alpine countries in the last century, and inbreeding in isolates may have similar effects. Such factors cannot account, however, for wide variations between large and essentially similar samples. Perhaps the most remarkable divergencies are to be met with in Brugger's own publications from four German and Swiss-German studies over the decade from 1928 to 1938, all conducted by the same authors and therefore presumably comparable. In 1928, using the proband method, Brugger finds an uncorrected rate of 3.3 for siblings of schizophrenics in the city of Basel and age-

corrects this to 4.3 [49]. It may be compared with M. Bleuler's study four years later [38] in the Basel countryside (Kanton Basel-Land), again by the proband method, using 200 relatives of somatic patients in a general hospital, among whom he found 4 oligophrenics = 20 per 1000. But Brugger published in 1933 a census study from the Bavarian Allgäu [51] with the to our knowledge unsurpassed age-corrected figure of 54.9, which declines to "merely" 22.2 when he counts only imbeciles and idiots. From Rosenheim, also in Bavaria, Brugger reported in 1938 [52] an age-corrected rate of 25.3 for oligophrenia, but of 5.8 when restricted as in the Allgäu to severe cases. Strotzka's [188] 18 per thousand in "Kleinburg" lies not far below Rosenheim. Shepherd found in London only 2 per thousand but justly remarks that his sample from general practices certainly contains less "feeble minded" than would have been found in a thoroughly representative study of the metropolitan population.

In Table D IV 11 we see the distribution of the 29 cases by ICD rubrics, degrees of pathology, etiology (where known or suspected) and sex. The severity of the total psychopathology does not necessarily correspond to that of the oligophrenia, since the former can and often does include other symptoms and deviations besides the latter. Our intentional parsimony in the diagnosis of questionable or border-line cases is reflected in the small number – four only – that fell into the ICD rubric 317. The gravest cases (ICD 318.2) are by nature few. The bulk are to be found in the middle zones corresponding to ICD 318.0–1, whereas the number of P_3 cases is substantially larger than those of "profound mental subnormality" for the reasons given.

The mean IQs for the sub-groups whether by ICD or our own P_{1-3} ratings did not exhibit the expected drop parallel to the clinical diagnoses, but clustered around 70–80. Several factors working together explain this at first sight dismaying finding. Out of 58 possible scores (since each subject should have taken two tests) 28 were zero. These include two subjects who could not be tested at all because of their inattentive and obstreperous behavior and whose performance even with better co-operation certainly would have been low. As we could not be sure that the other zero scores represented an absolute bottom, we omitted them when calculating means, even though the conversion tables in some instances yield a positive weighted score and an IQ for zero

Table D IV 11. Oligophrenias

ICD	m	f	m + f	
317	3	1	4	"mild mental retardation"
318.0	6	7	13	"moderate mental subnormality"
318.1	6	4	10	"severe mental subnormality"
318.2	2	0	2	"profound mental subnormality"
	17	12	29	
P_1	6	3	9	
P_2	7	5	12	
P_3	4	4	8	
	17	12	29	
Cryptogenetic	10	7	17	
Genetic	1	3	4	2 Down's syndrome, 2 Turner's
Early acquired	6	2	8	
	17	12	29	

raw score. Furthermore, some children's positive raw scores could not be converted into weighted scores or IQs because the number of subjects in the respective standardizing categories was too small (all illiterate boys below 15, block design test for illiterate girls below 15). In the adult range, for example, the zero raw score of a 20 year old illiterate male on the block design test corresponded to a weighted score of 7 and an intelligence quotient of 81, the inference being that the test for illiterates of this age class does not differentiate below IQ 80 (cf. Part C, Chap. I 2). The maximum range of 20 weighted score points per test also limits by itself the number of levels that can be distinguished. As a similar result appears in several other instances and as the mean IQs of the sub-groups, as mentioned, hardly fall below 70, it seems prudent to regard an IQ of 80 or below as already suspicious of, but by no means as demonstrating, oligophrenia and as an indication for further investigation. The concurrence of all these factors leaves us with so few scoreable test results for each sub-group that the calculation of means for them becomes illusory.

The importance of clinical considerations can be illustrated by a note on the two cases of "profound mental subnormality" classed 318.2 by the ICD. One was a nine year old boy who scored zero on both tests. The other achieved a weighted score of 7 (= IQ 72) on the arithmetic test and of 12 on the block design, the latter corresponding to a respectable and in this case startling IQ of 105! The following information was gleaned from his mother. According to her the patient had fallen out of the cradle at the age of six months and been unconscious for perhaps half an hour, remained ill for a long time thereafter and in the course of the illness suffered an icterus. He began to walk at a year and a half but did not speak a word until he was twelve. After a pilgrimage, contrary to the doctor's and everyone else's expectations, he began to talk, learned to do so slowly and with great difficulty and when seen by us at the age of 29 still spoke like a little child with difficulty in articulating some letters (r and s). At interview he first tried to hide, then came forward and behaved politely. The skull was small, the brow and hairline were low, the facial expression lacked differentiation, the tongue was large and deviated to the right. The man was left-handed. He reacted slowly throughout, had never been able to attend school, could not form a correct full sentence, knew coins but could not tell time by the clock although he was in general temporally and spatially orientated. He was able to help with simple housework, iron smooth pieces and sew on buttons so that he had tried working with a tailor but was mocked so much that the attempt had to be given up. He was said and appeared to be good natured but easily became excited and then threw things about or even destroyed them. His hobby was the cinema. In view of his modest accomplishments a diagnosis of imbecility might have been nearly as well justified as that of idiocy, but we were moved to the latter by the emotional complications, the inability to make use of what he had learned and the evident total dependence upon the surroundings – one of our criteria for P_3. His relative success with the block design test was a surprise to everyone but accorded with his better acquisition of manual than abstract abilities as just described. To round off the picture we may mention that the Z Test produced a scanty but not typically oligophrenic result with 3 responses in 10 minutes as follows:

I.	Flower	WF–	Pl
II.	Rejection		
III.	Human beings	WM+	HP
	Blood	DC	Blood

The simplicity of the responses and the pure color response fit well with the oligophrenia, less so the movement response (though a popular) and the rejection of Card II.

With the diagnosis of psychopathy we find ourselves upon the most uncertain ground of all. In Marvdasht, our first survey, it appeared superfluous. In Khuzestan, our second, we applied it to four cases that seemed not only convincing but also did not fit into any other category. As described in [28] one, the only woman, aged 35, had been a quarrelsome shrew from her childhood days and was the bane of the village where she lived, a sufferer from a gastric neurosis or psychosomatic gastritis as well, incessantly demanding new and more medicines against her vociferously proclaimed ills. One could almost hear her strident voice upon entering the village gate. One of the three men was a schizoid psychopath aged 44, probably in remission from a paranoid-hallucinatory schizophrenia as described in Chap. B II 4. A 50 year old psychopathic hypochondriac and a 41 year old "sociopath" completed the brief register. The latter was a ne'er-do-well who could stick to no job and carry no task to its conclusion as the histories of his relatives and townsmen confirmed, not "anti-social" as the ICD would have it, but the very prototype of the *haltlos* or tieless psychopath of German psychiatric terminology. The mean age of the four was 42 years.

The 11 persons from Shiraz diagnosed as psychopaths turned out in retrospect to be much younger, having a mean age of only 24 years. The two eldest were both 40 years, and there were five aged less than twenty. Below this age the clinical psychiatrist is reluctant to make a diagnosis of psychopathy at all and wisely contents himself with a descriptive title or a diagnosis of pubertal crisis or of neurosis until the course of the mature patient's history disillusions him. In all the present younger cases we weighed and rejected the diagnosis of a pubertal crisis. The anamneses showed that they were not crises, but conditions of long standing. All but one of the younger segment were poor, the majority were illiterate, and none had more than primary schooling. They tended to belong to the pathological family clusters upon which we have commented before. How much of their own pathological condition was referable to social and environmental damage in a wider sense or was induced by the family constellation and example in the narrower sense was well-nigh impossible to ascertain. A genetic component seems not improbable, but we emphasize again that our designation of such disorders as "constitutional" is not meant to imply more than the word denotes: a constitution, forged by various forces, that responds with typically pathological emotional reactions to inexcessive, ordinary stimuli and situations and promises little capacity for alteration. We do not exclude that certain of the younger or even of the elder cases might have been diagnosed character neuroses with some, though we believe not with equal justification, for this alternative was ever in our minds also and was not rejected lightly. If we subtract the less than twenty-year-old from the psychopaths in the Shiraz psychiatric sample the discrepancy between city and country still does not vanish, but it diminishes noticeably (6 cases out of 928 probands in Shiraz, 4 out of 482 in Khuzestan or out of 482 + 497 = 979 in Khuzestan + Marvdasht. Moreover, we did not discover any psychopath among the 144 in Qalandari).

The diagnostic table discloses that of 15 psychopaths altogether seven were irritable, two "anti-social", two schizoid, one of the two having almost certainly sustained episodes of schizophrenia and the other being strongly suspect even at the time of examination as described in Chap. B IV 3. Among the four "other" we count one each as "hysterical" in the wider sense of exaggerated, appelative behavior, as hypochondric, asthenic and insecure.

As conceptions and criteria of psychopathy vary enormously, comparisons with other epidemiological studies do little but to emphasize this troublesome point. Published prevalence rates range between Uchimura's of 0.4 per 1000 for Japan and Lin's of 0.9 for Taiwan up to Bremer's of 76.2 per 1000 for Norway. Ours of 6.7 per 1000 lies somewhere in between. If we disregard the five cases aged less than twenty it sinks to 4.3. Looking at newer European investigations in which the concept of psychopathy probably approximates more closely to that we have used, we presume Essen-Möller's "major personality deviation", which he distinguishes from neurosis, to be its rough equivalent and find a very high prevalence rate of 7.5 per 100 or 75 per 1000 for men and 36 per 1000 for women, practically identical with Bremer's. Both psychiatrists came of the same Scandinavian school. Shepherd, like Essen-Möller, avoids the word psychopathy in his tables, though it has slipped once or twice into the text of his book. In his Table 14 giving "Patient consulting rates per 1000 at risk for psychiatric morbidity, by sex and diagnostic group" [178, p. 81] we find non-neurotic "personality disorder" in 5.5 per 1000 for both sexes, 7.2 per 1000 for males and 4.0 for females. His London rates thus lie very close to ours. Both with Shepherd and with Essen-Möller one notes that the rates for men tend to be roughly double those for women, and our own findings agree with this. That is the more worthy of remark in the light of the circumstance that other psychiatric troubles discussed above, notably depression, hysteria and psychosomatic migraine, are found significantly more often in the female sex. The sex difference for our small number of psychopathies is not statistically significant, but both the trend and its similar dimensions in other surveys are in suggestive agreement. Finally, Strotzka in his group of 100 psychiatric patients registers 14 psychopaths, about thrice our percentage of 5.3, but admits multiple diagnoses, which might raise our rates substantially.

V. Discussion and Conclusions

The authors have been asked two questions so often during their field work and the decade devoted to the preparation of this book that it is appropriate to commence this final chapter with them and with their answers.

The first has been regularly: "Have you encountered any forms of mental disturbance that were peculiar, indigenous to Iran or to the Middle East and do not occur in Western psychiatry?" The answer is a simple No. This implies that familiar Western categories of psychopathology and of psychiatric diagnosis could be applied without essential difficulties or, as we believe, falsifications to our Iranian findings. Here lies no occasion for surprise. These categories are structural, not contentual, and the structure of the human mind, like that of the human body, is essentially the same throughout the world. Allowance naturally has to be made for differences in content and in ways of expressing it, and this can hardly be done without a more than superficial acquaintance with the culture and the people.

The second has been: "Is the frequency of mental disturbance or psychiatric illness the same or different in Iran and in Western countries?" With an important reservation we can answer that by most indications it seems to be very nearly the same, and that the agreement is even closer than we or anybody else had anticipated. The exception concerns the two tribal samples of the Qashqai: the nomads and the sedentary residents of Qalandari. We shall return to these below. Leaving these and Marvdasht for the moment aside, it is a striking fact that the total prevalence rates for environments as diverse as the city for Shiraz and the cluster of villages in Khuzestan lie very close together with about 15–16 % and that these lie equally close to total rates from environments as different from them and from each other as London, a Polish town and city, and the small Austrian city that Strotzka has named "Kleinburg". The agreement was altogether unexpected. By the time Gnat and Henisz had published in 1966 [83] we had completed the tabulation of the findings we gathered in Khuzestan at the end of 1965. They were not published because of technical delays until 1969, the same year in which Strotzka's "Kleinburg" appeared, and it was from this book that we first learned of the work of Shepherd and his collaborators published in 1966. Shepherd jestingly called us all the "fifteen percent club". Shiraz came later. During and after this survey we did what we could to avoid any conscious bias, worked to the same standards, did not even count our cases until we had finally left the field, then did so in Switzerland as objectively as possible, first evaluating and classifying the cases singly and totaling them only after we had fixed their diagnosis and classification by degree of severity. Their close agreement with Khuzestan was unforeseen.

Though the total prevalence rate for Marvdasht was lower than that for Khuzestan and Shiraz, the rate for $P_2 + P_3$ together corresponded well with the equivalent rate for both. These all lie around 7–8 %. For reasons explained in the body of the book (cf.

Chaps. B 1, D III) we have cause to believe that too few P_1 cases were identified in Marvdasht, and that the true prevalence is probably very similar to that in the other surveys just mentioned. At all events, the combined rates for medium and severe cases do agree so well at all three highly diverse sites that no statistically significant difference, not even a tendency to such, can be demonstrated between them. Comparison with other epidemiological surveys, the total prevalence rates of which lay on approximately the same level, suggested that their authors had counted mainly or exclusively the medium and severe cases such as we have denominated with P_2 and P_3 and that a statistical comparison could be made legitimately between them and our combined $P_2 + P_3$ figures for Shiraz, Khuzestan and Marvdasht, the purpose of the combination being to obtain as broad a basis for comparison as possible. Yet other surveys seem to have dealt only with the severest cases corresponding more or less to our P_3.

Since we have, with some reservations, stated rates for all surveys combined in Table D IV 4, it is natural to take these as a basis of reference. We have seen in Chap. D IV 1 that the male:female and rural:urban proportions are not substantially different from those of the country as a whole. A question remains about the tribal component, which constitutes 15 % of our subjects. The number of tribal people was estimated in 1963 as three to four million, the total population as some 26 million (in 1966 25.9), i. e. the share of the tribes at about 11–15 %. Though our figure coincides neatly with the upper limit, the possibility cannot be excluded that tribal subjects were somewhat over-represented and that this diminished the general prevalence rate. If so, it was in any case not by much; and it must be borne in mind that the estimates are rough. With due caution the combined rates can be taken as a reference, but they are not necessarily the best and certainly not the only one.

We can thus define three bases, each with its advantages and disadvantages, as follows:

Base A: combined results of all five surveys (Shiraz, Khuzestan, Qalandari, Marvdasht, nomadic Qashqai) including all degrees of severity;

Base B: combined results of the Shiraz and Khuzestan surveys, including all degrees of severity;

Base C: combined results of the Shiraz, Khuzestan and Marvdasht surveys, including only the medium and severe cases ($P_2 + P_3$) but omitting the mild cases (P_1).

A fourth base comprising the severe cases (P_3) only was tried but abandoned. It seemed a priori likely that comparison of the severe and thus presumably obvious cases only would result in a least moderate consensus. It did not, and the scope of diversity was disconcerting. As mentioned in the Introduction, not many authors have attempted to classify their cases according to severity at all (Essen-Möller being a notable exception). Many, however, employ a rubric called "psychosis", where we expected to find mainly P_3 cases. "Psychosis" turned out to be such an heterogeneous designation that it was of no help whatever. For some authors it implied schizophrenia plus manic-depressive psychosis; others included epileptic psychoses, yet others both defined and undefined additional organic psychoses, and still others omitted any definition. Rates for "psychosis" danced between 2 and 109 per thousand. We therefore gave up any attempt to use this now stringent, now liberal category and compared, where possible, rates for single more or less defined psychoses. These comparisons are to be found under Special Psychiatric Epidemiology in Part D, Chap. IV.

Iranian prevalence rates to all three bases have been compared with those from a large number of epidemiological surveys from various parts of the world, first by inspection, then, where roughly similar rates could be observed or expected, by the usual statistical criteria. Where these indicated conformity within the commonly accepted limits the results have been tabulated in Table D V 1. Eleven surveys showed agreement within a 95 % confidence range to at least one of the three bases. Two (Baasher's and Giel and van Luik's) were from the Eastern Mediterranean Region of the WHO; two were from India (Nandi's and Thacore's). The extremely divergent and mostly incomparable findings from other surveys in the Middle and Far East are listed in Annex III, yet others from Europe, America and also the East by Lin and Standley [122].

Though we have pointed out in Annex III the immense difficulties in the way of comparing reactive disorders and have expressed some doubts whether any valid comparisons could be drawn for these, we have nevertheless made the attempt for this diagnostic category and this only in Table D V 1. This right-hand section of the Table might have been included in the previous section, but can be presented here more compactly. The reactive disorders (abbreviated Dr as in earlier chapters) are not subdivided here into simple, neurotic and psychosomatic. The data of other authors, where they indicated such subdivisions, have been recombined, sometimes rather generously. A sharp division could not always be made, as when at least one writer comprehended under his heading "depression" explicitly both the endogenous and reactive. As the latter are far more numerous we have treated, in this case, all "depressions" as reactive, well aware that an error is involved but assuming it to be marginal. Some writers present no data on reactive disorders: here we have set a dash in the appropriate space; others give only rates per hundred or thousand but no absolute numbers: here we set a question mark. As the significance of differences could only be calculated in such cases with the help of the critical ratio, we have employed this method, for the sake of consistency, throughout. Strotzka gives rates only, which are derived from a sample of 100 consecutive primarily psychiatric cases in a general practice and thus can be projected upon any population. His "Kleinburg" is said to have about 5000, but it would be altogether unsuitable to use this as an actual reference number. No significances could be calculated, therefore, but the good agreement with our total figures on both Bases A and B cannot be overlooked. For the reactive disorders, to our mild surprise, it does not seem to hold, unless it be affirmed that his rate of 130 per 1000 be not too far from ours of 94 per 1000 to Base B. The data of Roth and Luten are quoted from Lin and Standley [122], all the rest from the original publications.

After this preface the display of the data should not present great difficulties. In the top four lines come our own: first the base or reference population, second the absolute number of cases (to the left all diagnoses, to the right reactive), third the corresponding prevalence rate per thousand and fourth its standard deviation. Below follows the comparison with other authors' data line by line. Since we are looking here for indications of similarity, not of difference, the use of chevrons as hitherto did not seem suitable. The zero hypothesis is now our aim. It cannot be proved, but its probability can be indicated. One cross indicates that it has a probability of 95 %, two crosses a probability of 99 % or, in other words, that the numerical differences, now assumed to be false rather than true, have an improbability of the same dimensions. For Strotzka we have chosen the customary signs of near equality by inspection.

Table D V 1. Comparison of Selected Psychiatric Epidemiological Surveys[a]

		All diagnoses					A	B	C	Reactive (Dr)		A	B	C
Bash and		Population					2243	1410	1910	Population		2243	1410	1910
Bash-Liechti		of which pathological					283	226	145	Dr		173	133	57
		prevalence per 1000					126	160	76	Dr/1000		77	94	30
		standard deviation					7.01	9.76	6.06	SD		5.63	7.77	3.90
Author	Place	Year	Ref.	Pop.	Path.	Path. p. 1000				Dr	Dr p. 1000			
Baasher	Wadi Halfa, Sudan	1961	10	1860	117	63			++	?	46			+
Bremer	Finmark, Norway	1951	47	1080	251	232				76	70	++	+	
Essen-Möller	rural Sweden	1956	70	2550	350	137	++	+		—	—			
Giel & v. Luik	Bonga, Ethiopia	1969	82	384	33	86			++	22	57	++	+	
Gnat & Henisz	Poland	1966	83	1671	253	151	+	++		132	79	++	++	
Nandi et al.	West Bengal, India	1975	156	1060	109	103	+			91	86	++	++	
Roth & Luton	Tennessee, U.S.A.	1938	171	24804	1721	69			++	?	36			++
Shepherd	London, England	1966	179	14697	?	140		+		?	134			
Strömgren	Island Rø, Denmark	1935	187	913	80	88			++	—	—			
Strotzka	"Kleinburg", Austria	1969	188	*	*	150	~	≈		*	130			
Thacore et al.	North Bengal, India	1975	189	2696	220	82			++	108	40			+

[a] For explanation see text.

Looking down the columns we find, as anticipated, agreement to all three bases – for the total cases more often separately, for the reactive disorders not seldom to both A and B, with which C nowhere overlaps. Study of the corresponding texts confirms our suspicion that different authors have been working to different standards which they have only partly, and sometimes not at all, defined. Essen-Möller is again the outstanding exception, and it is the more regrettable that his determinedly Scandinavian nosology and classification render any comparison by diagnostic categories, even by such broad ones as reactive disorders, well-nigh impossible or at least so highly questionable that we have not felt ourselves justified in attempting it. Rather the same holds for Strömgren's detailed study of the Island of Rø within the much larger framework of his genetic investigations. Although he does give rather minute data for non-psychotic cases, we have not succeeded in translating them with any confidence into otherwise current terms and have therefore left the Dr columns blank. It seems probable that a substantial proportion of the cases that both authors have classified as deviant personalities would be assigned by others to the reactive category.

Agreement for total cases is most noticeable to the Base C and regularly reaches a high level of statistical probability. The assumption seems justified that these investigators and a great many others beside have tended to disregard the fringe cases such as fall into our P_1 group. There are good and valid reasons for doing so, but it would seem preferable to explicate them rather than to throw up one's hands in despair over the apparently chaotic disagreement between epidemiological findings. The same holds, of course, when mild or marginal cases are deliberately included. There we find, as with Shepherd and Strotzka, high prevalence rates for reactive disorders – so high that the difference to ours becomes statistically significant. It is noticeable and hardly a matter of chance that both authors gleaned their data from general practices in countries with a psychiatric tradition. Working upon deliberately similar lines in Switzerland Agosti [3] has found that 190 out of 1000 patients in a general practice showed neurotic or psychosomatic disturbances.

The rejoinder is at close hand that, if one culls enough surveys, one will stumble upon agreements more or less by chance. Yet a rough estimate of the number to be expected is possible. The standard deviations of our bases multiplied by the factor of 1.96 define the 95 % two-sided range of confidence. This is to say that, if the survey were repeated in identical fashion (which is not possible) 95 % of the prevalence rates found on repetition would fall into that confidence range, 5 % outside of it. The apparent differences are all, by assumption, false, but only 5 % of the false difference would fall outside of the range, and by convention we should accept differences outside of it as "true" with a likelihood of error equivalent to 5 %. Prevalence rates falling within the range of confidence could be accepted by the same convention as agreeing with the empirical rate, the likelihood of agreement being 95 %. Let us now consent to treat other surveys as repetitions of our own. The assumption is empirically false, for not even one's own survey can be repeated because of practice effects, chronological changes etc., and it is altogether unlikely that any other survey will cover precisely the same number of subjects unless by prior arrangement (such as is possible e.g. in practice surveys, where workers may agree to take, 100 or 1000 consecutive patients consulting the practice). Nevertheless, Table D V 1 shows a number of surveys of roughly the same order of magnitude, i.e. 1500 to 2500 subjects. If they were (hypothetical) repetitions of our own surveys and were endless in number (which of course they are not), we should expect about 5 % of them to be in true agreement with our findings, for the other 95 % of agreements are false. Actually, we have reviewed some 40 surveys, nearly all of which are mentioned either in Chap. D IV or in Annex III. Five percent of these would amount to two surveys. Confidence limits are for:

Base A 126 ± 19 i.e. 107 – 145
Base B 160 ± 45 i.e. 115 – 205
Base C 76 ± 17 i.e. 59 – 93.

To each of these bases we find four to five surveys out of the forty whose prevalence rates do fall within these bounds, not two as expected by chance, and the like holds for the reactive disorders. It holds, moreover, even though certain surveys such as Giel's and Strömgren's are based on much smaller, others such as Roth and Luton's and Shepherd's on much larger numbers, so that our theoretical assumption does not appear too bold. By this criterion the agreements found are better than chance.

The internal agreement between our three more extensive surveys is good. This obtains at all levels for Shiraz and Khuzestan, although the latter was performed by the census method and the former by random sampling, and it extends to Marvdasht for the levels of medium and severe impairment. Even if it be postulated that two surveys could arrive at essentially the same prevalence rates by chance, albeit they involved very different populations, the fundamental correspondence with the third hardly can be referred to mere coincidence. This carries implications both for the reliability and validity of the method and for the interpretation of the results. We take the reliability to be indirectly confirmed, with the further implication that the divergent rates obtained elsewhere by the same method are real. The interpretation demands caution. If total prevalence rates are so similar in town and country, what makes them so? Not simply human nature, for in yet other socio-cultural environments we encounter presumptively true rates that are significantly lower. Do uniform or at least very similar psychological conditions in the city and the two village clusters explain the nearly identical psychiatric morbidity? They cannot, for they are not in fact uniform, as we have observed when discussing differential psychology. Without recapitulating needlessly all that was said in Chap. D I, itself a recapitulation, we can remind ourselves of the differences most easily by a glance back to Table C II 18, in which the mean numbers of affirmative responses to items from the psychiatric questionnaire are stated by place, age class and sex and look first only at the overall numbers. They are high and very nearly equal in Shiraz and Marvdasht, only half as high in Khuzestan, which had the same rate for total psychiatric morbidity as Shiraz. One deduction seems ineluctable: such complaint scales as this, of which dozens are in use and upon which psychiatric epidemiologists tend more and more to rely, cannot be taken blindly as indicators or predictors of psychiatric morbidity. Complaints are neither frustrate symptoms nor diluted diagnoses, and they do not in general (though they may in special cases) reliably prefigure either. Endless confusion arises when a naive complaint or self-rating is confounded with a pathological symptom. It is the special science and art of the psychiatrist to discriminate between them. Such confusion may be responsible in part for the not altogether happy state of psychiatric epidemiology. In rejecting diagnoses made by psychiatrists as too subjective, epidemiologists have flown from the

Devil into the Deep Sea by accepting at face value even more subjective statements made in answer to contextless printed questions by lay subjects. Such statements possess meaning and value beyond doubt, but their meaning is often different from the word, and their value is that of an index of professed discomfort. This is far from being identical with psychiatric illness. Nowhere among the adults, though occasionally among the children, and for the well and unremarkable in Khuzestan in both sexes and age classes, does the complaint score in Table C II 18 fall below 1.0, implying that practically every adult person (a correction must be allowed for Q 7) registered some subjective uneasiness, disequilibrium or outright complaint. Had we taken these at their face value, we should have arrived at nigh upon one hundred percent morbidity. The Midtown Survey stopped not far short of this. While we do not deny that such information is in itself meaningful, we do consider its relation to clinical psychiatry to be tenuous and very much in need of definition.

Khuzestan has not only a low complaint rate, in fact the lowest of all, but it also exhibits another peculiarity: the overall rates for both sexes are equal, whereas elsewhere the women lead. The possible objection must be considered that in Khuzestan we had only male examiners, and that the women might have been more reticent toward them. In Shiraz the great bulk of the work was performed by female examiners, and the complaint rate was high, but it was no less high in Marvdasht, where we had roughly equal numbers of male and female field workers, and the women's was higher than the men's. It is our impression, based on intensive direct observation, that this factor was not decisive, but we have no conclusive proof for it. Have the men more objective reason to complain? With all due caution we can only answer: none that struck our eye. This was struck rather forcefully, however, by another sex difference in Khuzestan such as did not subsist elsewhere: female maturation did not lead for the most part into pseudo-extraversion as it did in Shiraz. The female sex in Khuzestan acquires in womanhood increased, not diminished capacities for genuine introversion. Introversion implies reticence. Fewer complaining utterances may be referred to this. We have hypothesized the girl's schooling in Shiraz and their lack of it in Khuzestan as a cause. Whether the hypothesis be correct or not, the facts of introversive tendencies and relatively low complaint scores remain. Be it noted also that the complaint rates for boys and girls in Khuzestan are nearly equal. The boys grow up for the larger part into extraverts, the girls do not. Thus Shiraz boys also grow up into extraverts, but their sisters rather into pseudo-extraverts. The psychiatric consequences can be read off in Table D III 4, from which it is apparent that the Shirazi females have very significantly more reactive disorders than the males in relation to total disorders, while for these the sex difference in Shiraz is trifling and in Khuzestan nonexistent. From the same table it appears that the Khuzestani females likewise exceed the other sex in their share of reactive out of total disorders, but only in P_2 and there with a significance of 5 % as opposed to 1.0 – 0.1 % in Shiraz. The significance of the difference can be calculated more directly by means of a fourfold table in which the reactively and otherwise disordered of the two places are compared: it turns out both by X^2 and by critical ratio for one-sided comparison to be about 7 %. Fifty-eight percent of the pathological Khuzestani females are reactively disordered, but 72 % of the Shirazi. By a different computation we can compare the reactively disordered of both sexes in both places and arrive again by X^2 at $0.10 > p > 0.05$, by critical ratio of 1.62 at so close to 5 % (for which 1.65 would be required) that we may accept this level of confidence. The pattern lends a conviction that the statistical measures do not quite succeed in providing. Paradoxically, the total morbidity rates remain the same for both sexes in Shiraz and Khuzestan (Table D III 3). As we have observed above and as is evident again from Table D III 4, the difference is made up for the Shirazi men by an excess of symptomatic disorders, their rate for such being about double that of the women. Why is it not higher also in Khuzestan? The common explanation that the adult male is more exposed does not avail. We suspect rather that the difference lies in that the Shirazi men are not more, but the women less exposed than in Khuzestan, for in Shiraz there is a notable proportion of middle class and even well-to-do families whose womenfolk undoubtedly enjoy on the whole both better home and environmental sanitation and less outdoor exposure than do the peasant women of Khuzestan. The suspicion is borne out by Tables B IV 3 and B IV 30. In some part the urban males are likewise less exposed or endangered, but probably in less. We possess no strictly comparable data on somatic morbidity in the two localities, but such as we do have support the hypothesis. Thus Gremliza [87] reports that the frequency of several endemic diseases in Khuzestan is practically equal for the sexes except where greater occupational exposure, as in the case of schistosomiasis, leads to a higher rate among the men. From Shiraz we have a tabulation of the ten major causes of death in the city during 1971 [150]. The total mortality for the males from these causes was 1468, for females 1095, giving an m:f ratio of 57:43. The male rate was higher in most categories, most strikingly in that of accidents, poisoning and suicide with 74:26, than in diseases of the digestive system with 68:32 and in cancer and other tumors with 64:36. For infectious and parasitic and for genito-urinary diseases the rates were approximately equal. The women lead by far in the group of endocrine, nutritional and metabolic diseases with 32:68, but in this group alone. As tenth and last group were listed "psychotic disturbances", which were held responsible for 32 male and 25 female deaths, or a ratio of 56:44, approximately that of the total.

Constitutional disorders tend to be recorded somewhat oftener among men than women in Khuzestan, but the numbers are small, and it remains doubtful whether the difference is real. It does not appear in Khuzestan.

It is in consonance with the enhanced frequency of reactive disorders among the women of Shiraz that this manifests itself especially in the simple reactions and developments (lower half of Table D III 4). Intellectual or pseudo-extraversion need not lead over into reactive disorder, but is a matrix favorable for it. Thus we may expect from it primarily cases in which dissociation is not involved.

The tribal groups now claim our attention. They are the exceptions. Their prevalence rates for psychiatric morbidity are very much, and very significantly lower than elsewhere, and their complaint scores are also low – only a trifle above Khuzestan. As this holds for both groups, living under quite different environmental circumstances, we have no hesitation in taking their common socio-political tribal structure as the explanation. Their psychiatric cases are so few that we can draw no conclusions from an analysis of them. In respect to complaints the women, just as in the city and the non-tribal villages except Khuzestan, surpass the men. Their generically typical forms of reaction are quick (sometimes at the cost of accuracy), global, emotionally tinged, intuitive among the true nomads and rather less so in the village. Here we meet with an undertone of probably nostalgic melancholy, especially among the men, while the boys seem untouched by it. Belief in magic is high among the true nomads, weak among those who have settled down. The Qashqai women of both tent and town appear as congenital extraverts, the men somewhat less so, and these retain certain reserves of introversion as do the likewise mostly unschooled girls of Khuzestan. Since tribal schooling was moving apace seventeen years ago, present-day findings might turn out quite differently.

In the case of the tribal groups low complaint scores and low psychiatric prevalences coincide, as they do not in Khuzestan. It is anything but self-evident that the complaint scores of the nomads, victims of drought and harassed by both robbers and the military, should be low. Neither were they, in spite of what was said above about the men, on the whole reticent introverts. One cannot but suspect a higher level of tolerance, abetted by a less deviant pattern of maturation for both sexes. Inner tensions, instead of being accumulated, were discharged freely as both the Z Tests and direct observation showed. Concerns were more immediate, as the memories indicate. It is notable that within this framework the almost never openly confessed, but covertly manifested nostalgia of the Qalandari men for the old ways did not result, in spite of neurotoid signs such as chiaroscuro responses and shocks, in psychiatric disturbance, which did not even rise to the level of the other surveys. Whether the manner of life, of reaction and behavior that we have tried to depict and for which we have an abundance of direct and indirect evidence, be the most effective for coping with different environments is beside the point and constitutes a question that it is not in our province to answer. Under the given circumstances it was conducive beyond doubt to mental health. As its common denominator was the tribal structure of both Qashqai groups the corollary seems evident that, where such structure still exists and serves a purpose, i.e. is not degraded to an artifically preserved relict or a tourist attraction, it should be conserved and even encouraged.

The Qashqais are a conspicuous exception, but Shiraz has some claim to be considered an exception also, being the single city that we have been able to survey. By most recent census projections the proportions of rural and urban inhabitants of Iran were taken to be roughly equal, but at the time of the actual survey in 1970 they were not. Iran was essentially an agricultural country, though not without metropolitan centers, and the rural population was the true standard of reference. How does Shiraz compare with it? Summarizing the many details of Part B, Chap. IV, we can say first of all that we have no shred of evidence that urban life, as represented by Shiraz at that time, exercised any detrimental influence on the whole upon mental health. As it is quite commonly assumed, often on inadequate evidence, that city life is somehow detrimental, this point deserves emphasis. When we were given to understand that it was a fool's errand to look for psychiatric disorder in the countryside it was with the unspoken implication that it was to be found in the city. It was, but in the country no whit less. This is true, moreover (cf. Table D III 3), for all degrees of severity and on the whole for both sexes, but a difference emerges between them for the poor. The poor women in the city, but not the poor men, have a distinctly higher total prevalence rate, which is so compensated by the lower rate among the urban women of the middle and upper classes that no significant overall sex difference results. We recall that there was no sex difference in Khuzestan, and that the apparent difference in Marvdasht was very probably an artefact. Not a few of these pathological poor females in the city were immigrants from villages, more often by their husbands' choice than by their own – uprooted, confused and forlorn in a strange environment. Looking at their husbands as well we come upon indirect negative evidence concerning the supposedly detrimental influence of city life: the great majority of the poor immigrants to the city had brought their psychopathology with them. It would be hazardous to generalize. Investigations in Tehran or even in the more industrialized cities such as Isfahan or Tabriz might have led to different results and conclusions, but we possess no evidence at all for such.

While we do encounter a sex difference in Shiraz and to a lesser degree in Khuzestan also in regard to categories of psychopathology, the females having significantly more of the reactive type, and while the female poor in Shiraz do have more pathology than the male poor, there is no support outside this limited group for the frequently advanced thesis that poverty in itself contributes significantly to psychopathology of one or another variety. Neither does the converse hold. No pattern of psychopathology typical for poverty (within the rather wide boundaries of our principal categories) can be demonstrated. Within the group it is still debatable whether poverty be cause or effect, but our data on migrants and our own observation of such in the city speak more for the latter.

In still another respect the Shiraz findings do not correspond with the expectations of Western sociology: the poor urban women, whether normal or pathological, are neither more fecund nor do they have more living children than their better off sisters. The middle class pathological females, but not the unpathological, have both (Table B IV 7). Nevertheless, families with pathological members tend to be larger than those without, and such members tend to cluster within the specific families. As the taking of detailed family histories under survey conditions was out of the question, we cannot even venture a guess whether this was referable more to heredity or to environment.

This leads into the larger question of epidemiological sex differences. On the whole we do not find any (though there is a somewhat uncertain indication of a female excess of medium and severe cases in Khuzestan: cf. Table D III 3). The greater inclination of the female sex to reactive, of the male sex to symptomatic disorders has been noted. Within the reactive disorders the women far outnumber the men in respect of the anxious and depressive simple developments. Yet the true anxiety neuroses (as opposed to the simple developments) are the men's domain, the hysterias and hypochondrias the women's, specifically the urban women's. Among the psychosomatic cases no sex difference appears in Khuzestan, but in Shiraz somewhat more men, especially the lighter cases, are classified as such. The men are prone to tension headaches, the women by a large margin to migraine.

In regard to other disease categories, we must mention again that all three patients diagnosed as endogenous-depressive were female, which may be mere chance. Among the schizophrenias we encountered no sex bias. In the symptomatic category, where the men significantly exceeded the women, the decisive diagnoses were those of post-infectious and post-traumatic conditions (including symptomatic epilepsies) and of addiction (no females). On the other hand, the female senile and arteriosclerotic cases outnumbered the male by more than two to one.

While literacy is certainly no cure for psychopathology either reactive or symptomatic as its prevalence in highly literate Western countries proves, a relation nevertheless is to be found. In Shiraz the poor exhibit more pathology than the non-poor, the illiterate poor still more. Again, many of them come from the poor, often already pathological immigrants to the city. The question is discussed in more detail in relation to Table B IV 20. Corresponding thereto we meet some indication, but no satisfactory statistical proof, that the members of unskilled occupations, who are also for the most part poor and illiterate, are more subject to psychiatric disturbance than the skilled and semi-skilled.

Such relationships as we have just discussed are dynamic and subject to change and circumstance. The importance of the circumstances has been shown over and over again as we have passed from one survey to another, covering periods of drought, want and persecution, of social change, of relative prosperity and of forced development. Findings that hold under one set of circumstances may be altered and even transformed under another. In only one instance could we study a direct sequence: in Qassemabad. The socio-economic condition had changed radically between 1963 and 1976. The rates of evil memories and of complaints fell. Those for psychiatric prevalence did or did not according to the criterion that one chose. Overall prevalence was lower in 1976, but not to a statistically significant degree. It was strikingly lower, however, when one counted only the medium and severe cases (the latter had in fact disappeared, though we cannot assume this to be a lasting condition). Several of the old P_2 cases had recovered, and nearly all the new cases were of degree P_1. Though they were mild, it would seem imprudent as well as unjust to pass them over, for they carry in them propensities to P_2 as well as to improvement. So do the neurotoid matrices we observed in Qassemabad in 1976 and in Khuzestan in 1965.

We arrive at a few final reflections. Iran is no less subject to psychiatric disturbance than other nations of the East or West, and the Iranian countryside no less than the cities. This implies a need for psychiatric services, to meet which it is exceedingly difficult. In Iran as elsewhere psychiatrists congregate in the cities, but the problem created thereby is less in a small country with a close network of transportation than in a country with the vast distances of Iran. Though we are partial to out-patient treatment as far as this is reasonably possible, the question seems at least deserving of debate whether in Iran not mental hospitals, but residential centers for psychiatric patients in the cities might serve a valuable function (we have seen a good example in Khartoum). Since there is practically no skilled nursing staff, mental hospitals are the poorest solution and should not be multiplied.

What can be done in the way of amelioration or prevention? The WHO strives rightly for the integration of mental health into public health, but this is a vast and still somewhat vague aspiration. We have found rather high rates of symptomatic disorders, particularly among the men. Improved sanitation and much stricter accident prevention could accomplish something here. Within our day poliomyelitis has been nearly, smallpox wholly eradicated, and malaria, though still recurrent, has become relatively rare. Their hapless residues will tend to decrease and, we hope, vanish. But the implication of a greater life expectancy in better physical health must not be forgotten: the psychiatric disorders of old age, for which scant provision has been made. These are problems common to most developing countries. Three at least remain that seem more specifically, though not exclusively, Iranian.

One is that of the women. On the whole they are less afflicted by symptomatic disorders, and a reduction of these will affect them less. Their marked surplus of reactive disorders remain, especially in the city. The illiterate poor urban women are the worst sufferers. We European psychiatrists rated their sufferings even higher, as appears from Part D, Chap. II, than our female Iranian co-workers on the whole did. At this point psychiatry becomes inseparable from culture. Whose ratings are to be accepted and what consequences are to be drawn from the culture ultimately will decide. We must content ourselves here with stating the question.

A second is that of the schools. By our evidence it seems altogether likely that formal schooling in Iran leads not seldom, more among the girls than among the boys, to a forced or pseudo-extraversion that is scarcely conducive to mental health, although it does not necessarily result in mental disturbance. Advocating a return to ignorance and even illiteracy would be equivalent to the prescription of decapitation for headache. How the problem is to be met – and not in Iran only – is a matter for pedagogues to decide.

The third is that of the tribes. One of the best established and for us most noteworthy findings of our surveys was that mental health flourishes within a tribal structure, and that this is not dependent upon a nomadic way of life. One obvious measure of prevention is to conserve such structures where they are still existent and viable and even to encourage them. In this lies an invitation to our colleagues in ethnology.

Books could be written on any of these topics. We wish their authors well and now close ours.

Annexes

Annex I

Survey Form from the Shiraz Mental Health Survey

Persian complete; English translation of Page 1 (personal and family data) only, as test records and questionnaire are discussed in the relevant chapters.

Page 1 — No. _ _/ _ _ _ _ /_ _

Shiraz Mental Health Office — Date ____________
Shiraz Mental Health Survey 1969/70

World Health Organization – Ministry of Health – Pahlavi University

Address ______________________________ Number of persons in household ☐☐

Relationship of respondent to head of household ______________________

Forename ____________________ Family name ______________________

Father's name ______ Father's No. _ _/_ _ _ _ _ _/_ _ Date of father's death ________

Mother's name ______ Mother's No. _ _/_ _ _ _ _ _/_ _ Date of mother's death ________

Age ________ years Sex: male ☐ 1 female ☐ 2

Occupation ____ ☐☐

Marital status:	Single	Married	Widowed	Divorced	Separated
	☐ 1	☐ 2	☐ 3	☐ 4	☐ 5

Name of spouse ____________________ No. _ _/ _ _ _ _ /_ _

Date of spouse's death ________________

Orphanism:	☐ 1	☐ 2	☐ 3	☐ 4

Father's occupation at time of respondent's marriage ____________________

Number of live-born children ☐☐ Number of children now living ☐☐

Place of birth ____________________ Years resident in Shiraz ☐☐

Religion:	Moslem	Jewish	Zoroastrian	Christian	Other
	☐ 1	☐ 2	☐ 3	☐ 4	☐ 5

Literacy and Education:	Illit.	Pre-S.	Prim.	Sec.	Univ.	Old	4 Cl.	6 Cl.	9 Cl.	12 Cl.	Univ.
	☐ 01	☐ 02	☐ 03	☐ 04	☐ 05	☐ 06	☐ 07	☐ 08	☐ 09	☐ 10	☐ 11

Menstruation:	yes	no	pregnant	stilling	Clay eating:	yes	no
	☐ 1	☐ 2	☐ 3	☐ 4		☐ 1	☐ 2

شماره --/-----/-- صفحه ۱

اداره بهداشت روانی شیراز

تاریخ ....

مطالعات بهداشتی شهرشیراز ۴۸- ۱۳۴۹

سازمان بهداشت جهانی - وزارت بهداری - دانشگاه پهلوی

آدرس .... تعداد خانوار در منزل ☐☐

نسبت پاسخ دهنده ....

نام .... نام فامیل ....

نام پدر .... شماره پدر --/-----/-- تاریخ فوت ....

نام مادر .... شماره مادر --/-----/-- تاریخ فوت ....

سن سال - جنس مونث ☐ ۲ مذکر ☐ ۱

شغل .... ☐☐

تاهل .... مجرد ☐ ۱ متاهل ☐ ۲ بیوه ☐ ۳ مطلقه ☐ ۴ جدا ☐ ۵ نام همسر شماره --/-----/--

☐ ☐ ☐ ☐ ☐ تاریخ فوت همسر

قرابت .... ☐ ۱ ☐ ۲ ☐ ۳ ☐ ۴ ☐☐

شغل پدر موقعیکه شما ازدواج کردید .... ☐☐

چندطفل بدنیاآورده اید ؟ ☐☐ چند نفرآنها زنده اند ؟ ☐☐

محل تولد .... چند سال است بشیراز آمده اید ؟ ☐☐

مذهب مسلمان ☐ ۱ کلیمی ☐ ۲ زردشتی ☐ ۳ مسیحی ☐ ۴ دیگری ☐ ۵

سواد بی سواد ☐ ۰۱ طفل ☐ ۰۲ دبستان ☐ ۰۳ دبیرستان ☐ ۰۴ دانشگاه ☐ ۰۵ قدیمی ☐ ۰۶ ۴ کلاس ☐ ۰۷ ۶ کلاس ☐ ۰۸ ۹ کلاس ☐ ۰۹ ۱۲ کلاس ☐ ۱۰ دانشگاه ☐ ۱۱

قاعدگی بله ☐ ۱ نه ☐ ۲ حامله ☐ ۳ شیرده ☐ ۴ گل خوردن بله ☐ ۱ نه ☐ ۲

صفحه ۲

شماره --/-----/--

حساب الــف

سکه ها : میشناسد و تشخیص میدهد ________

۷ ________

۱۹ ________

حساب ذهنـــــی

۵ + ۳ = ________

۷ + ۸ = ________

۱۹ + ۱۲ = ________

۳۳ + ۲۸ = ________

۴۸ + ۷۴ = ________

۸ ـ ۵ = ________

۱۲ ـ ۷ = ________

۳۴ ـ ۱۸ = ________

۱۲۳ ـ ۷۸ = ________

۲ × ۳ = ________

۳ × ۶ = ________

۷ × ۸ = ________

۹ × ۱۲ = ________

۱۳ × ۱۳ = ________

۱۲ : ۳ = ________

۳۲ : ۴ = ________

۶۴ : ۸ = ________

۷۲ : ۱۲ = ________

۱۱۰ : ۱۰ = ________

۱/۲ ÷ ۱/۴ = ________

۱/۲ + ۱/۳ = ________

جمع .

نام و امضاء تکمیل کننده

صفحه ۳

شماره --/-----/--

محدودیت وقت (ثانیه)	شماره سئوال		جواب	زمان انجام کار	جمع نمره وامتیازها
۱۵	۱	مردی چهارسیگارداشت و ۲ عدد دیگر خرید حال روبهمرفته چند سیگار دارد ؟	--	--	--
۱۵	۲	پسری ۱۲ روزنامه داشت ۵ عدد آنرا فروخت حال چند روزنامه دارد . ؟	--	--	--
۱۵	۳	اگر هربسته سیگار ۷ ریال باشد ۳ بسته سیگار چند میشود ؟	--	--	--
۳۰	٤	یك شیرفروش ۲۵ شیشه شیر داشت و ۱۱ شیشه آنرا فروخت . چند شیشه برای او باقیمانده ؟	--	--	--
۳۰	۵	کارگری ۲۸۸ تومان بدست آورد . درصورتیکه حقوق او ۳۲ تومان درروزباشد وی چند روزکارکرده است ؟	--	--	--
٦۰	٦	چنانچه شما ۳کیلوپرتقال راازقرارکیلوئی ۳۰ریال بخرید و ۱۰۰ ریال بفروشنده بدهید چقدر ازپول شما باقی خواهد ماند	--	--	--
٦۰	۷	اگر ۳عدد مداد ۵ ریال شود قیمت ۲٤ عدد مداد چقدر میشود ؟	--	--	--
۱۲۰	۸	چنانچه یك تاکسی برای یکربع کیلومتراول ۲۰ ریال بخواهد و برای هریکربع بعدی ۵ ریال برای ۲کیلومترونیم چقدر باید داده شود .	--	--	--
۱۲۰	۹	اگر دو نفر تیرانداز بتوانند دریك دقیقه ونیم ٦ پوکه فشنگ را پرکنند پنج نفرتیرانداز درنیمساعت چند پوکه را پر خواهندکرد . ؟	--	--	--
۱۲۰	۱۰	پرویزو بهرام باهم ورق بازی میکردند . درابتدای بازی هرکدام ۲۷ تومان پول داشتند . قرار براین گذاشتندکه درهردست هرکس بازنده میشود فقط یك سوم موجودیش رابه برنده بدهد . حالا اگرپرویزهرسه دست اول رابرنده بشود معلوم کنید بهرام دراول بازی دست چهارم چقدر پول موجود دارد ؟	--	--	--
		جمع کل			--
		جمع سنجیده شده			--
		بهره هوشی			--

نام و امضاء تکمیل کننده

شماره --/-----/---　　　　صفحه ٤

طرح کعب

الف :

ب :

	شماره طرح	حدودیت وقت (ثانیه)	زمان انجام کار (ثانیه	امتیاز بدست آمده	نمره خام
طرح	اولین مرتبه	٦٠			
نمونه	دومین مرتبه	٤٥			
	١	٧٥			
	٢	٧٥			
	٣	٧٥			
	٤	٧٥			
	٥	١٥٠			
	٦	١٥٠			
	٧	١٥٠			
				جمع	

جمع منجیده شده ____________

بهرهوشی ____________

نام و امضاء تکمیل کننده

صفحه ٥

شماره --/-----/--..

زی تست

۱ــ ساعت شروع ساعت دقیقه
زمان آغاز ثانیه

II- ختم و برگرداندن کارت ساعت دقیقه
زمان آغاز ثانیه

III - ختم و برگرداندن کارت ساعت دقیقه
زمان آغاز ثانیه

ختم و برگرداندن کارت ساعت دقیقه = ساعت پایان تست

مشاهدات ــ طرز رفتا رو سلوك

نام و امضاء تکمیل کننده

صفحه ٦

شماره --/-----/--

پرسشهای شخصی

۱ــ هیچوقت فلج شده ای (بدنت لمس شده) ؟

ــ

۲ــ گاهی حمله غشی کرده ای ؟

ــ

۳ــ گاهی ناخوشی داشتی، که خیلی سرت درد بکنه و پشتش هم خیلی بخوابی ؟

ــ

٤ــ چه چیز توی زندگی برات بهترین خوشیها را آورده (بهترین خاطره) ؟

ــ

٥ــ چه چیز توی زندگی بزرگترین درد سر و زحمت را برات پیش آورده (بدترین خاطره) ؟

ــ

٦ــ گاهی شده آنقدر بارغم رو دلت بوده که دست و دل کارکردن نداشته باشی ؟

ــ

۷ ــ گاهی شده که اززور شور و خوشحالی دست و پات را گم کنی و نتوانی کارکنی ؟

ــ

۸ ــ گاهی شده که دل شوره و ترس داشته باشی اما ندونی چراو واسی چی ؟

ــ

۹ ــ گاهی شده که فکر کنی همه دنیا میخوان اذیتت بکنن ؟

ــ

۱۰ــ گاهی شده که دنیا عجیب و غریب پیش چشمت بیاد یا آنکه چی بنظرت بیاد ؟

ــ

۱۱ــ گاهی شده که چی بشنوی ــ مثل اینکه بهت حرف میزنند اما کسی نباشد ؟

ــ

۱۲ــ گاهی شده که حس کنی جادو و جمبلت کرده اند و سحر شده ای یا آنکه چیزی اطرافت سحرشده باشد یا آنکه معجزی بشه ؟

نظر مصاحبه کننده درباره وضع روانی پاسخ دهنده :

احتیاج به مطالعات بعدی دارد

" " " ندارد

نام و امضاء تکمیل کننده

Annex II

Psychiatric Facilities in Iran

The information in the accompanying Table cannot claim to be either accurate or complete. Nevertheless, it seemed better to furnish the reader at least with some notion of the clinical psychiatric facilities in Iran than to leave him wondering whether there were any such outside the capital or indeed any at all. All numbers are approximate at best.

The tabulation is based principally upon the first author's personal knowledge, embodied in many internal reports to the WHO and the Iranian Ministry of Health and brought up to date as far as possible, then upon two papers by Dr. T. A. Baasher, WHO Regional Adviser on Mental Health, Regional Office for the Eastern Mediterranean: "Report on Mental Health Activities in Iran" [11] and "National Statistics of Mental Health Services in the Eastern Mediterranean Region" [12]. They were rendered in 1973 and 1974 respectively. The first of these shows little change since I terminated my assignment in 1964. On my return visits in 1974 and 1976 I could observe directly some major alterations: at Razi Hospital in Rey near Tehran the opening of several large wards that had been under construction and the closing of others, so that total capacity did not greatly differ but could not be determined exactly as it was changing almost from month to month; in Shiraz the opening of the new Hafez University Hospital with a psychiatric division; and in Tabriz the construction of the 400 bed Shagoli Psychiatric Hospital, since opened and functioning. In 1979 a colleague's letter announced that the desolate Kaveh Hospital in Isfahan had been demolished and replaced by a modern clinic. He did not state the number of beds: the Table contains the former number with a question mark. All requests for further information have remained unanswered except for East Azerbaijan.

The history of mental hospitals in Iran goes back at least to the foundation of the Daru'sh Shafa in Yazd, a general hospital with a psychiatric division, in A. H. s.666/ A. D.1446. It is silent for centuries thereafter. The present Razi Mental Hospital in Rey was founded in Tehran under the name of Aminabad in 1917. Other mental hospitals were founded successively in the years between the two World Wars or after. Most of the public ones are used as teaching hospitals.

It may come as a surprise to some readers that it is not possible to assert with any assurance which public authority is administratively and financially responsible for which psychiatric hospital. These have changed too often and too rapidly. The Ministry of Health and its divisions, the Ostans, semi-official and religious foundations (waqf), regional and local health councils, the universities, even the Municipality of Tehran (in the case of Razi Hospital) all have been involved, seldom happily, and have passed the mental hospitals with changing legislation back and forth like hot potatoes into each other's unwilling hands.

The number of patients in mental hospitals that are declared as such is not equivalent to the number of psychiatric patients in hospital or custodial care. Other institutions which care for them are special clinics for addicts (the larger with about 200 beds in Tehran, a smaller one with some 40 beds in Isfahan), military hospitals, hospitals belonging to the Laborers' Insurance and above all the work camps of the Ministry of the Interior, in which, beside all manner of the homeless and the derelict, not a few chronic psychiatric cases could be found. There are no data on the number of these.

In earlier years I have tried to list the psychiatric out-patient facilities, but it is now impossible to do so even roughly. They have multiplied substantially since 1960, when there were only a handful, but they have opened, closed, changed their names, locations and even their supporting agencies so much that it is hopeless to try to trace them from a distance.

There is or was no register of medical specialists in Iran. For years the number of psychiatrists, most of them both in government service and private practice, stagnated at an estimated 30–50. Nearly all were in Tehran. The number mounted swiftly in the seventies, and lately I have been informed of psychiatric practices in secondary centers where one would not have dreamed of looking for them a decade or two ago. For a recent estimate see below. Psychiatric nursing hardly exists despite efforts of the WHO to further it.

Table X II 1. Psychiatric Hospitals in Iran

Ostan	City	Name	Beds		Character
0 Central	Tehran	Rousbeh	100		1
Central	Tehran/Rey	Razi	1500		1
Central	Tehran	Military	40		2
Central	Tehran	Tcherazi	100		3
Central	Tehran	Rezai	80		3
Central	Tehran	Mehmanat	80	1900	3
3 East Azerbaijan	Tabriz	Mental Hospital	80		1
East Azerbaijan	Tabriz	Shahgoli	400		1
East Azerbaijan	Tabriz	Khajavi	30		3
East Azerbaijan	Tabriz	Ordoobadi	25	535	3
5 Kermanshah	Hamadan	Gharb	220	220	1
6 Khuzestan	Abadan	National Iranian Oil Co. Hospital	25	25	2
7 Fars	Shiraz	Hafez	40		1
Fars	Shiraz	Salami	100	140	3
9 Khorasan	Meshed	Hejazi	250	250	1
10 Isfahan	Isfahan	University	300?		1
Isfahan	Isfahan	Tcherazi	25		3
Isfahan	Isfahan	Dorché	25	350	3
Total				3420	

Key: 1 = public; 2 = restricted; 3 = private.

Based on official statistics, Baasher has given the following information for Iran in 1974:

Psychiatric hospitals	18
First admissions to these per year	10000
Total admissions per year	22000
Psychiatric out-patient services (policlinics)	115
First visits to these per year	112500
Total visits (consultations) per year	345000
Psychiatric beds per 10000 population	1.2
Psychiatrists	120
Psychiatric nurses	15

Annex III

Crude Rates per Thousand for Psychiatric Morbidity in the Middle and Far East

In the Table on p. 403 we have utilized only data from field surveys, none based on hospital or out-patient statistics. They are limited to geographical and ethnological regions somewhat comparable to our own and therefore include two studies from North Africa. No pretension is made to completeness. Several investigations which we should have liked to include were inaccessible; others have had to be quoted at second hand. A thorough survey of the existing literature would have required a treatise to itself and thus far exceeded our present scope.

All prevalence rates are given to the basis of one thousand. They vary discomfortingly, even distressingly. The demonstration of this fact alone may justify the tabulation. The comparison for which we were looking usually can be drawn only with difficulty if at all and is only permissable when the methods employed for case identification and examination, furthermore the diagnostic criteria and those of distinction between "ill" and "well" are adequately described. Rates cannot be compared without reservation. The total prevalence rates for psychiatric disorders in this table alone range from 5 to 433 per thousand. Rates are most likely to be comparable when they stem from the same investigator or the same team. Besides this there exist more or less comparable, recognizable levels of thoroughness and exactitude that afford a still rather uncertain assistance. Surely real differences are not to be denied, but when figures differ by the order of 10^2 one must first ask whether different measures have been used or even different things measured.

The extremely diverse manners in which epidemiological authors present their data constitute another difficulty of hardly less magnitude. Some count only manifest cases, others such as have remitted or recovered (most commonly in regard to the functional psychoses), some inform the reader about the age structure of the population, others not, and not even the sexes are always treated separately. Elder authors are more inclined to apply an age correction, younger less, and when one is applied there is little agreement, especially in recent non-European publications, about the age of risk. Even this would not be too disastrous if one could recalculate the data. Often, however, the way in which they are collated, organized or tabulated renders this impossible. If one writer begins his age classes at 15, another at 10 or 20, and if both count, as is usual, by decades, no comparison can be made. Different kinds of data require different forms of presentation, to be sure, and we do not argue that they should be restricted to only a single one, but we do consider it essential that in psychiatric epidemiology no less than in the natural sciences the comparability of findings should be assured. It will be a difficult, but in the near future inescapable task for epidemiological research to set up standards for this.

In regard to the column headings of the Table the following is to be remarked:

Author indicates the principal author from whose publication the data have been taken. The author is often, but not always (particularly in case of Japanese surveys) identical with the main investigator.

Place means the area, region, city or town within the respective country, the latter being shown in *italics* as heading.

Year means the year or years in which the survey was conducted, so far as this can be ascertained. Where it cannot, the year of publication has been inserted. Dates of publication, sometimes several years after the field work, can be found from the references in the bibliography (cf. column *Ref.*).

m stands as an abbreviation of "manifest". Some authors have counted only active, i.e. manifest cases and are indicated in this column by *a* (= active). Others have included both inactive and active cases and are designated here by *i* (= inactive besides active). The difference, when rates have to be computed, is far from trivial, as can be seen from the data of the single author who has quoted both.

c stands for age *c*orrection. In this table only crude rates are given. Where the original publication allows age-corrected rates to be calculated or where the author has actually applied an age correction at least to some of his data, a plus sign (+) stands in this column, where not a minus (–). As Lin has already re-calculated the findings of a number of his Japanese and other colleagues with a uniform age correction and has published them [121, 122], whereas most of the other studies quoted here do not permit such a correction, we have refrained from any systematic attempt to do so. Where we have nevertheless re-calculated certain data for comparison with ours this is mentioned in the text or in the notes below, not in the Table.

Under the following six principal headings we have ordered and arranged the data so fas as possible to conform with the scheme we have used for Iran. Where no relevant data were presented or where it seemed seriously doubtful whether they could be accommodated to the heading in question we have put a question mark (?). In a number of cases the respective authors' data could be regrouped to fit more or less our headings. We have done this rather liberally without, we hope, doing violence to any investigator's findings, as our aim throughout has been comparability. We have done so here even more freely than in an earlier version of this Table published in *Psychopathologie im Kulturvergleich* [24] as experiments with recombinations according to our own concepts have shown that better agreement between field reports could be attained in this way than appeared at first glance: cf. Table D V 1. For this reason the rates stated in the Table will not always be identical with those in the original publications. Where the differences are of moment they will be explained in the notes below.

Schiz. = schizophrenia is the one disease that all authors mention. Most refer to the definition of the ICD. Comparative tabulation met with hardly any difficulties. Once more it may be mentioned that rates can differ substantially according to whether point or lifetime prevalence is intended.

MD = manic-depressive or affective psychosis. Most authors seem to comprehend under this heading both unipolar and bipolar endogenous affective psychoses including involutional depressions. A few do not distinguish sharply enough for a tabulation, or do not distinguish at all between endogenous, organic, reactive and neurotic depressions.

Epi. = epilepsy in all its variants. Where only epileptic psychoses were meant we have omitted the rate as scarcely comparable. Prevalence rates for epilepsy in general have been included only when the epilepsies were distinguished clearly enough from other neurological and psychiatric diseases.

SAD = senile-arteriosclerotic dementia, again quoted only from the rather few publications that differentiated it clearly from other organic brain diseases.

React. = reactive psychopathological and psychiatric disorders. These data are the least comparable of all, partly because of the enormous, but by no means always or even usually explicit differences in their conception and definition, partly because of the inclusion or exclusion of related categories such as disorders of behavior and adjustment, undefined "personality disorders", psychogenic depressions, psychosomatic disturbances etc., partly because of the now stricter, now laxer criteria of diagnosis, partly because of the very methods of investigation. As our own policy has been to include the distinctive groups of the simple, neurotic and psychosomatic disorders under one principal heading, we have endeavored to regroup other authors' data so far as possible in the same manner. Thus we include under it simple reactions, manifest neuroses together with such usually neurotic disturbances as enuresis or misbehavior (well aware that not all cases belong here), also the psychosomatic illnesses that some writers keep separate, but not "personality disorders", which we assume to correspond in the majority of cases with rubric 301 of the ICD and for which we have retained the designation of psychopathy. They are presumed to be mainly congenital, not reactive. As just mentioned, the shifting categories of the depressions complicate the task. Although certain cautious comparisons do appear possible after such studied reclassification, we must confess regretfully that they are few and at best rather uncertain – a circumstance that is the more unfortunate because this category is one of the largest and practically most important. To render such comparisons truly and fairly reliably possible will be another of the thorny, but inescapable tasks of future psychiatric epidemiology.

Olig. = oligophrenia, mental debility or feeble-mindedness. Again the rates vary to a discomforting and even alarming degree, the more so when one reflects upon the practical consequences. So far as we could ascertain none of the authors quoted here has employed standardized intelligence tests.

Total = total psychiatric morbidity or prevalence as the respective authors have stated it. It is not always and not even in the majority of cases equal to the cross sum of the six main classes because some categories that the authors themselves have used are not included in this tabulation. We have not thought fit to exclude them from the total, which in itself is intended as a general index of prevalence. How little comparable these indices are remains a disconcerting fact, a challenge to the future.

Ref. = reference number from the general bibliography of the source from which the tabulated data have been extracted.

Table X III 1. Crude Rates per Thousand for Psychiatric Morbidity in the Middle and Far East

Author	Place	Year	Pop.	m	c	Schiz.	MD	Epi.	SAD	React.	Olig.	Total	Ref.
Taiwan													
Lin		1946–48	19931	i	+	2.1[1]	0.7	1.3	0.3	1.2	3.4	10.8[2]	121
Lin et al.		1961–63	29184	i	–	1.4[3]	0.5	?	0.4	7.8[4]	4.9[3]	17.2[4]	123
Japan													
Uchimura[5]	Hachijo	1940	8330	i	+	3.8	1.0	0.6	0.2	?	0.6	6.8	192, 193
Kato	Hachijo	1961	12207	i	–	4.7	0.8	1.4	?	?	?	?	111
Akimoto[5]	Komoro	1941	5207	i	+	2.1	2.5	2.5	2.3	2.5	10.0	26.5	4
Tsugawa[5]	Tokyo	1941	2712	i	+	2.2	0.7	2.6	0.4	?	9.6	30.8	191
Min. of Health[6]	Nation	1954	22993	a	–	2.3	0.2	1.4	0.86	3.0	7.0	15.1	111
Min. of Health[6]	Nation	1963	44092	a	–	2.3	0.2	1.0	0.36	2.8	4.2	12.9	111
India													
Dube	Agra	1970	29468	a	–	1.49	0.51	2.24	?	9.40[7]	3.70	18.0	63
Dube	Agra	1970	29468	i	+	2.17	1.26	3.19	?	12.63[7]	3.70	23.8	63
Elnagar et al.	West Bengal	1969	1383	a[8]	–	4.3	2.8[9]	4.3	?	1.4[10]	1.4	27.5	67
Nandi et al.	West Bengal	1972	1060	a	+	2.8	?[11]	10.4	?	85.8[12]	2.8	102.8	156
Thacore et al.	North Bengal	1975	2696	a	–	2	2	?	?	40.1[13]	14	82	189
Carstairs and Kapur	Kota	1972	1233	a	–	8.1	0	5.7	1.6	353	?	369[14]	54
Sri Lanka (Ceylon)													
Jayasundara	Aluthgama	1960	2506	a	–	5.2	1.2	?	?	1.6[15]	?	10.0	107
Jayasundara	Seeduwa[16]	1961	2212	a	–	2.3	0.90	?	?	0.45[15]	?	5.0	107
Ethiopia													
Giel & v. Luijk	Bonga	1967	384	a	–	2.6	0	5.2	?	57.3	2.6	85.9	82
Sudan													
Baasher	Wadi Halfa	1960	1860	a	–	6.98	5.91	?	?	46.2[17]	3.76	62.9	10
Iran													
Bash and Bash-Liechti	Nation	1963–70	2243	a	+	1.78[18]	1.34	5.80	7.1	77.1	12.9	126.2	
Davidian	Roodsar	1975	488	?	–	6.1	6.0	?	?	278[19]	?	433	61

Notes to Table X III 1

[1] In a later publication from 1969 [123] Lin et al. give this rate as 2.2 rather than 2.1.

[2] In the same later publication we find this rate as 9.4 rather than 10.8.

[3] The differences for schizophrenia between 2.2 in 1948/53 and 1.4 in 1963 and for oligophrenia between 3.4 in 1948/53 and 4.9 in 1963 are significant with $p < 0.05$.

[4] The differences for reactive disorders between 1.2 in 1948/53 and 7.8 in 1963 and for total morbidity between 10.8 in 1948/53 and 17.2 in 1963 are significant with $p < 0.01$.

[5] Quoted from Lin [121].

[6] Quoted from Kato [111].

[7] Combining Dube's categories of hysteria (11 male, 250 female cases) and other psychoneuroses (53 m, 58 f), under which latter he subsumes the apparently infrequent psychopathies, for which no separate figures are given.

[8] Apparently only active cases, but the brief text leaves room for question.

[9] All kinds of depressive states, not only psychotic.

[10] "Persons suspected of suffering from psychosomatic disorders were found; but because of difficulties in differential diagnosis they were not included in the study."

[11] Nandi et al. state the very high figure of 40 cases of "depression" or 37.7 per 1000 but make it clear that "endogenous depression, depressed type of MDR, reactive depression and involutional depression have all been included." As it seems probable that the great majority are reactive, we have counted them under our corresponding heading. No data for endogenous depression are to be found.

[12] We combine here a list of presumably reactive disorders, including the "depressions" mentioned in Note 11, as follows:

Depression	40 cases
Neurotic depression	5
Anxiety	13
Hysteria	18
Phobia	1
Obsession	1
Psychosomatic	10
Enuresis	3
	91 = 85.8 per 1000

[13] Including 55 neuroses (= 20 per 1000), 9 "psychophysiological disorders" (psychosomatic cases? 3 per 1000) and 6 "transient situation reactions" (2 per 1000). Besides these Thacore et al. mention 50 "personality disorders" and 2 cases of "social maladjustment referable to habitual excessive drinking."

[14] Defined as "anyone with one or more symptoms" as determined by the subject's answers to the Indian Psychiatric Survey Schedule with its 124 items or by the answers of informants replying to the same Schedule. This includes many somatic complaints, which Carstairs and Kapur regard as psychologically co-determined and which we have therefore included under "React.". They constitute 100 per 1000.

[15] Only severer cases.

[16] In his publication Jayasundara gives data for two other villages as well but expresses such doubts himself about their reliability that we omit them.

[17] Including 5.4 per 1000 psychosomatic disorders, the rest neurotic.

[18] Four cases, three with definite, one with probable diagnosis. Cf. Part D Chap. IV 2.

[19] Of which 208 per 1000 were simple or reactive neurotic depressions in nearly equal shares, 35 per 1000 other neuroses and also 35 per 1000 psychosomatic disorders. Besides these, Davidian mentions 94 per 1000 personality disorders, 8 per 1000 organic disorders including mental subnormality and 12 per 1000 opium addictions.

References

1. Adams RN (1962) Agricultural and urban life in early southwestern Iran. Science 136: 109–122
2. Adham M (1963) Health statistics for Iran. Ministry of Health, Tehran
3. Agosti E (1973) Psychisch Kranke in einer Allgemeinpraxis. Diss Zürich
4. Akimoto H (1942) Demographische und psychiatrische Untersuchung der abgegrenzten Kleinstadtbevölkerung. Psychiatria et Neurologia Japonica 47: 351–374
5. Alter M, Hauser W A (eds) (1972) The epidemiology of epilepsy: A workshop. NINDS Monograph No. 14. DHEW Publication No. 73–390. US Government Printing Office, Washington D.C.
6. Anastasi A, Foley J P, (1949) Differential psychology, revised edn. Macmillan, New York
7. Angst J (1966) Zur Aetiologie und Nosologie endogener depressiver Psychosen. Springer, Berlin Heidelberg New York
8. Anon (1963) Zinc deficiency in man. Lancet, February 10
9. Arberry AJ (1960) Shiraz. University of Oklahoma Press, Norman, Oklahoma
10. Baasher TA (1961) Survey of mental illness in Wadi Halfa. World Mental Health 13:1–5
11. Baasher TA (1973) Report on mental health activities in Iran 29 January to 10 February 1973. WHO, Regional Office for the Eastern Mediterranean EM/MENT/ 51 IRAN 5401. Stencilled, 18 p, Alexandria
12. Baasher TA (1975) National statistics of mental health services in the Eastern Mediterranean Region. Int Symp on Epidemiological Studies in Psychiatry Tehran 1974. World Psychiatric Association and Psychiatric Society of Iran, Tehran
13. Baraheni MN (1975) A psychometric study of the Eysenck Personality Inventory on a sample of Iranian college students. Internat Symp on Epidemiological Studies in Psychiatry Tehran 1974. World Psychiatric Association and Psychiatric Society of Iran, Tehran
14. Barth F (1961) Nomads of South Persia. Oslo University Press, Allen and Unwin, London
15. Bash KW (1953) Ueber die Bestimmung und statistische Verteilung der Introversion und Extraversion im Rorschach-Versuch. Rorschachiana-Zeitschr 1:333–343
16. Bash KW (1955) Einstellungstypus und Erlebnistypus: Jung CG and Rorschach H. J Projective Techniques 19:236–242
17. Bash KW (1964) First preliminary report on neuropsychiatric epidemiology. Marvdasht Mental Health Survey, Province of Fars, Iran. In: Petrossian A, Shayan K, Bash KW, Jessup B.: The health and related characteristics of four selected village and tribal communities in Fars Ostan, pp. 73–95. Shiraz
18. Bash KW (1964) Die Psychiatrie und das Glück. Schweiz Med Wschr 94:970–974
19. Bash KW (1966) Psychotherapeutische Erfolgsstatistik. Deutsche Med Wschr 91:2089–2094
20. Bash KW (1967) Untersuchungen über die Epidemiologie neuropsychiatrischer Erkrankungen unter der Landbevölkerung der Provinz Fars, Iran. In: Petrilowitsch N(ed.) Beiträge zur vergleichenden Psychiatrie, pp. 162–178. Karger, Basel
21. Bash KW (1967) Psychologische Prüfungen in Iran. I: Intelligenzprüfungen bei der Bauernbevölkerung von Marvdasht. Schweiz Zschr Psychol 26:217–233
22. Bash KW (1969) Epilepsia sine ictu. Schweiz Arch Neurol Neurochir Psychiatr 103:351–353

23. Bash KW (1972) Patterns of drug abuse in Iran. In Drug abuse. Non-medical use of dependence-producing drugs, Btesh S (ed). pp. 118–122. Plenum Press, New York London
24. Bash KW (1980) Prävalenzraten psychischer Erkrankungen im Mittleren und Fernen Osten. In: Psychopathologie im Kulturvergleich, Pfeiffer WM und Schone W (eds), pp. 42–47. Enke, Stuttgart
25. Bash KW Ein Vergleich dreierlei Meßmethoden für die Introversion-Extraversion. Schweiz Zschr Psychol 40
26. Bash KW, Bash-Liechti J (1969) Studies on the epidemiology of neuropsychiatric disorders among the rural population of the province of Khuzestan, Iran. Social Psychiatry 4:137–143
27. Bash KW, Bash-Liechti J (1970) Psychologische Prüfungen in Iran. II: Z Test findings among Iranian peasants and nomads. In: Rorschach Proceedings. VIIth international congress of Rorschach and other projective techniques London August 5–8, 1968. Rorschachiana IX, pp. 244–251. Huber, Bern Stuttgart Wien
28. Bash KW, Bash-Liechti J (1970) Psychologische Prüfungen in Iran. III. Intelligenzprüfungen bei der Bauernbevölkerung von Chuzestan und bei den Qashqai-Nomaden. Schweiz Zschr Psychol 29:137–143
29. Bash KW, Bash-Liechti J (1972) Psychiatrische Epidemiologie in Iran. In: Perspektiven der heutigen Psychiatrie, Ehrhardt HE (Hrsg), pp. 313–319. Gerhards, Frankfurt
30. Bash KW, Bash-Liechti J (1973) Psychological testing and psychiatric morbidity in Iran. International Mental Health Research Newsletter 15:2
31. Bash KW, Bash-Liechti J (1974) Studies on the epidemiology of neuropsychiatric disorders among the population of the city of Shiraz. Social Psychiatry 9:163–171
32. Bash KW, Bash-Liechti J (1978) Psychiatrisch-epidemiologische Nachuntersuchung eines iranischen Dorfes nach dreizehn Jahren. Nervenarzt 49:713–719
33. Beck SJ (1944/1946/1962) Rorschach's Test. Vol. I 1944, Vol. II 1946, Vol. III 1962. Grune and Stratton, New York
34. Beck SJ, Robin AI, Thiessen WG, Molish HB (1950) The normal personality as reflected in the Rorschach Test. J Psychol 30:241–298
35. Binder H (1947) Der Begriff der Neurose. Schweiz Med Wschr 77:157–177
36. Binder H (1979 [original 1960]) Die psychopathischen Dauerzustände und die abnormen seelischen Reaktionen und Entwicklungen. In: Binder H: Ausgewählte Arbeiten in 3 Bde Bd I: Klinische Psychiatrie. Bash KW (Hrsg), pp. 577–600. Huber, Bern Stuttgart Wien
37. Binder H (1979 [original 1932]) Die Helldunkeldeutungen im psychodiagnostischen Experiment von Rorschach. In: Binder H: Ausgewählte Arbeiten in 3 Bde Bd II: Der Rorschach-Versuch, Bash KW (Hrsg), pp. 33–154. Huber, Bern Stuttgart Wien
38. Bleuler M (1932) Psychotische Belastung von körperlich Kranken. Zschr Ges Neurol Psychiatr 142:780–810
39. Bleuler M (1972) Die schizophrenen Geistesstörungen. Thieme, Stuttgart
40. Bleuler M, Bleuler R (1935) Rorschach's ink-blot test and racial psychology. Character and Personality 4:97–114
41. Bohm E (1972) Lehrbuch der Rorschach-Psychodiagnostik, 4th edn. Huber, Bern Stuttgart Wien
42. Bohm E (1975) Psychodiagnostisches Vademecum. 3rd edn. Huber, Bern Stuttgart Wien
43. Bourguignon E (1979) Psychological anthropology. An introduction to human nature and cultural differences. Holt, Rinehart and Winston, New York
44. Bratt-Østergaard N (1959) Gibt es charakteristische Rorschach'sche Formkonstellationen bei den sogenannten psychosomatischen Kindern? Rorschachiana V, pp. 305–324. Huber, Bern
45. Braun CM, Bonta JL (1979) Cross-cultural validity, reliability and stimulus characteristics of the Lüscher color test. J Personality Assessment 43:459–461
46. Bräutigam W (1974) Pathogenetische Theorien und Wege der Behandlung in der Psychosomatik. Nervenarzt 45:354–363
47. Bremer J (1951) A social psychiatric investigation of a small community in northern Norway. Munksgaard, Copenhagen

48. Brewis M, Poskanzer DC, Rolland C, Miller H (1966) Neurological disease in an English city. Acta Neurol Scand 42 [Suppl 24]:9–89
49. Brugger C (1929) Zur Frage einer Belastungsstatistik der Durchschnittsbevölkerung. Zschr Ges Neurol Psychiatr 118:459–488
50. Brugger C (1931) Versuch einer Geisteskrankenzählung in Thüringen. Zschr Ges Neurol Psychiatr 133:352–390
51. Brugger C (1933) Psychiatrische Ergebnisse einer medizinischen, anthropologischen und soziologischen Bevölkerungsuntersuchung. Zschr Ges Neurol Psychiatr 146:489–524
52. Brugger C (1938) Psychiatrische Bestandsaufnahme im Gebiet eines medizinisch-anthropologischen Zensus in der Nähe von Rosenheim. Zschr Ges Neurol Psychiatr 160:189–207
53. Burney LE (1963) Report and Recommendations on the Administration and Organization of the Ministry of Health. US AID Tehran
54. Carstairs GM, Kapur RL (1976) The great universe of Kota. Stress, change and mental disorder in an Indian village. Hogarth Press, London
55. Cattel RB, Eber HW (1962) Handbook for the sixteen personality factor questionnaire. Institute for Personality and Ability Testing, Champaign, Ill.
56. Ceylon Mental Health Association (1961) Mental Health Survey of Alutgama – Bandaragama, September 1960. Probation and Child Care Journal 1:1–17
57. Cohen D, Schmidt JP (1979) Ambiversion: Characteristics of midrange responders on the introversion-extraversion continuum. J Personality Assessment 43:514–516
58. Cotte S (1955) Etude statistique sur les réponses zoomorphique (A) dans le test de Rorschach des infants impubères. Bull Group Franc. de Rorschach 7
59. Cremerius J (1962) Die Beurteilung des Behandlungserfolgs in der Psychotherapie. Springer, Berlin Göttingen Heidelberg
60. Cremerius J (1968) Die Prognose funktioneller Syndrome. Enke, Stuttgart
61. Davidian H, Izadi C, Motabar M, Nahapetian V (1975) Prevalence of psychiatric disorders in the Caspian Area, Roodsar. Iranian Journal of Public Health 3. In Persian with English summary
62. Donaldson BA (1938) The wild rue. A study of muhammedan magic and folklore in Iran. Luzac, London
63. Dube KC (1970) A study of prevalence and bio-social variables in mental illness in a rural and urban community in Uttar Pradesh, India. Acta Psychiatr Scand 46:327–359
64. Dube KC, Kumar N (1973) An epidemiological study of manic-depressive psychosis. Acta Psychiatr Scand 49:691–697
65. Dutz W (1971) Das Gebet des Königs. Privately printed, Tehran
66. Elgood C (1957) A medical history of Persia and the Eastern Caliphate. Cambridge University Press, Cambridge
67. Elnagar MN, Promilla M, Rao MN (1971) Mental health in an Indian rural community. Br J Psychiatry 118: 499–503
68. Enke W (1927) Die Konstitutionstypen im Rorschach'schen Experiment. Zschr Ges Neurol Psychiatr 108:645–674
69. Ernst K, Kind H, Rotach-Fuchs M (1968) Ergebnisse der Verlaufsforschung bei Neurosen. Springer, Berlin Heidelberg New York
70. Essen-Möller (1956) Individual traits and morbidity in a Swedish rural population. Munksgaard, Copenhagen
71. Eysenck HJ (1947) Dimensions of personality. Routledge and Keagan Paul, London
72. Eysenck HJ (1952) The scientific study of personality. Routledge and Keagan Paul, London
73. Eysenck HJ (1958) A short questionnaire for the measurement of two dimensions of personality. J Appl Psychol 42:14–17
74. Eysenck HJ (1959) Das "Maudsley Personality Inventory" (MPI). Hograefe, Göttingen
75. Eysenck HJ (1975) The Eysenck personality questionnaire. Educational and Testing Service, San Diego, Calif.

76. Eysenck HJ, Eysenck SGB (1963) Manual for the Eysenck personality inventory. Industrial Testing Service, San Diego, Calif.
77. Eysenck SGB, Eysenck HJ (1968) The measurement of psychoticism. A study of factor stability and reliability. Br J Soc Clin Psychol 7:286–294
78. Eysenck SGB, Eysenck HJ (1969) Scores on three personality variables as a function of age, sex and social class. Br J Soc Clin Psychol 8:69–76
79. Fahrenberg J, Selg H (1970) Das Freiburger Persönlichkeitsinventar (FPI). Hograefe, Göttingen
80. Flückiger M-L (1975) Introversion und Schulerfolg. Arbeiten zur Psychologie, Pädagogik und Heilpädagogik, Montalta E (Hrsg), Bd 30. Universitätsverlag, Freiburg (Schweiz)
81. Fremming K (1947) Morbid risk of mental diseases and other mental abnormalities in an average Danish population on the basis of a catamnestic study of 5500 persons born 1883–87. Munksgaard, Copenhagen
82. Giel R, van Luijk JN (1969) Psychiatric morbidity in a small Ethiopian town. Br J Psychiatry 115:149–162
83. Gnat T, Henisz J (1966) Current developments in social psychiatry in Poland. Soc Psychiatry 1:53–56
84. Goldmann-Eisler F (1953) Personality. Knopf, New York
85. Good B (1977) The heart of what's the matter. The semantics of illness in Iran. Medicine and Psychiatry 1:25–58
86. Gremliza FGL (1956) Bejel in Deschteh Mischan, Khuzestan (Iran). Zschr Tropenmedizin und Parasitologie 7:438–464
87. Gremliza FGL (1962) Ecology of endemic diseases in the Dez Irrigation Pilot Area. Development and Resources Corporation, New York
88. Gremliza FGL (1965) A method for measuring the quality of village conditions in less developed areas. Am J Public Health 55:107–115
89. Griffiths R (1935) Imagination in early childhood
90. Gudmundsson G (1968) Epilepsy in Iceland. A clinical and epidemiological investigation. Acta Neurol Scand 43 [Suppl 25]:1–124
91. Harris DB (1963) Children's drawings as measures of intellectual maturity. A revision and extension of the Goodenough Draw-A-Man Test. Harcourt, Brace and World, New York
92. Harrower-Erickson M, Steiner E (1945) Large scale Rorschach techniques. Thomas, Springfield, Ill.
93. Harvald B (1972) Genetik der Epilepsien: Häufigkeit der Epilepsien. In: Psychiatrie der Gegenwart, Kisker KP, Meyer J-E, Müller M, Strömgren E (Hrsg) 2. Aufl Bd II/2, pp. 691–713. Springer, Berlin Heidelberg New York
94. Hauser WA, Kurland LT (1975) The epidemiology of epilepsy in Rochester, Minnesota, 1935 through 1967. Epilepsia 16:1–66
95. Heim AW (1967) AH4 group test of general intelligence manual. National Foundation for Educational Research, The Mere, England
96. Heim AW (1968) AH5 group test of high-grade intelligence. National Foundation for Educational Research, The Mere, England
97. Helgason T (1964) Epidemiology of mental disorders in Iceland. Munksgaard, Copenhagen
98. Henrysson St, Haseloff OW, Hoffmann HJ (1960) Kleines Lehrbuch der Statistik. de Gruyter, Berlin
99. Heydarian S. Uncompleted thesis for licentiate in psychology, University of Bern. Quoted by permission
100. Hosseini AA, Mehryar AH, Razavieh A (1973) Extraversion, neuroticism and psychoticism as measured by Eysenck's inventories in Iran. J Genet Psychol 122:197–205
101. Ionescu-Tongyonk J (1971/1972) Depressions in Thailand in the perspective of comparative transcultural psychiatry. J Psychiatric Association of Thailand 16:337–354 (1971) and 17:44–65 (1972)

102. Ionescu-Tongyonk J (1977) Transcultural psychiatry in Thailand: a review of the last two decades. Transcultural Psychiatric Research Review 14:145–162
103. Ionescu-Tongyonk J (1978) The social perspectives of depressions in Thailand. Thai Medical Journal 2:213–217
104. Ionescu-Tongyonk J (1978) Depressive somatization of Far East orientals and occidentals. Thai Medical Journal 2:270–272
105. Janz D (1972) Die Anfalls-Syndrome: Epidemiologie. Psychiatrie der Gegenwart, Kisker KP, Meyer J-E, Müller M, Strömgren E (Hrsg), 2. Aufl Bd II/2, pp. 565–630. Springer, Berlin Heidelberg New York
106. Janz D, Scheffner D (1980) Ueber epileptische Anfälle bei Kindern von Eltern mit Epilepsie. Nervenarzt 51:226–232
107. Jayasundara MG (1969) Mental health surveys in Ceylon. In Mental Health Research in Asia and the Pacific, Caudill W, Lin TY (eds). East-West Center Press, pp. 54–65, Honolulu
108. Jung CG (1958 [original 1929]) Ziele der Psychotherapie. In: Gesammelte Werke, Niehaus-Jung M, Hurwitz-Eisner L, Riklin F (Hrsg), Bd 16, pp. 38–56. Rascher, Zürich und Stuttgart
109. Jung CG (1960 [Original 1920]) Psychologische Typen. In: Gesammelte Werke, Niehaus-Jung M, Hurwitz-Eisner L, Riklin F (Hrsg), Bd 6. Rascher, Zürich und Stuttgart
110. Jung CG (1968 [original 1945]) Medizin und Psychotherapie. In: Gesammelte Werke, Niehaus-Jung M, Hurwitz-Eisner L, Riklin F (Hrsg), Bd 16, pp. 90–99. Rascher, Zürich und Stuttgart
111. Kato M (1969) Psychiatric epidemiological studies in Japan. The problem of case finding. In: Mental Health Research in Asia and the Pacific, Caudill W, Lin TY (eds), pp. 92–104. East-West Center Press, Honolulu
112. Keyhan International (1973). Tehran, September 8
113. Klar H (1968) Farbpsychologische Untersuchungen von 1000 Persern (Vergleich mit Europäern in Persien). Acta Trop 15:234–240
114. Klar H (1959 [20 Avril]) L'ivresse de l'opium à la lumière du test des couleurs. Médicine et Hygiène 427:206–207
115. Klemperer J (1933) Zur Belastungsstatistik der Durchschnittsbevölkerung: Psychosenhäufigkeit unter 1000 stichprobenmäßig aus den Geburtsregistern der Stadt München (Jahrgang 1881–1890) ausgelesenen Probanden. Zschr Ges Neurol Psychiatr 146:277–316
116. Kloos G (1952) Anleitung zur Intelligenzprüfung in der psychiatrischen Diagnostik, 3rd edn. Piscator-Verlag, Stuttgart
117. Kraus G (1954) Report on Mental Health Survey in Iran 8 December 1953 – 14 January 1954. WHO, Regional Office for the Eastern Mediterranean EM/MENT/7. Stencilled, 32 pages, Alexandria
118. Kurland LT (1959) The incidence and prevalence of convulsive disorders in a small urban community. Epilepsia 1:143–161
119. Läufer H-E (1964) Assignment report on the communicable eye disease control project in Iran 25 August 1963 – 29 February 1964. WHO, Regional Office for the Eastern Mediterranean EM/TRACH/42. Stencilled, 15 pages + 3 annexes, Alexandria
120. Lauter H (1974) Epidemiologische Aspekte alterspsychiatrischer Erkrankungen. Nervenarzt 45:277–288
121. Lin T-Y (1953) A study of the incidence of mental disorder in Chinese and other cultures. Psychiatry 16:313–337
122. Lin T-Y, Standley CC (1962) The scope of epidemiology in psychiatry. WHO, Geneva
123. Lin TY et al (1969) Mental disorders in Taiwan, fifteen years later: a preliminary report. In: Mental health research in Asia and the Pacific, Caudill W, Lin T-Y (eds), East-West Center Press, Honolulu pp. 66–91
124. Lindzey G (ed) (1961) Projective techniques and cross-cultural research. Appleton-Century-Crofts, New York

125. Löffler R, Friedl E (1967) Eine ethnographische Sammlung von den Boir Ahmad. Beschreibender Katalog. Archiv für Völkerkunde 21:95–207
126. Löwy M. Ueber eine Unruheerscheinung: Die Halluzination des Anrufes mit dem eigenen Namen. Vortrag vom 22. November 1910 in der medizinisch-biologischen Sektion des "Lotos" in Prag. Brochure of 131 pages without publisher, place or date.
127. Loosli-Usteri M (1952) L'homme "normal" vu à travers le Test Rorschach. Rorschachiana-Journal 1:24–36
128. Loosli-Usteri M (1958) La femme "normale" vu à travers le Test Rorschach. Rorschachiana Supplement VI. Huber, Bern Stuttgart, pp. 12–29
129. Loosli-Usteri M (1961) Praktisches Handbuch des Rorschach-Tests. Huber, Bern
130. Lüscher M (1949) Psychologie der Farben. Test-Verlag, Basel
131. Luxenburger H (1928) Demographische und psychiatrische Untersuchungen in der engeren biologischen Familie von Paralytikerehegatten. Zschr Ges Neurol Psychiatr 112:331–491
132. Mahloudji M (1967) Familial and congenital simple anhidrosis. Archives of Diseases of Children 113:477–479
133. Mahloudji M (undated) Preliminary report on a total population study in a village near Shiraz. Stencilled, 13 pages
134. Mashayeki MB, Hayes GS (1952) Some demographic and health characteristics of 173 villages in a rural area of Iran. Rockefeller Foundation, New York
135. Mathai KV, Dunn DP, Kurland LT, Reeder FA (1968) Convulsive disorders in the Mariana Islands. Epilepsia 9:77–85
136. Maugham S (1966 [original 1921]) Of Human Bondage. Collected Edition. Heinemann, London
137. Mehryar AH (1970) A cross-cultural investigation of Eysenck's hypothesis regarding the relationship between personality and attitudes. Br J Soc Clin Psychol 9:216–221
138. Mehryar AH (1970) Some data on the Persian translation of the Eysenck Personality Inventory. Br J Soc Clin Psychol 9:257–263
139. Mehryar AH (1972) Fathers' education, family size and children's intelligence and academic performance in Iran. Int J Psychol 7:47–50
140. Mehryar AH (1972) Some socio-demographic correlates of measured intelligence in Iran: In: Determinants of behavioral development. Academic Press, pp. 303–310, New York London
141. Mehryar AH (1972) Personality patterns of Iranian boys and girls on Cattel's 16 personality factor test. Br J Clin Psychol 11:257–264
142. Mehryar AH (1973) The application of the GATB tool matching scale to a group of Iranian workers and its correlations with age and literary achievement. Int Revue Appl Psychol 22:105–112
143. Mehryar AH, Khajavi F, Razavieh A, Hosseini A (1973) Some personality correlates of intelligence and intellectual attainment in Iran. Br J Educ Psychol 43:8–16
144. Mehryar AH, Khajavi F, Hosseini A (1973) Some correlates of psychoticism in a normal group of Iranian youth. Psychology 10:1–9
145. Mehryar AH, Shapurian R (1970) Some normative data on a Persian form of the New Junior Maudsley Inventory. Psychol Rep 26:743–746
146. Mehryar AH, Shapurian R (1970) The application of a high-grade intelligence scale (AH5) in Iran. Br J Educ Psychol 40:307–311
147. Mehryar AH, Shapurian R (1972) A preliminary report on a Persian adaptation of Heim's AH4 Test. J Psychol 80:167–180
148. Merian D (1956) Ueber freches Verhalten im Kindesalter. Huber, Bern
149. Meulen EEC van der (1959) Vulgaer Deutungen bij de Z-Test in Indonesia. Nederlands Tijdschrift voor de Psychologie, Nieuwe Reeks, 14:218–231
150. Ministry of Health, Iran: Department of Public Health, Ostan of Fars. Personal commmunication
151. Mitscherlich A (1954) Zur psychoanalytischen Auffassung psychosomatischer Krankheitsentstehung. Psyche 7:561:578

152. Moayed E (1961) Rural health organization in Iran. Ministry of Health, Tehran
153. Mofidi CMH (1961) Health status of Iran. Institute of Malariology Publication 1110, Tehran
154. Mombour W (1972) Verfahren zur Standardisierung des psychopathologischen Befundes. Psychiatria Clinica 5:73–120, 137–157
155. Nahapetian W, Khezaneh H (1977) Mizanhayi hiyati Iran (Vital Statistics of Iran). University of Tehran Press, Tehran. In Persian
156. Nandi DN et al (1975) Psychiatric disorders in a rural community in West Bengal – an epidemiological study. Indian J Psychiatry 17:87–99
157. National Census of Population and Housing (1966), Vol. 34, Shiraz Sharestan. Iranian Statistical Center, Tehran.
158. McNemar Q (1949) Psychological statistics. Wiley, New York, and Chapman and Hall, London
159. Nowparast N, Tarighati Sg (1974) The Rorschach behavior of non-psychiatric Iranian college students. Internat Symp on Epidemiological Studies in Psychiatry, pp. 261–273, Tehran
160. Oberholzer E (1931) Zur Differentialdiagnose psychischer Folgezustände nach Schädeltraumen mittels des Rorschach'schen Formdeutversuchs. Zschr Ges Neurol Psychiatr 136:596–629
161. Oedegaard O (1946) A statistical investigation of the incidence of mental disorder in Norway. Psychiatric Quarterly 20:381–399
162. Okhowat V (1973) An investigation on the diagnostic value of the MMPI short form in Iran. Tazahai Ravanpezeschki 3. In Persian
163. Okhowat V (1974) A study on the applicability of the MMPI short form in Iran. International Symposium on Epidemiological Studies in Psychiatry, Tehran 1974. pp. 242–247, Tehran
164. Olfat M, Acting Director-General, Health Statistics and Survey. Ministry of Health, Tehran. Personal communication
165. Overseas Consultants Inc (1949) Report on seven year development plan for the Plan Organization of the Imperial Government of Iran. Tehran
166. Petrossian A, Shayan K, Bash KW, Jessup B (1964) The health and related characteristics of four selected village and tribal communities in Fars Ostan, Shiraz, Iran
167. Pfister M (1951) Farbpyramiden-Test, Heiss R, Hiltmann H (Hrsg), Huber, Bern
168. Prasad AS, Halsted JA, Madimi M (1961) Am J Med 31:532
169. Reid DD (1960) Epidemiological methods in the study of mental disorders. WHO, Geneva
170. Rorschach H (1972) Psychodiagnostik. 9th revised edn. Huber, Bern Stuttgart Vienna
171. Roth WF, Luton FH (1943) The mental health program in Tennessee. Am J Psychiatry 99:662
172. Sahebo'z-Zamani MH, Bash KW (1968) Notizen zur Geschichte der Psychiatrie in Iran. Schweiz Arch Neurol Neurochir Psychiatr 101:396–401
173. Salomon F (1954) Erfahrungen mit dem Z-Diapositiv-Test. Zschr Diagn Psychol 2:12–32
174. Salomon F (1962) Ich-Diagnostik im Zulliger-Test. Huber, Bern Stuttgart
175. Schepank H (1974) Erb- und Umweltfaktoren bei Neurosen. Tiefenpsychologische Untersuchungen an 50 Zwillingspaaren. Unter Mitarbeit von PE Becker, A Heigel-Evers, CO Köhler, Helga Schepank und G Wagner. Springer, Berlin Heidelberg New York
176. Schulte W, Tölle R (1971) Psychiatrie. Springer, Berlin Heidelberg New York
177. Schultz-Hencke H (1951) Lehrbuch der analytischen Psychotherapie. Thieme, Stuttgart
178. Shepherd M, Cooper B, Brown AC, Kalton GW (1966) Psychiatric illness in general practice. Oxford University Press, New York Toronto
179. Shepherd M, Brooke EM, Cooper JE, Lin T-Y (1968) An experimental approach to psychiatric diagnosis. Munksgaard, Copenhagen
180. Silverman C (1968) The epidemiology of depression. Johns Hopkins Press, Baltimore
181. Sjögren T (1948) Genetic-statistical and psychiatric investigations of a West Swedish population. Munksgaard, Copenhagen

182. Skalweit W (1934) Konstitution und Prozeß in der Schizophrenie. Thieme, Leipzig
183. Slater E, Beard AW (1963) The schizophrenia-like psychoses of epilepsy. Br J Psychiatry 109:95–150
184. Spindler LS (1962) Menomini women and culture change. American Anthropological Association Memoir 19
185. Spindler LS, Spindler GD (1967 [original 1958]) Male and female adaptations in culture change: Menomini. In: Personalities in cultures: Readings in psychological anthropology, Hunt R (ed). Natural History Press, Garden City, New York
186. Srole L et al (1962) Mental health in the metropolis. The Midtown Manhattan Study. McGraw-Hill, New York
187. Strömgren E (1938) Beiträge zur psychiatrischen Erblehre. Munksgaard, Copenhagen
188. Strotzka H (1969) Kleinburg. Österreichischer Bundesverlag, Wien
189. Thacore VR, Gupta SC, Suraiya M (1975) Psychiatric morbidity in a North Indian community. Br J Psychiatry 126:364–369
190. Tooth GC (1958) Report on a visit to Iran (Mental Health) February–April 1958. WHO, Regional Office for the Eastern Mediterranean EM/MENT/16 IRAN 28. Alexandria. Stencilled, 7 pages
191. Tsugawa T (1942) Ueber die psychiatrische Zensus-Untersuchung in einem Stadtbezirk von Tokyo. Psychiatria et Neurologia Japonica 46:204–218
192. Uchimura Y et al (1940) Ueber die vergleichend psychiatrische und erbpathologische Untersuchung auf einer japanischen Insel. Psychiatria et Neurologia Japonica 44:745–782
193. Uchimura Y et al (1942) Eine weitere vergleichend psychiatrische und erbpathologische Untersuchung auf einer japanischen Insel. Minzokueisei 10:1–51. In Japanese
194. US Department of Labor (1962) Guide to use of the General Aptitude Test Battery, Section III: Development. US Government Printing Office, Washington D.C.
195. Valentine M (1959) Psychometric testing in Iran. Journal of Mental Science 105:93–107
196. Vatankha H-M (1970) Psychoneurotische Störungen bei Frauen im Bezug zu ihrem Sozialstatus. Confin Psychiatr 13:50–66
197. Vernon PE, Allport GW (1931) A test for personality values. J Abnorm Social Psychol 26:231–248
198. Vernon PE (1969) Intelligence and cultural environment. Methuen, London
199. Wagner D (1969) Elektroenzephalographisch gekennzeichnete Psychosen. Schweiz. Arch Neurol Neurochir Psychiatr 103:377–397
200. Wajsbort J, Haral N, Alfandary I (1967) A study of the epidemiology of chronic epilepsy in Northern Israel. Epilepsia 6:105–116
201. Wechsler D (1946) The Wechsler-Bellevue Intelligence Scale. Form II. Manual for administering and scoring the test. Psychological Corporation, New York
202. Wechsler D (1944) Measurement of adult intelligence. 3rd ed. Williams and Wilkins, Baltimore
203. Weinberg W (1925) Methoden und Technik der Statistik mit besonderer Berücksichtigung der Sozialbiologie. In: Handbuch der sozialen Hygiene und Gesundheitsfürsorge 1, Berlin
204. WHO Visiting Team of Medical Scientists to Iran October 1957 (1958) Report WHO/AS/28.58/Rev. 1. WHO, Regional Office for the Eastern Mediterranean. Alexandria. Stencilled, 150 pages
205. WHO (1960) Technical Report Series 185. Epidemiology of mental disorders. Eighth Report of the Expert Committee on Mental Health. WHO, Geneva
206. WHO (1973) The international pilot study of schizophrenia. Geneva
207. WHO (1978) Mental disorders: glossary and guide to their classification in accordance with the ninth revision of the international classification of diseases. WHO, Geneva
208. Zulliger H (1941) Einführung in den Behn-Rorschach-Test. Huber, Bern
209. Zulliger H (1948) Der Z-Test. Ein Formdeutverfahren zur psychologischen Untersuchung von Gruppen. Huber, Bern
210. Zulliger H (1954) Der Tafeln-Z-Test. Huber, Bern

211. Zulliger H (1962) Der Zulliger-Tafeln-Test, 2nd edn. Huber, Bern Stuttgart
212. Zulliger H (1969) The Zulliger individual and group test. Salomon F (ed), trans. Dusya T Dubrovski. International Universities Press, New York

MIX
Papier aus verantwortungsvollen Quellen
Paper from responsible sources
FSC® C105338

If you have any concerns about our products,
you can contact us on
ProductSafety@springernature.com

In case Publisher is established outside the EU,
the EU authorized representative is:
Springer Nature Customer Service Center GmbH
Europaplatz 3, 69115 Heidelberg, Germany

Printed by Libri Plureos GmbH
in Hamburg, Germany